The Medical Works of Moses Maimonides

The Medical Works of Moses Maimonides

New English Translations Based on the Critical Editions of the Arabic Manuscripts

By

Gerrit Bos

BRILL

LEIDEN | BOSTON

Cover illustration: Ms Paris, BN, héb. 1103, fol. 45v, the beginning of Maimonides' *Talkhiṣ K. Ḥīlat al-Bur'* (*Summary of Galen's "De Methodo Medendi"*). The illumination hails from the workshop of Ferrer and Arnau Bassa in Barcelona. Cf. M. Garel, *D'une main forte*: *Manuscrits hébreux des collections françaises*, Paris 1991, no. 48. The cover design is a copy of the original design by Brigham Young University Press.

Library of Congress Cataloging-in-Publication Data

Names: Bos, Gerrit, 1948- author.
Title: The medical works of Moses Maimonides : new English translations based on the critical editions of the Arabic manuscripts / by Gerrit Bos.
Description: Leiden ; Boston : Brill, 2021. | Includes bibliographical references and index.
Identifiers: LCCN 2021044549 (print) | LCCN 2021044550 (ebook) | ISBN 9789004498877 (hardback) | ISBN 9789004498884 (ebook)
Subjects: LCSH: Medicine, Arab. | Maimonides, Moses, 1135-1204.
Classification: LCC R128.3 .B67 2021 (print) | LCC R128.3 (ebook) | DDC 610.917/4927–dc23/eng/20211108
LC record available at https://lccn.loc.gov/2021044549
LC ebook record available at https://lccn.loc.gov/2021044550

Typeface for the Latin, Greek, and Cyrillic scripts: "Brill". See and download: brill.com/brill-typeface.

ISBN 978-90-04-49887-7 (hardback)
ISBN 978-90-04-49888-4 (e-book)

This book is printed on acid-free paper and produced in a sustainable manner.

To D. Morgan Davis,
co-traveller on the road to the publication of
The Medical Works of Moses Maimonides

Contents

Preface XI

Introduction 1

1 *On Asthma* 13
Chapter One: *On the best regimen in general* 16
Chapter Two: *On the provision of rules concerning the foods to be eaten or avoided in relation to this disease* 17
Chapter Three: *On the different kinds of food that should be avoided or consumed, selected from those foods that are readily available and common among us* 19
Chapter Four: *On the composition of different dishes which are beneficial in this disease* 23
Chapter Five: *On the quantity of food* 26
Chapter Six: *On the times of day for the consumption of food* 29
Chapter Seven: *On beverages* 31
Chapter Eight: *On the proper regimen in connection with the air and movements of the soul* 33
Chapter Nine: *On the proper regimen for retention and evacuation* 35
Chapter Ten: *On the proper regimen regarding sleep and waking, bathing, massage, and sexual intercourse* 41
Chapter Eleven: *On the provision of rules for the treatment of this disease* 45
Chapter Twelve: *On the composition of drugs necessary for every different kind of this disease, according to the scope of this treatise* 49
Chapter Thirteen: *On the provision of rules, few in number but of great help for people in general, concerning the regimen of health and the healing of diseases; in hortatory form* 57

2 ***On Poisons and the Protection against Lethal Drugs*** 77
The First Chapter of the First Part: *Concerning the regimen of someone bitten in general* 81
The Second Chapter of the First Part: *Concerning the simple and compound topical remedies that are put on the site of the bite* 83
The Third Chapter of the First Part: *Concerning the simple remedies that are beneficial for the bite of all kinds of vermin* 84
The Fourth Chapter of the First Part: *On the compound remedies beneficial against bites and stings* 87

The Fifth Chapter of the First Part: *Concerning the specific treatment of someone bitten by a certain animal* 89
The Sixth Chapter of the First Part: *Concerning the foods to be given to bite victims in general and in particular, and certain remedies with specific properties which are fitting for this purpose* 95
The First Chapter of the Second Part: *On the prophylaxis against deadly poisons* 97
The Second Chapter of the Second Part: *Concerning the regimen in general of someone who took a deadly poison or who suspects that he took it* 99
The Third Chapter of the Second Part: *Concerning the simple and compound remedies that are generally beneficial for someone who took poison* 100
The Fourth Chapter of the Second Part: *On the regimen for someone who knows which poison he took* 101

3 ***On Hemorrhoids*** 105
Chapter One: *A general discussion of the improvement of the digestions* 106
Chapter Two: *On the food from which one should refrain because of this illness* 108
Chapter Three: *On the foods that one should aim for because of this illness* 110
Chapter Four: *On the simple and compound drugs that one should regularly take* 110
Chapter Five: *On topical remedies which should be taken repeatedly as well* 112
Chapter Six: *On that which one should rely upon when this disease flares up* 113
Chapter Seven: *On the fumigations that should be prescribed for this illness* 115

4 ***On Rules Regarding the Practical Part of the Medical Art*** 117

5 ***Medical Aphorisms*** 142
The First Treatise: *Containing aphorisms concerning the subject of the medical art, by which I mean the form of the organs of the human body and their functions and faculties* 146
The Second Treatise: *Containing aphorisms concerning the humors* 160
The Third Treatise: *Containing aphorisms concerning the principles of the art and general rules* 166

The Fourth Treatise: *Containing aphorisms concerning the pulse and the prognostic signs to be derived from it* 186
The Fifth Treatise: *Containing aphorisms concerning the prognostic signs to be derived from the urine* 194
The Sixth Treatise: *Containing aphorisms concerning the other prognostic signs* 198
The Seventh Treatise: *Containing aphorisms concerning the causes of diseases which are often not known or which are discussed in a confused way* 215
The Eighth Treatise: *Containing aphorisms concerning the correct regimen for the healing of diseases in general* 231
The Ninth Treatise: *Containing aphorisms concerning specific diseases* 245
The Tenth Treatise: *Containing aphorisms concerning fevers* 270
The Eleventh Treatise: *Containing aphorisms concerning the periods and crisis of a disease* 285
The Twelfth Treatise: *Containing aphorisms concerning evacuation by means of bloodletting* 290
The Thirteenth Treatise: *Containing aphorisms concerning evacuations by means of purgatives and enemas* 299
The Fourteenth Treatise: *Containing aphorisms concerning vomiting* 309
The Fifteenth Treatise: *Containing aphorisms concerning surgery* 311
The Sixteenth Treatise: *Containing aphorisms concerning women* 324
The Seventeenth Treatise: *Containing aphorisms concerning the regimen of health in general* 330
The Eighteenth Treatise: *Containing aphorisms concerning physical exercise* 337
The Nineteenth Treatise: *Containing aphorisms concerning bathing* 340
The Twentieth Treatise: *Containing aphorisms concerning foods, beverages, and their consumption* 346
The Twenty-First Treatise: *Containing aphorisms concerning drugs* 360
The Twenty-Second Treatise: *Containing aphorisms concerning the specific properties of remedies* 382
The Twenty-Third Treatise: *Containing aphorisms concerning the differences between well-known diseases and the elucidation of technical terms that are well known to the physicians but whose exact meanings are sometimes unknown to them* 392
The Twenty-Fourth Treatise: *Containing curiosities, which feature and are related in the medical books, and unusual, rare occurrences* 412
The Twenty-fifth Treatise: *Containing some doubts that befell me concerning Galen's words* 423

6 *On Coitus* 460

7 ***On the Regimen of Health*** 468

Chapter One: *On the regimen of health in general, with respect to all people, in a few words* 469

Chapter Two: *On the regimen of sick people in general, when no physician can be found, or when the available physician is such that one cannot rely upon his knowledge* 475

Chapter Three: *On the regimen of my Master in particular, according to the symptoms he complains about* 480

Chapter Four: *Consisting of sections in the form of hortatory rules that are useful in general and in particular for healthy and sick people in all places and all times* 488

8 ***On the Elucidation of Some Symptoms and the Response to Them* (Formerly Known as *On the Causes of Symptoms*)** 499

9 ***Commentary on Hippocrates'* Aphorisms** 518

The First Part of the *Commentary on Hippocrates'* Aphorisms 522

The Second Part of the *Commentary on Hippocrates'* Aphorisms 537

The Third Part of the *Commentary on Hippocrates'* Aphorisms 549

The Fourth Part of the *Commentary on Hippocrates'* Aphorisms 557

The Fifth Part of the *Commentary on Hippocrates'* Aphorisms 573

The Sixth Part of the *Commentary on Hippocrates'* Aphorisms 586

The Seventh Part of the *Commentary on Hippocrates'* Aphorisms 598

Glossary of Technical Terms 609

Glossary of Weights and Measures 614

Sigla 615

Index of Quoted Physicians, Philosophers, and Their Works 616

Index of Diseases and Afflictions 621

Index of Medicinal Products, Dishes, and Their Ingredients and Components (Including Poisons and Antidotes) 659

Preface

I am very pleased to offer the current volume to the reader. The medical works composed by the famous Jewish physician and philosopher Moses Maimonides (1138–1204) have been consulted by physicians and interested laypeople throughout the ages. From the thirteenth century on, manuscripts of his medical writings, both original works in Arabic and translations into Hebrew and Latin, were copied and commented upon time and again. After the invention of the printing press in the second half of the fifteenth century, his works belonged to the earliest books to be printed. His *Regimen of Health* was printed in 1477 or 1481 and reprinted five times until 1535. The *Medical Aphorisms* were printed in Bologna in 1489, followed by a new edition in Venice in 1497, which was reprinted again in Venice only a few years later in 1508.

In spite of the interest in these works also in our times, reliable editions and translations have been a desideratum until recently. The first publication of Maimonides' medical works in English translation, published by the Maimonides Research Institute, Haifa, in seven volumes as *Maimonides' Medical Writings* between 1984 and 1995, is unreliable as, for the most part, it is not based on the Arabic original texts but on uncritical editions of the Hebrew translations, replete with errors. These cannot be considered to reflect the original words of the author.

This unfortunate situation has changed drastically with the publication of *The Medical Works of Moses Maimonides* (MWMM) in seventeen volumes by Brigham Young University Press, Provo/UT (vols. 1–10), and Brill, Leiden (vols. 11–17) between 2002 and 2021. These volumes include critical editions of the original Arabic texts and the medieval translations into Hebrew and Latin as well as modern translations into English, which can now also be consulted in an online edition.

The current volume is intended for a general public. It includes all English translations of Maimonides' medical writings collected in the aforementioned MWMM series, with a minimum of explanations of specific technical terms. In order to make the consultation of these works easier—especially with regard to the use of certain plant medicines—an alphabetical index of medicinal ingredients has been added. Common English plant names as well as their Latin scientific nomenclature were harmonized and updated throughout according to Marwān ibn Janāḥ, *On the Nomenclature of Medicinal Drugs* (*Kitāb al-Talkhīṣ*) (eds. and trans. Bos/Käs/Lübke/Mensching, Leiden 2020) and/or the accepted names in the ITIS (Integrated Taxonomic Information System, https://www.itis.gov) database. Furthermore, this volume also features indexes of mentioned diseases and afflictions as well as quoted physicians, philosophers, and their works, which were at times added to the text following Maimonides example in his *Medical Aphorisms*. Those additional references, as long as they were not explicitly or completely mentioned by Maimonides himself, are enclosed in square brackets.

Thanks go to Felix Hedderich and Jessica Kley for their help in the completion of this volume and to Teddi Dols and Maurits van den Boogert at Brill Publishers for their enthusiastic support of its publication.

Introduction

Abū ʿImrān Mūsā ibn ʿUbayd Allāh, usually called Moses Maimonides, one of the greatest philosophers and experts in Jewish law (*halakhah*), was an eminent physician as well. After settling in Fusṭāṭ, the ancient part of Cairo, Maimonides started to practice and teach medicine. Thus, he became the physician of al-Qāḍī al-Fāḍil, the famous counselor and secretary to Saladin. Later on, he became court physician of al-Malik al-Afḍal, after the latter's ascension to the throne in the winter of 1198/1199. As a teacher of medicine, he taught his sister's son Abū l-Riḍā, surnamed *al-tilmīdh al-zakī* ("the brilliant student"). The Cairo Genizah (a storeroom of old manuscripts and manuscript fragments found in the Ben Ezra synagogue in Old Cairo) has preserved a letter in which Meir ibn al-Hamadānī implores Maimonides to admit his son as his pupil.

Next to being a physician and philosopher, Maimonides is the author of a rich and varied corpus of medical works. Of his ten known medical writings, four are held to be his major works, namely,

1. *Medical Aphorisms*;
2. *Commentary on Hippocrates'* Aphorisms;
3. *On Poisons and the Protection against Lethal Drugs*; and
4. *Epitomes from the Works of Galen.*

The mentioned texts were only available in corrupt editions of the medieval Hebrew translations and in flawed modern English translations based on the Hebrew.

Additionally, Maimonides composed six minor treatises, namely,

1. *On Coitus*;
2. *On the Regimen of Health*;
3. *On the Elucidation of Some Symptoms and the Response to Them*;
4. *On Hemorrhoids*;
5. *On Asthma*; and
6. *On Rules Regarding the Practical Part of the Medical Art.*

Of these minor works, some have been edited in the past by Hermann Kroner, a German physician living and working in Bopfingen, Southern Germany, in the 1920s. But these editions suffer from mistakes as well and were edited on the basis of only one or two manuscripts.

Since Maimonides' medical works had been so sorely neglected by scholarly research, the project *The Medical Works of Moses Maimonides* (MWMM) was set up, aiming at providing first-time critical editions of all the unedited medical works as well as new critical editions of the already available but flawed editions. The project was initially started in 1995 at the University College Lon-

 | DOI:10.1163/9789004498884_002

don and supported by The Wellcome Trust. It was continued at the University of Cologne, Germany in 1997 with the support of the Deutsche Forschungsgemeinschaft (DFG) and the Institute for the Study and Preservation of Ancient Religious Texts (ISPART, renamed the Neal A. Maxwell Institute for Religious Scholarship in 2006) at Brigham Young University, Provo/UT. The project was eventually finished in 2021 with the publication of the seventeenth volume of the MWMM series.

The published volumes, comprising nine original medical works by Maimonides, from which the English translations are presented in this volume in a harmonized form, are:

1. *On Asthma*, vol. 1 (2002);
2. *Medical Aphorisms*, vol. 1 (Treatises I–V) (2004);
3. *Medical Aphorisms*, vol. 2 (Treatises VI–IX) (2007);
4. *On Asthma*, vol. 2 (2008);
5. *On Poisons and the Protection against Lethal Drugs* (2009);
6. *Medical Aphorisms*, vol. 3 (Treatises X–XV) (2010);
7. *On Hemorrhoids* (2012);
8. *On Rules Regarding the Practical Part of the Medical Art* (2014);
9. *Medical Aphorisms*, vol. 4 (Treatises XVI–XXI) (2015);
10. *Medical Aphorisms*, vol. 5 (Treatises XXII–XXV) (2017);
11. *On Coitus* (2018);
12. *On the Regimen of Health* (2019);
13. *On the Elucidation of Some Symptoms and the Response to Them* (Formerly Known as *On the Causes of Symptoms*) (2019);
14. *Commentary on Hippocrates'* Aphorisms (2 vols.) (2020);
15. *Medical Aphorisms*: Hebrew Translation by Nathan ha-Me'ati (2020);
16. *Medical Aphorisms*: Hebrew Translation by Zeraḥyah ben She'altiel Ḥen (2020); and
17. *Medical Aphorisms*: Glossary & Indexes (2021).

In the end, one of Maimonides' mentioned medical works, the *Epitomes from the Works of Galen*, was not included in the MWMM series because it is merely a collection of Galenic quotes written down by Maimonides, as he said so himself both in the introduction to his *Commentary on Hippocrates'* Aphorisms:

> Every explanation that I will mention anonymously is that of Galen, according to its sense (figuratively), for I do not envisage (intend) to be meticulous in quoting his words as I did in the *Epitomes* [*from the Works of Galen*];

and in the introduction to his own *Medical Aphorisms*:

> In these aphorisms I have not adhered to the method that I followed in the *Epitomes* [*from the Works of Galen*], in which I quoted Galen's very words.

Furthermore, his *Glossary of Drug Names* was also not included because it was already exquisitely edited and translated into French by Max Meyerhof in 1940 and can be consulted in the English translation by Fred Rosner. Only the common English plant names and their Latin scientific nomenclature should be updated to modern standards, as it was done with this edition.

Maimonides' medical works are a rich source of information for the following aspects of his medical biography:

1. His medical training;
2. his medical theoretical knowledge;
3. his medical practice;
4. his attitude towards remedies belonging to the so-called *Dreckapotheke*; and
5. his critical attitude towards the works of other physicians.

As to his medical training, one should distinguish between formal training during a longer period and informal short contacts. It is certain that Maimonides did receive some sort of formal medical training, that is, he studied with senior physicians. In *On Asthma* XIII.33, he informs us explicitly that he studied with one of them while he was still in the Maghreb. He states that he turned to a *shaykh* (senior physician) under whom he studied since he wanted to find out more about a notorious medical incident in which a young man, a glutton, weakened by indigestions and suffering from continuous choleric fever, died as a result of the wrong treatment he received from the hand of the attending physician. And in *Medical Aphorisms* VIII.69, he remarks about diabetes that neither did he see it in the Maghreb nor did anyone of the senior physicians under whom he studied inform him that he had seen it. Formal medical training usually took place in this way. One or several students would receive what we would call private tutoring from a physician of established fame and would also practice under his or another's supervision.

As to informal short contacts, Maimonides repeatedly informs us how he met with senior physicians in order to obtain more information about the composition of certain drugs and about certain medical incidents. Thus, in *On Asthma* XII.9, 10, he tells us that in his presence the best physicians repeatedly tested the composition of certain purgatives; and having listed them, he remarks that he received all these formulas as personal instruction from the senior physicians in the Maghreb.

In *On Poisons and the Protection against Lethal Drugs* 83, we hear how he turns to the senior physicians to find out more about the reason why in every city he passed through some men suffer from suppurating elephantiasis, which results in the limbs falling off. He remarks that those senior physicians informed him that these men had been poisoned by their adulterous wives by means of menstrual blood, which they took from the beginning of the menses and put into the food and which then caused the observed afflictions. Maimonides wonders what to do with this information as this is something that is not mentioned in any medical book that he read with this end in view; how then could one devote a chapter to the treatment of such a kind of poisoning? And in the same treatise—when speaking about rabies—Maimonides entreats the reader to be careful and to distinguish—as it is done in the medical books—between the bite of a mad dog and that of a dog that is not mad, for people have died because of that, as he was informed by the senior physicians whom he met. That failing to do so could lead to disaster is then illustrated with the following account in which he tells us about his contact with a senior well-known physician who related to him that

> he once saw in the city of Almería a young silk weaver bitten by a dog, and that it was not accompanied by any of the symptoms of the bite of a mad dog. The physicians then decided that it was a domesticated dog and let the wound close up after a month or so and the boy recovered. He stayed healthy for a long time and carried out the activities of healthy people. Later, the symptoms of the bite of a mad dog became apparent in him, he got hydrophobia and died. [*On Poisons* 63].

This discussion by Maimonides shows us in an enlightening way how the medical theory formulated by him draws on two sources, both theoretical, that is, what he learned from the medical books, and practical, what one can learn from everyday life.

An important motive for contacting senior physicians was his interest in pharmaceutics and pharmacology. As noted above, in *On Asthma* Maimonides describes the preparation of certain purgatives that the most skillful physicians have tested repeatedly in his presence while he was in the Maghreb and adds that he received all these formulas as personal instruction from them and that only a few of them are written in books, while they are unknown among the people. In his *Glossary of Drug Names* 6, he relates that French lavender, Arabic *usṭūkhūdus*, which is employed by the physicians in the Maghreb and Egypt, is the same plant that the people of Maghreb call *al-ḥalḥal* and that he has learned from eminent scholars who study plants in a learned and diligent way that it is not the same lavender as that mentioned by Galen but something that possesses the same medicinal properties. Maimonides remarks that the real lavender has larger leaves and thicker inflorescences and that it grows in the vicinity of Toledo. In *On Poisons* 23, Maimonides informs us how he consulted a learned botanist to find out the identity of the serpent root, that is, the root of a plant that can be found in the vicinity of the Temple in Jerusalem and which is effective—as experience has shown—against poisons, a recipe taken from the *Kitāb al-Murshid fī jawāhir al-aghdhiya waquwā l-mufradāt mina l-adwiya* by al-Tamīmī, a physician who hailed from Jerusalem and moved to Egypt in 970 to serve the vizir Yaʿqūb ibn Killis. The learned botanist told him that it is "a species of melilot that is called 'the scorpion-like.'" We see how Maimonides tries to make the theoretical information gleaned by him from the *Kitāb al-Murshid* fit for practical application by finding out the identity of this plant in the region where he lives. In his *Glossary of Drug Names* 7, he states in more general terms that this species is called "the scorpion-like melilot" and that he has learned that the roots that are imported from Palestine are useful as a theriac against the bites of vermin. In his *On the Regimen of Health* III.3, Maimonides remarks that his advice to his client to use barberry seeds, which are known for their constipating qualities in a laxative preparation with purging cassia, is based on information he received from the senior physicians, namely, that the barberry seeds prevent the possible distress and abrasion caused by purging cassia. We may conclude that next to a formal training limited to a certain period in his life he was always looking for opportunities to supplement and update the training he received with fresh information from reliable informants.

As to his theoretical medical knowledge, a study of his medical works shows above all his thorough command of the medical corpus composed by the famous physician Galen from Pergamum (c. 139–217), who was active as a personal physician to the Emperors in Rome. As for all his predecessors and contemporaries, Galen was the physician and medical authority *par excellence*. Being a physician was in a way following in his footsteps, which meant appropriating the wealth of material incorporated in his medical works. Maimonides was no exception to this. Repeatedly he expresses his veneration for Galen the physician. Thus, he calls him the master (*imām*) of the art of medicine in his *Medical Aphorisms* XXV.1. And in the context of his devastating critique of Galen as a philosopher in his *Medical Aphorisms* XXV.59, Maimonides hails him as the greatest physician and anatomist that ever lived, who unfortunately overstepped his boundaries and ventured out to speak about things in which he is very deficient, that is, philosophy. Maimonides must have studied Galen in depth and known large parts of his works by heart.

Another ancient physician he was familiar with was Hippocrates of Kos (c. 460–370), the father of medicine. After Galen, he is the second most quoted author in Maimonides' *On Asthma*. More than his other writings, Maimonides favored his *Aphorisms*, as he remarks in the introduction to the commentary he composed to this work:

> And since I consider Hippocrates' *Aphorisms* to be the most useful of the books he composed, I decided to explain them; for these are aphorisms that every physician should know by heart. I have even seen how non-physicians have schoolchildren memorize them, so that subsequently people who are not physicians know many of these aphorisms by heart from learning them as young children at school.

Next to these ancient physicians, Maimonides was profoundly familiar with the works of Arab physicians such as Ibn Sīnā (Avicenna, c. 980–1037) and al-Rāzī (Rhazes, 865–925), and especially with those of authors from al-Andalus, such as Ibn Wāfid (c. 997–1074) and Abū Marwān ibn Zuhr (Avenzoar, c. 1090–1162). Ibn Sīnā's *Kitāb al-Qānūn fī al-ṭibb* (*The Canon of Medicine*) is a primary source for the composition of his *On Hemorrhoids*, as the many close parallels to Ibn Sīnā's discussion of this illness suggest. It is also one of the sources explicitly mentioned and consulted by Maimonides in his *Medical Aphorisms* XXI.67, *On Poisons* 18, 38, and *On Coitus* 6, 7. In this last treatise, Maimonides remarks that he has consulted Ibn Sīnā to compose an *ʿujja* (omelet; egg fritter) for strengthening the sexual lust and that a patient who used it found it greatly beneficial. Next to Ibn Sīnā, al-Rāzī features prominently in Maimonides' *On Hemorrhoids* IV.5, 7; VI.7 and *On Poisons* 13, 33, 35. Of the Andalusian physician Ibn Wāfid from Toledo, Maimonides consulted a list of drugs in his *Medical Aphorisms* XXI.67–89, namely of 265 drugs to be applied internally and twenty drugs to be applied externally, which are common in all places and which every physician should know by heart. However, Maimonides most appreciated Ibn Zuhr. He regarded him as an authoritative source he could rely on for recommending certain recipes as he had gained so much experience. Maimonides says so explicitly in his *Medical Aphorisms* XXII.35 when quoting a long list of remedies belonging to the so-called *Dreckapotheke* with the following words:

> Abū Marwān ibn Zuhr has mentioned many specific properties of remedies that he tested. He was one of the great empiricists. His son told me amazing things about his precision and diligence in matters depending upon experience. Therefore, I thought it a good thing to mention

> them in his name, although some of them have been mentioned by others before. However, he is the one who verified these experiential matters.

The intimate knowledge of the medical literature—ancient and contemporary—exhibited by Maimonides suggests lifelong study and devotion to the subject, as Maimonides bears witness to in his well-known letter to his student Joseph ben Judah ibn Shimʿon:

> When I come home to Fusṭāṭ, the most that I can do during what is left of the day and the night is to study that which I may need to know from the medical books. For you know how long and difficult this art is for someone who is conscientious and fastidious and who does not wish to say anything without first knowing its proof, its source in the literature, and the type of reasoning (*wajh al-qiyās*) involved.

Private study was common practice in the medieval Middle East. One famous Egyptian physician called ʿAlī ibn Riḍwān (d. 1061) even held that studying from books was preferable to working under the supervision of teachers. This opinion, however, was not generally accepted. The actual subject matter of the medical studies can be reconstructed from the inventories of physician's libraries as well as from actual remnants of medical books preserved. The main impression we get from these lists is that of the paramount authority of the Arabic translations of the works of Hippocrates and Galen. Studying medicine meant in the first place memorizing selected writings of Hippocrates and—even more—of Galen. Next to these classics, a serious student would study their pre-Islamic and Islamic commentaries as well as the later Greek physicians and the renowned physicians of the Islamic period. Maimonides' theoretical and practical training thus fits well within the general pattern of his time and society. But in spite of his lifelong studies, Maimonides was deeply aware of the fact that for one physician it was almost impossible to master the entire medical art, to memorize its different parts, and to apply this theoretical knowledge to every individual case. Comparing his generation with Galen, he exclaims in his *On Asthma* XIII.19:

> And if Galen—with his excellent intellect and long experience in the practice of medicine, his devotion to this art, and his strong aspirations to excel in it—casts doubts on his own practice and is tentative about it, how much more should this be the case in our generations, in which physicians have only very little experience, while at the same time much memorizing

> is needed, since the different parts of medicine have become so lengthy! Consequently, a lifetime is too short to attain perfection in even one part of it.

One way in which Maimonides tried to solve the conflict between the high demands set by the medical art and human imperfection to master the entire art is by limiting the information that a physician should have at hand to the essential. Thus, he provides a selective list of drugs taken from Ibn Wāfid, mentioned above. In the same vein, Maimonides remarks in *On Poisons* 6 that he will only mention a few remedies, small in number but large in benefit, because an accumulation of medicines necessarily causes that they cannot be remembered and that one has to rely on books to look them up when one needs them. Another way to solve the conflict is through the combined effort of a number of physicians. In his *On Asthma* XIII.49, Maimonides says so explicitly when he remarks that if the physicians gather together as in the case of kings and rulers and debate and argue until they have come to a decision about what should be done, it is most appropriate and best. For then the patient benefits from the sum of their correct judgements, since no single physician can remember everything that he has learned, and this art is difficult for most scholars not with respect to understanding it but with respect to remembering it, because it requires a very good memory. Maimonides' remarks about rulers consulting more than one physician was common practice in the world he lived in.

Our information about his own medical practice and experience, about his actual treatment of certain patients is scant. In most cases, he bases the treatment he recommends on the experience gathered by other physicians. Only once in a while do we get an impression of his practical experience as a physician, especially in the context of certain recipes he composed or certain medicines he tested. An example is a quotation in his *Medical Aphorisms* XIII.49 from one of the "rules in hortatory form" (*wasāyā*) (advice) gleaned from the *Waṣīya*, a lost work composed by Abū al-ʿAlāʾ ibn Zuhr (d. 1131) for his son Abū Marwān (d. 1162). For when Abū al-ʿAlāʾ remarks:

> It is a mistake to use musk as a part of purgatives, and, similarly, to drink it with wine. Those who compound this remedy and administer it are mistaken, because they want to strengthen the organs and let the medicine rise to the head; but they forget that the effect of these purgatives is carried to the major organs, and sometimes such an organ cannot tolerate this, and the patient is killed,

Maimonides comments:

> This is correct if the purgation is done by poisonous drugs, such as pulp of colocynth or St. Thomas lidpod, because of their poisonous effect; or by strong drugs, such as bay laurel, because of its strength. But safe drugs—and especially agarikon, which is good for poisons—are very beneficial if imbibed in wine. I have done so several times and used such a drug in order to cleanse the head, and I saw that it is very effective and that it cleanses the brain to a degree any other drug is incapable of. Moreover, the patient taking this drug found new energy and dilation of the soul. Therefore, consider the specific properties of the drugs that you administer.

And in his *Medical Aphorisms* IX.57, Maimonides remarks that

> it is my practice to heat the oils in a double vessel because their strength is lost if they are heated in any other way,

when he comments upon Galen's statement that

> if someone suffers from indigestion and the like and from a burning in the stomach that is so severe that one imagines that there is an inflamed tumor there, he will benefit from a salve prepared with quince oil.

This example shows us that at least occasionally, Maimonides prepared his own salves and medicaments. As we know from the Cairo Genizah, even famous physicians did so. In *On Poisons* 21, Maimonides relates that he has tried the mineral bezoar—a stone about which wondrous things are related in the books of later physicians—but that none of them was found to be true. For he tried all the different types of this mineral stone against scorpion bites but they were not beneficial at all. In *On Coitus* 8, Maimonides recommends a compound remedy consisting of forty *dirhams* of manna dissolved in one *raṭl* of fresh milk to increase sexual vigor, taken from the works of other physicians, but adds that he has personally mixed it with a quarter of a *dirham* of pounded clove and that it had a good effect. In a unique case, Maimonides tells us in his *On Asthma* XII.5 about his successful treatment of a young woman suffering from asthma attacks through the administration of an electuary for cleansing the lungs and the brain that he composed himself. In a certain stage of his medical profession, Maimonides clearly felt confident enough to compose and apply his own medications instead of those recommended in the medical literature.

Worthy of discussion is also his recommendation of or—perhaps one should say—reference to remedies belonging to the so-called *Dreckapotheke*, that is, remedies consisting of different parts of animals, their droppings, and urine. These remedies feature as part of a long list throughout his *Medical Aphorisms* XXII and are derived from Galen, Abū Marwān ibn Zuhr, and al-Tamīmī (d. 990) and seem at first sight to be completely misplaced in Maimonides' medical system and therapy. For instance, quoting from Galen's *De theriaca ad Pisonem*, he states in his *Medical Aphorisms* XXII.2:

> Mouse heads, burned and kneaded with honey, and rubbed on the spot affected by alopecia, stimulate hair growth. Similarly, mouse excrement, if pulverized in vinegar, is beneficial for alopecia. Viper skin is also good for alopecia, if it is grounded with honey.

Even more amazing is the following recommendation derived from Galen's *De simplicium medicamentorum temperamentis ac facultatibus* in his *Medical Aphorisms* XXII.27:

> I know someone in our times who treated patients by giving them burned human bones to drink without informing them about this, lest they turn away from taking it. This man used to cure with these burned bones many patients suffering from epilepsy and pain in the joints.

The question arises how to reconcile Maimonides' listing of these remedies, which we would classify as working through some sort of magic and/or superstition, with his opposition to and condemnation of magic and superstition and his reputation of an eminently rationalist philosopher and physician. A possible answer to solve the apparent contradiction between the application of these "magical" ingredients and Maimonides' rationalist attitude lies in the fact that for Maimonides these remedies do not belong to the realm of magic, that is, are not effective through some sort of supernatural force. For with Galen, he holds that these ingredients operate through the whole of their substance and are effective through their specific property contrary to "natural" remedies that operate either through their matter or through their quality or power.

While the pharmacological action of remedies that operate through their matter or quality can be assessed by a physician, this is not the case with the remedies effective through their specific property which lack a pharmacological basis. Thus, their effectivity can only be learned through experience. Although Maimonides was an eminent rationalist philosopher and physician, he allows the application of these remedies since as he says "experience has shown them to be valid even if reasoning does not require them." One is reminded of his statement in *The Guide of the Perplexed* III.37 about practices that the sages allowed:

> You must not consider as a difficulty certain things that they have permitted, as for instance the nail of one who is crucified and a fox's tooth. For in those times these things were considered to derive from experience and accordingly pertained to medicine and entered into the same class as the hanging of a peony upon an epileptic and the giving of a dog's excrements in cases of the swelling of the throat and fumigation with vinegar and marcasite in cases of hard swellings of the tendons.

For Maimonides, experience, that is, the repeated successful application of these kinds of medicines by reliable ancient or contemporary physicians, is the ultimate criterion to allow or disallow them.

Maimonides was a physician with an open and independent mind who did not hesitate to criticize physicians he otherwise held in high esteem. This may be inferred from a statement in the introduction to his *Commentary on Hippocrates'* Aphorisms, where he rebukes Galen for refraining from criticizing Hippocrates and for explaining certain statements in the exact opposite of their intended meaning in order to justify the correctness of the statements. Thus, Maimonides does not hesitate to criticize Hippocrates and remarks that among his aphorisms are some which are doubtful and require explanation, some which are self-evident, some which are repeated, some which are not useful for medical therapeutics, and some which are absolutely erroneous viewpoints. Another more contemporary physician Maimonides was critical of is al-Tamīmī. But it was especially Galen who was the target of his criticism, both in medical and philosophical issues. His critique of Galen is largely concentrated in his *Medical Aphorisms* XXV. This treatise actually consists of two parts, the first part consisting of aphorisms 1–58 and 69–72 and the second part covering aphorisms 59–68. The first part contains Maimonides' critique of the medical inconsistencies found in Galen's works and the second part contains Maimonides' refutation of Galen's denial of the Mosaic doctrines of God's omnipotence and creation of the world.

Although Maimonides' critique of Galen in medical issues is largely concentrated there, it is certainly not lacking in the other treatises of his *Medical Aphorisms*. For instance, in I.34, he criticizes Galen for not having solved the question of how the will of someone who is asleep or absent-minded can be abolished and yet he carries out voluntary movements.

At times, Maimonides criticizes Galen severely and in an ironic tone, as in the case of Galen's belief in the superiority of the testicles over the heart, where Maimonides exclaims in XXV.26:

> Consider then, ye who possess insight, whether this is correct, because if the heart would be excised from a living being, could he remain alive to live a good life? That is, could he have sexual intercourse and show his male sexual potency and not lack any vital function? But if his testicles are cut off, he remains alive as we see in the case of eunuchs. Are then the testicles more eminent than the heart?

Summarizing the information we can glean from his medical works concerning his medical biography, one gets the impression that his cautiousness and reluctance to actually treat patients do not stem from a lack of experience in the actual treatment of patients, as he has been accused of, but from a deep awareness of the inadequacy of the physician to master, to memorize the entire medical art. Therefore, he was liable to make mistakes in both diagnosis and therapy. While such mistakes could be corrected in the case of a mild treatment, they were often fatal in the case of a more drastic treatment, as he knew from his own experience. Hence his repeated warnings against the application of such drastic means of treatment, especially purgation and bloodletting. On the other side, it is important to point out that although Maimonides stresses the need of continuous theoretical study and is cautious to actually treat patients, he was at the same time very interested in gathering practical information, mostly of a pharmaceutical nature, and often tried out certain medicines he knew from medical literature but was not sure whether they were reliable and composed new ones if necessary.

Gerrit Bos
September 2021

The introduction is based on "Maimonides' Medical Works and their Contribution to his Medical Biography," *Maimonidean Studies* 5 (2008): 243–266.

BOOK 1

On Asthma

First published in:

Maimonides
On Asthma

A Parallel Arabic-English Text,
Edited, Translated, and Annotated
by Gerrit Bos.

Provo/UT (Brigham Young University Press) 2002
MWMM 1

∴

(N.1) Says Mūsā ibn ʿUbayd Allāh the Israelite from Córdoba: My honorable, esteemed, beloved, and successful Master—may God grant him everlasting greatness and grace—has informed me about this chronic disease from which he suffers which is called asthma. He has ordered me to write for him something about the foods that he should avoid and those that he should take and about the kind of regimen which is best for this disease, according to the explanations of the esteemed physicians. It is well known among the physicians that this disease can have many causes and that the regulation of the healing of diseases differs according to the different causes. And it is well known among the physicians that one cannot treat a disease in a proper way unless one has first examined the temperament of the patient in general and the temperament of every organ in particular, and especially the temperament of the ailing organ itself and of those organs that share in its pain. Then one should examine the fatness or leanness of the body of the patient, which to some extent also falls under the category of temperament. And then one should examine his age, the condition of his town or country, his habit, the time of the year, and the temperament of the weather at that moment. If my intention in the composition of this treatise were to be all-embracing—namely, to impart knowledge about the treatment of this disease for every individual case, place, time of the year, and cause—it would become very lengthy and it would be necessary to examine all the aforementioned issues in detail. But this is not the purpose of this

 | DOI:10.1163/9789004498884_003

treatise, since the physicians have already laid down for every disease all that is necessary in this respect. Also, this disease is not so uncommon and its causes are not so obscure that a special treatise should be devoted to it. And I do not have anything to propound that is so unusual that I should devote a treatise to it, especially composed for the sake of that unusual interpretation. Rather, the purpose of this treatise is specific: namely, to deal with the requirement brought forward by my exalted Master—may God cure him of every affliction.

(N.2) I know from what I have witnessed with my own eyes and from what my Master has described to me that the cause of this asthma from which he suffers is a defluxion that descends from the brain at certain times of the year, but mostly in winter. And I know that the orthopnea and distress do not cease through the night for days on end, according to the length or brevity of the attack, until the defluxion decreases and until that fluid which has reached the lungs has been cocted so that the latter have become clean. This is what I know about the cause of this disease. You have also informed me that from sheer necessity you resort to purging once or twice a year, with that whose property it is to expel the phlegm and cleanse the brain and lungs. And I know that you often take a purgative in the case of an attack and by that means you then get rid of it. I also know that you are middle-aged and that your body is intermediate between leanness and heaviness and that your general temperament is very close to the balanced type, though it tends somewhat toward heat, and that the temperament of your brain is hotter than it should be. I inferred this from the fact that you are harmed—as you told me—by the odors of hot ingredients, that you cannot stand their smell, that your hair feels very heavy for you, that you find relief only by shaving it very frequently, and that you are made very uncomfortable by covering your head with a large turban. All these symptoms indicate excessive heat of your brain.

(N.3) You told me—may God heal you—that the air of Alexandria is very harmful for you and that you go to Cairo whenever you expect the onset of an attack of asthma because the air of Cairo is lighter and calmer so that it is easier for you to bear that attack. You also told me—may God give you everlasting glory—that a number of physicians have treated you as they thought necessary but that this has not eliminated the disease. After this introduction, which may be my apology to a physician who looks into this treatise and finds in it partial rules based on tendentious terms, I will begin to answer that which you, my exalted Master, have asked me.

(N.4) I thought it appropriate to arrange this treatise in general chapters which may be very useful to everyone in adherence to the regimen of health, in the prevention of the occurrence of diseases, and in the healing of most diseases. I have gleaned these chapters from the words of Galen and others as I remembered them during the composition of this treatise. I have not cited them literally but have adapted them in order to encourage their practical application. Similarly, at the end I have written down general beneficial rules concerning the regimen of health and the healing of diseases. My intention in all this is to be useful to people in general as much as I can so that you—may God give you everlasting glory—may benefit from this entire treatise and others may benefit from part of it. I thought it a good thing to divide it into chapters to make it easy to remember or to find what one wants to know.

Chapter one: On the warning about the best regimen in general.
Chapter two: On the provision of rules concerning the foods to be eaten or avoided in relation to this disease.
Chapter three: On different kinds of food that should be avoided or consumed, selected from those foods that are readily available and common among us.
Chapter four: On the composition of different dishes which are beneficial in this disease.
Chapter five: On the quantity of food.
Chapter six: On the times of day for the consumption of food.
Chapter seven: On beverages.
Chapter eight: On the proper regimen in connection with the air and movements of the soul.
Chapter nine: On the proper regimen for evacuation and retention.
Chapter ten: On the proper regimen regarding sleep and waking, bathing, massage, and sexual intercourse.
Chapter eleven: On the provision of rules for the treatment of this disease.
Chapter twelve: On the composition of drugs necessary for every different kind of treatment of this disease, according to the scope of this treatise.
Chapter thirteen: On the provision of rules, few in number but of great help for people in general, concerning the regimen of health and the healing of diseases; in hortatory form.

Having set forth the division of these chapters, I will now start my explanation of the contents of every chapter in a concise way, God willing.

Chapter One
On the best regimen in general

(I.1) Everyone who looks into this treatise should know that all chronic diseases which occur in cycles—such as gout, arthritis, stones in kidneys and gallbladder, asthma, migraine and the headache called *khūdha* (helmet) in Arabic, and other similar diseases—are impossible or difficult to heal. In the case of each of these diseases, if one adheres to a good regimen and abstains from everything from which one should abstain and relies on that on which one should rely, one necessarily prolongs the interval between the cycles, diminishes the occurrences of attacks in a cycle, alleviates the suffering and pain which they cause, and makes it easier to bear them. But when one adheres to a bad regimen and gives in to one's lusts and habits without abstaining from anything, it necessarily reduces the time between the cycles and increases the occurrence and severity of the attacks during the cycle; in time the pain will become so severe that the patient will die. And if an organ is weak by nature—by its very formation—and continuously receives the body's superfluities because of its weakness, a good regimen will diminish these superfluities and their bad effect; but a bad regimen will increase the superfluities and their bad effect. We have already drawn attention to this very useful rule, which informs all that is good in this art.

Galen said: What proves our words with absolute clarity is that we find that some people suffer from diseases in the weak organs of their bodies every six months or more. And if the cause were only the weak organ that is overcome by the disease, this weak organ would always be ill. But, since we do not find it to be always affected, it is clear that there is another factor which, in addition, brings about the occurrence of the disease in it. And this factor is nothing other than the bad superfluity, with respect to either its quantity or its quality. [*De sanitate tuenda* VI.13].

(I.2) Says the author: Galen has proven to us that the weak organs become ill because of an excess of humors, even when these humors are good; because of the badness of the humors; and because of a change in their quality, even when they are small in quantity. And when they are plentiful and bad, the damage is greater. Galen also informed us that he cured many people of the diseases from which they had been suffering for many years simply through a good regimen and proper exercise. [*De sanitate tuenda* V.1]. Galen further stated that one's moral qualities are also damaged by being habituated to bad things, such as bad kinds of food and drink, but that a good regimen greatly improves the moral qualities. [*Quod animi mores corporis temperamenta sequantur*]. These are very useful general rules which should be applied in the case of both healthy and sick people.

(I.3) It is well known that the regimen of healthy and sick people in general has been summarized by the physicians in seven categories, six of them essential and one occasional. The six essential categories are:

1. the air that surrounds us;
2. food and drink;
3. physical exercise and rest, which is opposite to it;
4. movements of the soul;
5. sleeping and waking; and
6. excretion and retention.

The occasional factor is that which affects the body occasionally, except for the air in the bathhouse and massage.

(I.4) Sexual intercourse has not been included as a category in the regimen of health by any ancient physician. But Hippocrates and Galen have said in the context of the healing of diseases that it is sometimes necessary to scatter the sperm through intercourse in the case of a bad temperament. [*Epidemics* VI.5.15; *In Hippocratis Epidemiarum commentarius* VI.6.5]. Mostly, however, men have sexual intercourse not because it is necessary but for mere pleasure. It therefore seems appropriate to consider it in this seventh category. I will discuss the regimen for each of these seven categories in a very concise and abbreviated way in accordance with the scope of this treatise.

∴

Chapter Two

On the provision of rules concerning the foods to be eaten or avoided in relation to this disease

(II.1) Every kind of food which produces thick or sticky humors should be avoided, and similarly everything that is very nutritious, even if it is good. Every kind of food which is rich in superfluities should be avoided, but one should take that kind of food which is moderate or somewhat less in its quantity of superfluities and which is neither sticky nor thick in quality, but is somewhat fine. The reason for this is clear—namely, that, when foods are digested in the organs and when the superfluity from the third digestion is minimal and is not sticky or thick, they are dissolved in a concealed way and leave the body through evaporation and perspiration. And if some superfluity remains of this, it can be easily expelled from the organ through the fine passages of the body and excreted with the feces and the urine and the like. But if there is much superfluity or if it is thick or sticky, it is not easily dissolved and does not pass easily through the fine passages; the superfluity cleaves to the organ and is difficult to expel from it. When the organ is extremely powerful, it overcomes the superfluity and expels it to another weaker organ, where the superfluity then becomes settled and fixed and becomes even more corrupt.

When a physician wants to dilute and dissolve the superfluity which is stuck in the weak organ, he needs strong drugs or a long period of time for treatment or both, according to the thickness, viscosity, or quantity of the humor; according to the narrowness or wideness of the passages in that organ; and according to the weakness or strength of that organ and of that which surrounds it. This is what makes it so difficult to change a humor or to make it respond to the will of the physician; for it remains firmly in its place, where it corrupts everything that comes in contact with it until the damage that is caused is so great that the organ or the entire body is ruined. For this reason, a thickening regimen is a mistake for everyone in general when adhered to in the extreme, and a great danger for some people. One's intention should be that all the veins and passages are open and clean and free from obstructions and constriction so that the pneumas and humors stream through them freely and the superfluities are expelled.

(II.2) Galen has made the following statement, and these are his very words: One acts with prudence and firmness if one takes care that the passages or channels which carry the food from the liver are open and clean, not only in the case of the sick but also in that of the healthy. [*De alimentorum facultatibus* II.8]. In another chapter, he said the following: Therefore, I advise everyone to abstain from all the foodstuffs that produce bad humors; even if someone digests them easily and quickly, he should not be deluded by this, for in the process of time one of these bad humors will collect in his veins while he does not notice it. And when the slightest cause occurs to this humor and causes it to putrefy, it putrefies and gives rise to malignant fevers. [*In Hippocratis De alimento commentarius* III.26].

(II.3) Says the author: This is a very useful rule and great advice for everyone to beware of coarse, sticky foods in general. As for the personal disease we are speaking about now, a thickening regimen is disastrous for it, while a thinning one is very beneficial, according to what we have explained. But one should not pursue it to the extreme—and this is according to what we mentioned about the equilibrium of the body in leanness and fatness. Similarly, one should avoid every kind of food which produces vapors and fills the head with them, and especially when these vapors are very hot. For the weakness of the brain increases through hot things, since heat is the cause of its weakness, as Galen has explained. The strength of all the organs deteriorates when they deviate too much from their equilibrium in whatever quality. Moreover, any organ, when it becomes hot, attracts superfluities. And when the brain becomes filled with superfluities, they stream in a large quantity—as is usual in this disease—toward the lungs and fill the bronchial tubes, which part from the trachea. Consequently, the lungs are saturated and soaked with those superfluities.

One should also avoid those foods which are hard to digest; for, when something is difficult to digest in the stomach, it stays there for such a long time that some of the vapors resulting from its coction ascend to the brain, make it heavy, and fill it, so that the brain weakens. This is the information that I considered necessary to mention in this chapter, according to the scope of this treatise.

∴

Chapter Three

On the different kinds of food that should be avoided or consumed, selected from those foods that are readily available and common among us

(III.1) Galen has explained that every kind of food prepared from wheat flour that has been thoroughly sifted is thick and sticky and digests slowly, but it is very nutritious. [*De alimentorum facultatibus* I.2]. Its harm is only eliminated when flour is used that is not sifted as much, when the leaven is still recognizable in the bread, when the bread is well salted and the dough well kneaded, when it is baked in a *tannūr* (circular earthen oven), and when it is well done. Any bread prepared in this way is better than that prepared from whole grains. After bread baked in a *tannūr* comes bread baked in a *furn* (regular oven); and next in excellence after flour which is not sifted as much comes flour prepared from wheat which has been neither soaked in water nor peeled. Instead, the flour is sifted lightly so that not all the bran is removed, and it should be well ground. For, when this flour is kneaded and made into bread, as we have mentioned, it is good regular food, easy to digest, with a moderate nutritional effect. Anything made from wheat prepared in a different way is bad and harmful for people in general and for my honorable Master in particular, such as that food prepared from wheat itself—as, for instance, *harīsa*, or *ḥarīra*. Neither should it be prepared from flour which is boiled, such as *wetiqa* is. Nor should it be that which is prepared from the dough, such as noodles and vermicelli and the like. Nor should food be made from that flour which is mixed with oil or fried, since this increases its stickiness and makes it hot—such as *kaʿk* mixed with oil and sweet pancakes. *Qaṭāʾif* are also very bad because they are unleavened and sticky and are a poor-quality bread. If, in addition, they are covered with sugar or eaten with honey, this is a serious cause of diseases developing in healthy people—and even more so in sick people, whose humors we want to thin and the stickiness of whose humors we want to remove. Since all these different kinds of bread are thick food (food producing thick humors), oil increases their stickiness, as we mentioned. When one adds honey or sugar to them, they cause great harm to the liver and increase its obstruction, because the liver favors this kind of food and is so susceptible to it that it penetrates to the ends of the liver until the veins are obstructed by sticky humors. Be aware of this, and avoid it above anything else. The worst of all these kinds of bread is that which is made from the very fine flour prepared from the innermost pure grain of the wheat.

(III.2) Galen said: Anything made from this very fine flour of wheat produces a thick humor, is slow in passing, obstructs the food passages from the liver, hardens and enlarges the spleen when it is weak, and causes kidney stones. [*De alimentorum facultatibus* I.4]. Galen also said: Unleavened bread from coarse barley meal is unfit and not beneficial for anyone. [*De alimentorum facultatibus* I.2.7].

(III.3) Says the author: Similarly, one should avoid all the pulses which produce flatulence, such as broad beans and peas, for instance, Indian and black-eyed peas; and those which are thick, such as rice and lentils; and everything which sends vapors to the brain, such as nuts; and that which produces next to it extreme heat, such as garlic, onions, and leek. One should also avoid all the different kinds of thick meat, such as that of cows (beef), goats (chevon), and grown sheep (mutton). Galen said that these latter are worse than the meat of cows. [*De alimentorum facultatibus* III.1.7].

(III.4) It is well known that cheese is a thick food, and when it is old it is very bad. All the usual kinds of milk fill the head and harm the brain; avoid them. Similarly, all waterfowl are thick, such as geese and ducks, which contain many corrupt humors. Of the different kinds of meat, one should choose the meat of fowl which is not fat, because it contains little superfluity and is quickly digested, such as francolin, pigeon, and partridge; and all the smaller kinds of fowl—such as small birds—are beneficial for this disease, especially when they are fried or roasted with barley gruel. Soup prepared from old roosters acts like a beneficial drug for this disease. But as for the yolks of the eggs laid by hens, although they are good, moderate food—and especially poached eggs—I do not think that you should use them because of their moisture. But small saltwater fish with little fat and white flesh which has a pleasant taste, and which falls apart easily because it is not sticky, is good food for you because it digests quickly and has little superfluity. Freshwater fish are not harmful when they come from a large river with streaming, clean water.

(III.5) Besides these kinds of fish which, as I explained to you, are beneficial for this disease, pickled fish are also recommended because they have a purgative and attenuating effect. But one should not take too much of them, so that they do not make the phlegm sticky. I also recommend that you partake of the kind of fish which is called mullet and of fish which has been cooked and recently pickled; it is good to take this once or twice a month.

(III.6) You should mostly partake of mutton, because it is common food with us. Since this is the case, the best thing to take is a yearling or an animal at the beginning of its second year. But do not take an animal which has completed two years. And take that animal which is grazing in the field, but not that which is stall-fed, for the latter contains many superfluities, especially fat animals. However, the meat of the female of this species is very bad for people in general and for this disease in particular because it is sticky and hard to digest and contains many superfluities. All the intestines of any species whatever are bad; the heads contain many superfluities; and, while the legs are free from superfluities, they do contain stickiness. In general, you should not eat anything from the male of this species except for the meat from the front part and the meat which is attached to the bone, such as the shoulder, the chest, and the ribs around the heart; all this is of the same kind. All the fats of the abdomen are, in general, bad for all people because they are sticky and spoil the digestion. And since they satiate and spoil one's appetite, they have a deadly effect in the case of this disease because of their increased moisture. None of your dishes should be very fat; when one of the kinds of meat which we described has much fat on it, the fat should be removed so that nothing of it is left with the meat except for that which gives it a pleasant taste—but nothing else.

(III.7) Know that the meat of gazelles, deer (venison), and rabbits is good and recommendable for this disease, even if it is not good in general. Similarly, the fats of rabbits are recommended for this disease. The same holds good for those things which have the same effect as remedies, even if they are normally bad foods, such as the meat of foxes, and especially their lungs. Also, the meat of wild hedgehogs is very beneficial, it is said, for this disease, because it thins those corrupt substances (humors) and corrects what can be corrected. Hedgehogs' lungs are beneficial, especially for this disease.

(III.8) Among the vegetables recommended for this disease are chard and asparagus, even if they are hard to digest. Although fennel, celery, peppermint, mint, oregano, garden cress, and radish are all bad foods, they act like remedies for this disease. All the moist vegetables—such as cultivated lettuce, garden orach, mallow, *qarʿ* (field pumpkin or winter squash), and the like—are bad for this disease; avoid them. Similarly, vegetables with a thick substance—such as wild taro, wild carrots, cabbage, eggplant, and turnips—should all be avoided because of their thick substance, although they contain refining moisture. There is no way for you to use any of these, because they combine the qualities of both bad and thick foods.

(III.9) Among the fresh fruits, there are some which are juicy, such as *biṭṭīkh* (common melon or watermelon), peach, apricot, mulberry, and cucumber. These are bad, because all the fresh fruits are bad food for everyone in general, and those which we mentioned are especially bad for someone with this disease. Fresh dates are especially bad, because they are thick and sticky and cause headache. The same holds good for grapes, because they cause flatulence; and everything that causes flatulence—said the physicians—fills the head and makes digestion more difficult. But if someone sips some grape juice in the morning on an empty stomach and then eats an astringent dish seasoned with peppermint, I have no objection to it. It is not necessary to avoid the consumption of fresh figs, although one should not eat them continuously; for, although they cause flatulence, a small amount of them is not harmful, because they rapidly leave the stomach. But one should eat them on an empty stomach, like the other fruits; their peels should be removed, and one should eat them very ripe. And if one eats them with barley gruel or vinegar or salt mixed with common rue, peppermint, or cumin, it is like a medicine with a thinning effect. And if one does not like to immerse the figs in one of these ingredients and then eat them, one may eat them as they are; but one should take a little bit of one of these ingredients after one has finished eating the figs. On that same day—once the figs have left the stomach—one should have a light meal, such as young chickens, pigeons, or small birds cooked in vinegar or lemon juice and seasoned with peppermint. And if one sips some pomegranate juice, it is beneficial for the chest.

(III.10) To suck quinces after the meal is beneficial, but one should not take too much of them, because all the astringent things such as quinces, *nabiq* (fruits of Christ's thorn jujube), and common medlars are harmful for this disease; apples are also bad because they are astringent and produce flatulence. Among dried fruits, raisins are very beneficial for this disease because they coct and thin the humors and alleviate heartburn, but one should first remove their seeds. Dried figs are also beneficial when one takes them after they have been immersed in pounded and sifted anise. And for dessert one should take pistachio nuts and almonds, especially the bitter nuts, which one may mix with sweet nuts until one becomes accustomed to eating them. For this is an excellent remedy for this disease, because it thins the humors, opens all the obstructions, cleans the lungs, and helps expectoration; keep it in mind. Large pine nuts are also beneficial, since they clean the lungs, especially when they are soaked for some hours in hot water and are eaten when the water is cool. As for hazelnuts, I have no objection to their limited use. But we have warned against the use of walnuts because of the vapors arising from them to the brain. The dried kernels of all these nuts should be taken with sugar or *fānīdh* or a little bit of one of the different kinds of dried sweets that does not contain starch (amylum) or sesame.

∴

Chapter Four

On the composition of different dishes which are beneficial in this disease

(IV.1) I have explained the properties of the foods which should be avoided or consumed by someone suffering from this disease, and I have mentioned the simple types of these foods. According to this, one should prepare various dishes selected from those which are well known and common among us. Among them are *isfīdabāj* (stew) with beetroots, chicken, or mutton, as we have stipulated. If this dish is cooked with chickpeas and you do not want to eat any of the chickpeas themselves, but you prepare the stock for the dish with the water in which the chickpeas have been soaked, it is nevertheless beneficial.

(IV.2) Another dish is that prepared from raisins: It is extremely beneficial and very tasty and is like a remedy. Its preparation is thus: Boil mutton or fowl that has been roasted in the same way as other foods and spices that I will describe further on. Then remove the meat and set it aside. Then take the raisins, remove their seeds, and soak them for two hours in vinegar. After this, pulverize them in a stone mortar with peeled almonds equal to one-quarter of the amount of the raisins, and strain this through a sieve until the skins of the raisins are removed. Add this to the roasted meat stock and put it on a low fire until it is well cooked. This is a dish that I have seen being prepared in Egypt; I strongly recommend its preparation because it thins and cocts the humors and it is of a moderate heat with a tendency to dry. It also opens obstructions and is good for all healthy people, but it is the best thing for this disease.

(IV.3) A benefit of this compound dish is that the raisins fatten the liver and agree with it very well, and they take away the heartburn and the burning from the passages of the lungs and have an alleviating effect. It has been said that, if one eats them frequently, they burn the blood, and that the vinegar, although it thins and dilutes the humors and opens the obstructions, is harmful for the liver and irritates it; whitens the blood; and is also harmful for the windpipe, because it dries and hardens it and thereby impedes coughing. But, when the raisins and the vinegar are mixed together, each ingredient protects against the harmful effect of the other, so that they retain their combined beneficial effects. This is especially the case when they are mixed together in chicken stock with almond kernels. I have not seen anything better than this compound dish.

(IV.4) Similarly, *maṣūṣ* and *zīrbāj* are beneficial, but one should use little vinegar in them. It is also good to cook the meat with lemon, sugar, almonds, or safflower seed. Similarly, it is good when this dish is prepared with rose preserves and used constantly in the wintertime. So, too, when one cooks it with skimmed honey or sugar or a little vinegar or lemon juice seasoned with peppermint, it is a good preparation. Another dish which one should take in wintertime is that prepared with fresh fennel. Remove its leaves, take its hearts, cut and boil and roast them separately. Then pour chicken stock which is not very fat over it and add the roasted chicken to it and leave it on a low fire until it is well cooked. And if one takes the shoots of the fennel once they have grown large and peels them and cuts their hearts and cooks them with it as we have described, it is a dish beneficial and helpful for expectoration. This dish is well known and very common among us in the Maghreb and is beneficial. Similarly, if one prepares the dish which we call the "mixed one" by adding to the soup barley gruel, one quarter of all of the mentioned things meaning the chicken stock and fennel, and a little lemon juice and spices that are not too aromatic, and by leaving it until it is well cooked, it has a delicious taste and is easy to digest.

(IV.5) Among the foods also eaten by the people of Egypt is bread seasoned with vinegar and skimmed honey or with vinegar and sugar and barley gruel. One should always have on one's table, especially in wintertime, sea squill vinegar,

(IV.6) and one should dip some morsels of bread in it. Similarly, one should sometimes dip them in mustard. Among us in al-Andalus, the mustard is prepared as follows: Take one *mudd* of Syrian mustard, soak it in hot water overnight, and let the water cool off. Put the mustard in a stone mortar and add carded cotton to it so that it sticks together and is not scattered during the pounding. Pound it extremely well with strong vinegar. Pour fragrant, sweet olive oil over it little by little until the *mudd* of mustard has absorbed one *raṭl* of the fragrant olive oil and has become very soft. After this, macerate it in white vinegar, then take one *raṭl* of sweet almonds and peel them and pound them until they become like marrow and macerate this substance in the same vinegar as that in which the mustard was macerated. Strain the entire substance through a piece of cloth or sieve until it has the consistency and color of milk of a cow and only differs from it in taste. This mustard preparation is very good for the digestion; it dissolves the phlegm, cleans the lining of the stomach, dissolves the stickiness of the humors, and does not heat excessively.

(IV.7) Know that the hot and dry ingredients are extremely harmful for this disease, especially for the temperament which we mentioned because they make the fatty humors sticky and thicken and coagulate those humors which have no fatness. Because of all this, no spices should—in my opinion—be apparent in the food, especially not those spices which are exceedingly hot, as we are used to in most of these countries. One should limit oneself to the following compound: Half an ounce of black pepper, two ounces each of cinnamon bark and caraway, half an ounce of ginger, three *dirhams* of spikenard, two *dirhams* of mace, six ounces of dry coriander. Pulverize all these ingredients and add from this an amount to the food which is sufficient to season it but which does not have a heating effect. As for the dishes prepared with vinegar, we do not object if one adds to the ingredients which we mentioned two ounces each of bitter ginger and clove wood, because, in combination with the vinegar, they increase the thinning and dilution process of the humors. And concerning every dish to which one is accustomed to adding saffron, one should adhere to that custom and not decrease the amount, because the saffron cocts and thins the humors without a strong heating effect.

(IV.8) As for the different kinds of sweets, everything that contains starch (amylum) or anything prepared from wheat, such as *khabīṣa* and *qāhiriyya* and the like—all this is very bad, because it causes obstructions. I have already said that the different kinds of dried sweets should be used in combination with the shelled nuts which I mentioned. For instance, if one coats pine nuts with *fānīdh*, just as one coats pistachio nuts, they are excellent.

Chapter Five
On the quantity of food

(V.1) Since I have spoken about the quality of the food to be ingested, I should also speak about its quantity, which varies according to the different individual characteristics of people. For people with a large stomach and strong digestion can tolerate a large amount of food, while those with a small stomach and weak digestion by nature can tolerate only a small amount. It is well known that this art of medicine is devised only for rational beings. Therefore, every human individual should calculate the amount which he should eat when he is healthy and know the amount which, if he consumes it in the springtime, can be easily tolerated and well and easily digested. That amount should be taken as one's basic portion; one should reduce it gradually as the heat increases and increase it gradually as the cold increases. The main principle in this entire matter is to avoid harmful satiation and distension of the stomach, because when any organ is distended, its functions are necessarily impaired. For distension is a dissolution of continuity. When the stomach distends more than is natural for it, all its functions weaken and it can no longer contain the food, which then becomes a burden to it and so loathsome that it requires water—although there is no thirst—so that the food can be discharged from it and its burden be relieved as the food is dissolved in water. This explains the reason for the urge to drink large amounts of water after satiation.

(V.2) The physicians have fixed appropriate rules in this matter by stating that a person should stop eating before he detests it, preferably at a time when most of his appetite has been satisfied and only a little appetite remains. If, in the case of dumb animals—such as horses, donkeys, and camels, whose regimen is fixed according to the standard of rational beings—man measures out their regimen in such a way that they eat only a fixed amount of fodder and do not eat at random, why would not man determine his own food intake in such a way that he eats according to his appetite and not according to what he can tolerate to the point that the food reaches the lowest part of the esophagus?

(V.3) I have sometimes seen certain gluttons belching and thereby returning the food from their stomachs to their mouths, just like ruminating animals. This is the main cause for most diseases, because good food—even the best there is—necessarily corrupts one's digestion if one takes too much of it, and bad humors originate from it which are the origin and source of diseases. When there is an overabundance of humors, indigestion occurs; and indigestion is one of the extremely acute diseases. Galen said that indigestion kills within one day when it is severe, and when it is not severe it can kill within two or three days or at least cause illness. Indigestion which accompanies diarrhea is followed by well-known symptoms; one among these is a burning pain of the cardia of the stomach, causing fainting. [*In Hippocratis De acutorum morborum victu commentarius* II.47]. But it is not our intention in this chapter to give medical advice for the different kinds of indigestion. Rather, its intention is simply to warn against them and to advise on the great harm they cause, so that they will be avoided.

(V.4) The physicians have forbidden the consumption of many dishes during a single meal and commanded limiting oneself to a single dish. The reason they give for this is that the stomach has various ways of digesting different dishes. Since there is only one stomach, if it contains different dishes, the humors in the stomach would of necessity either be unable to digest all the different dishes or would digest only one dish in an excessive and extreme way. They have also urged that one not fail to consider the sequence in which one takes the dishes, because the digestion of food is corrupted in many ways. It can be corrupted because of its quality or because of its quantity, as we have mentioned, or because of the sequence of dishes; for the food which is coarser should be eaten first, and then the food which is finer, according to some views. Galen thinks that the food which is finer should be eaten first, and then that which is coarser. [*De alimentorum facultatibus* II.11]. Similarly, one should first eat that which has a diluting effect and then eat that which is astringent, according to the opinion of all physicians. And if there is one dish, one does not have to pay attention to this sequence as they mentioned it. It is evident to me that this regimen of one dish has a very great advantage over the other two regimens mentioned, for the presence of many dishes prompts someone to take much food, because the appetite is stimulated with every dish one takes. But in the case of a single dish the appetite is satisfied with it, so that in most cases one does not eat more thereof than is necessary unless—and this is the worst case—someone is very gluttonous. In any case, when one eats from one dish, one eats less than when one eats from many dishes. A basic rule to be observed in the regimen of health is to eat as little as possible so as not to reach the point of satiation.

(V.5) Hippocrates has said the following, and these are his very words: The preservation of health consists of being on one's guard against satiation and giving up laziness for exertion. [*Epidemics* VI.4.18]. Concerning this matter, Galen has given a useful recommendation which, in my opinion, it is advisable to quote here in his very words: Rest is very bad for the preservation of one's health, whereas moderate movement is very good. [*De bonis malisque sucis* III]. For a person does not fall ill if he takes care to ensure that bad digestion never befalls him and that he does not move vigorously after eating. This is because, just as exercise before a meal is more beneficial than anything else for the preservation of health, so movement after a meal is worse than anything else because the food leaves the stomach and spreads through the body without having been digested, so that many humors accumulate in the veins. And these humors tend to produce different diseases, if they are not dissolved previously by strenuous effort or digested or converted into blood through the faculty which is in the liver and the veins.

(V.6) Says the author: Resting after a meal is, in my opinion, of great benefit. And from this it may be clear to you that going to the bathhouse, having sexual intercourse, and allowing venesection after having a meal are a great mistake, because all these are movements of the body; on the contrary, one should maintain absolute rest after the meal. Consider also the degree of benefit gained when one guards oneself against bad digestion, which is without any doubt a cause of indigestion. Galen has enumerated a number of symptoms, and these are his very words: In all such cases, we observed with our own eyes that it occurred to him whose food is not digested. It is clear to us that Galen does not mean by this that all these symptoms happen to everyone whose food is not digested, for one or more of these symptoms may occur to every individual person according to the different temperaments of people, their age, their bodily dispositions, and the different kinds of foods which are corrupted. And the symptoms mentioned by him which develop from bad digestion are flatulence; burning pain; a soft or excessive stool; nausea; loss of appetite or excessive appetite; indolence; a slow and sluggish mind; a heavy head; insomnia; heartburn; epilepsy; derangement; dullness of mind; lethargy; melancholic distress or any kind of distress; pain in the colon, intestines, spleen, liver, or joints; indisposition; shivering fit; shivering; or fever. [*De symptomatum causis* III.12].

(V.7) Says the author: Intelligent healthy people should consider and conclude logically whether the pleasure they derive from eating makes up for the anticipation of all those afflictions which Galen has enumerated and which can be avoided if one limits oneself to eating a single good food, does not fill oneself with it, and does not exercise after eating it, as mentioned previously. If this kind of precaution is indispensable for healthy people, how much more should they be obligatory for chronically ill people, and especially for someone who suffers from a weakness of one of the major organs, either inherently or as a result of illness. They should become accustomed to adhering to the good alimentary regimen whose principles and types we have mentioned above.

∴

Chapter Six
On the times of day for the consumption of food

(VI.1) People have different habits concerning this. Most of them eat in the morning and evening, some people eat three times in two days, and some once a day. I do not know the habit of my honorable Master in this regard. The general rule to be followed is that strong people may feed themselves with what they need in one sitting. But if weak people, such as the elderly and convalescents, take their food in one sitting, it is a grave mistake. Their food should be divided in proportion to their strength, and they should take it little by little so that their strength does not wane and their innate heat does not become extinguished.

(VI.2) With regard to the general regimen of the elderly, Galen said the following: The best advice for them when their strength is weak is to feed the body little by little at short intervals, and when their body is strong, they should take much food at long intervals.

(VI.3) Says the author: This subject is repeated many times in Galen's books, and the essential point—whatever the context—is that one should not consume one meal after another and that one should eat only when the stomach is empty and not as the fools do, who fix a certain invariable time of the day to have their meal, as if it is an obligatory prayer. Instead, one should let it depend on the emptiness of the stomach, and this varies according to the kind of food one eats, according to the length or brevity of the day, or according to external factors. The moment after which one may partake of food is that wherein the food eaten earlier has left the stomach, when there is no aftertaste from eructation, when there is a real appetite, and when saliva begins to flow to the mouth—and, even then, one should wait half an hour. The physicians said that no one should wait more than two hours after the moment when food leaves the stomach and that someone should determine the right time according to the fatness or leanness of the body, the large or small amount of humors, and their hotness or coldness; for someone with a lean body and a small amount of hot humors should wait half an hour and then eat, while someone opposite in every aspect should wait for two hours. This is the criterion of the emptiness of the stomach which they mentioned. But hunger is not the only criterion to be considered, because people suffering from indigestion often have a false sensation of hunger originating from bad humors which irritate the cardia of the stomach. It has been explained that those who are accustomed to eating in the morning and evening should, in the winter, eat in the second or third hour of the day, depending on the length of the night and the strength of the digestion, and that in the summer they should eat in the fifth hour, because then the stomach is empty. Similarly, the time for eating in the evening is earlier or later, according to the criteria which we have mentioned. Know that it may happen to someone who eats once a day that one winter night he will wake up at the beginning of the night with a stomach that has been empty for many hours. And in the summertime, it may happen that someone takes a light dish earlier than normal, because of the length of the day, and then has an empty stomach when he goes to bed. These things happen frequently.

(VI.4) This theoretical observation is confirmed by personal experience. For, when I take some bread—even a small amount—at an unusual time, I am harmed by it and my digestion is spoiled. And if I spend the night with an empty stomach, my humors are burned and my stomach is heated by bad humors flowing toward it, as happens to everyone who is fasting. I have found that the best thing to do is to have the stomach occupied with light tasty foods which are easy to digest. Sometimes I drink soup made from young roosters, when it is available, and then go to sleep; and sometimes I boil five or six eggs and eat their yolks with some cinnamon and salt sprinkled on them. Sometimes I eat some pistachio nuts and raisins without their seeds, or raisins and almonds with *fānīdh*, and drink a beverage of sugar or honey—whichever is available. During the winter I take a glass of wine when it is cold. In general, one should not spend the night in a hungry state except when the stomach contains crude, raw, and thick humors whose coction is desired.

(VI.5) I advise my Master to do all this, but to take, instead of a glass of wine in the winter, between a third and a half *raṭl* of refined hydromel. For I have seen that this regimen has a very good effect.

Chapter Seven
On beverages

(VII.1) Since we have mentioned the proper regimen concerning the consumption of food, we should follow that with the regimen concerning beverages, although most of this regimen does not apply to Muslims, since wine is prohibited to them and the different kinds of *nabīdh* are prohibited to most of them. God has already so safeguarded you against it that there is no need to warn you about it. Although wine and all the different kinds of *nabīdh* fill the head and are harmful to the brain and heat it and cause serious and grave diseases, and while they are especially harmful in the case of this disease (asthma), that which effects all this is the consumption of a large quantity of it, especially to the point of drunkenness. But, when one takes a small quantity of wine—such as three or four glasses—when the food is digested and leaving the stomach, it is of very great benefit for the regimen of one's health and for the healing of diseases. One of its benefits is that it improves digestion and increases the innate heat and expels the superfluities by means of perspiration and urine. But it is useless to enumerate the benefits of something the consumption of which is impossible for my Master. In general, if one takes a little bit of wine at the appropriate time, it is very beneficial for body and soul under all circumstances, and especially for the elderly, for whom it has been proven that it is indispensable and irreplaceable for them. But a large quantity of it is very harmful to both soul and body for all people of all ages.

(VII.2) But since the consumption of both a large and a small quantity of wine is forbidden under Islam, the physicians have taken pains to find a beverage that can replace it to a certain degree. This beverage is that consisting of honey seasoned with spices, for it can substitute for most of the excellent qualities of wine, except for the gladdening of the soul and the removal of the turbid, gaseous superfluity from the pneumas which they deposit in everyone according to his age and temperament. I will give my Master the recipe of such a drink which was composed by elders whom I observed and which is of the highest degree of perfection and is in accord with reason. And I will add thereto those spices which fit your temperament and disease. Take half a *mudd* of chickpeas, preferably the black ones, wash them from their dust, and macerate them in five Egyptian *raṭl*s of pure water overnight. The next morning, boil the chickpeas until their firmness is gone, but do not wait until they are completely done. Sieve the liquid into a *raṭl* of the finest white honey, put it on a low fire and let it simmer and remove the froth little by little. And when there is no froth left, add to it half an ounce of borage, three stalks of peppermint, and spices according to the age of the patient, his temperament, and the conditions of his organs.

What is, in my opinion, proper for my Master according to his disease and according to what I know of the temperament of his organs is that one adds to the chickpeas, once they are macerated, half an ounce of maidenhair fern. After removing the froth, one should put a finely woven piece of cloth which contains two *dirham*s of cinnamon bark; half a *dirham* each of pounded ginger, mastic, mace, and spikenard; and a quarter of a *dirham* of saffron into the beverage. Do not remove the piece of cloth, but squeeze it out with a spoon several times until the liquid assumes the consistency of the finest julep. Take it from the fire and do not make more than a *raṭl* of it at a time, for, when it is left for a long time, it ferments and turns sour. This beverage, of fine consistency, is the best in that one does not have to mix it. But if one prepares it in this consistency and puts it in a pitcher and then every time that one takes some of it, mixes it with water to drink it, its excellent qualities are impaired. But if it is necessary to mix it because one has to go on a journey, one should mix it with cold water in the summer and with warm water in the winter. And one should not drink it immediately after it has been mixed but take it one hour later, so that everything is well mixed and blended by the effect of time. Similarly, it is my opinion that, instead of peppermint, water mint should be taken, or the amount of peppermint should be increased so that it helps my Master to expectorate and remove the superfluities from chest and lungs.

(VII.3) Regarding water, most people know that, if one drinks it with a meal, it keeps the food crude because it forms a barrier between it and the stomach so that the food floats and is poorly digested. But if one has a fixed habit of doing so, one should take as little as possible and delay taking it as long as possible. The best time to drink water is about two hours after a meal. One should select water that is sweet, pure, light, free from any change in odor, drawn on the same day from running water. One should boil the water a few times, let it cool off, and then drink it, for this dispels much of its harm and corrects much of the corruption inherent to its kind. If one arranges to add some peeled licorice during the boiling, the taste of the water will not change; and, if one adds some mastic, the taste and odor of the water will be savory. One should boil the water in a new, polished pot, for this kind of water is the very best for all healthy people in both winter and summer: It strengthens all the internal organs, it is beneficial for the stomach, and even a small amount of it quenches one's thirst. If someone complains about some ailment, one should prescribe a diet for him of the appropriate water.

Know that the consumption of tepid water—that which is not truly cold—is very harmful for the digestion of all people; it weakens the stomach, and even a large quantity of it does not quench one's thirst. But cold water which is not so cold that a person shies away from drinking it and which is not as cold as ice is the choicest type of water, which one ought to drink when thirsty—and especially someone with a warm temperament.

(VII.4) The physicians have enumerated the excellent properties of this water when one drinks it in a moderate amount and not excessively. They have said that it is beneficial for the digestion, draws the body of the stomach together for digestion of the food, increases and strengthens the appetite, reddens the complexion, prevents one from falling victim to fevers and acute diseases, and prevents inflammation of the heart and stomach and putrefaction of the blood in the veins, and they note that even a small amount of it quenches thirst.

However, tepid water has the opposite effect: It causes swelling, corruption of the temperament, and the beginning of dropsy. Therefore, they said: We find that most people who drink warm water—that is to say, water which is not cold—have a greenish yellow complexion; are lean; suffer from abscesses in the spleen and liver; have weak appetites; are lacking in fat and in pleasantness and brightness of expression because their blood is bad and susceptible to inflammation and putrefaction. Therefore, one should be extremely careful to avoid it.

(VII.5) Since we have completed discussing the part of the regimen that concerns food and drink—which also includes the regimens of bodily movement and rest, as was our plan with this treatise—let us now discuss the rest of the seven categories, also according to the scope of the treatise.

∵

Chapter Eight

On the proper regimen in connection with the air and movements of the soul

(VIII.1) It is well known that it is necessary to correct and improve the air and to prevent its putrefaction in the case of all healthy people. As for sick people, the air should counteract the disease. The same holds good for the seasons deviating from the middle course—that is to say, that, in the summer, one should regulate the air with running, fragrant, pure waters; with those flowers and leaves which provide coolness; and with ventilation. Similarly, one should heat the air in winter with those fragrant plants and perfumes which provide heat and with a fire and drying fumigations. In the case of my Master, cold, moist air is very harmful. You should be extremely careful to avoid cold and hot defluxions.

(VIII.2) The case of the movements of the soul influencing the body is well known—that is to say, that one sees that one's soul and its psychical, vital, and natural functions can be so weak that one loses one's appetite, as, for instance, when one is sad, afraid, worried, and distressed. And if such a person wishes to raise his voice, he cannot do so, but he can only sigh deeply because his respiratory organs are too weak to function properly and because of an excess of gaseous superfluity. He is also unable to stand erect because he is not strong enough to raise his limbs. If this condition continues for a long time, he necessarily becomes ill; and if it becomes chronic, it will kill him. These facts are so well known that we do not have to discuss them at length.

But joy and pleasure have an effect opposite to all these things because of the dilation of the soul and the movement of the blood and pneuma to the outside of the body so that the functions of the organs seem to be at their very best. But if this emotion becomes very strong and the enjoyment of it very intense, as happens to those who are misled by their ignorance, it makes one ill; and sometimes it kills, due to the dissolution of the pneuma and the movement of the pneuma to the outside, so that the heart becomes cold and the person dies.

(VIII.3) The cure for these two kinds of movements of the soul and their prevention, so that one does not fall victim to them, is not effected by foods and drugs only, nor by the physician in charge of this medical art. Rather, the cure of these cases belongs to other arts—namely, ethical philosophy, or theoretical considerations, or the disciplines and admonitions of the Law. There is no doubt that all these disciplines provide a better way to get rid of these symptoms and protect a person against their occurrence; for by means of theoretical considerations one will learn the common nature of what exists and of what is intrinsically connected to this, the world of generation and corruption. Similarly, by means of ethical philosophy a person keeps away from passions and is not influenced by mere anger or pleasure, as is the case with beasts and as happens to the multitude. Rather, the movements of his soul follow the demands of human counsel and not mere physical passion, such as gentleness and harshness and the like. Similarly, by means of the refining constraints and admonitions of the Law a person will attach little importance to this world and its imaginary fortune and misfortune, all of which are momentary. Do not be deluded or troubled by them, for all these things are only important for us at a collective first sight. But, after true consideration, all of them are nothing but momentary amusement and pleasure.

(VIII.4) I have mentioned this, although it is not within the scope of the treatise, because I know—may God give you lasting, true happiness and save you from real misfortune—that you are at this moment in a condition of great distress and worry, and for this one cannot prescribe a proper regimen of health nor provide complete medical treatment of an illness. A person such as you should take an example from the righteous and the prophets of blessed memory and follow in their footsteps by casting away excessive distress over the dead, by subduing your natural tendencies and conceding that God's judgment in that matter is just, and by occupying yourself with that which is useful instead of that which is not useful. May God give all of us true knowledge.

∴

Chapter Nine

On the proper regimen for retention and evacuation

(IX.1) A good regimen for all people, and especially for someone in whose body bad humors have accumulated, is that the stools always be soft or nearly soft. When the stools are dry at a certain moment and stay like that for some days, one should soften them. Abū Marwān ibn Zuhr has recommended softening them with the following drug: Macerate ten *dirham*s of tamarind in sufficient warm water to cover them, and then soak three-quarters of a *dirham* of ground Chinese rhubarb for twenty-four hours, and strain this into one ounce of *utrujj* (citron or lemon) juice.

(IX.2) Says the author: I approve of this drug for someone with thin humors, for young people, and for those living in hot countries. However, for someone with thick or viscous humors or for old people—and especially for those who suffer from this disease, for whom I composed this treatise—the best thing to do, in my opinion, is to soften their stools with the remedy mentioned by Galen, which is prepared from the hearts of dried figs and safflower hearts and from raisins or field bindweed. This remedy should be prepared with the following amounts and in the following manner: Take five *dirham*s of safflower hearts, one-eighth of a *dirham* of salt, and twenty *dirham*s of the hearts of dried figs; pound all these ingredients in a stone or wooden mortar; once it is completely mixed, take it with some sips of warm water. For this remedy is extremely softening and is of the utmost benefit for the elderly, as Galen stated.

Another remedy: Pound the field bindweed, press it out, and strain half a *raṭl* of it with two ounces of honey, for it is very softening. Similarly, if one swallows one hazelnut (weight) of turpentine resin, it softens the stools without harm and cleans and purifies all the internal organs—the liver, spleen, kidneys, urinary bladder, and lungs. These remedies should be taken by turns.

(IX.3) Says the author: Similarly, if beetroot is seasoned with barley gruel and much olive oil—and the juice should not be discarded—it softens the stools. The same applies to the dish, well known in Egypt, which is prepared with lemon juice, safflower hearts, and beetroot. It is a preparation good for the softening of the stools for most people. Similarly, hydromel softens the stools; and if it is boiled with sebesten (Assyrian plum), licorice, and common marshmallow and strained with sugar and sweet almond oil, it softens the stools and expels the residues by making them smooth. One should select from these remedies what is suitable for one's bodily condition, one's age, and the season of the year.

(IX.4) But if the stools become softer than necessary and this lasts for two or three days, then one should take less food and consume one of the common astringent dishes such as those prepared from tanner's sumach (*summāqiyya*), unripe sour grapes, dried raisins with their seeds and pomegranates with beetroot ribs. This should be cooked in quinces and rose water.

(IX.5) In general, it is desirable that one return one's stools to their normal condition by means of the foods to which one is accustomed. One may also sip some of the usual syrups and robs, such as apple syrup and quince rob and other similar astringent robs. One should likewise take whichever of these is suitable according to one's age and the season of the year. For these kinds of things, one does not need to consult a skilled physician, nor should one be sparing in the amounts to be taken, because the matter is well known to most intelligent urban folk in those countries where medical practice is a common phenomenon. But when one wants to apply strong attracting purgatives—such as the pulp of colocynth, St. Thomas lidpod, scammony and the like—one should be extremely careful, never deem it an easy thing, and only do so on the advice of a skilled physician, especially in the case of the elderly, whom Galen warned very strongly against purging with these drugs. [*In Hippocratis De humoribus commentarius* I.12; *De sanitate tuenda* V.9]. Similarly, stopping diarrhea by means of strong drugs should not be attempted by anyone except upon the advice of a skilled physician who can ascertain the circumstances of a disease.

(IX.6) For the preservation of health and the healing of diseases, evacuation by means of enemas is one of the best regimens and is of very great merit, because it evacuates the humors. For, an enema with which one wants to attract the humors does not harm the principal organs and does not cause distress, as purgatives do. One can be assured that they are safe for one's health. If one wants to use the enema to soften and expel the dry stools, it is the most appropriate thing for the preservation of health and does not harm the nutritive organs. But one should not resort to taking decoctions and the like for softening these stools because they loosen the lining of the stomach and cause nausea, as most laxatives do when taken.

Galen has mentioned a number of enemas, some of which are good for the preservation of health and others which one needs only for healing a disease. I will mention those which are especially good for this disease of yours in this treatise. Those enemas which all or most people should take for the preservation of health when the stools are solid and dry and when it is nearly impossible to evacuate them are the following: Take two ounces of honey, half a *raṭl* of water, one ounce of fine olive oil, and one *dirham* of natron; heat all these ingredients; and use them as an enema. If you want to soften the dry residues or to make them smooth, you should increase the amount of olive oil; and if you want to expel the viscous humor, you should increase the amount of honey and natron. [*In Hippocratis De humoribus commentarius* I.12].

(IX.7) Another enema: Take half a *raṭl* of beetroot juice and two ounces of fine olive oil, heat this, and use it as an enema. Another enema: Take wheat bran, soak it in an amount of water sufficient to cover it, cook it until one-third of the water has evaporated, strain it until you have a sticky mass, add olive oil to it, and use it as an enema; it is good for the evacuation of hard stools. These three enemas I have chosen from among all the preparations mentioned by Galen, for they are, in my opinion, very good for the preservation of health. Similarly, enemas prepared with the mucilage of flax and fenugreek—both with olive oil, chicken fat, and beetroot juice—are preparations good for the evacuation of the stools in a smooth way without causing irritation or harm. And if, in the case of the elderly, one adds some honey or virgin honey thereto, it is beneficial. This is the opinion of Galen as well.

(ix.8) And Galen said that the application of an enema with mucilage of flax is beneficial for those suffering from hectic fever and mitigates the bad humors. [*In Hippocratis De humoribus commentarius* i.12]. Know that regular use of enemas thoroughly cleanses the brain incidentally and purifies the senses; it delays aging, improves the digestions, and prevents many diseases because it cleanses and flushes the lower organs so that the upper organs find open vessels to expel the superfluities according to the intention of nature to expel them through these passages. And thus, it is necessary to do as we have mentioned.

(ix.9) Know that nothing is more harmful to the preservation of health and more likely to cause disease than the retention of the two prime superfluities. Galen has explained that if the feces are retained, they corrupt the humors through the ascension of vapors to the brain and make all the pneumas turbid; and that they cause the beginning of putrefactions, corruption of the digestions, and the beginning of serious diseases. The same occurs from the retention of the urine. We have mentioned only some of the harm caused by them as related by him. Therefore, one should be very much aware of this problem.

(ix.10) Vomiting is necessary for the preservation of the health of all people and may also be applied for the actual healing of diseases. I will mention the mode of its application to heal the disease of asthma. One should only desist in the application of vomiting for the preservation of health when someone is not used to it, when it is very hard on him, or when he suffers from a brain or eye disease. The reason vomiting is necessary in the preservation of health is that phlegmatic superfluities unavoidably develop in the stomach and intestines. And when superfluous phlegm, which is viscous by its nature, remains in these organs—meaning those of the first digestion (the stomach and the intestines)—, it forms a barrier between the food and the stomach itself and the intestines and thus impedes digestion, so that some of the food is corrupted. But the intestines have been shown the mark of Divine Providence, for, when superfluous yellow bile streams into them, the yellow bile cleans out the phlegm and thus constantly cleanses the intestines and purifies them. But not even a small amount of this bile should stream to the stomach, since this would cause the great detriments enumerated by Galen, who relied in this event on man's artifice to cleanse the stomach through vomiting. [*De usu partium* v.4].

(ix.11) Galen says again—and these are his very words: The cleansing of the stomach can be accomplished very easily. The ancient physicians were right when, along with their other precepts for the preservation of health, they prescribed the application of vomiting after a meal once every month. Some of them thought that the stomach should be cleansed twice a month, and all of them advised that before vomiting one should take food with a sharp taste and the power to clean and purge. This should be done in order to cleanse all the phlegm from the stomach without harming the body by the bad effect of this food; for cleansing, sharp foods produce yellow bile and are all bad. [*De usu partium* V.4].

(IX.12) Says the author: The fact is that one can see that most people crave sharp, bad foods such as salted cheese, *murrī*, and *ṣīr*, even if they are evil-smelling—as, for instance, *kawāmikh*, garlic, the different kinds of congealed milk, radish, onion, and the like. The reason for all this is the phlegm which collects in the stomach over many days, so that a person craves something that can dilute and cleanse the phlegm from it. And when the stomach is cleansed through vomiting—as Galen mentioned—or through a purgative or through remedies which saturate the stomach and dissolve the phlegm therefrom when there are no humors stuck in its layers, it will not crave any of those bad foods, unless my Master is accustomed to vomiting them, since he has already long been in such a condition that his stomach is unclean.

(IX.13) I do not know the habit of my Master concerning vomiting. If it is easy for you, do it in your usual manner. Our common way of purifying the cavity of the stomach and vomiting the superfluity it contains is this: Take two or three peeled white radishes and cut them to the size of hazelnuts, cook one ounce of dill in one *raṭl* of water, and add this to the cut-up radishes with two or three ounces of honey and one ounce or more of very acid vinegar, depending on its strength. Let it all stand overnight. The next morning, shortly before the usual noon meal time, the one who wants to induce vomiting should eat unleavened bread together with different kinds of food—namely, salted fish, *murrī*, *biṭṭīkh* (common melons or watermelons), apricots when in season, radishes, onion, leek, honey, broth of crushed broad beans, and barley broth with the husks. All these and their like and what is easily prepared from them are among the various foods which induce vomiting. One should fill oneself with food and wait a little until the stomach is disturbed by its heaviness, then one should bandage one's eyes, tighten one's belly with the lower stomach, drink all of that previously prepared juice while it is lukewarm, wait a little while, and then vomit everything from a raised position and not leave anything in one's stomach. This should be done at noon. When it is winter, one should do the vomiting in the bathhouse, rest afterward, and not eat anything for a long time until one is really hungry. When one is thirsty, one should drink apple juice but nothing else. When one is very hungry, one should eat young chickens, small birds, or pigeons as *zīrbāj*. One should eat good foods for some days after the vomiting so that the stomach is strengthened.

Some people find it easy to vomit; after vomiting those foods, they should cleanse their stomach with oxymel and hot water. Other people who vomit from barley broth alone or from taking one of the different kinds of *nabīdh* or wine should drink a large quantity of one of these at one sitting and then vomit. All this is good. However, for someone who finds vomiting difficult and is not used to it or who is prevented from it by the weakness of particular organs or should be wary of vomiting because of his disposition, I deem it proper for him to take every fifth day one ounce of rose preserves with one ounce of syrup of oxymel of seeds. Then he should wait a while and take acidic food, for that purifies his stomach from the phlegm and relieves him from the need to vomit.

(IX.14) If he has a moist body and his temperament is phlegmatic, he should drink one ounce of oxymel of sea squill with one ounce of honeyed rose preserves. If he is extremely phlegmatic and his stomach is cold, one should add to it a little of the honey of thickened ginger juice or half a *dirham* of the ginger itself. And if he has a warm temperament or is a young person, he should take one ounce of rose preserves and one ounce of lemon juice every fifth day. All these ingredients cleanse the stomach of phlegm and relieve him of the necessity of vomiting when something prevents him from doing so, as we have mentioned above.

(IX.15) I experimented upon myself and took one ounce of white sugar pulverized with half a *dirham* of anise in the wintertime; in the summertime I drank it with a little lemon juice every third or fourth day, according to what was appropriate. I found that it purifies the stomach from the phlegm and cleanses it well. The same can be achieved by the ingestion of oxymel of quinces or of lemon juice with a quince-like astringency, when taken regularly. After just a few days it is beneficial in improving the digestive processes and purifying the stomach from phlegm. Its composition is thus: Take some fine, slightly astringent and acidic quinces and cook them in water until one-half of the water is left; remove its froth and then take one *raṭl* of the water, half a *raṭl* of vinegar, and four *raṭl*s altogether of sugar and skimmed honey. Put all this on a low fire and add to it one *dirham* of white pepper and two *dirhams* of ginger. This small amount does not arouse a distaste; you can add to either one of these amounts according to the coldness of your temperament and country, and according to the same criteria you can also add to both together. One may take lemon juice instead of vinegar; for, although it falls short of the effectiveness of vinegar in thinning the humors, opening obstructions, and resisting putrefaction, its detrimental effect on the nerves and sinewy parts is less than that of vinegar.

(IX.16) The maintenance of health through evacuation by means of bloodletting or the ingestion of purgatives is a grave mistake and is not part of the advice of an eminent physician, unless mistakenly. One should resort to bloodletting and the use of purgatives only when diseases occur that require such action, as in the case of someone whose body is so full of accumulated humors that his blood cocts and boils because of a bad constitution or a continuously bad regimen. For such a person this is necessary. If someone is accustomed to bloodletting or to the ingestion of purgatives at fixed times, he should watch his habits and see if he can gradually increase the intervals between the fixed times and gradually decrease the evacuated amounts, so that when he reaches old age his habit of bloodletting and using purgatives has ceased.

∴

Chapter Ten

On the proper regimen regarding sleep and waking, bathing, massage, and sexual intercourse

(X.1) Sleep is often harmful in this disease, especially during an attack and immediately after a meal. Someone suffering from this disease should therefore sleep as little as possible. Know that sleeping immediately after a meal is in general harmful for all people, and especially for my Master because it fills the brain with vapors. But if you have a habit of doing so, you should gradually busy yourself after the meal until there is an interval of three or four hours between the meal and the sleep. For then the sleep helps the completion of the digestion and cocts the superfluities of the food remaining in the stomach. One should adhere to one's habit in the complete regimen of one's body even if it is bad; one should not give it up unless in an imperceptibly gradual way so that nature is deceived, like someone who steals from her while she does not notice it. This holds good in the case of the regimen of health. But in the case of the healing of diseases, one should not consider changing the habit in any manner or for any reason. Instead, it should be observed with utmost attention, as Galen explained to us in his helpful instructions; and Galen has this to say in his discussion of one's habit, and these are his very words: All people are used to different types of regimen, and giving up one's habit in this is very dangerous, not only in the case of the regimen of convalescents and their like but also in that of the healing of diseases.

(X.2) Taking a bath is not fitting for my Master. Cold water is often harmful in this disease because it closes the pores of the body and prevents the dissolution of phlegm, which is the main aim in treating this disease. Similarly, entering the bathhouse is also very harmful for this disease; it has been forbidden by the physicians, and especially around the time of an attack of this disease or during its actual occurrence. Beware of habitual recourse to it. You should try to increase gradually the intervals between bathing sessions on one day and reduce the time spent in the bathhouse. Be extremely careful to avoid a cold draft when leaving the bathhouse and to enter it only when the stomach is empty. And sleep for an hour immediately after leaving the bathhouse, for that is very beneficial for everyone who wants to coct crude, viscous humors, and especially for this kind of disease.

(X.3) Galen said the following, and these are his very words: You should know that nothing compares to sleep immediately after a bath for cocting what can be cocted and dissolving the bad humors themselves. [*De sanitate tuenda* IV.4].

(X.4) Says the author: Since I have come to know about this, I have not bathed except at the time of sunset, and I go directly from the bathhouse to the deep and beneficial sleep of the night. I was very happy with its effect on me. One should not go into a bathing basin or tub filled with cold water in the bathhouse. Rather, the water should be so hot that its heat almost hurts a little bit. And if the water is salted, it is very good, because the intention here is to dry the body and not to moisten it. Know that, for people in general, frequent bathing is bad because it putrefies their humors or prepares them for putrefaction. Physicians in our time have stated that the proper measure for this is to go to the bathhouse every ten days at the most, depending on the different countries, temperaments, and habits. About habits we have already said what is necessary.

Pouring lukewarm water over the head is very harmful in the regimen of health of people in general, because doing so increases the moisture of the brain and makes it soft so that its strength is diminished. Similarly, pouring cold water over the head is extremely dangerous because it cools the brain and causes it to retain its superfluities. One should accustom oneself to water that is so hot that the skin of the head almost turns red, because this warms the brain with a balanced heat so that its activities improve and its superfluities are reduced. It also makes the skin of the head firmer and stronger so that it is not affected anymore by the slightest cause. One should also mention the force of habit in all this.

(X.5) Massaging the entire body at the beginning of the day, upon waking, and massaging the arms and legs at bedtime is a good regimen for all people when they are healthy. The physicians have given many directives about the different kinds of massage and its times and ways of application which are not suited to this treatise, for then I would also have to mention everything that must be mentioned about the different kinds of exercise. Moreover, our way of preserving one's health as we know it today does not require everything which Galen has mentioned concerning the different kinds of exercise and massage in his treatise *De sanitate tuenda* [II]. The most one can possibly do is that which I have mentioned in this treatise. Physicians in our time have mentioned the importance of massage of the chest for this disease about which you complain, but I have not seen that they describe it in detail or stipulate its conditions. But, from all the rules concerning massage, I will mention the main point and rule referred to by Galen. Then I will mention to my Master when massage of the chest is beneficial and when you should be careful to avoid it and to beware of it.

(X.6) Galen has said the following, and these are his very words: One should beware of applying massage to weak limbs at times when their diseases are stirred up in them. But when they are healthy, it may be necessary to apply massage to them more frequently than in the case of the other limbs, and especially to apply dry massage. In the case of pains which occur to some of the limbs in cycles, one should apply this kind of massage in order to prevent their occurrence, especially when one applies it in the quiet times two or three hours before the attack. The reason is that these limbs are strengthened thereby and that the usual influx of superfluous matters into them is reduced. These things are equally beneficial to old people and to anyone else. [*De sanitate tuenda* V.3]. In the case of old people with weak limbs, I recommend the application of exercise to a lesser degree than in the case of others, because the best thing for the bodies of the elderly is rest for their weak limbs.

(X.7) Says the author: It will already be clear to you that massage of the chest during the course of an attack or shortly before it is very dangerous. But one should apply massage in the quiet time or two hours before the attack. One should never exercise the weak limbs of old people.

(X.8) As for sexual intercourse, it is well known—even to the masses—that it is very harmful to most people and that excessive indulgence in it is harmful to all people. Emission of sperm is only exceptionally part of the regimen of health—namely, for those people who have bad varying temperaments. For, along with the sperm, vital fluids and innate heat are necessarily emitted, so that the vital organs turn dry and cold. However, young people may tolerate a mistake in this very well, although some of them cannot avoid becoming ill because of it. On the other hand, sexual intercourse is fatal for old people, because they need that which increases their heat and moistens their vital organs, whereas sexual intercourse dries their organs and exhausts their remaining heat, as we have mentioned. A man should therefore decrease his accustomed sexual activity as he becomes more advanced in years. This is necessary with respect to the regimen of the body and, moreover, with respect to the purity of the soul and the ethical qualities of tranquility, modesty, and chastity which he is bound to acquire.

And although sexual intercourse is harmful for all the organs in general, it is most harmful for the brain to the degree that most of the evacuation of the seminal fluids occurs from the brain. This was mentioned by Hippocrates. Therefore, someone whose brain is weak for whatever reason should abstain from sexual intercourse. If you observe those who have frequent sexual intercourse, you will see that they are overcome by forgetfulness, mental debility, and stupidity, in conjunction with a yellow complexion, a loss of the prime of life, and leanness of the cheeks. One's habit in this matter is of great consequence. And equally important is the fact that people have different temperaments. The physicians have said that some people who suffer from laziness, depression, and weak digestion become cheerful and energetic and develop a good appetite when they have sexual intercourse, while in the case of others the opposite occurs. The conditions of people vary greatly in this regard.

Galen has referred to a bad bodily disposition and said the following, and these are his very words: There is another bodily disposition which is also very bad—namely, that in some people much hot sperm originates which stimulates and arouses them to expel it. And when they expel it through having sexual intercourse, the cardia of their stomach becomes flaccid, and their whole body likewise; they become weak and dry and lean, their complexion changes, and their eyes become sunken. But, if they abstain from sexual intercourse on account of its effects on them when they engage in it, their head becomes heavy and they suffer from heaviness and pain in their stomach. Abstinence does not benefit them very much. The reason for this is that they suffer from nocturnal emissions, so that the same harm occurs to them as that which results from sexual intercourse. [*De sanitate tuenda* VII.14].

(X.9) Says the author: My intention with this quotation is to point out the various conditions of people in this regard; but it is not the intention of this treatise to provide a cure for everything which might happen to every individual, since that would involve the entire art of medicine. In short, one's habit should be observed and it should be diminished only gradually, with respect to this disease in particular and with respect to age in general, as I have stated earlier. Know that sexual intercourse is not good for anyone immediately after leaving the bathhouse, nor immediately after physical exercise, nor for some days after bloodletting, nor for some days after the ingestion of a purgative; for joining one discharge to another destroys one's strength. One should also not carry out this activity when one is hungry, nor when one is satiated, but when the food has left the stomach and before hunger has set in. The harm resulting from carrying out this activity when one is hungry is greater than that resulting from carrying it out when one is satiated. Sexual intercourse is fatal for someone recovering from a disease which has exhausted him. I personally observed, and others also observed and told me, that someone who had sexual intercourse while recovering from acute fever lost his strength that very same day, lost consciousness at the end of that day,

and died that night. The reason this happened only became known to them when he had begun to faint. If they had known earlier to what extent he had engaged in sexual intercourse, then, according to some of them, this problem could have been corrected.

(x.10) Now that we have set forth these chapters as a preface, which constitute a sort of regimen of health and precautionary dietary prescriptions and other types of regimen, we should proceed to a description of the regimen of this disease, the different kinds of drugs, and that which should be relied upon shortly before and after the attack.

∴

Chapter Eleven

On the provision of rules for the treatment of this disease

(xi.1) The care provided in treating this disease should consist of cleansing the body in general by means of compound drugs whose property is to expel different coarse humors, and of cleansing the lungs in particular. One should also take care to cleanse the brain so that it neither receives nor produces nor discharges superfluities. One should strengthen every other individual organ—unless it is affected by a disease—through evacuating superfluities it might contain and through balancing its temperament (restoring its natural temperament). For when any organ is free of superfluities so that it has its natural temperament, it is strong, unless it is affected by a disease. To strengthen any organ and to restore its natural temperament, it is unavoidable that we use astringent drugs in accordance with what is appropriate to each organ. A detailed description of these would be too lengthy and is not within the scope of this treatise.

(XI.2) The physicians have mentioned as part of the treatment of some types of this disease—and it is well known to every physician—the application of rubefacients, or even blistering drugs, to the head. Their intention with this is the prevention of defluxions. But nothing of this is good for my Master, because your brain is hot; and the more one heats it, the more one weakens it, even if that heat dries up the superfluous matter, or what is left of it within the brain, and prevents it from draining. The physicians have also mentioned powders and liniments which strengthen the brain in this disease. However, all these have a warming effect, and for you anything that has a strong warming effect is not good.

It is also impossible to strengthen the brain with only cooling drugs because of the nature of the disease. And this kind of incongruity makes it difficult to heal this disease; for this reason, error is introduced because of the necessity of compounding drugs with opposite powers. Galen and all his successors, however, have forbidden strengthening the lungs with drugs which thin and cut the thick and viscous humors because these drugs are exceedingly warm and do not have an extremely thinning effect. Their application would thus cause the humors to congeal in the lungs; only the thin humors would be dissolved, but the coarse ones would coagulate and congeal even more so that their elimination would be difficult. It is thus necessary that any drugs used to treat this disease include moisture in order to ease expectoration. The same holds good for defluxions. Sometimes that which causes agitation and sleeplessness is that which streams and descends from the brain, while that which causes a feeling of pressure is that which is already there in the lungs. Sometimes the descending secretion is hot and fine and nevertheless needs something to thin and cut it even more. This increases the descending flow, when there is still something left of it to stream down. At other times that which descends from the head is cold and of a thick substance, although the brain is hot. This can occur in any organ—that is to say, that sometimes it happens that the superfluity in an organ is contrary to the temperament of the essential or incidental organ itself. Again, occasionally the matter which arrives in the lungs is of a thin and fine consistency but does not leave the lungs and cannot be expectorated until it is of a thicker consistency and becomes somewhat viscous. And this is similar to what happened to you, according to your description. And since these conditions—upon which we physicians can act only once we comprehend them—are so varied, you should be under the constant observation of an expert physician. For then he can consider the matter in a careful and deliberate way, until he knows how to proceed: Whether he should tend toward one way of treatment or follow two different ways and prepare a compound drug accordingly. All these subtle things are avoided by practitioners; it is thus easy for every one of them to offer treatment, for, as you know, they rely on all that is mentioned in the books of medicine. However, all that is mentioned is the generic kind of disease, not the specific variations of one disease, which vary according to different conditions.

(XI.3) And hence in these kinds of things the empiricists, who do not employ analogical reasoning, commit errors, so that sometimes their treatment is successful by mere chance and at other times it is not successful. Therefore, someone who places himself in the hands of an empiricist-physician who does not know the rules of analogical reasoning is like a sailor who surrenders himself to the blowing of the wind, which does not occur according to analogical reasoning. Sometimes the blowing of the wind makes the sailor arrive at his destination in the best possible way, but at other times it is the cause of his drowning. I have drawn your attention to this merely because people are often duped by the empirical treatment of the empiricists. Some of them escape unharmed, but others die, all entirely by chance.

(XI.4) Hippocrates said: *Experiment (experience) is dangerous.* [*Aphorisms* I.1]. And so, Galen and very eminent physicians after him wrote down a number of drugs which were compounded according to reason and human thought and which are good for these different conditions and for others. One can also treat this disease with enemas, which should be administered during the attack in order to attract the superfluous humor in the opposite direction, or with a fumigation, which should be inhaled to strengthen the brain and to dry any moisture it contains in order to prevent its streaming down. I will select two, three, or more drugs from every particular kind of treatment of this disease, all of them appropriate for my Master and good for your temperament, which I know well, so that you can alternate between them. Sometimes you should take one and sometimes you should take another, for this is something recommended and advised by the most eminent physicians for diseases in general, and it is also mentioned for this disease in particular—that is to say, to alternate between one drug and another, although the powers and effects of those compound drugs are very similar. To describe the reason for this is not within the scope of this treatise.

The order of treatment upon which you should rely is this: You should persist in strengthening the brain with those drugs which I will describe for you when I mention their composition. Then you should empty your body with a purgative—I will describe to you a number of its formulas—twice a year if you find your body very full of humors and once a year in the springtime if you find it only lightly filled with humors. The same holds good for the ingestion of other remedies, if you feel very full. And I hope that, if you adhere faithfully to the regimen which I have mentioned, you will need only a light drug once a year in the springtime. When an asthma attack occurs, begin by drinking one of the decoctions which I will describe for you. Begin with the least diluting decoction and dilute your food very well, contenting yourself with sugar beverages and soup made from young chickens and licking one of the linctuses which I will describe and which assists in expectoration. For the night, take refined barley broth if you have fever, or soup of very old roosters if you do not have fever. If this is sufficient and the lungs are cleansed and the attack subsides, you do not need anything else. But if the attack does not subside with this treatment and the lungs are not cleansed, you should turn to another more powerful decoction. If the decoctions are not sufficient, you should take one of the enemas which I will describe, beginning with the mildest of them. And if you get relief from it, do not drink a purgative. But if that is not sufficient, then, in the proper seasons of the year, begin to drink one of the purgatives by which the whole body is cleansed.

(XI.5) You should start with the lightest of them and take small amounts. If this is sufficient, fine; and, if not, drink a stronger one. Besides all these you should take care to strengthen the brain with aromatic substances, and to fumigate with incenses which I will describe, and to lick those linctuses which cleanse the lungs when the defluxion is light and its flow ceases. As long as the defluxion remains and you feel it streaming, you should not concern yourself with anything else before you have stopped it with that which I will describe, unless the lungs are so filled with superfluities that breathing is difficult because of them. In that case, the lungs should be cleansed gradually with all that which I have outlined above. But if the disease becomes worse and the matter becomes difficult—God forbid—it becomes unavoidable to apply vomiting time and again. In all these conditions, be careful not to sleep too much, especially during the daytime. By no means should you lie down to sleep, but you should endure it; and when you cannot endure it any more you should sleep for a little while in a sitting position, supported by cushions on all sides. Be careful not to drink your fill of water, but take only as much as you need to quench your thirst. Similarly, be careful about bathing and exercise. But mild gradual movement is beneficial in this condition or during the peak of an attack.

Chapter Twelve

On the composition of drugs necessary for every different kind of this disease, according to the scope of this treatise

Decoctions with which one wishes to coct the superfluities and to ease expectoration and to clean the lungs, and which should be used before the purgatives:

(XII.1) The first decoction with which one should start in the beginning of the attack is the following: Two *dirhams* each of peeled and crushed licorice, common marshmallow, and borage, three *dirhams* of maidenhair fern, and five to six hearts of fresh fennel. This should be cooked and strained into a julep.

Another similar decoction: A fistful of fresh fennel, ten *ḥabbas* of dried figs, and four *dirhams* of maidenhair fern. This should be cooked, macerated, strained, and drunk with sugar or honey or their like.

Another decoction stronger than it: Four *dirhams* of maidenhair fern, three *dirhams* of the skin of the fennel root, two *dirhams* each of licorice and common marshmallow, one *mithqāl* each of pounded Florentine iris root and *utrujj* (citron or lemon) peel, and half an ounce of seedless raisins. All these ingredients should be cooked, macerated, and strained into sugar or julep; and, if you want to increase its thinning effect, you should strain it into a beverage of lemon and oxymel.

Another decoction stronger than this one, which powerfully cleanses the lungs from the coarse humors: Three *dirhams* each of licorice and maidenhair fern; two *dirhams* of dry hyssop; one *mithqāl* each of French lavender, elecampane—that is, *al-rāsan*, which the druggists in Cairo know as *al-janāḥ*—and common centaury; and six *ḥabbas* of figs. This should be cooked and strained into honey. But one should not take this in the case of fever.

Another decoction stronger than this one: One *dirham* each of *ḥāshā* (lesser calamint or creeping thyme), Florentine iris root, white horehound, and common madder; half a *dirham* each of the seed and wood of the Mecca myrrh (balsam wood) and of spikenard; four *dirhams* each of maidenhair fern and licorice root; two *dirhams* each of mint, *bābūnaj* (German or Roman camomile) root, and common centaury; five *dirhams* each of dried figs and seedless raisins. All these ingredients should be cooked, macerated, and strained into
… as a strong cleansing effect and prevents defluxions from
… hould not take it when one suffers from fever. But even
… sharp and fine defluxion, one should not give up mak-
… ecoctions. To these belong the simple drugs—namely,
… ce root, borage, *hindibāʾ* (endive or chicory) seed, fresh

fennel, fresh or dried *nīlūfar* (blue Egyptian, European white, or yellow water lily), seed of different kinds of cucumber, sebesten (Assyrian plum), and common jujube, according to what is available. There is no need to be sparing with the amounts of the drugs, but when one uses them in the form of a decoction one should macerate manna (exudation of camelthorn) or violet preserves in it. One may also add to the decoctions dried or fresh violets, according to the opinion which the physician has about the condition of the patient. These are the drugs that may be employed when there is a fever. When the fever is mild, there is no objection to adding seedless raisins or figs to the decoctions. Al-Rāzī said that, if one administers to those regularly suffering from this disease one *dirham* of *sqūlūfandriyūn* (rusty-back or hart's-tongue fern), which is also called *al-ʿuqrubān*, with fig juice, it expels a large quantity of coarse, stinking phlegm. It is a wonderful remedy. [*Kitāb al-Ḥāwī fī al-ṭibb* IV.8].

(XII.2) Says the author: This remedy, which al-Rāzī has tested and praised, finds support in logic. For we in the Maghreb have a well-known habit of taking the following drug under various circumstances for cleansing the lungs, cocting the superfluities, easing breathing, and taking away cough: We soak wheat bran in hot water for one night, macerate and strain it, add sugar and almond oil to the strained substance, cook it until it assumes the consistency of julep, and drink it when it is lukewarm. If one adds to it the hearts of bitter and sweet almonds after they are well pounded, it is very beneficial. One may also soak licorice root with the bran. All these compounds are beneficial and widely used for this disease. There is no need to be cautious in their application—not even in the case of fever.

(XII.3) The following are some of the linctuses which also cleanse the lungs, coct the superfluous humors in them, ease one's expectoration, are clearly beneficial for shortness of breath, and can be taken throughout the disease and at any time during the day or the night: Cook two equal parts of seedless raisins and fenugreek in pure water, strain the water, allow it to stand, and administer it continuously after rewarming it. This medicine has been mentioned by Galen, who said that it is very beneficial. [*De compositione medicamentorum secundum locos* VII.6]. Other later physicians mention another compound drug: Cook fenugreek and figs, strain the water, add honey to it, and thicken this until it becomes a linctus.

Another stronger linctus mentioned by Galen: Take sea squill, press it out, add to the juice a similar amount of honey, thicken it until it becomes a syrup, and take one ounce of it before and after meals. [*De compositione medicamentorum secundum locos* VII.6].

Another extremely strong linctus mentioned by Galen: Take equal parts of mountain mint, *ḥāshā* (lesser calamint or creeping thyme), roots of Florentine iris, dried water mint, white pepper, and roasted anise; pound these, strain them through a fine sieve, and knead them in boiled honey; and take a portion the size of a hazelnut.

Another very strong linctus mentioned by later physicians: Take three ounces each of smearwort and fenugreek flour, two ounces of myrrh, one ounce of common madder, and one ounce of saffron; pound all these ingredients; and take a portion the size of a hazelnut.

Another beneficial but mild linctus mentioned by later physicians which my Master should rely upon: Take large pine nuts which contain much resin, cook them with fresh white horehound, halve the quantity of the nuts, strain this, and mix the resulting liquid with a similar amount of pure honey; cook this until it assumes the consistency of the honey, and use this, for it cleanses all that is in the chest in a wonderful way.

Another common drug which may be taken in different conditions: Take one ounce of the thickened juice of pounded, strained licorice and two ounces each of the hearts of peeled bitter almonds and *fānīdh*; pound the hearts of the almonds until they become soft; dissolve all this in fennel juice; and thicken it into a linctus on a low fire. In the case of this recipe, I personally prepared lemon juice with a quince-like astringency instead of *fānīdh*, and I added to it a decoction of maidenhair fern and almond oil; and this resulted in a very beneficial all-purpose linctus.

(XII.4) One of the drugs which my Master should have ready with him is the opium poppy syrup mentioned by Galen, because it prevents defluxions, puts one to sleep, and thickens the thin sickening matter and helps in its expectoration. [*De methodo medendi* V.13]. Its composition is thus: Take ten *dirhams* of crushed licorice root and ten *ḥabbas* of fresh, ripe white opium poppy; cut this as it is, with its seed; macerate it for one night in hot water; cook it the next morning; strain it into one *raṭl* of thickened grape juice, or one *raṭl* of sugar, or one *raṭl* of honey; and let it thicken so that it becomes a syrup from which you should sip when you need it. The syrup prepared from honey is stronger and cleanses better but is not suited for the treatment of the hot, thin defluxion. The syrup prepared from thickened grape juice is better to prevent the defluxion, and the one prepared from sugar is intermediate between them. When the defluxion becomes lighter and it ceases streaming down and nothing remains except for that which is in the lungs, you should not use any kind of syrup unless the matter which is in the chest is so thin that it cannot be expectorated and you need something to thicken it. For, then, the procedure for you should be to take gum tragacanth and gum Arabic; pulverize them; dissolve them, in the syrup just mentioned, over a low fire; and sip from it little by little. And take equal parts of Iraqi opium poppy seed, sugar, and starch (amylum); pulverize and pound everything with mucilage of fleawort seed; and partake of this little by little—or else knead these three ingredients with quince mucilage. You may add violet preserves.

(XII.5) I once personally compounded an electuary for a woman about whose case I was very concerned. My intention was to cleanse the lungs and the brain, to prevent defluxions, and to ensure that the brain would not be exceedingly hot; because this disease afflicted her when she was a young woman, and her brain was neither hot nor unusually cold, and her body was lean. This drug was very beneficial during attacks. And as she continued to take it when she was healthy, the attacks became less frequent until she reached the point where an attack came upon her only once a year, and sometimes the attacks left her alone for two years, and then only a mild attack came upon her. In the composition of this drug, I followed the opinion of Galen, who said that very beneficial drugs are those compounded from medications which differ not only in their nature but also in their strength.

This is how I compounded it: I took maidenhair fern, macerated it in hot water, and cooked it at random, without regarding its weight. I strained it and put into the strained substance a similar amount of maidenhair fern, without weighing it. I cooked this and strained it once again, until the juice acquired some sort of color. I prepared this separately. I did the same with licorice root: I crushed it, macerated it, and cooked it alone. Then I strained it, returned it to a low fire until it assumed the consistency of honey, and set it aside. Then I took two glasses from the maidenhair fern decoction, one glass from the licorice root decoction because of its thicker consistency, one glass of fresh fennel juice, and two glasses of thickened grape juice with the consistency of honey. I mixed everything, put it on a low fire, cooked it, skimmed the foam from the top of it, and took it from the fire. This is a good linctus with the consistency of honey and a delicious taste. This linctus alone is, without doubt, very beneficial for this disease.

Subsequently, I assembled the following ingredients: Three ounces of Roman nettle seed; one ounce each of macerated, washed pine nuts and roasted flax; one ounce each of opium poppy seed, starch (amylum), peeled bitter almonds, and ground fenugreek; half an ounce each of Florentine iris root, smearwort, elecampane, spikenard, wild carrot seed, white horehound, and common madder; ten *dirhams* each of *sqūlūfandriyūn* (rusty-back or hart's-tongue fern) and Massilian hartwort; two *dirhams* of saffron; and three *dirhams* of myrrh. The total number of ingredients is eighteen, and the total amount is about seventeen ounces. I pounded and strained everything that could be strained, and I pulverized the seeds and hearts of that which could not be strained until they became soft as marrow. I kneaded everything over a low fire with four *raṭl*s of the aforementioned linctus which has the consistency of honey and then applied it. I have not seen this compound drug described by any of the earlier or later physicians, but it has been compounded according to the rules of analogical reasoning. I have already described to my Master what I have observed from my experience with it, and I advise my Master to have it with him and to use it regularly both in times of health and in times of an attack of asthma, unless you suffer from a high fever, God forbid.

(XII.6) We have already said that soups prepared from old roosters are beneficial for the coction of the crude superfluities and for their expectoration. As for drugs which strengthen the brain in this disease, Ibn Zuhr has remarked that he found powders better for this than ointments. [*Kitāb al-Taysīr fī l-mudāwāt wa-l-tadbīr*]. As I informed you, excessive heating is not appropriate for this disease, nor is unlimited cooling. In my opinion, the following is appropriate: Take three *dirham*s of mace; two *dirhams* each of spikenard and *maqāṣīrī* (good pieces of) sandalwood; one *mithqāl* of myrrh; and one-quarter of a *dirham* of old camphor. Pulverize this mixture thoroughly, strain them, knead them with rose water, and make pastilles of the paste. From it, take one pastille after another, pulverize them, and apply the powder to a spot where the hair of the head parts. In the summer this should be done with rose water, while in the winter the middle of the head should be rubbed with quince oil and then that powder should be sprinkled on it. The preparation of quince oil is as follows: Take one ounce of fragrant rose oil, squeeze a quince into it, add half a *dirham* of turpentine resin and a quarter of a *dirham* of spikenard, and put it on hot ashes. Leave it there until the liquid has evaporated, then collect the oil and store it.

Know that crude ambergris strengthens the hot or cold brain. We have also heard from the elders—who knew this by experience—that *hindibā'* (endive or chicory) is beneficial for a hot or cold liver. Therefore, I advise my Master to use this continuously as an errhine and to use nothing but this for fumigation, for it strengthens the brain and prevents it from receiving and producing superfluities.

Another remedy: Take four *dirhams* of simple ben oil that has been neither flavored nor processed; dissolve in it one *mithqāl* of crude ambergris, half a *mithqāl* of pulverized and strained *maqāṣīrī* (good pieces of) sandalwood, and a quarter of a *dirham* of old camphor; prepare an unguent from this; and rub the middle and front part of the head with it about half an hour after leaving the bath. Do this continually in the winter and less often in the summer, but do not abandon it.

As for the time of an attack, physicians in our time have mentioned fumigations which strengthen the brain and dry its superfluous moistures and prevent them from streaming. One of these is aloe; they have said to cast it onto a fire so that its vapor enters the nostrils and the mouth, for it is a tried and true remedy. Another drug: Take one part each of costus, liquid styrax, red arsenic, galbanum, and mastic. Mix all these ingredients and put the mixture on a fire so that its vapor arises and enters the mouth and nostrils and fills the chest and the head. They have said that this medicine is entirely beneficial. Another drug: Take arsenic and long birthwort, pulverize and knead them with oxen fat, and use this as a fumigant.

(XII.7) As for enemas, the composition of the mildest is thus: Take half a *raṭl* of beetroot juice and four ounces of sesame oil, cook this, add one *dirham* of borax to it, and use this as an enema. A stronger enema is: Take olive oil in which common rue was cooked, add a little natron or borax, and use this as an enema. A yet stronger purgative is: Take a fistful each of mint and dill, half a *raṭl* of beetroot juice, and one *raṭl* of fine olive oil; boil this; add a little borax to it; and use it as an enema. An even stronger enema is: Take a fistful each of dill, mint, and common centaury; cook all these in water; and add to it two ounces of fine olive oil and the sweet, honey-like pulp of purging cassia; and use it as an enema when it is lukewarm. If the patient has flatulence, add half an ounce of cumin to it. It is a good thing to add duck fat or chicken fat to the olive oil in the case of all these enemas.

An even stronger enema is obtained when one adds to the enema from half a *dirham* to two *dirhams* of the pulp of colocynth, which should be cooked with the aforementioned ingredients and then used as an enema. And if one adds to it sagapenum, opopanax, and castoreum, according to the condition at hand, one gets an even stronger enema. None of these hot enemas should be used in the summer, nor in the case of fever. One should not resort to any of them except in a case of very thick humors or severe obstruction.

(XII.8) Galen has forbidden the application of hot enemas to old people under any conditions. [*De sanitate tuenda* V.9]. Know that the application of very hot enemas is like the application of strong purgatives and should be used only on the advice of an expert physician who is in attendance himself and not giving advice from afar. Among the purgatives commonly used for expelling phlegmatic humors and cleansing the head is the following: Take one *mithqāl* of *hiera picra*, half a *dirham* each of agarikon and St. Thomas lidpod, and a quarter of a *dirham* of ginger, and sip this with hydromel.

Another purgative, stronger in cleansing the lungs than this one: Take half a *mithqāl* of agarikon, half a *dirham* of birthwort, and a quarter of a *dirham* of anise. Another purgative stronger than this: Take half a *mithqāl* of opopanax, one *dirham* of *hiera picra*, and one-quarter of a *dirham* of pulp of colocynth prepared with an equal amount of shelled pistachio nuts and gum tragacanth, and drink this with hydromel.

Another purgative, which is stronger than this and which is a good compound drug that should be used for emptying the body during all seasons and during a strong attack: Take half a *dirham* each of agarikon and St. Thomas lidpod; one *dirham* of *hiera picra*; one-quarter of a *dirham* each of myrrh, root of Florentine iris, and white horehound; one-quarter of a *dirham* of sarcocolla; one-eighth of a *mithqāl* each of pulp of colocynth, anise, gum tragacanth, and blue bdellium; and knead these ingredients with thickened grape juice.

Another purgative stronger than this one: Take one *mithqāl* each of St. Thomas lidpod, agarikon, and absinth wormwood juice; one *dirham* of *hiera picra*; one-quarter of a *dirham* each of pulp of colocynth and gum tragacanth; one-eighth of a *dirham* each of scammony and mastic; and half a *dirham* of blue bdellium. Knead all these ingredients with fennel juice and make pills from it, using almond oil. Another purgative stronger than this one which cleanses the lungs very well: Take one-eighth of a *mithqāl* each of pulp of colocynth and gum tragacanth and half a *dirham* each of anise, dodder, sagapenum, and birthwort, and knead this with hydromel.

Another purgative stronger than this one: Take one *dirham* each of Roman nettle seed and common polypody, half a *dirham* of the juice of squirting cucumber, one-quarter of a *dirham* of pulp of colocynth, and three *ḥabba*s of shelled pistachio nuts; knead these ingredients with celery juice and make pills from them, using almond oil. This purgative expels the many thick, viscous, and bad humors.

Know that these strong purgatives are beneficial in this disease if they are applied correctly. But by no means can one apply the different kinds of myrobalans to purge the body in the case of this disease. And if only a relaxing treatment is needed, a mild and light purgation with purging cassia and rhubarb does not do any harm. But neither purging cassia nor rhubarb has any effect in cleansing the head or the lungs.

(XII.9) Description of the preparation of all the purgatives which the most skillful physicians in the Maghreb have tested repeatedly in my presence. The description of the preparation of such a purgative is as follows: Agarikon should be ground over a sieve until it is sifted. St. Thomas lidpod should be peeled at the top, ground, and sifted; similarly, *hiera picra* should be sifted thoroughly.

Colocynth should be cut as fine as possible with scissors; one should take only the pure white part from the largest possible fruit. And one should be very careful to avoid putrefied St. Thomas lidpod. Gum tragacanth should be macerated and then taken from the pieces of cloth in which it has been macerated.

Every purgative which contains the pulp or leaves of colocynth should be prepared as follows: First, pound the blue bdellium and add it to the cutup pulp of the colocynth or to its crushed leaves; then pulverize pistachio nuts that have been shelled with a knife and add them to it. Then take the gum tragacanth from the pieces of cloth in which it was macerated, knead it with the pulp of the colocynth and its shells, and pound everything until it becomes loaf-shaped. Then add *hiera picra* and the other strained ingredients. The scammony and mastic should be coarsely ground; similarly, the other purgatives which we did not mention should be coarsely ground but not sifted. This is especially the case for the different kinds of myrobalans, since these should be coarsely ground but not sifted. All this should be kneaded with that which is used for kneading liquid things, and pills should be made from it, using almond oil. If you want to cleanse the rest of the body, the pills should be small and moist and should be taken at daybreak. If, as a result of taking the medicine, one experiences cramps and pain in the stomach, one should boil three *dirhams* of borage, one *mithqāl* of French lavender, and half a *dirham* of the edible oregano and take it in sips or strain it over sugar and drink it, because it alleviates the pain and cramps in the stomach so that the medicine can have a proper effect.

(XII.10) All these formulas we received as personal instruction from the elders in the Maghreb. Only a little of it is written in books, and these are unknown among the people. I have written all of this in order to provide as much benefit as possible to all people. However, to describe the reactivation of every purgative medicine when it has stopped from being active—or its discontinuation when its effect is too strong—or to describe how to counter act accompanying bad symptoms is a major subject in the art of medicine, but one beyond the scope of this treatise. For all these things vary according to the different medicines ingested and the different ages, temperaments, places, and seasons of the year.

If one resorts to emetics, one should start by consuming radish and then take two *dirhams* of borax with only half a *raṭl* of hydromel. Another emetic stronger than this one: Take some pieces from the root of white false hellebore or from its stalks and stuff the radish with it and leave them for a day and a night, then remove the white false hellebore and consume the radish, drinking hydromel with it, and you will vomit. Another emetic stronger than this one:

Take one *dirham* each of mustard and salt, half a *dirham* of Armenian borax, and two *dāniqs* of natron; dissolve this in three ounces of water and one ounce of honey, then drink it, and it will make you vomit.

(XII.11) It is clear that the intention of this treatise is not to mention all the different kinds of treatment for this disease, but merely to select those medicines which are easily prepared and which are usually taken by most people and applied by most physicians. In my opinion, I have recorded for my Master more of those medicines than you requested, God willing—may he be exalted.

∴

Chapter Thirteen

On the provision of rules, few in number but of great help for people in general, concerning the regimen of health and the healing of diseases; in hortatory form

(XIII.1) One should first pay attention to the improvement of the air, then to the improvement of the water, and then to the improvement of the foods we take. This is so because what the physicians call "pneumas" are fine vapors found in the bodies of living creatures. Their origin and most of their substance come from the air inhaled from outside. The vapor of the blood found in the liver is called "natural pneuma," and the vapor found in the heart and the arteries is called "vital pneuma," and the vapor found in the ventricles of the brain and that which is transmitted from it into the cavities of the nerves is called "psychical pneuma." All these pneumas and most of their substance originate from the air inhaled from outside; and, if the air is putrid, evil-smelling, or turbid, all these pneumas are altered and their condition becomes the opposite of what it should be.

(XIII.2) Galen said: Pay attention to the matter of the essence of the air which reaches the body through inhalation so that it will be utterly balanced and free from all that might pollute it. [*De methodo medendi* VIII.6].

(XIII.3) Says the author: The finer the pneuma is, the more it changes with changes in the air. The natural pneuma is coarser than the vital pneuma, while the vital pneuma is coarser than the psychical pneuma, so that with the slightest change in the air the condition of the soul changes perceptibly. Therefore, one sees that many people notice a deterioration in their psychical functions with the corruption of the air—that is to say, that they suffer from dullness of understanding, lack of comprehension, and loss of memory, although their vital and natural functions are not perceptibly changed.

(XIII.4) The relationship between the air in cities and the air in deserts and steppes is comparable to the relationship between water of a coarse, turbid substance and fine, pure water. In the city, because of its high buildings and narrow streets, the refuse and waste of its inhabitants, their dead and the carcasses of their animals, and the putrefaction of their food, the air becomes stagnant, turbid, thick, misty, and foggy. The pneumas gradually become like that as well, although a person might not realize what has befallen him. If we cannot escape from this, since we have grown up in cities and are used to them, one should at least choose a city with open horizons, especially toward the north and the east, high on the mountains or hills, sparse in trees and waters. If you have no choice in this—that is, if you cannot choose to move to another city—you should at least try to live on the outskirts of the city, facing the east and the north. The dwelling place should be a tall building with a wide court, so that the north wind can traverse it and sunlight can enter it; for sunlight dissolves the putrefied air and makes it fine and clear. One should strive to put the toilet as far as possible from the place where one lives. And one should endeavor to improve the air and dry it with fragrant odors, vapors, and fumigation, as is proper according to the changes in the air. This is a fundamental rule with which every regimen of body or soul should start.

(XIII.5) Even if you are careful as much as you can be, there is no escape from minor ailments constantly occurring in the human body. For instance, sometimes the stools become a little bit soft and sometimes a little bit dry, or one finds a feebleness in his digestion one day, or suffers from a mild headache or a mild pain in some part of his body. There are many minor ailments like these. One should be extremely careful, then, not to be hasty in treating this minor ailment by taking medicines to eliminate it. The most eminent physicians have warned against it, because one's nature alone is sufficient in things such as these and does not need the assistance of medicines; rather, one should adhere to a healthy, good regimen. For once you start to treat that minor ailment, you do one of two things: Either your action is a mistake and contrary to the tendency of your nature, so that you confuse it and aggravate the ailment; or your action is correct and you restore the natural functions of your nature but at the same time you teach your nature passivity and you accustom it not to do what is required except with external assistance. You can compare this, as they say, to someone who accustoms his animal not to move except with a spur, for the animal stands still forever until it is spurred. It is also similar to the situation that you find when the stools have softened in an unusual way even though you did not change your regimen in any way; this may last for two or three days without pain or weakening of your stamina. And if you hasten to use astringents and thus stop this diarrhea, your nature returns to its normal condition by means of medication. But sometimes the cause of this is a natural movement of the expulsive power, which moves to expel that which should be expelled, so that the stools become soft. But when nature is restrained in such a case, it is confused, its proper activity is suspended, and that which should have been expelled is retained, so that harm is being done. At other times, that softness of the stools is caused by the weakness of the retentive power, and if it had been left alone it would have awakened and the organ would have returned innately to its natural function. But when this power is strengthened by means of drugs whenever it is weak, this will become its custom and habit; whenever this power is weakened, it will need an external stimulant. Thus, it is clear that the correct thing to do is to refrain from interfering with nature. This should be done in every case where there is no danger to life.

(XIII.6) Abū Naṣr al-Fārābī has mentioned in this connection that, in the art of medicine, in seamanship, and in agriculture, the outcome does not necessarily depend upon the efforts invested. For the physician may do whatever is necessary in the best possible way, without any error committed either by him or by the patient, yet he may not attain the cure which is the ultimate goal. The reason for this is clear, for the active factor in us is not medicine alone, but medicine and nature. Sometimes nature does not react for a number of reasons, some of which have been mentioned in this treatise. Similarly, the farmer may do all that is necessary, but the seed may not prosper. Similarly, the seaman may navigate his ship in the best possible manner, build it with the best construction, and sail the sea at the usual time, yet the ship may perish. The reason for all these failures is that the goal is achieved only through the action of two agents, one of which does all that is necessary, while the other falls short in its action.

(XIII.7) If you consider the contents of the preceding chapter, you will realize that sometimes the disease is mild and that nature is stronger than it and has begun to remove it and to do all that should be done; yet the physician may err in his treatment, or the patient may err, and the actions of nature come to nothing. This happens in the majority of cases in all places and at all times.

(XIII.8) In one of his aphorisms, al-Rāzī makes a statement with the following meaning: When the disease is more manifest than the strength of the patient, medicine is of no use at all; and when the strength of the patient has the upper hand over the disease, there is no need for a physician in any wise. But when they are equal, then the physician is needed to support and promote the strength of the patient against the disease. [*Kitāb al-Murshid aw al-fuṣūl*].

(XIII.9) Says the author: From the words of this man, who is perfect in his art, one can also learn that, when one draws an analogy with all the diseases, one can do without a physician more often than one needs him, even when he is excellent and knows how to support nature and does not confuse it and divert it from its proper way.

(XIII.10) Careless physicians often commit very grave errors against people; yet the sick do not die, but recover. I have seen several times how someone administered a strong purgative to a person who did not even need a weak purgative. As a result, this person lost much blood from below, which condition lasted for several days, and he suffered from severe dysentery; yet he recovered afterwards.

I have also seen how someone bled a person suffering from indigestion at a time when he did not know about his indigestion. As a result, the patient lost consciousness, his strength diminished, and his illness became protracted and worsened; yet he recovered in the end. However, this should not mislead one into thinking that physicians' errors do little harm. Nor should one say: If they commit such grave errors and the patient does not die, why should he die if the physician errs in determining the correct amount of nutrition or of mild decoctions? The matter is not so, however; for the case of these preceding internal causes of illness is rather like that of the following external causes. You see with your own eyes people whose arms are cut off below the elbow or whose legs are cut off below the knee, or whose eyes have been extracted, or who have been stricken in battle with severe blows in the cavity of the body and who do not die, but live, as God wills. And on the other hand you see a person pricked by a thin needle or thorn that hits one of his nerves, and he has spasms and dies. The same applies to errors by physicians: A physician may commit a grave error, and yet the patient is saved; or he may disregard something which both he and the patient consider a minor thing, and yet it becomes the cause of the patient's death. This should be taken into consideration by every thinking person.

(XIII.11) It is well known that all men suppose that eating the usual food, drinking the usual water, bathing in cold water for one who is used to this, or bathing in the bathhouse are all matters which are not very dangerous for the sick, even if done improperly. But this is not so. Galen has explained to us that, among those suffering from fever, there are some in whom the drinking of cold water—which they are allowed to drink—causes their humors to become crude and fires their fever, so that they perish. And there are others for whom the drinking of cold water is a cure: It softens their stools and extinguishes the fire of their fever, and they recover; if water is withheld from them, they perish. Similarly, some patients with fever recover and are saved when one lets them enter cold water, while others perish by it. Similarly, bathing in the bathhouse cleanses the body of some of those with fever and enables their complete recovery, while in the case of others it increases their putrefaction, gives them a bad fever, and kills them. The same holds true for food: Withholding it from a patient can be the cause of his recovery or the cause of his death; and giving it freely to the patient can be the cause of his recovery or the cause of his death.

The rules for all these matters and the conditions under which every single one of these actions should be allowed or prohibited have already been given and explained, and proof has been given for the reasons behind them. Understanding all this from books is very easy for everyone who is in full possession of his faculties, but applying it in an individual case is very difficult for a conscientious scholar. But, for those who are ignorant of the basic principles of this art and for those who are reckless with this art, nothing seems difficult, and they do not see that there are diseases which require consideration.

(XIII.12) In one of his aphorisms, al-Rāzī has said: Medicine is a studied art and is subject to claim by the riff-raff among physicians; but how difficult is its attainment for the skilled physician!

(XIII.13) Says the author: Concerning the matter discussed by al-Rāzī in this aphorism, Galen has remarked many times in his books that the crafty find this art easy and insignificant, while Hippocrates finds it difficult and time-consuming. But do not think, dear reader, when you consider my words, that this is unique to medicine. If you look into the natural sciences, or the conventional ones, or the ones on the religious law, you find the same. The more accomplished a person is in that science, the more precise his investigation becomes: Doubts and difficult questions arise in him; he becomes deliberate in his investigation and hesitant in some of his answers. The less a person knows, the more he considers all that is difficult to be easy and holds all that which is distant to be near. Such a person makes many nonsensical and pretentious remarks and gives prompt nonsensical answers to that which he does not understand.

But let me return to my subject and reiterate what I said about the ease with which the medical art is understood by those who have a good intellect, and about the difficulty they have in practicing it, which has already been mentioned by Galen in a statement with the following words.

(XIII.14) Galen said: Therefore, it is easy to say that it is correct to rub the elderly with oil and massage them, but to do this properly is a most difficult thing. [*De sanitate tuenda* V.4].

(XIII.15) Says the author: Consider, O possessors of fair judgment: If the procedure of rubbing with oil and massage is, according to Galen, one of the most difficult things to put into practice—that is to say, its practical individual application—and likewise the drinking of water or abstention therefrom, as we explained, how much more so is this the case for bloodletting; for evacuation by means of pulp of colocynth, juice of squirting cucumber, and the two hellebores (black and white false hellebore); for the enemas with castoreum and opopanax; for cautery, lancing, and cutting! Are all these procedures really easy for a physician, or difficult?

(XIII.16) Ibn Zuhr has said in one of his extant and well-known books: I have never administered a purgative without thinking about it for days before and after. [*Kitāb al-Tadhkira*].

In one of his well-known books, Hippocrates has made a statement to which I would like to draw your attention, dear reader, in this treatise. To this end, I will quote Hippocrates' statement itself and Galen's commentary on it in their very words, so that you can consider both of them carefully, with heart and mind, word for word. After that, I will describe what follows from it.

(XIII.17) Hippocrates has said: One who is a physician should devote himself to two things: one is to benefit the patient, and the other is not to harm him. [*Epidemics* I.2.11].

(XIII.18) Says Galen: I once thought that this was a small matter, not important enough for Hippocrates to mention. For I thought that nobody doubts that the physician should, above all, intend to benefit his patients and that, if he is unable to do so, he should at least not harm them. I thought so in the beginning of my study of medicine, before I had actually given any sort of treatment or had been in the presence of another physician treating a patient. But, once

I was in their company, I saw that many famous physicians should be blamed for harming many of their patients by the way they treated them, whether by bleeding them, allowing them to go to the bathhouse, recommending the ingestion of a drug, or allowing them to drink wine or cold water. And I thought it only natural that some of this should have happened to Hippocrates, as it happened, without any doubt, to many of his contemporaries. From then on, I was extremely careful, whenever I started to give a patient a strong kind of treatment, that I myself first understood the effect of such a treatment. And I would not be content until I saw the extent of the harm I would cause the patient if I were wrong in the treatment I intended to give him. I would not do anything, under any circumstances, unless it was clear to me that, if I were not able to reach my goal of curing the patient, I would at least not harm him so much that his condition would grow worse. [*In Hippocratis Epidemiarum commentarius* I.2.53].

(XIII.19) Says the author: Consider, dear reader, how, during the time of Galen, great and famous physicians were mistaken in allowing—as he mentioned—the drinking of cold water and bathing, whereby they caused serious harm to the patient; and how the same thing also happened to Hippocrates, who, for this reason, was cautious in this matter and told others to beware of it. For even Galen, with all his perfection in this art, declared concerning his own medical practice that, in any kind of case in which he had to treat someone, he would not rely upon his own analogical reasoning and conjecture and would not act upon his own opinion only, but would say to himself, for instance: The patient should be purged from such and such a humor with such and such a drug when the symptoms are such and such. Then he would consider and assess whether the purgation would be beneficial if the case is as indicated by the symptoms and whether it would not cause great harm if it is the opposite of what he thought; only then would he give the patient the purgative to drink. But if he concluded that, if the case was the opposite of what he thought, the purgative would cause serious harm, then he would not act according to his reason nor according to the symptoms. The same applies to bleeding and similar procedures, as he mentioned.

And if Galen—with his excellent intellect and long experience in the practice of medicine, his devotion to this art, and his strong aspirations to excel in it—casts doubts on his own practice and is tentative about it, how much more should this be the case in our generations, in which physicians have only very little experience, while at the same time much memorizing is needed, since the different parts of medicine have become so lengthy! Consequently, a lifetime is too short to attain perfection in even one part of it, as I explained in my *Commentary on Hippocrates'* Aphorisms. I have told you all this merely as a warning to beware of the physicians and not to surrender yourself hastily to whomever you find. Rather, be satisfied with a good regimen, whose principles and main requirements we have described in this treatise. For the errors of the physicians are much more frequent than their correct prescriptions.

(XIII.20) Aristotle has said the following in one of his famous books, and these are his very words: We should first examine the nature of the patient, both when he is healthy and when he is ill. Most physicians are subject to error in their assessment of this force, so that the patient dies as a result of their medical treatment. [*De sensu et sensibilibus*].

(XIII.21) Says the author: In another translation I saw that he said at this point: Most people die as a result of medical treatment. I think that Aristotle should be trusted in this assessment. As you know, in his time the medical sciences were in the prime of their youth, and scholars did not occupy themselves with anything else.

I have extracted for you important things which were extremely well hidden in books, in order to focus your attention on those things which are of equal benefit in the art of medicine as a whole.

(XIII.22) I know that you could say: The conclusion to be drawn from your words is to abandon medicine, because every effort and attention given to this art is given in vain. I will dispel the doubt for you. And if it has already been dispelled by the force of my words so far, I will nevertheless return to the subject once again. Know that medicine is an art that is very necessary for man at all times and in all places—not only when he is ill but also when he is healthy—almost to the point that one should never detach oneself from a physician. This holds true when the physician masters his art to perfection, for then one may deliver one's soul and body into his hands, that he may guide them with the regimen he prescribes according to his view. But such a situation is rare in all places and all times, so one should not rely upon an incompetent physician—which is the most common situation—in the way that one feeds oneself with bad food if one cannot find good food. For one cannot do without food, but one can manage without surrendering one's soul and body to an incompetent physician. Rather, one should leave the matter to nature, in combination with a good regimen that one has adopted according to a sound judgment.

We have already explained that the skilled physician who is perfect in his art, observes its principles, and uses examination and analogical reasoning knows which diseases should be ruled out, so that he leaves healing to the activity of the patient's nature and he does not accustom it to inactivity, as we said. And he knows which disease we should hasten to treat and to confront before it becomes so bad that it can no longer be treated. And he knows when there is reason for fear and concern and acts accordingly with care and precaution, as Galen said about himself. And he knows in which doubtful cases one should not do anything at all, so he will advise in these cases to refrain from medical treatment and to leave the patient to the activity of his nature. And even in cases where the physician does know what to do, he follows the activity of the patient's nature and goes in its footsteps, as Hippocrates and Galen informed us. The example of such a physician should be imitated, and his words should be remembered in all these cases. For if he makes a mistake in one of these cases, it is a rare and unusual occurrence. He is only rarely deceived and is slow to act in those things which demand much hesitation and unhurried deliberation.

On the other hand, the incompetent physician never stops rendering medical treatment and is always actively involved, although he is ignorant of all these subjects. Sometimes he is successful in his treatment, and sometimes he fails; but his failures are more frequent, while his successes are accidental and rare. Therefore, if one cannot find a physician other than this one, one should leave the matter to nature. For sometimes it is successful, and sometimes it fails; but its successes are more frequent and are part of its essence, while its failures are rare and accidental. Therefore, everyone who is intelligent and knowledgeable should prefer to stay with nature rather than rely on the regimen prescribed by the incompetent physician. But since no one does this, it is unavoidable that people seek healing through whatever they get from whoever is at hand. And since most physicians are incompetent, the result is as Aristotle has said—namely, that most people die as a result of medical treatment. For this reason, I have warned you and advised you and urged you to rely on nature, because it is quite adequate in most cases if left alone and undisturbed.

(XIII.23) Hippocrates has said the following: Nature cures diseases. He also said that nature finds and evaluates the proper ways to cure by itself, not through rational deliberation. And he further said: Nature does what should be done because it is well trained and educated. [*Epidemics* VI.5.1]. Consequently, through nature we learn and are educated.

(XIII.24) Says the author: He repeats this idea in a number of his books so that people would pay attention to it, and he instructed them to imitate the activities of nature, since all of these activities—there is no doubt about that—are appraised as wise by those endowed with justice.

(XIII.25) In one of his well-known treatises, Galen said the following: When the Greeks were in doubt about a disease, they left it to nature to expel it. Their argument for this was that nature looks after the health of living beings and treats them in the case of disease, and that it knows the temperament of their organs and sends to every individual organ the appropriate kind of nourishment, after first preparing sites for the superfluities of the food and humors appropriate to the body.

(XIII.26) Says the author: If you look at these words carefully, you will find that they confirm what I have pointed out—namely, that, if you cannot find a perfect physician and you are absolutely in doubt about the disease, then you should leave it to nature, as I said.

(XIII.27) Having heard my words, do not assume that I am the one into whose hands you should deliver your soul and body for treatment. May God be my witness that I know for certain about myself that I, too, am among those who are deficient in this art, who stand in awe of it, and who find it difficult to achieve its goal. There is no doubt that I know myself better than anyone else does and that I can criticize my own knowledge or the knowledge of others better than someone with less scientific insight. Again, may God be my witness that I do not state this out of modesty, nor in the customary manner of the erudite, who say about themselves that their knowledge is deficient even when it is perfect and that their deeds fall short even when they are very diligent. But I state the truth of the matter as it is. I have adduced this chapter strictly for fear that, when you look into it, you would suspect me of that of which I am innocent and would therefore find it difficult to accept my advice, since you would think that it is partly motivated by self-interest. Consequently, you would act according to my advice only rarely and would thus frustrate my intention. For this reason, I have written this section, and I will now return to complete what I wanted to write.

(XIII.28) It is known to anyone who has tried to practice the art of medicine—and, in fact, to most people—that it is an art which requires experience and analogical reasoning. And the things which are known through experience are far greater in number than those known through reason. Since people know this, they rely so much on experience that the multitudes have a well-known saying: Ask the experienced practitioner but not the theoretical physician. So, people die as they are deluded by old women and common folk and as they rely on anyone claiming medical experience. Any cheating, impudent, and insolent person can gain access to this art by saying: I have remedies which I have tested. And most of the noble people prefer physicians either because they hold them to be experienced or because they are advanced in age. Often, they say: So-and-so is not a learned physician; but he has experience, practical training, and skill. All these are errors which cause those eventualities against which we have warned.

(XIII.29) The greatest mistake is the belief that the experience which is mentioned and referred to in medicine is only the experience of the individual physician in his own era. But this is not so. Rather, medical experience is the sum of the experience acquired over the course of past generations even before the time of Galen—namely, those things which have been written down in the medical books. Some of the drugs and compound remedies were tested for hundreds of years and were then written in books. But the individual practitioner of this art can in no way be qualified as experienced, since the right conditions for acquiring experience are missing; for not even an eminent physician carries out experiments, because Hippocrates said: *Experiment* (*experience*) *is dangerous*. [*Aphorisms* I.1]. But, in our times, experience is claimed only by pseudo-physicians, who make people believe in something which has not been proven in order to cover up their lack of experience.

(XIII.30) A second mistake is to imagine that one can have experience in the practice of medicine without knowledge. On the other hand, it is truly possible for a person to have knowledge of the medical art and to understand its principles and various branches without having practical medical experience, if he studied from books but did not see the elders of this art practicing it and did not try to practice it himself. But it is impossible for a person to be experienced in the medical art because he observed and saw it being practiced, although he has no theoretical knowledge of it. For the art of medicine is not like the craft of carpentry or weaving, which can be learned through observation and can be mastered through repetition, because the practice of this art of medicine is subordinate to theoretical speculation and reflection. Every person who falls ill necessarily requires renewed speculation and reflection. One cannot say: This disease is similar to that disease, and this is how it is usually treated. Nor can one say: I have seen how my elders treated it in this or that way. This matter has absolutely no foundation in the medicine of Hippocrates and Galen, because according to their medical theory the physician should not treat the general kind of a disease, but, rather, the individual case of the disease itself. However, to discuss these matters in a detailed and exhaustive way is not the intention of this chapter; rather, my intention is that you will not be misled by these delusions and will rely only upon those physicians who are committed to theoretical speculation. For knowledge is the root and practice is the branch, and there is no branch without a root. However, one can find roots which have not yet grown branches, as we have explained.

I have mentioned to you in this treatise that someone who surrenders himself into the hands of an empiricist physician who does not employ analogical reasoning but acts according to his observation is like a sailor who survives or dies by pure chance. Galen has written much and elaborately about this in many places in his books. [*De simplicium medicamentorum temperamentis ac facultatibus* VI.0; *De libris propriis* 5]. One of his statements about experimentation and the empiricist is the following: Analogical reasoning demonstrates for you the existence of the things for which you search. But if one experiments without any logical reasoning, one is like a blind man who is not shown the right way.

(XIII.31) Says the author: If you reflect on his comparison of the empiricist with a blind man, you will find that it is similar to the comparison of a patient who surrenders himself into the hands of the empiricist physician with a sailor. This is also something that one should know, and one should take care not to succumb to it.

(XIII.32) What I have mentioned before—that a physician may make a mistake in allowing or forbidding the drinking of cold water or bathing and thereby cause great harm—is indeed true as I quoted it for you in the words of Galen, but it is an unusual and rare occurrence. But my warning in general is simply that you should not rely on someone who is deficient in the art of medicine for a strong treatment. There is no stronger treatment in the medical art than bloodletting and the ingestion of a purgative, and next comes the application of vomiting and sharp enemas. For these, one should not rely upon whoever happens to be available. Nevertheless, you find people, both healthy and sick, who rely on barbers for bloodletting and on young pseudo-oculists for the ingestion of purgatives.

Galen has explained and clarified that there is a medical rule according to which one should bleed a patient although there are no symptoms indicating an overfilling. The same rule applies to purgation of the belly and the application of vomiting. The reason for undertaking such action is, as he said, the severity and gravity of the disease considered together with the abundance of the patient's strength. He explained to us what such severity and gravity of a disease together with the abundance of the patient's strength means. [*De meth-*

odo medendi IV.6]. He also explained to us that sometimes a healthy person can show symptoms of overfilling together with great strength, and yet we are not obliged to let blood, nor to purge, nor to apply vomiting. Rather, it is sufficient for one individual patient to fast and for another to eat less. For another patient, it is sufficient to soften the belly (to administer a mild laxative), which is not the same as purgation; and for another, to take a bath. For another patient, physical exercise alone is enough; and, for yet another, only frequent and firm massage. [*De methodo medendi* IV.6]. All these are very important matters. Therefore, examine and consider, dear reader, whether we need a skilled physician in all these cases or whether someone who learned medicine from mere observation is sufficient.

(XIII.33) In the Maghreb, I once saw a young man, who was very strong but clearly suffering from overfilling, who became afflicted with continuous choleric fever. The physician bled him on the second day of his disease, and when he had drained around fifty *dirham*s of blood the patient's strength declined. The physician became frightened and closed the place of the bleeding and ordered the patient to drink rose syrup and oxymel and to rest until the next day so that he could give him the appropriate treatment. However, the patient died that very night. This incident became notorious among the physicians and the people. A learned physician under whom I studied told me: Do you know the nature of the mistake of that physician in bleeding that patient? I answered him: O Master, do you also say this as if he made a mistake? He laughed and said: Yes, So-and-so—meaning that patient—was one of those who love luxury. He was a glutton who often suffered from indigestions which weakened the cardia of his stomach so much that it became worn out and a choleric humor was produced in his stomach. Galen has forbidden bloodletting in the case of someone in this condition or anyone in a similar condition, because the patient will quickly faint during the act of bloodletting. [*De methodo medendi* IX.5]. The right thing to do would have been to strengthen the cardia of the stomach with such and such and to dress it on the outside with such and such after the evacuation of that which might have irritated the cardia. Only then should bloodletting have been applied, if it was unavoidable. But since the physician bled the patient before doing that, he should have strengthened the cardia of his stomach immediately. But he became alarmed and went away, so that the irritation of the cardia of the stomach became even worse and the humors streamed toward it, so that the patient was overcome by fainting and died. This is what that teacher told me.

(XIII.34) Says the author: Since I see how many dangers may attend such cases, I advise you not to rely in these cases on whoever happens to be there. I also consider it advisable to cite the words of Galen in this matter; for, when he ordered the application of bloodletting and the extraction of blood in the case of a continuous fever to be carried out without mercy until the patient faints [*De methodo medendi* IX.4], he informed us about those cases in which one should avoid bloodletting—such as this fever (continuous choleric fever), and all the more so in other cases. As such, he mentioned indigestion in which a residue remains in the belly, or a decline of the strength of the patient, or considerations of the patient's age or temperament or of the current weather. Similarly, he said that someone with a cardia of the stomach in which bilious juices are produced or with a weak and very sensitive cardia should not be bled. [*De methodo medendi* IX.5]. This was succeeded by the following statement, and these are his very words:

(XIII.35) As for the bleeding which I said should be done until the patient faints, and which aims at extinguishing the heat and the blaze of the continuous fever, which is occasioned by the impossibility of dissolution, and at allaying its vehement force, it often causes no small harm when it is performed at the wrong time or in an inappropriate amount.

(XIII.36) I know of two men whose deaths were caused by physicians on account of fainting that overcame them due to bleeding. They died immediately. Others did not die immediately, but eventually perished because of the exhaustion and weakness overcoming their strength. If they had not been bled so oppressively that their strength declined, they would not have died. Many people fell victim to a chronic illness because they lost their strength as a result of excessive bleeding. Still others suffered a change in the temperament of their body and acquired a cold temperament which they could not improve by any means, and they remained thus for the rest of their lives. This was caused by excessive bloodletting. In some of them, that coldness was the cause of a change in their complexion and a deterioration of their bodily constitution to such a degree that they rapidly fell ill from the slightest cause. And others were afflicted because of this by different diseases, such as fatal dropsy, orthopnea, weakness of the liver and the stomach, paralysis, and hemiplegia. [*De methodo medendi* IX.10].

(XIII.37) Says the author: Consider the dangers of bleeding when it is not performed at the right time, or when it is at the right time but excessively, and its consequences. Therefore, I must advise you not to act recklessly in this matter and not to trust whoever happens to practice medicine. This is also the case—as Galen said—with all the forms of evacuation of the body when applied in an exaggerated way.

(XIII.38) These great medicines such as the "snake theriac", the Mithridates, the Theodoretus, and many similar compound medicines, which Galen calls beneficial in many ways, have a strong effect on patients. Therefore, one should not administer any such thing to a patient in particular except on the advice of a skilled physician. When these medicines are applied at the right time, they cure serious and grave diseases that same day. But if one fails in one's diagnosis of these diseases and these medicines are applied at the wrong time, they kill or cause a very serious disease.

There is a well-known story which once circulated in the Maghreb about what happened to the successor of ʿAlī (ibn Yūsuf ibn Tāshufin), commander of the Muslims—may God have mercy on him. He had been ill for some time—I have not heard what he suffered from—and he was older than twenty years of age and, as they said, of a very strong bodily constitution. It was wintertime, and the city where he lay ill was the seat of the king of the Maghreb—namely, the city of Marrakesh. When he recovered from his illness, he did not gain his full strength, but became a convalescent with a corresponding lifestyle. His physicians prescribed for him a regimen normal for a convalescent. These physicians, who were four in number and who were very learned in this medical art, were Abū al-ʿAlāʾ ibn Zuhr; Sufyān (Abū al-Ḥasan Sufyān al-Andalūsī); Abū al-Ḥasan ibn Qamniel of Saragossa, the Israelite; and Abū Ayyūb ibn al-Muʿallim of Seville, the Israelite (Solomon ben Joseph ibn Ayyūb). When they saw that his body was clean but that he was not fully recovered and that his digestion and innate heat were weak, they decided, since he drank no wine, to give him half a *dirham* of the great theriac to drink so that his innate heat would be revived, his digestion would be strengthened, and all the natural functions would return to their normal state according to the effect which the great theriac is known to have. They also agreed that the patient should take it in the last third of the night because, if he then ate as usual at three o'clock in the afternoon, the theriac would have left his stomach and dissipated and had the desired effect and would not mix with the food—a necessary condition for its success. The physicians spent the night in the palace, and in the last third of the night they came and brought the theriac sealed with the seal of the sultan from the royal treasury. They gave him the amount agreed upon and went away to their quarters in the palace, intending to return to him at the appropriate time. About three hours later, just before the morning prayer, a loud cry was heard in his residence.

The physicians were roused to come to him immediately, but he died—may God have mercy upon him—before or shortly after their arrival, as the story goes.

Abū Yūsuf the physician, the son of the aforementioned Abū Ayyūb, told me, on the authority of his father, that the mistake lay in the amount of the theriac, for the patient could tolerate only a quarter of a *dirham* or a quarter of a *mithqāl*. The vizier Ibn Abī Bakr, the son of Abū Marwān, who in turn was the son of the aforementioned Abū al-ʿAlāʾ, told me that his father, Abū Marwān, thought that his grandfather, Abū al-ʿAlāʾ, had erred in the amount of the theriac, saying that his death was due specifically to an insufficient amount and that he should have taken half a *mithqāl*. I did not hear from any of them whether they themselves thought that the cause of his death was either an insufficient or an excessive amount. For I asked every single one of them about it in order to learn something useful from it. But they kept silent so that I could not profit from it.

(XIII.39) Much later on, while I was looking into this and other matters, I found Galen stating the following, and these are his very words: All drugs which are antidotes for fatal drugs, when taken in an overdose, will in most cases cause great harm to the body. Therefore, for all those drugs with such an effect, one should calculate an amount which is not so large that it harms the body and not so small that it is too weak to resist the fatal drugs and is overwhelmed by them. [*De simplicium medicamentorum temperamentis ac facultatibus* V.18].

(XIII.40) Says the author: It seems to me that those physicians who closely followed this story to this point might think of a text by an ancient author other than the text with which I dealt. I have heard many things explaining the cause of that incident, but it is of no use to mention them here. For the intention of this chapter has been achieved—namely, to warn patients to resort to a strong drug of that kind only at the advice of an eminent physician, and even then with great caution, and only if there is no other way.

(XIII.41) The following medical procedure is well known among the Egyptians; and, if the matter is true, they do not apply medicines in most cases but divert the attention of their patient until his nature is strengthened so that the patient is healed, or until it becomes even weaker so that the patient dies. I praise this method for various reasons; I will first describe their method in detail and then explain my reasons for praising it. It is clear to me from their method that they are so cautious that most of the simple and compound drugs which are well known to all physicians are not used by them. They content themselves with a small number of mild drugs. When they want to dilute thick humors or to coct a thick humor, they do so by applying drugs with a weak power which do not exceed the first degree of heat, or sometimes the second degree. For purging, they use mostly purging cassia, rhubarb, agarikon, and the myrobalans. Of the different kinds of *hieras*, they use only *hiera picra*. Most of their compound drugs consist of well-known flowering plants and of robs prepared from common fruits. Only rarely do they use drugs with many different beneficial effects; they use neither theriac nor any kind of electuary. In their opinion, they exceed the proper bounds when they prescribe the rose electuary. They never purge with a strong purgative. This is the gist of their method, and I praise it for four reasons.

(XIII.42) The first reason, which is the most important already mentioned by us in these sections, is the deficiency of the physicians in this art. If they limit themselves to this mild treatment, the effectiveness of the physician—when this treatment is correct—will be delayed and the disease will only be prolonged. And if they are mistaken and give a mild treatment which is wrong, the patient will not die. But if they give a strong treatment with the wrong effect, it will kill the patient.

(XIII.43) The second reason is that their country is hot. The land of Egypt is counted among the hot countries. But since this matter has a natural cause, it is inappropriate to discuss it lengthily in this treatise. However, the constitution of its inhabitants is weak, and one should not apply a strong treatment either in hot countries or in the case of those who have weak bodies. Perhaps this was the reason the theriac killed that convalescent; for a strong drug first of all undermines one's powers, and once they are weakened, they decline and are thus unable to return to their former state and to overcome what undermined them.

(XIII.44) The third reason is that most of their diseases are hot because of the thinness of their humors and the leanness of their bodies. These hot diseases do not need strong drugs. It is well known that Hippocrates and Galen treated hot diseases with oxymel and barley broth and the like.

(XIII.45) The fourth reason is that they follow the rules laid down by the physicians—namely, that anything which can be healed by means of a dietetic regimen should not be treated by other means. If this is not possible, one should administer food with medical properties; and if this is not possible, one should administer mild drugs. Anything which can be treated with a simple drug should not be treated with a compound drug, and even then one should choose the least compound one. If this works, we have what we wanted. All these things have been advised by the most eminent physicians in general. The Egyptians mostly follow this method. There is no doubt that sometimes at least chronic diseases occur to them which need a strong treatment, but they recoil from applying it because of their lack of experience with strong treatments. For this reason, nothing of their usual treatment produces any harm; in general, their method succeeds more often than it fails.

(XIII.46) But that for which they should be strongly criticized in particular is that they are terrified to use the theriac of four ingredients and similar multi-beneficial drugs, or to take the cumin electuary or mint electuary and similar healthy drugs. Another point of criticism is that they apply continuous bloodletting and evacuation of large quantities of blood and administer purgatives in the different seasons of the year as a regimen for the elderly. Even if they do so only in the case of the elderly, all these things are obviously wrong. One should point this out.

(XIII.47) Concerning both prominent and ordinary people, I have regularly seen in the land of Egypt that only rarely would a single physician be entrusted with the treatment of a patient from the beginning to the end of his disease. They would rather go from physician to physician. A patient will consult a number of physicians, according to his preference, for one disease, while one physician does not know about the others and the patient lets every single physician believe that he is relying only on him. The patient or the person in charge of his affairs takes the prescription of every single physician, compares them, and chooses from among them the one that seems to be most appropriate in its claim. He thinks that all this can be a precaution, protection, and guard against the errors of the physicians.

But I would like to point out to you that this course of action has some harmful effects. In the first place, there is the patient's own confusion, since he does not know which physician is correct. If he prefers one of them, it is based merely on a fancy and not on the medical expertise required for a sound judgment. Secondly, there is the confusion of the physician. If he carries out the treatment of the patient from its beginning until its end, he will stick to his method when it was clearly successful; and, if he sees the opposite, he will change to another method. But when he is interrupted in his treatment by another physician, the other has to rely on his own method of treating the patient and that of his colleague. In the third place, there is the harm which the physicians inflict on each other, for every one of them speaks badly of his colleague and accuses him of committing an error. In the fourth place, there is the indifference of the physician, his lack of determination, and his reliance on others because he knows that, if he makes a mistake, he will not be the only one to be blamed for it, and, if the treatment is successful, he will not be the only one to be thanked for it. He will not exert himself to do what is necessary, because he knows that he will not be the only one to be relied upon.

(XIII.48) Al-Rāzī said: If someone receives medical treatment from two physicians, he should suspect that he will suffer from their combined errors.

(XIII.49) Says the author: This is correct when he is treated by them separately, as in the case of all the harmful effects which we enumerated above. But if the physicians gather together for treating a patient, as in the case of kings and rulers, and debate and argue until they have come to a decision about what should be done, it is most appropriate and best. For then the patient benefits from the sum of their correct judgements, since no single physician can remember everything that he has learned; rather, this art is difficult for most scholars not with respect to understanding it, but with respect to remembering it, because it requires the command of a very large amount of memorized material. It may happen that that which a physician does not remember at a certain moment is exactly what he needs in the case of that particular disease. But if there are some physicians gathered together and they remind and assist each other in reaching their goal, together they will achieve the perfection for which they strive.

But if you see them quarreling, and if each one of them wants to come out glorious and victorious and to demonstrate to the patient his perfection in the art and the deficiency of his colleague, the correct thing to do is to be on one's guard and to avoid all of them. For the patient might die if the physicians disagree merely because each one wants his opinion to prevail. When physicians are afflicted by this disease, every one of them unavoidably makes mistakes because of his disregard for what is right, even if he is perfect in this art. Therefore, I advise you to dismiss all of them and to rely upon the activity of nature alone, as we have stated above. The astrologers have said: Love and hatred turn one's judgment away from the right path.

(XIII.50) Alexander of Aphrodisias has said: There are three causes for dissension about something:

1. the love of leadership and victory, which prevent man from grasping the truth as it is;

2. the subtlety and obscurity of the object of apprehension in itself—its inscrutability and the difficulty of apprehending it;
3. the ignorance of him who apprehends and his inability to grasp that which can be apprehended. [*Maqāla fī al-qawl fī mabādiʾ al-kull ʿalā raʾy Arisṭaṭālīs al-faylasūf*].

(XIII.51) Says the author: There is a fourth cause of dissension greater than the three mentioned by Alexander, but he was right in not mentioning it since it did not exist in the time of the Ancients and was thus not part of their way of life. What I mean is that a person is used to certain ideas, since he has been brought up according to them. For a person has a natural tendency to adhere to certain habits, irrespective of whether these are practical or theoretical. A person is inclined to the ideas according to which he was reared, to which he grew accustomed, and which he acquired in a natural way; and he shies away from opposite ideas, even if they are more correct. Thus, he prefers bad foods to which he is accustomed over good foods to which he is not accustomed. However, this is not the intention of this treatise. For I wanted only to discuss the first cause mentioned by Alexander, according to the goal which I set myself in this chapter.

(XIII.52) I have explained in this chapter how one can avoid many mistakes which are detrimental to the preservation of one's health and the treatment of diseases.

May God, in his grace and forbearance,
guide us on the right way to salvation in both worlds.
Praise be to God forever and ever.

BOOK 2

On Poisons and the Protection against Lethal Drugs

First published in:

Maimonides
On Poisons and the Protection against Lethal Drugs

A Parallel Arabic-English Edition,
Edited, Translated, and Annotated
by Gerrit Bos,
with Critical Editions of Medieval Hebrew Translations
by Gerrit Bos
and Medieval Lation Translations
by Michael R. McVaugh.

Provo/UT (Brigham Young University Press) 2009
MWMM 5

In the Name of God,
the Merciful, the Compassionate.
O Lord, make my task easy by Your grace

(1) Says Mūsā ibn ʿUbayd Allāh from Córdoba: The conduct of our Master (ʿAbd al-Raḥīm ibn ʿAlī al-Baysānī), the most honorable and eminent Judge—may God grant him a long time—is well known in our time and in our country and even in some other countries. Equally well known is his endeavor in this world to share any good that God has bestowed on him with all people in general, to keep them from harm, and to constantly provide them with benefits, through his wealth, his rank, his wise words and his consideration of a certain matter. With his charity he satisfies the needs of the poor and indigent, raises orphans and redeems prisoners, builds houses of study in the cities and increases the number of scholars and students. He uses his high position—may God elevate it even more—to satisfy the needs of people of eminent position and rank and to provide sustenance to heads of families and to protect men of honor against disgrace. With his eloquent and pure speech and wonderful elocution which

 | DOI:10.1163/9789004498884_004

God has bestowed upon him, and with which he surpasses all those known to have preceded him, he prevents kings and rulers from mostly judging according to their natural inclinations, with which they believe the first statement they hear at the expense of the statement they have not yet heard, and with which they hasten to take revenge on and to extirpate a criminal, and with which they pursue their passions to achieve their goal in whatever way that happens to be. He has inclined their hearts to behave in a noble, moral way, and thus he has saved highly esteemed people from death, not only certain individuals, but many groups and large cities. He has watched over people to guard their riches from soldiers who only waged battle in order to seize these riches. He has protected women against those who seized power and whose only intention was to disgrace them. And how many fires of feuds have broken out between the believers (the Muslims) and he extinguished them, and how many fires of wars against the polytheists he has lighted and kindled until he opened their minds and the word of God's Unity spread through all their countries and the holy cities were freed from uncleanness and the word of God's Unity spread in them.

(2) All this was accomplished by him with God's will with his tongue and pen. With his noble way of thinking, he acted with extraordinary ingenuity in guiding the kings of those countries so that he fixed principles of justice and fairness for them to act upon. As a result, their reputation has been elevated, their word has become widely known, the condition of their subjects has improved, and the behavior of the inhabitants in this country who follow the advice of our master is better than the behavior of the inhabitants of all the other countries we have heard about. These things are so well known that there is no need to describe them here. It is also not the purpose to which I now speak. The tongues of the poets of our time are too feeble and their intellect too weak to describe the conduct of our Master, they would never achieve their aim. But what prompted me to write this treatise—what I am going to mention—also prompted me to start with this introduction to this work which I am making an effort to write now.

(3) For our Master—may God preserve his power—in putting his noble thoughts to the welfare of the people, ordered the physicians in Egypt to prepare the great theriac and Mithridates. The preparation of these two electuaries in the city of Cairo was extremely difficult since none of the herbs used for the preparation of the theriac grows in this land, except for the opium poppy. As a result of the execution of your order, these ingredients were brought from the most distant lands in the West and East. Then the two electuaries were prepared and were made available to anyone who might benefit from them,

according to the opinion of the physicians, for these two remedies cannot be found in the treasury of most kings, let alone in the public markets. And whenever the supply of these two electuaries was exhausted or nearly so, you would take care that more was prepared. All this is done quickly, thanks to the interest you would take in everything that is right and beneficial for human beings.

(4) But in this time, in the glorious month of Ramadan of the year 595 (1198), you said to your most humble servant: It occurred to me yesterday that someone could be bitten by a poisonous animal and that the poison would spread through his body before he could reach us and take the theriac, and so he would die, especially if he was bitten during the night and would only reach us in the morning. It also occurred to me that these two remedies that are so difficult to prepare would be used up for minor cases, such as scorpion or *rutaylā'* (tarantula) stings, for which the theriac of four ingredients and the like would suffice. Therefore, I command you to compose a treatise, short and concise, that deals with the treatment that the bitten person should be given promptly, and to mention the medications and foods that he should take and some of the theriacs that are generally beneficial for bitten people, apart from these two theriacs, so that these are saved for cases in which the other antidotes are of no avail. Undoubtedly our Master knows that all the ancient physicians, as well as the modern ones, composed books on this subject and dealt with it in length, and that most of the things they said passed by your eminent intellect during the study of the medical books. But his intention—may God lengthen his days—was to select the simplest and closest remedies from what they said so that they can be easily remembered and made and so that the information about them could spread among all people.

(5) I hastened to comply with your command—which I cannot but obey—and composed this treatise and called it "Treatise for Fāḍil," thus called after al-Qāḍī al-Fāḍil ('Abd al-Raḥīm ibn 'Alī al-Baysānī). I did not intend to present something extraordinary or rare that had not been recorded or mentioned before. Rather, my intention in obeying your sublime command was to select some statements, small in number but large in benefit. Therefore, when I mention the simple, beneficial remedies in this treatise, I will not mention all those that have been cited. This I avoided since an accumulation of medicines necessarily causes that they cannot be remembered and that one has to rely on books to look them up when one needs them. But a small number of medicines can be easily remembered.

(6) With this in mind I will strive to mention those remedies which are most potent and which are most easily available in these regions. Many times, the physicians mention a simple drug and say that it is beneficial against deadly poisons but do not mention the way in which it should be prepared nor the appropriate dose that one should take, on the assumption that the attending physician will be familiar with the general methods of the application of these medicines. Therefore, I will explain them clearly in this treatise so that one will not need the attendance of a physician as well. Similarly, I will only mention those compound remedies that can be easily composed and that are most beneficial.

(7) I have divided this treatise into two parts:

The first part: Concerning the bites of vermin and some poisonous animals.
The second part: Concerning someone who took a deadly poison.

The first part consists of six chapters:

The first chapter: Concerning the regimen of someone bitten in general.
The second chapter: Concerning the simple and compound topical remedies that are put on the site of a bite.
The third chapter: Concerning the simple remedies which are beneficial against the bite of all kinds of vermin.
The fourth chapter: Concerning the compound remedies beneficial for that case.
The fifth chapter: Concerning the specific treatment of someone bitten by certain animals.
The sixth chapter: Concerning the foods to be given to bite victims in general and in particular, and certain remedies with specific properties, which are fitting for this purpose.

The second part consists of four chapters:

The first chapter: Concerning the prophylaxis against deadly poisons.
The second chapter: Concerning the regimen of someone who took a deadly poison or who suspects that he took it.
The third chapter: Concerning the simple and compound remedies that are generally beneficial for someone who took any type of poison.
The fourth chapter: On the regimen for someone who knows which poison he took.

In this chapter I will only mention some of the substances which a person can consume without knowing their specific nature or with which it is easy to assassinate someone because they can be found in many places. As I said, all this I am doing with the intention to abbreviate the extent of this treatise.

May God direct me to what is right.

The First Chapter of the First Part
Concerning the regimen of someone bitten in general

(8) When someone is bitten, one should hasten to immediately tie the spot above the bite as tightly as possible so that the poison does not travel and spread throughout the body. While the site of the bite is being tied, someone else should make an incision in the site of the bite and suck it with his mouth as hard as he can and spit out all that he sucks. But he should first rinse his mouth with olive oil, or with wine and olive oil, and then suck. He may also smear his lips with violet oil, if available, or with olive oil. The person who is sucking should take care that he does not suffer from any illness in his mouth or from decayed teeth. Some physicians stipulate that the sucking person should be fasting, whereas others stipulate that he should not be fasting but should eat something and then suck. It seems to me that it is more beneficial for the bitten person if the sucking person is fasting, but that it is more dangerous for the latter. And if the sucking person has eaten something, it is less dangerous for him but also less beneficial for the bitten person, for the saliva of a fasting person heals the sites of bites of vermin and most virulent ulcers. If sucking is impossible, one should hasten to apply cupping glasses, with or without fire. The ones with fire are stronger and more effective because they combine attraction of the poison and cauterization of the wound. Then one should empty the stomach with a mild emetic. If vomiting is difficult for the patient, let him vomit with olive oil or clarified butter, but be careful not to cause severe vomiting. Then the patient should take the great theriac, if available, or Mithridates if the theriac is unavailable or one of the great electuaries that are generally beneficial against deadly poisons if these two are unavailable; or if these are unavailable one of the simple remedies that generally save from the bite of vermin. I will describe all these and the manner of their administration below.

(9) Then one should put on the site of the bite one of the remedies that attract the poison, either simple or compound, whatever is available. Then the bitten person should rest for a while and one should observe his symptoms. If his pain subsides and his pulse becomes stronger and his complexion improves, nothing further should be done. However, one should take care that he does not fall asleep. For if the bite victim falls asleep, the innate heat and the superfluous matters penetrate the interior of the body and the poison reaches into the depths of the body. It may even reach the vital organs and have a fatal effect. Therefore, one should always take care that the bite victim does not fall asleep and that his wound does not close, but that the site of the bite stays open so that the poisonous matters can stream out of it and he is safe from that disastrous poison. If you see that he is in pain because of the tightness of the bandage, loosen it somewhat.

(10) When the remedy has left his stomach and made its therapeutic effect and not less than eight hours have passed, feed him with foods that are appropriate for bite victims. But if you see that the pain of the bite increases and becomes more severe before you feed him, remove the remedy that you put on the site of the bite, slaughter a young pigeon, slit open its abdomen immediately after the slaughtering, and put it on the site of the bite. When the bite victim feels the heat of the flesh of the young pigeon diminish, remove it and put another one on. If there are no pigeons available, take young chickens, roosters or hens, and apply them once you have slaughtered them, one after the other. It is said that the application of a weasel has a strong effect in this case; that is, one slits open its abdomen and puts it on the site of the sting or bite. Continue to slaughter these animals, one animal after the other, slitting open their abdomens and applying them to the site of the bite until the pain subsides, because this regimen alleviates the pain and attracts the remaining poison. Some physicians first apply these slaughtered animals and then the topical remedies, simple or compound, that attract the poison.

(11) If none of these animals that should be slaughtered is available, pour hot vinegar on the site of the bite or put a poultice with flour boiled in olive oil on it. These are some of the ingredients that alleviate his pain. If the pain does not subside after all of this was done but becomes more severe, and the condition of the patient worsens and he faints, these things require a treatment whose description does not fit the scope of this treatise. Rather, the attendance of a skilled physician is required, who will act according to the circumstances, the general rules mentioned in the extensive medical books, and the personal temperament of the bite victim.

∴

The Second Chapter of the First Part

Concerning the simple and compound topical remedies that are put on the site of the bite

(12) Amongst the simple remedies that attract any poison from the body if they are put on the site of the bite are the following: Water mint, which is "crocodile mint," pigeon dung, duck dung, sulfur, asafetida, goat's dung, blue bdellium, cooking salt, garlic, and bitumen. Whichever of these is available should be pulverized, kneaded with honey, and smeared on the spot of the bite after it has been sucked with the mouth or cupping glasses have been applied; it will draw out the poison. Similarly, rubbing the site of the bite with the gall of a cow draws out the poison. *Utrujj* (citron or lemon) seed, whether sour or sweet, if pulverized and applied as a poultice to the site of the bite, saves from death because it has a specific property that is very effective in resisting any poison.

(13) Amongst the compound remedies are the following: Pulverize equal parts of garlic, salt, and pigeon dung, and put it as a poultice on the site of the bite. Another one: Pulverize common marshmallow seed, fresh or dried, with vinegar and olive oil, and rub it on the site of the bite. Another one with a strong attractive power: Equal parts of mustard, *qilyun*, and quicklime; mix these ingredients with tar and hurry to apply it to the site of the bite before the poison spreads in the body. Another one: Equal parts of salt, ashes of the wood of the fig tree or of the grapevine, and borax; knead these ingredients with vinegar and gall of a cow and rub it on the site of the bite. Another remedy is mentioned by al-Rāzī, who said that it is a proven remedy for alleviating the pain of any bite and for attracting the poison. Its composition is thus: Take equal parts of sagapenum, castoreum, asafetida, sulfur, pigeon dung, mint, and Cretan dittany; mix these ingredients with ancient olive oil into which pitch has been dissolved; pound them well; and hold it ready for the time that you need it; and then rub it on the site of the bite.

(14) Says the author: If Cretan dittany is not available or hard to obtain, one may take in this case sharp cinnamon bark instead of it. It is also good to boil mint in vinegar and to foment the site of the bite with it. All these are remedies that are easily found and that can be obtained from a nearby place and that are greatly beneficial for this dangerous matter.

∴

The Third Chapter of the First Part

Concerning the simple remedies that are beneficial for the bite of all kinds of vermin

(15) The physicians have mentioned many remedies that may be ingested on their own, each of which is beneficial for the bite of any poisonous animal. Your servant has examined them all and found them to be hot. I have not found any cold remedy to be beneficial against bites in general, except for the mandrake root. It cannot be denied that a hot or cold remedy can be beneficial for any poison, whether hot or cold, because the action of these remedies that save from fatal poisons is not dependent upon their quality but upon their whole substance, as the physicians declare, or upon their specific property, as they say. This means, as the philosophers have explained, that these remedies are effective through their "specific form." Some of the remedies mentioned by the physicians should, as they order, be imbibed in wine, some in water, some in vinegar, and some in milk.

(16) As for myself, I advise anyone who was bitten or stung by an unknown sort of animal to examine his condition. If he feels a strong heat as occurs in someone bitten by a viper, the most appropriate thing for him to do is to choose from those remedies, which are taken in milk or in vinegar or in water. If he feels a severe cold, as someone feels who was bitten by a scorpion, he should choose from those remedies which are taken in wine. If someone is not allowed to take wine, he should take what he selects from them in an anise decoction, because all the physicians agree that anise is beneficial against all animal poisons.

(17) After this introduction, I am going to mention those simple remedies, which are most frequently found with us and which are most effective and have been proven by experience.

(18) Amongst them is *utrujj* (citron or lemon) seed: It is good against any poison which is fatal to the human body, whether the poison was ingested or absorbed through a bite. It should be prepared as follows: Clean the *utrujj* seeds from their peels, take their kernels, pulverize them, and ingest them in a dose varying from one *mithqāl* to two *dirhams*. Ibn Sīnā said that one should take two *mithqāls* in wine or cold water. [*Kitāb al-Qānūn fī al-ṭibb* (*The Canon of Medicine*)]. There is no difference between sweet or sour *utrujj* seed.

(19) To these also belongs emerald: A condition for its successful application is that it is to be a lustrous green and transparent. It should be well pulverized

and taken in a dose of nine granules in cold water or wine. The venerable Abū Marwān ibn Zuhr has said that this remedy has proven itself beyond any doubt. [*Kitāb al-Taysīr fī l-mudāwāt wa-l-tadbīr*]. It is good against all kinds of poison and eliminates them through emesis just as *terra sigillata* (sealed earth) does. It is a substitute for *terra sigillata* in theriac since *terra sigillata* is not available anymore.

(20) Bezoar: Galen does not mention the bezoar stone, nor the one which is called "animal bezoar" and which is a substance that has the form of an acorn, is a deep green color, and is formed by concretion, and therefore we find it as layer upon layer. Some say that it can be found in the inner corners of the eyes of stags in the countries in the East, and others say that it can be found in their gallbladder and this is more true.

(21) The mineral bezoar is a stone that can be found in the land of Egypt, namely, in Aydhāb. It has many colors, and wondrous things are related about it in the books of later physicians, but none of them was found to be true. Rather, I have tried all the different types of this mineral stone that can be found in our land against scorpion bites, and they were not beneficial at all. I gave many of them to bite victims, but to no avail. But what is stated about the beneficial effects of the animal bezoar has been proven by experience and confirmed empirically. It should be prepared in the following manner: Rub it in olive oil on a grindstone until it lacks no less than one *qīrāṭ* up to an eighth of a *mithqāl*. Let the person who has been bitten or who has ingested a poison lick this up. One should also rub some of it on the site of the bite, and the patient will recover and be saved.

(22) It has been proven by experience beyond any doubt that these three remedies—I mean *utrujj* (citron or lemon) seed, emerald, and bezoar—are effective against all types of animal, vegetable, and mineral poison.

(23) Serpent root, that is, the root of a plant that can be found in the vicinity of the Temple, is a plant well known for its pods, and its effectiveness has been proven by experience. It should be pulverized and imbibed in wine or cold water in a dose varying from one to three *dirhams* and the patient will be saved. It does not have the same strength as the emerald or animal bezoar, but, nevertheless, one should provide oneself with this remedy and always have it available. An expert on plants told me that this remedy is the root of a species of melilot that is called "the scorpion-like."

(24) Any type of rennet, especially that of a hare, if imbibed with vinegar in a dose varying from half a *dirham* up to one *mithqal*, saves from the fatal effect of animal and vegetable poisons.

(25) Another remedy that has been mentioned is Celtic spikenard. A dose of one *dirham* should be pulverized and taken in wine. Other remedies include the herb common agrimony and its seed; it should be pulverized and taken in a dose of two *dirhams* with wine.

(26) Oil of balsam of Mecca, half a *mithqāl*; it should be taken with fresh milk. Wood of the Mecca myrrh (balsam wood), six *dirhams*; boil it in one and a half *raṭl* of water until one third has evaporated, then imbibe it while it is hot. Garlic: All the physicians agree that it can replace the great theriac for all cold poisons and that it is also beneficial against hot poisons. It should be prepared as follows: Peel the garlic, crush it, and then take a dose varying from one up to two *mithqāls* and swallow it.

(27) Ginger preserve: Take two *dirhams* with hot water. Mandrake root: Pulverize and sieve it and take two *dirhams* of it with one ounce of honey. Cinnamon: Pulverize and ingest one *mithqāl* with cold water. Bitter costus: Pulverize and sieve it and take one *mithqal* with wine. One may also take, in the same composition, the same quantity of long birthwort on its own, or of agarikon on its own, or of great yellow gentian on its own, or of sweet flag on its own.

(28) Iris, that is, the root of Florentine iris: Pulverize two *dirhams* of it and take it with vinegar. Wild carrot seed: Take two *dirhams* of it with wine. Celery seed, three *dirhams*: It should be pulverized, sieved, and taken with wine.

(29) Cumin: Pulverize four *dirhams* and ingest it with water or wine. The same should be done with anise. River crabs: Boil them and drink the soup prepared from them.

(30) All these remedies can be found easily, except for oil of balsam of Mecca, but this is easily obtainable in Egypt. Hasten to take whatever is available from these remedies immediately after emesis, as I mentioned previously. And if a bite victim takes three ounces of heated honey and one ounce of rose oil and ingests it, it is greatly beneficial to him.

(31) All the aforementioned quantities are recommended for someone who has reached full maturity and is older than twenty years. Between ten and twenty

years the quantities to be taken should be calculated proportionately: The younger the patient, the smaller the quantity. I have not seen anyone younger than ten years survive who suffered from a sting or bite. Nevertheless, he should be given one-quarter of the above-mentioned quantity of the simple remedies and from one-quarter of a *dirham* up to one quarter of a *mithqāl* of the theriacs, according to the opinion of the attending physician. One should also consider the individual temperament and the current time of the year.

∴

The Fourth Chapter of the First Part

On the compound remedies beneficial against bites and stings

(32) The most important compound remedy is the great theriac: One should take from one-fourth of a *dirham* up to one *mithqāl*. Next is Mithridates: One should take from one-quarter of a *mithqāl* up to one *mithqāl*. Next is the theriac of four ingredients: One should take from one *dirham* up to four *dirham*s. Its composition is: Take equal parts of myrrh, peeled laurel berry, Roman gentian, and long birthwort, and knead this with skimmed honey in a quantity that is three times as large as that of the other ingredients. Each of these four ingredients is like a theriac against all poisons. It is the first compound remedy which the ancient physicians made, against poisons in general.

(33) Also, the asafetida theriac, which al-Rāzī recommends against all cold poisons, is a theriac with which one should provide oneself. Its composition: Take one ounce each of myrrh, leaves of dried common rue, costus, dried mint, black pepper and pellitory, and one and a half ounces of asafetida; dissolve the asafetida in wine and pulverize; sieve and knead the dry ingredients with skimmed, well-thickened honey. Take from one *dirham* up to two *dirhams* in hot countries and from two *dirhams* up to four *dirhams* in cold countries.

(34) Likewise, the walnut theriac, which is a great theriac, is a theriac with which one should provide oneself and to which one should accustom oneself for constant use. It is said that if someone constantly takes it before meals, poisons will have no effect on him. It consists of four ingredients: Figs, walnuts, salt, and common rue. As to their quantities, Galen mentions the following: Twenty parts of common rue leaves, two parts of the heart of walnuts, five parts of salt, two parts of dry figs [*De remediis parabilibus* III]; all these ingredients should be mixed through squashing them.

(35) Al-Rāzī prefers the following composition: One part of peeled dried walnuts, one-sixth of a part of coarsely ground salt and of leaves of dried common rue, and white figs in a quantity equal to all the other ingredients. One should divide it into rather large portions like walnuts, and the patient should take one portion of it. [*Kitāb al-Ḥāwī fī al-ṭibb*].

(36) The venerable Abū Marwān ibn Zuhr, may God have mercy with him, mentions the garlic theriac, and experience has proven for him that it is beneficial against any bite of a poisonous animal. Its composition is four ounces of peeled garlic; one ounce each of strawberry tree fruit, great yellow gentian, black pepper, white pepper, long pepper, and ginger; half an ounce each of the female species of agarikon and French lavender; and two *dirhams* of opium. Steep the opium in wine until it becomes soft, pulverize the dry ingredients, and knead everything with skimmed, well-thickened honey. The dose to be taken is from one up to three *dirhams*. [*Kitāb al-Taysīr fī l-mudāwāt wa-l-tadbīr*]

(37) All these theriacs should be taken with wine or an anise decoction, as I noted above. The calculation of the quantities to be taken of each theriac, from the smallest to the largest, should be according to the age, severity of the symptoms, time of the year, and country. In cold seasons and in cold countries human bodies tolerate strong medications while in hot seasons and countries the opposite is the case.

(38) Ibn Sīnā mentions an electuary that is good for any bite; its composition is three *dirhams* each of black cumin, Syrian rue seed, and cumin; one and a half *dirhams* each of great yellow gentian and smearwort, one three-quarters of a *dirham* each of white pepper and myrrh. All these ingredients should be kneaded with skimmed honey and then one should take a dose of half a *dirham*. [*Kitāb al-Qānūn fī al-ṭibb*].

(39) Galen mentions a remedy which is beneficial against all fatal animal bites, extremely severe pains, and hysterical suffocation: Take four *mithqāl*s each of poison hemlock juice and black henbane and one *mithqal* each of castoreum, white pepper, costus, myrrh, and opium; pulverize all these ingredients; and pour three ounces of sweet wine over them. Pound this in the sun and leave it there until it solidifies. Prepare pastilles from it with the size of an Egyptian bean. Take a dose of one pastille with three ounces of sweet wine.

(40) Says the author: Using the earlier and later physicians' writings, I have selected from the generally beneficial compound remedies those that can be prepared with the least effort and that are most beneficial. One should provide oneself with whatever one wishes.

∴

The Fifth Chapter of the First Part

Concerning the specific treatment of someone bitten by a certain animal

(41) The scorpion: One should begin with the general treatment which I mentioned above: incision, suction, and ligature, and then applying a poultice with one of the simple remedies specific for scorpion bites to the site of the bite. Also let the patient ingest one of the simple or compound remedies which are specific for scorpion bites, whatever is available of those I will mention in this chapter.

(42) Leaves of lemon balm: One should ingest three *dirhams* of this remedy and rub the spot of the bite with it. *Utrujj* (citron or lemon) seed: One should drink two *dirhams* of it. Colocynth root is an extremely powerful remedy for scorpion bites. The maximum amount to be ingested is two *dirhams*; it should also be applied as a poultice on the spot of the bite. If it is fresh, it should be pounded and rubbed on the spot of the bite; and if it is dried, it should be pulverized, kneaded with vinegar and honey, and applied as a poultice to the spot of the bite. Asafetida: It should be dissolved in olive oil and applied as a poultice to the spot of the bite. Seed of *nānakhwāh* (bisnaga or ajowan): One ounce should be boiled in two *raṭl*s of water until its strength is extracted and applied as a fomentation to the spot of the bite. Also sulfur and pine tree resin: One part of each should be kneaded with vinegar and applied as a poultice to the spot. Similarly, salt and flax, one part of each, and two parts of garlic should be pulverized and applied as a poultice to the spot. The theriac of four ingredients is most effective against scorpion bites; one should take one to four *dirhams* thereof.

(43) Galen mentions a theriac which is especially effective against scorpion bites and stings by the *rutaylā'* (tarantula). One makes it by taking four *mithqāl*s of birthwort, two *mithqāl*s of black pepper, one *mithqal* of opium, and three *mithqāl*s of pellitory; knead this with honey and make pastilles from it the size of an Egyptian bean. One should take two pastilles of this theriac with three ounces of pure wine. [*De antidotis* II.123].

(44) One should not take any of these remedies for scorpion bites, whether simple or compound, except with strong pure wine, because scorpion poison is a very cold poison that kills through its coldness. If someone cannot take it with wine, he should take it with an anise decoction, as I mentioned before.

(45) Another proven remedy is to take one *mithqāl* of frankincense, pounded and sifted, with one *raṭl* of wine. Another remedy tried by later physicians is the following: Take the green alkali plant, pulverize and sift it in silk, mix this with clarified butter of a cow and knead it with honey, and administer an amount of two *mithqāl*s to someone stung by a scorpion, and it alleviates the pain immediately. In the same manner, Ḥunayn says: If one smears white naphtha on the spot of the bite, it alleviates the pain immediately. [*Kitāb al-Tiryāq*].

(46) Says the author: The poisonous animal that is mentioned in the medical writings and called *al-jarārāt* is a kind of scorpion that has a small body and does not bend its tail over its body as scorpions do, but drags it over the earth. Therefore, these scorpions are called *jarārāt*. It is found in Eastern countries, and it is—as is said—more harmful than the scorpions found in our region, but anything beneficial against the latter is also beneficial against the former.

(47) *Al-rutaylā'* (tarantula): This name applies to many species of animals. Some say that there are six species of it, and according to others there are eight. All of them are different species of spiders. According to the physicians, the worst species of them all is the Egyptian one. As for the two species which are found in the houses in most districts—and one of which is the spider with long legs and a short body which spins many black webs between walls and ceilings, while the other has a larger body and shorter legs and spins thick white webs similar to a cloth prepared from silk and linen on the ceilings—the harm caused by these two species is minor; sometimes one does not feel the bite of either of them, and often one is bitten by one of them during the night without feeling it. However, in the morning the affected spot is swollen and red. But if one puts chewed bread or flour boiled in olive oil and salt on it, it dissolves the swelling on the same day.

(48) The other species of the *rutaylā'* are found in the countryside. It is said that one of them has downy hair, namely, the species which is called *abū ṣūfa* ("father of wool") in Egypt. The treatment of the bite of all these species is similar to the treatment of the bite of the scorpion. Anything that is beneficial for the sting of the scorpion is also good for the bite of the different species of the *rutaylā'*.

(49) I have found some specific remedies against the bite of the *rutaylāʾ*. Amongst them is asparagus root: Take five *dirhams* of it and boil it in six ounces of wine and drink it. Likewise, the leaves of lemon balm: Drink one to four *dirhams* of it and apply it as a poultice to the spot of the bite. Fruit of the French tamarisk: Drink from two to six *dirhams* of it. Mulberry leaves: Crush them and press out their juice and drink ten *dirhams* of it. All these should be consumed in wine or an anise decoction. Likewise, one *mithqāl* of black cumin, pulverized, in cold water. A poultice to be applied to the site of the bite may also be prepared from myrtle extract in wine. Equally, milk of cultivated lettuce. Whatever of these is available should be applied promptly after the incision and sucking of the wound.

(50) Honey bees and wasps: Good against their sting is the ingestion of five *dirhams* of marshmallow seed; it should be boiled in half a *raṭl* of water and one ounce of wine and then ingested. Another remedy is broad-leaved thyme: One should drink one *mithqāl* of its leaves in two ounces of the oxymel beverage. Also good is an equal amount of dried coriander and sugar: One should pulverize one *mithqāl* of this and take it with cold water. One may also take cold vegetables such as cultivated lettuce, *hindibāʾ* (endive or chicory), common purslane, and cucumber. All these ingredients are beneficial. It is also good to drink a pomegranate beverage or a beverage of unripe, sour grapes.

(51) A remedy to be rubbed on the site of the sting of honey bees and wasps is that prepared with clay in vinegar. Likewise, common duckweed in vinegar. Also, a piece of cloth soaked in vinegar, and camphor, and rose water, applied to the site. One can also apply a poultice from mallow, or fresh coriander, or *ḥayy al-ʿālam* (common houseleek or tree aeonium), or leaves of Christ's thorn jujube, or honey, vinegar, and salt.

(52) Snakes: It is well known that there is nothing more effective than the great theriac for all deadly poisons and for the bite of all kinds of vermin, especially for the bite of vipers. Because of their extreme danger to man, ancient philosophers and physicians have devoted much attention to their case and gathered so much experience over the years that they were finally able to compose the great theriac. Should it not be available, one should hasten to take Mithridates, and if this is not available, hasten to take bitter vetch pastilles. Its composition: Take equal parts of lotos (*ḥandaqūq*), smearwort, wild rue and bitter vetch flour; knead this with vinegar, and prepare pastilles from it. Let the patient take one *mithqāl* in one ounce of old wine. It is said that it can serve as a substitute for the great theriac for viper bites; for this reason, one should have it at hand. It

is said that maidenhair fern, if boiled with wine and then ingested, is beneficial for viper bites. It is also said that six *dirhams* of the root of the white grapevine, boiled with wine and ingested, is beneficial for viper bites. It is said that agarikon acts as a theriac against viper bites; one should take one *mithqāl* sieved in half a *raṭl* of old wine, and it saves from viper bites. A remedy especially for the site of the bite once it has been incised and sucked out is to take cabbage juice, to mix it with wine, and apply it as a poultice to the site of the bite.

(53) Galen mentions a poultice for viper bites which has the following composition—in his own words: Take one *mithqāl* each of sagapenum, asafetida, and opopanax, and two *mithqāl*s each of galbanum and sulfur untouched by fire; pulverize the dry ingredients; sieve them in a fine sieve; then dissolve the resins in wine and mix this with the dry ingredients until it assumes the consistency of a salve. Apply this as a poultice to the site of the bite; then cover it with fig leaves or Roman nettle leaves. [*De antidotis* II.14].

(54) Mad dogs: The physicians have mentioned many symptoms of mad dogs; all these are correct and there is no need to mention them at length in this treatise, because a human being instinctively flees from them when he sees them, just as he flees from a scorpion and a viper. Even healthy dogs flee from them. One always sees them walking alone, stumbling and sticking to walls, without barking. There is no doubt that people everywhere hasten to kill them when they recognize their condition. But sometimes a mad dog bites before being recognized. And sometimes someone is bitten in the dark by a dog and cannot tell if it was a mad dog or not. Every remedy that we find mentioned for the bite of a mad dog is only beneficial if it is applied before hydrophobia sets in. If it is applied after the onset of hydrophobia, no one has ever been seen to survive. A person bitten by a mad dog does not suffer greater pain than the pain of the bite of any other dog. Rather, the serious symptoms which indicate rabies only begin to appear in most cases after eight days, and sometimes only appear after a long period. Therefore, anyone bitten by a mad dog or by a dog whose condition is unknown should promptly receive the general treatment that I mentioned: Ligature, incision, suction, copious bleeding from the site of the bite by means of cupping glasses, emesis, and ingestion of the theriac. He should also be treated with whatever is available of those remedies that are specific for the bite of a mad dog, both ingested and topical, that I am going to mention now in this chapter, according to the aim of this treatise.

(55) One of these is Indian lycium: One should drink half a *mithqāl* in cold water every day. Another remedy is pulverized and sifted black cumin: One should

ingest two *dirhams* every day in cold water. Another remedy is asafetida: One should ingest half a *dirham* every day in cold water. Another remedy is pulverized and sifted great yellow gentian: One should drink one *mithqāl* of it every day in cold water. More effective than all these are burnt river crabs: they should be pulverized and sifted; their ashes should be sprinkled on water and then be taken daily in a measure of one *dirham*.

(56) According to Galen and others (for instance, Al-Rāzī), of the compound remedies whose efficacy was proven by experience is the following theriac for the bite of a mad dog; its composition is thus: One part of frankincense, five parts of great yellow gentian, and six parts of the ashes of river crabs. [*De simplicium medicamentorum temperamentis ac facultatibus* XI.24; *Kitāb al-Manṣūrī*]. Grind these into a powder, drink two *dirhams* of it in cold water on the first day, and increase the dose ingested by half a *dirham* every day until it reaches six *dirhams* on the ninth day. Thereafter only increase the dose by small amounts. Another compound remedy proven by experience: One *dirham* each of great yellow gentian and myrrh and two *dirhams* of the ashes of burnt river crabs; this should be ingested every day in cold water.

(57) From the simple remedies to be applied as a poultice for the bite of a mad dog after the application of general remedies that attract the poison, I will mention the following: Flour of bitter vetch, to be kneaded with wine and applied as a poultice. Another remedy: Bitter almonds, to be pounded with honey until it becomes like a salve and to be applied as a poultice. Another remedy: Leaves of fresh peppermint with salt; this should be pulverized and applied as a poultice. Another remedy: Take asafetida, moisten it in wine, and fill the spot of the bite with it after enlarging it. Another compound remedy: Equal parts of walnut kernels, salt, and onion; they should be crushed in honey until all of it becomes like a salve and then it should be rubbed on the bite. One should hasten to apply whatever of these remedies is available.

(58) One should continue the treatment of the bite victim with beverages and poultices applied to the spot of the bite for a minimum of forty days. Similarly, one should leave the site of the bite open; one should not let it close in any way prior to forty days. If it becomes almost closed up, it should be opened and enlarged by the salves composed to this end. It is well known that, of necessity, accidents happen within these forty days according to the individual temperament and corporeal disposition of the bite victim, and one must resort to different kinds of treatment, such as purgation, bloodletting, or enemas, and different foods and poultices. But this is not within the scope of this treatise. Rather,

what I have mentioned is only meant as a first aid until a skilled physician is present to attend to the patient, or it may suffice in the case that no accomplished physician can be found who can adequately treat these difficult cases.

(59) As for the bite of domestic dogs and similarly of human beings or other animals that are not poisonous, it is sufficient to submerse the site of the bite in heated olive oil time and again until the pain subsides. Then put raw broad beans that have been chewed until they become like a salve and apply this as a poultice to the site of the bite. The same can be done with chewed wheat. And if the person who chews the broad beans or wheat has not yet eaten anything, and the chewing is being done in the beginning of the day, and the chewer is a boy or a young man, it is more effective.

(60) Another remedy: Pulverize onions, mix them with honey, and apply this as a poultice. Another remedy: Flour of bitter vetch; knead it with honey and apply it as a poultice. Another remedy: The soft part of leavened bread; chew it and apply it as a poultice. Whichever of these one prepares and applies is sufficient.

(61) Know that the worst bite is that of a non-poisonous animal that has an empty stomach, and if the biting animal has a temperament that is bad for that kind of animal or feeds itself with food that is bad for that kind of animal and it is still hungry, its bite is nearly as dangerous as that of a poisonous animal, especially if the bitten person is replete with food, or his body contains bad humors, or the bitten limb is weak. For such a limb may putrefy and lead to increased danger for his life. But the treatment of such exceptional cases does not fall within the scope of this treatise.

(62) As for bites that happen frequently and are common, and likewise for the bite of those animals that are frequently found in the cities and countryside around them and that we have mentioned above, what we have mentioned in this treatise is sufficient for their treatment, God willing.

(63) But beware of not heeding the distinction made in the medical books between the bite of a mad dog and that of a dog that is not mad, for people have died because of that, as the elders whom I met informed me. Rather, you should know as a precautionary measure that only once you have verified that that biting dog was a domestic one, you should treat it in the way mentioned above and let the wound close. If you are not sure about the dog in question, you should treat the bite victim in the way you treat someone bitten by a mad dog.

A senior, well-known physician told me that he once saw in the city of Almería a young silk weaver bitten by a dog, and that it was not accompanied by any of the symptoms of the bite of a mad dog. The physicians then decided that it was a domestic dog and let the wound close up after a month or so and the boy recovered. He stayed healthy for a long time and carried out the activities of healthy people. Later, the symptoms of the bite of a mad dog became apparent in him; he developed hydrophobia and died. Be cautious in such things, for analogical reasoning cannot be applied in the case of evil poisons.

∴

The Sixth Chapter of the First Part
Concerning the foods to be given to bite victims in general and in particular, and certain remedies with specific properties which are fitting for this purpose

(64) All persons who have been bitten and all those who have imbibed whatever poison should be nourished with different kinds of *tharīda* with olive oil and clarified butter. One should give them fresh milk to drink, and they should eat large quantities of figs, walnuts, pistachio nuts, hazelnuts, garlic, onion, and common rue. All these should be consumed separately or compounded. If one takes only one of these, one should eat it as a seasoning with whatever bread is available. Do not let them have any kind of meat, not even fowl, because the blood produced by meat tends to putrefy because of the gaseous substances of the poison that remain in the blood of the person who has been bitten or who has consumed poison. Otherwise, all his blood will putrefy and serious complications will afflict him. Put much salt in their dishes, for it will burn and dry out the poison. Honey is not bad either, especially with clarified butter. As for the widespread belief among the people that every bite victim should only eat unleavened bread, I do not know any basis for it, neither rational nor traditional. Let them drink as much wine as they can tolerate and mix it in their dishes, especially in the case of someone who was bitten by a scorpion, for the intoxicating effect of wine alone is enough to cure him. Someone bitten by a scorpion should also fill himself with walnuts, figs, garlic, common rue, and strong wine, because this immediately relieves his pain so that he does not need any other regimen. This is the regimen for any bitten person who feels extreme cold or tolerable heat.

(65) If you see that someone who has been bitten or who has consumed poisoned food is burning hot and asks for large quantities of water, hasten to only feed him with sour milk and some fresh butter, and let him suck sour apple,

sour pomegranate, and pomegranate juice. And if you see that the sensation of burning is extremely severe, let him take cooling vegetables such as *hindibā'* (endive or chicory), cultivated lettuce, and cucumber—especially the smaller variety; oxymel beverage is not bad either. Mix the water that they drink with a little wine; and garlic, walnuts, and figs are indispensable. But reduce their quantity in accordance with the intensity of the heat felt by the bite victim.

(66) As for someone bitten by a mad dog, all the aforementioned foods are good for him except for salt; for his food should only contain a very small quantity of it. But especially good for him is to eat young chicken soup and nutritious fowl, such as the turtle dove, partridge, francolin, and *ṭayhūj*. He should avoid young pigeon because it is bad foodstuff. He should feed himself with cabbage because it has the specific property of being beneficial against the bite of a mad dog. Feed him with large quantities of onion and garlic, both raw and boiled. Let him also eat salted fish, not continuously, however, but every other day. The best food for him is soup and meat of river crabs. They are, actually, both medicine and food and is also beneficial for any bite victim because of the specific property which God bestowed on them. Similarly, acorns, both raw and cooked, are good foodstuff for any bite victim because of their specific property.

(67) Amongst the medicines with specific properties whose effectiveness has been proven empirically for someone who has lengthy experience with them are boiled chicken brains, which are beneficial for any bite victim or for someone who took poison. They also improve the intellect of healthy people, just like soup of turtle doves, because such soup sharpens the intellect through its specific property. Lemon peel, if eaten, has the specific property of being beneficial against poisons. The leaves of the lemon tree, if imbibed as a decoction, have a similar effect.

(68) The physicians agree that fumigation with the horn of a stag chases away all kinds of vermin, and especially snakes. They say that fumigation with goat's hoofs, mustard, sulfur, black cumin, opium, or human hair has the same effect. When any of these is used as a fumigant, snakes and other kinds of vermin will flee from its smell. They also say that if one collects some scorpions and burns them in a house, all the scorpions in that house will flee from that smell.

(69) One should also take precautionary measures and fumigate with them the places where any kind of vermin may be found, because the excellence of the human intellect demands that one is constantly cautious and prudent and

takes every possible preventive measure to protect the body against afflictions, although there is no real protection but through God's benefactions.

∴

The First Chapter of the Second Part

On the prophylaxis against deadly poisons

(70) Says the author: It is appropriate that I first make some introductory remarks which are clear to the physicists but are not well known to the physicians, although Galen may have mentioned some of the remarks included in this introduction. But he mentions them only as far as required by the medical art and does not explain them in a general introduction. It is exactly such an introduction that I want to give now.

(71) It is well known that those bodies which are composed of elements possess color, taste, and smell. All these are undoubtedly accidental, but the rules concerning color are not the same as those concerning taste and smell. Color is an accident of something possessing color, and the perception of that accident by every observer is the same and never changes. So, for instance, the color black: A human being cannot perceive its black form, which effects a contraction of the eye, while another kind of living being perceives its white form, which effects dilation of the eye. Rather its form is perceived identically by all those who can see.

(72) As for taste and smell, this is not so—one and the same thing can be utterly sweet for one animal species and utterly bitter for another. I mean that for one species it would be sweet and pleasant—and this is the meaning of sweet taste for them—while another species would have an utterly unpleasant sensation when tasting it, and this can be bitterness, acridity, or astringency to them, as it is explained in the principles of natural science. Everyone knows that sea squill tastes extremely bitter to human beings, whereas pigs find it tasty and eat it greedily. The same applies to the different kinds of smell, because one and the same thing can have a pleasant smell for one species and a bad smell for another species. For a pleasant sensation of taste and smell depend upon the temperament of the animal species. Anything that suits a certain temperament tastes sweet and smells good for that species. Similarly, some plants are proper nourishment for one species but a deadly poison for another species, as is stated and illustrated by Galen. [*De simplicium medicamentorum temperamentis ac facultatibus* III.6].

(73) After this introduction I say that any plant or animal meat which a person finds tasty, that is, sweet and good smelling, is undoubtedly appropriate nourishment and may be eaten safely. But all the foods with different tastes, such as bitter, acrid, sour, and other tastes, and, similarly, all those with a bad smell, one should not taste them until one has verified what species they are. For there is a sharp-tasting plant that one may think that it is wild radish, while in reality it is a deadly poison, and, similarly, there is the fruit of a roundish plant that resembles truffles and changes its color into black and is fatal. One should beware of plants with these different kinds of taste and with a bad odor and of any plant whose species is unknown. One should also beware of different kinds of dishes which are common among us and that are thick and soupy, such as *maḍīra* and *laymūniyya*, and of dishes of changing colors such as *summāqiyya* and *rummāniyya*, and of food fried with *murrī*, and of any dish in which an apparent sour, astringent, or extremely sweet taste is predominant, and of dishes that smell bad such as *al-mutawakkaliyya* and *al-baṣaliyya*, and that which is cooked with garlic. One should eat nothing from these dishes unless they have been prepared by a reliable person about whom one does not have the slightest doubt, for assassinating someone artfully can only be done through these kinds of dishes because the taste, the smell, the color, or the consistency of the poison is hidden in them. Meat or fowl cooked in water only or roasted cannot be employed artfully because even the smallest tampering therewith changes its taste, color, consistency, or smell. Similarly, to use pure water artfully does not work out well. One should be especially careful not to drink water that was left uncovered. Poisonous creatures often drink therefrom and poison the water so that someone drinking from it is either killed or suffers from severe afflictions. I have personally observed such incidents and frequently heard about them.

(74) As for the idea that one can make a deadly poison that does smell horrible nor taste bad, and that does not change the color or consistency of the matter into which one throws it because of the small amount one uses, but that nevertheless has a deadly effect if one throws something of it, for instance, into water or chicken broth, this idea is extremely far from being part of the medical art and is widely spread only among the common people. Rather, the truth is that every lethal or harmful substance, whatever kind it is, tastes and smells bad, according to that particular kind. Similarly, all the substances which are harmful to man, even a small amount of them, change the color of that to which they are added. These substances are especially effective for assassination when they are added to those dishes of whose consumption I have warned, unless those dishes have been prepared by a reliable cook. Assassination can

also be easily effected by throwing poisons into wine, for wine is especially appropriate because it hides the color, taste, and smell of the poison put into it and also assists in the poison's reaching the heart. And if someone also takes wine when he knows that they want to assassinate him, he has undoubtedly lost his power of discrimination.

(75) But it seems to me that it is highly unlikely that bread can be used for such a trick. Nevertheless, someone who is afraid that they want to assassinate him with something that can be eaten or drunk should only take such things from someone whom he can completely trust. For it is far from difficult to take a poisonous liquid, simple or compound, with which one can carry out one's criminal plan, and to put it into any foodstuff or drink. Any poisonous liquid, even it does not kill, is harmful for the victim; there is no protection except by God.

The Second Chapter of the Second Part

Concerning the regimen in general of someone who took a deadly poison or who suspects that he took it

(76) Anyone who took poisoned food or suspects that what he took was poisoned should first of all hasten to vomit the food by means of hot water in which dill has been cooked and over which much olive oil has been poured. He should drink it lukewarm and purge everything that is in his stomach therewith. Then he should drink a large quantity of fresh milk and vomit it. Then he should wait awhile, drink some fresh milk, and vomit it. Then he should wait awhile and drink milk and fresh butter and vomit it. It is said that excrements of roosters have a specific property to eliminate every poison by vomiting. This also should be taken with hot water in a dose of two *dirham*s and it will induce vomiting. Then one should eat *thurda* (*tharīda*) with much clarified butter or fresh butter. And when the food has settled in his stomach for an hour, he should vomit it, for the oils, milks, and fat neutralize the harmful effect of the poison and form a barrier between the poison and the parts of the body.

(77) Then one should take the remedies that save from poisons (antidotes) in general, either compound or simple—one should hasten to take one of whatever is available—and I will describe their composition. And if the remedy leaves the stomach after some hours, as I have mentioned in the case of bite victims, you should feed him with exactly those kinds of food that I mentioned in the sixth chapter of the first part of this treatise. Let him follow that

regimen and prevent him from sleeping, as I mentioned to you previously, until his food is digested. And if you see his condition improve, delay his sleep even further and continue to feed him with those foodstuffs that I mentioned for two or three days. And then administer to him one of the life-saving remedies (antidotes), compound or simple, as a precautionary measure. When the remedy has left his stomach, nourish him with chicken and young chicken soup, and thus make him regain his normal state. But if, after all these efforts, the patient is afflicted by a severe pain in his stomach, or pain in the abdomen, or a colic, or easy vomiting, or diarrhea, the treatment of all these afflictions and other ones which tend to happen to him requires a very detailed and lengthy discussion, but that is not within the scope of this treatise.

The Third Chapter of the Second Part

Concerning the simple and compound remedies that are generally beneficial for someone who took poison

(78) Says the author: The simple or compound remedies that have the specific property of saving from any poison in all the possible varieties of poisons are those that are called "useful against poisons in general." They are also called "life-saving remedies" (antidotes), and they are also called *al-pādāzhariya*. It is well known that the best compound remedy which saves from all deadly poisons is the great theriac, followed by Mithridates, followed by the theriac of four ingredients. The best simple remedy is the emerald; it is an excellent theriac for every poison one takes and for every poisonous animal bite. Moreover, it has the specific property of strengthening the heart, if kept in the mouth, and it is good for pain in the stomach if it is hung on the stomach from the outside. It strengthens the teeth when it is held in the mouth. All this was mentioned and verified by the venerable Abū Marwān ibn Zuhr, may God have mercy on him, with his lengthy experience, because he was the greatest among men in testing drugs and one who devoted himself to this more than any other. He was able to do so more than any other because of his great wealth and his skill in the medical art. Everyone I met from his students and friends told me that, whether on the road or at home, he would always have at hand a silver bowl containing the great theriac and a piece of fine emerald, because he felt, may God have mercy on him, very suspicious about deadly poisons.

(79) After the emerald comes the animal bezoar, and after that *utrujj* (citron or lemon) seed, and then serpent root. I have already mentioned all of these and

have determined the dose that should be taken from them and with what they should be taken. And among the simple remedies that are useful for everyone who takes an unknown poison and that are common are the following: Wild caltrop, of which one should take two *dirhams* in wine; seed of wild or garden rue, of which one should take one *mithqāl* in wine; all the different mint varieties, whatever is available—if it is fresh, boil one ounce thereof in half a *raṭl* of wine and drink it, and if it is dry, pulverize it, sift it, and swallow three *dirhams* with wine—and all the different kinds of rennet, especially that of a hare: Take from whatever is available from half a *dirham* to one and a half *dirhams* in some sips of vinegar, for this also counteracts any poison. Moreover, all these remedies are easily available and extremely useful.

∵

The Fourth Chapter of the Second Part

On the regimen for someone who knows which poison he took

(80) I have already said before that I will only mention those substances of the kind that one can eat without knowing their specific nature or with which one can easily assassinate someone. Among these is oxen blood, and it is easy to assassinate someone with it if one mixes it into a dish to thicken it or into an omelet (egg fritter) prepared with meat; it is a deadly poison. And when someone knows that the substance with which they tried to assassinate him is oxen blood, he should hasten to induce vomiting by means of rennet and vinegar. and then he should vomit by means of two *dirhams* of natron and boiled vinegar. Then he should take two *dirhams* of cabbage seed; one *dirham* of asafetida, and one *dirham* of borax; he should swallow all of it in boiled vinegar. If he vomits it, that is good, and if it remains for some time in the stomach and then passes into the intestines, it is good as well, and it saves him. Then one should purge him with agarikon and *hiera picra*, according to his age and condition as observed by the physician. And then he should take one of the life-saving remedies (antidotes) which I mentioned in the previous chapter.

(81) Says the author: If a skilled physician thinks about the right treatment of a patient who has taken a poison that is necessarily fatal and with which one can easily assassinate someone, it becomes clear to him how difficult this is and how far he is from realizing his aspiration. A small quantity of the mineral poisons, such as litharge, verdigris, and arsenic, even if their smell is not perceptible in foodstuffs, changes the color of a large quantity of food, and the amounts that one needs of these poisons to kill someone are large.

(82) But a small amount of some vegetable poisons, such as opium, even if it does not change the color, greatly changes the smell, while other poisons belonging to those that do not perceptibly change the smell nor the color, such as the milk of latex plants and the honey of the marking nut, can by a small quantity produce a clear change in taste.

(83) Next to this difficulty for the physicians we find that some men are assassinated by their women by means of the food they take and die after one day or some days, or suffer from what is far worse than death, namely, suppurating elephantiasis, which results in the limbs falling off.

(84) In every city I passed through I have seen some men suffer from this illness. And what I and others have heard about it is too much to be summed up here. Those senior physicians whom I met told me in their own name and that of their teachers that they had looked into this matter thoroughly and carefully until they learned from those adulterous women themselves what substance they had used to assassinate so-and-so, and their stories are well known. And they learned from them that the substance with which they had tried to assassinate their husbands was menstrual blood that they took from the beginning of the menses— even a small amount—which they put into the food and which then caused the observed afflictions. This is something that is not mentioned in any medical book that I read with this end in view; how then could one devote a chapter to the treatment of such a kind of poisoning? Similarly, those physicians informed me that they had saved many men from this affliction in the beginning of their condition, after the general treatment, that is, the mentioned emesis, by means of the following simple and compound remedies: Rennet, borax, natron, asafetida, cabbage seed, ashes of the fig tree, and juice of the leaves of the mulberry tree. The physician should administer from these remedies, simple or compound, according to the age of the patient. I do not have experience in any of these things, but I saw it as my duty to mention what I know about it so that others may benefit from them and try them out to the best of their ability.

(85) Likewise, someone who wants to guard himself against someone else whom he suspects should not eat from his food until the suspect first eats a fair quantity from it. He should not be satisfied with eating only a mouthful, as I have seen done by the cooks of kings in their presence.

(86) It is also easy to assassinate someone with poison hemlock and black henbane. When a person knows that this is the case (that he has been poisoned

by one of these), he should hasten to take some bark of the mulberry tree, boil that in vinegar, and first induce vomiting with that and then with milk. Then he should finish his therapy with that which I mentioned above under the general treatment.

(87) Similarly, the weight of one *mithqāl* of the devil's trumpet is fatal, especially the Indian variety, which is cold. It is said that it kills the same day with cold perspiration and cold breathing. It is a common poison with which one can easily assassinate someone because it changes the taste or the smell or the color only in such a degree as is imperceptible in foodstuffs. If someone finds out that he has ingested it, he should hasten to induce vomiting with natron, hot water, and olive oil; then he should eat much clarified butter; and then he should drink much wine onto which he sprinkles pulverized black pepper and cinnamon.

(88) Mandrake: Some people suck its flesh and it does not harm them; its shell and seeds are harmful to all people. I have often seen women and children eat it in their greed and ignorance about its nature, and they suffered from the afflictions mentioned in medical literature, namely, redness and swelling of the body, itching, and a state of intoxication. Its treatment is the same as that of someone who was given to drink devil's trumpet.

(89) Spanish flies (cantharides): And among the things with which one can easily assassinate someone are Spanish flies; they cause ulceration of the urinary bladder and micturition of blood and a severe colic and inflammation and kill after some days. The treatment: Hasten to let the victim vomit with the general emetics as I mentioned before in the second chapter of this part. Then he should drink a decoction of dry figs, continuously. Then let him drink mucilage of fleawort seed—and common purslane juice with julep has a similar effect—until the inflammation subsides. Then he should be nourished with milk and *thurda* with fresh butter, as I mentioned in the sixth chapter of the first part.

(90) Among the substances that are eaten without knowing their nature are truffles and mushrooms. These two types of food are extremely bad and are eaten in large quantities by the people of the West (Maghreb/Spain) and Syria-Palestine (East). Each of them has a deadly variety, namely, the variety that has a black color, or a green color, or that smells bad. But even the safe variety of these two types, if used for a long time, produces angina, which leads to death or a severe colic. If someone eats this safe variety, he should add much black pepper and salt to it and drink much undiluted strong wine after it. As for the

fatal variety of these two types, someone who has eaten from it should—as soon as the symptoms develop in him—be quickly given to drink one ounce of barley gruel, two *dirham*s of borax, and half a *dirham* of Indian salt. He should wait until this has settled in his stomach and then vomit it. Then he should drink oxymel with juice of radish leaves and vomit it. And then he should be given to drink vinegar and salt and vomit it. Then he should drink a large quantity of milk, wait for an hour, and vomit it. Then let him drink pure wine little by little.

(91) To the substances taken by mistake belongs the soporific type of black nightshade, for we often prescribe black nightshade juice among the ingredients to be taken for diseases of the internal organs. One of its varieties that has black seeds and that is soporific is sometimes taken by mistake when the seeds are still green, before they turn black. Upon drinking, it immediately causes severe dryness, hiccups, and vomiting of blood. Its treatment: Hasten to let him vomit by means of the general emetics that have been described before. Then let him vomit for the last time by means of water and honey. Then let him drink a large quantity of water and honey. When he has digested something of it, he should take another drink of water and honey. He should do so for a day and a night. And then he should feed himself as usual. With this size of the treatise your servant has, in his opinion, sufficiently executed the order he was charged with. May it fulfill its purpose, God—Who is exalted—willing.

This is the end of the treatise,
by the grace of God,
praise be to Him.

BOOK 3

On Hemorrhoids

First published in:

Maimonides
On Hemorrhoids

A Parallel Arabic-English Edition,
Edited, Translated, and Annotated
by Gerrit Bos,
with Critical Editions of Medieval Hebrew Translations
by Gerrit Bos
and Medieval Latin Translations
by Michael R. McVaugh.

Provo/UT (Brigham Young University Press) 2012
MWMM 7

∴

In the Name of God,
the Merciful, the Compassionate

(N.1) Says Mūsā ibn ʿUbayd Allāh, the Israelite from Córdoba: There was a young man from a prominent and renowned family, from a noble house and of great power, whose case concerned me and whose service was incumbent upon me, who was affected by hemorrhoids at the anus, which irritated him at certain times. He received the customary treatment for them until their pain subsided and the excrescences that had emerged reentered and returned to the interior of the body, so that it reassumed its normal functions. But when the ailment recurred to him several times, he thought of cutting the hemorrhoids off in order to extirpate this malady from its root, so that it would not come back to him again. But I informed him about the danger inherent in such an operation, in view of the fact that I was not sure whether these excrescences were of the kind that may be cut off or not; because in some people they are cut off, but then other excrescences appear. This happened because the causes that produced the first ones in these people remained, and therefore new ones occurred

 DOI:10.1163/9789004498884_005

to them. I gave him sincere advice and told him about the right method to treat this illness and all similar chronic illnesses, or about that which diminishes these illnesses so that their burden becomes very light and only the slightest trace thereof remains.

(N.2) And this is the good regimen that he should adhere to, when he is healthy, without weariness or annoyance: To take only that which is beneficial insofar as it is necessary, and to refrain from everything that is harmful in the case of this disease. This way is so difficult for all ill and healthy people to follow that they return with criticism to the physician and claim that the medical art is deficient. He asked of me, when his pain became very severe to him, to prescribe for him a regimen that he could always follow. And so, I composed this treatise for him—small in its size but large in its benefit—because I intended to give a regimen therewith that is easy to bear for young people who love an easy life. It does not have as its purpose to provide a perfect and complete regimen of health, nor to include all the different aspects of the treatment of this illness. I have divided this treatise into seven chapters:

Chapter one: A general discussion of the improvement of the digestions.
Chapter two: A discussion of the foods that should be avoided because of this illness.
Chapter three: On the foods one should strive for because of this illness.
Chapter four: On the simple and compound remedies that one should take regularly.
Chapter five: On the topical remedies that should also be used regularly.
Chapter six: On the regimen that one should rely upon when this illness flares up.
Chapter seven: On the fumigations that should be prescribed for this illness.

Chapter One

A general discussion of the improvement of the digestions

(1.1) Know that most diseases, and the most severe ones in particular, occur especially because of a bad digestion by the stomach, because if the digestion of the food in the stomach is spoiled, this corruption also passes to the second digestion (in the liver) and to the third digestion (in the other organs). Corruption of the digestion occurs because of the consumption of foods in one of four infelicitous ways: Because of either their quantity, or their quality, or their wrong sequence, or the time of their consumption. We will explain them one by one.

(I.2) As to the quantity, it means the excessive amount that is eaten and drunk, because good foods, and even the extremely good ones, are badly digested if the stomach is overfilled with them. The best thing to rely upon in this matter is that one does not satiate the desire for food, but stops taking it while there is still some appetite left, and distracts the attention from the stomach so that it does not stretch until it protrudes like a tumor. For there are people whose appetite is so strong that their stomach is stretched to that proportion; and in spite of that, they still have appetite.

As to the quality, it means that the food should not have a bad quality; for bad foods, even if digested in the best possible way, will not produce good blood. The best thing to rely upon in this matter is that one should not consume foods whose heat is evident, such as mustard; or whose coldness is evident, such as cucumbers; or whose bitterness is evident, such as celery, eggplant, and wild taro; or whose acridity is evident, such as onions, and garlic, and radish; or that are as sour as vinegar and lemons.

In general, one should strive for foods whose taste is predominantly flat, sweet, or fat, such as the usual kinds of bread, the usual kinds of meat and eggs, honey and sugar, and the like. In the same way, one should avoid every food that has a putrid smell, such as *kāmakh*, *ṣīr*, and *kubab*, or similar putrid foods; one should also avoid dishes that have stood overnight and started to putrefy, and those fruits and oils that have started to putrefy. One should be extremely careful with these.

(I.3) Galen said in a similar vein, and these are his words: Putrefied foods and beverages produce corruption similar to that produced by lethal poisons. [*In Hippocratis De aere, aquis et locis commentarius* II.2.1].

(I.4) As to their wrong sequence, it means that a food is taken first which should be taken later. That is to say, the most preferable and best thing for someone to do is to take one dish only; but if it is unavoidable for him to take many dishes, he should first take a dish with lighter food and then one with heavier food. Thus, he should take steamed vegetables before eggs, eggs before poultry, and poultry before mutton; and similarly, that which softens the stool should be taken before that which hardens the stool. For instance, the dish called *laymūniyya* should be taken before the dish called *summāqiyya* or *rummāniyya*. The right time for drinking water also belongs to this chapter. That is, the drinking of cold water before the meal is very harmful; it produces serious diseases. Drinking it during the meal is less harmful, but it harms the digestion of the meal. The best time for consuming water is one hour after the meal.

(I.5) As for the proper time of the consumption of foods, one should eat only after feeling true hunger and should take care not to eat meal after meal. Likewise, one should not consume food except after exercise or movement that somewhat kindles the bodily heat; one should beware of bodily movement after a meal until the food is digested. Any movement after a meal is harmful to the digestion—I mean any movement—whether it is gymnastics, coitus, bathing, or movements affections of the soul. If someone relies upon this measure that we mentioned concerning the consumption of foods and beverages, it will certainly be sufficient to ensure a good digestion in general.

Chapter Two

On the food from which one should refrain because of this illness

(II.1) It is well known that these hemorrhoids mostly originate from a melancholic humor. Only rarely do they originate from a surplus of blood, and even more rarely from phlegm. What one always observes is that they are produced by black bile; for if melancholic humor increases in the blood, the blood becomes thick and turbid and the organs reject it. Then this superfluity is expelled from organ to organ until this residual and turbid blood sinks to the lowest parts of the body because of its heaviness and the thickness of its substance. The vessels of the anus become overfilled and stretched and widened. Then the heat and moisture of these spots overtakes these vessels, and those excrescences—that is, hemorrhoids—develop.

(II.2) Some of them are open and flow—they are the easiest ones—while others are obstructed and blind, and nothing flows out of them. One should not interrupt the flow of those that flow, because it is a protection against very grave diseases, such as insanity, the various types of melancholy, and epilepsy. And as for those that do not flow, one should make their blood flow or incise them, if possible. But none of this belongs to the scope of this treatise, because it was not composed so that one could do without the personal attendance of a physician, nor so that one could treat the subject of healing all the different kinds of this illness exhaustively.

(II.3) But we specifically mentioned what we mentioned so that our master—may his strength be permanent—knows that the main thing in the case of the different varieties of this illness is to beware of the consumption of foods that produce black bile, thicken the blood, and make it turbid—such as broad beans, lentils, Indian peas, cabbage, eggplant, tanner's sumach, beef, chevon, and salted, dried meat. Similarly, he should beware of thick foods, such as different kinds of *harīsa*, different kinds of *tharīda*, *zalābiyya*, dates, old cheese, *faṭīr*, and *qaṭā'if*. He should also beware of the foods that are rich in superfluities, such as waterfowl and the brains of animals, and of anything that blackens the blood or makes it dry, such as *murrī* and vinegar. You should not come near any of these things in any way. Know that among these aforementioned foods, three foods are the worst ones in the case of this disease, and they have a specific property to produce it and to incite its pains: Namely,

1. eggplant,
2. dates, and
3. brains.

The sum total of these foods that you should refrain from among the foods that are common among us here are the following eighteen foods:

1. Broad beans,
2. lentils,
3. Indian peas,
4. cabbage,
5. eggplant,
6. tanner's sumach,
7. beef,
8. chevon,
9. salted dried meat,
10. different kinds of *harīsa* and *tharīda*,
11. *zalābiyya*,
12. dates,
13. old cheese,
14. *faṭīr*,
15. *qaṭā'if*,
16. waterfowl,
17. brains of animals,
18. black-eyed peas.

And among that which is used to season the food, you should also refrain from vinegar and *murrī*. I have given them this visual arrangement so that it would be easy to look at them at all times in order to avoid them. The other foods that are common among us are allowed for consumption. One should always strive to have soft stools and be very careful that they do not become dry in the case of this disease. The composition of the foods should always be softening, such as *laymūniyya* with safflower seed; or that which is sweetened with sugar; or that which is cooked with vegetables that soften the stools, such as beetroot, mallow, and spinach. One should minimize that which is cooked with rice as far as possible, because it dries the stools and also contains thickness; and one should take care not to take a large quantity of salt or spices in the food, for this is one of the things which burn and thicken the blood.

∴

Chapter Three

On the foods that one should aim for because of this illness

(III.1) Fat chicken meat and soups prepared from it are the best kind of food with which sufferers from this illness should be nourished; similarly, they should eat one-year-old sheep cooked with yolk. The consumption of kidney fat and roasted fat tail is beneficial for them; and fat *isfīdabājāt*, *jūdhābāt*, and *zīrbāj* with almonds or pistachio nuts and sugar and a little bit of vinegar and leek are especially beneficial in the case of this illness. One should cook this, or eat it roasted with sesame oil, or make an omelet from it with yolk.

(III.2) In the same way, water from chickpeas is very beneficial, whether they are cooked with it alone or they are cooked with almond oil and that water is ingested. One should also rely on the following dessert: *Fānīdh*, coconuts, dried figs—figs that were dried with an incision are even better—and anise. One should take all these together or separately; and a few raisins with almonds are also a good dessert. As for the other foods that are common among us, one should neither strive for them nor avoid them in the same way that one should avoid those foods that are mentioned above, in the previous chapter.

∴

Chapter Four

On the simple and compound drugs that one should regularly take

(IV.1) For each of the five myrobalans (emblic, beleric, chebulic, Indian, and yellow (citrine) myrobalan), one should pulverize one *mithqāl* from one of them and add the same amount of sugar to it and take it with the water from chickpeas. Similarly, anise: One should take an amount of two *dirhams* of it pulverized with the same amount of sugar. Likewise, borage: One should cook an amount of three *dirhams* of it and filter it over sugar. Similarly, raw silk: One should cook an amount of one *dirham* of it and filter it over sugar. Similarly, a common jujube infusion: One should filter it over sugar or manna (exudation of camelthorn) and drink it. Whenever one suffers from hard stools, the best thing to soften them with is purging cassia because, besides its relieving effect, it clarifies the blood. To these remedies also belongs iron dross: One should take one and a half *dirhams* from it, wash it after pulverizing it, and steep it in half a *raṭl* of boiled-down wine and drink this. Likewise, mace is beneficial for hemorrhoids as a drink or inserted as a suppository in the rectum. Similarly, emblic myrobalan is beneficial for hemorrhoids when it is drunk or applied as a suppository.

(IV.2) Among the compound remedies beneficial for hemorrhoids are the small *iṭrīfal* in its different compositions, and an electuary of iron dross in its different compositions, and the bdellium pill in its different compositions.

(IV.3) I have composed an electuary for my master that should be taken constantly on consecutive days except during strong heat and strong cold, for then it is not necessary, as it is not effective. When it is consumed, it should be taken with hot water in which borage has been cooked, and one should take from four to three *dirhams* therefrom. Its composition is thus: Take one ounce each of Indian, chebulic, beleric, and emblic myrobalan and of anise, eight *dirhams* of blue bdellium, four *dirhams* of birthwort, three *dirhams* each of mastic and mace, two *dirhams* of spikenard, and four *dirhams* of *shīṭaraj* (pepperwort or garden cress). The remedies should be pulverized and mixed with four ounces of almond oil and kneaded with two *raṭls* of borage syrup.

(IV.4) The composition of borage syrup: Steep three ounces of borage in two *raṭls* of hot water for one day and one night; cook it the next morning and filter it over two *raṭls* of fresh rose syrup and put it on a fire. Let it attain the consistency of a syrup, and then knead the aforementioned ingredients with it. Similarly, I composed the following decoction which should be taken for three days during each week when it is cold. Its consumption should be on those days that he does not take the electuary; it may also be taken instead of the electuary—whatever is more convenient for our master. Its composition is thus: Take three *dirhams* of borage, half a *dirham* of raw silk, half a *dirham* of emblic myrobalan, one quarter of a *dirham* of mace, one *dirham* of anise, ten hearts of fresh fennel, and five flowers of roses in their season. Boil, macerate, and filter these ingredients over two ounces of sugar. In the summertime, these very remedies, except for mace and anise, should be steeped together with six *dirhams* of pitted and chopped tamarind in one *raṭl* of water. The next morning, this should be filtered over two ounces of sugar and ingested.

(IV.5) Al-Rāzī mentions a pill that should be taken repeatedly; he praises it exceedingly and guarantees its effectiveness. Its composition is thus: Take one part each of chebulic, emblic, and beleric myrobalan, one part of iron dross, and two parts of bdellium; put this together in leek juice; make pills of it; and take it repeatedly. [*Fī man la yaḥduruhu ṭabīb*].

(IV.6) Composition of an enema that is very beneficial for hemorrhoids: Take two ounces of leek juice; one ounce of celery; two ounces of butter of a cow; one ounce of walnut oil, turpentine tree oil, or oil of the castor oil plant; and one-half ounce of radish oil. Mix all these ingredients, boil them, and administer as an enema once every two or three months, for it may cure the hemorrhoids completely.

(IV.7) Al-Rāzī also mentions that one should take five *dirhams* of oleander leaves, pound this well, pour thirty *dirhams* of fragrant olive oil onto it, boil it several times, filter it, and administer it in a suppository if the hemorrhoids are internal, or smear it on them if they are external; for this is, as he says, a wonderful remedy for curing hemorrhoids, and one does not need anything else.

Chapter Five

On topical remedies which should be taken repeatedly as well

(V.1) The oils which should be applied constantly, either separately or compounded, are the following: Coconut oil, oil of the castor oil plant, spikenard oil, *yāsamīn* (white or Arabian jasmine) oil, and eggplant oil. All these oils are beneficial for hemorrhoids. Similarly, bdellium and lead extract make the hemorrhoids shrink.

(V.2) Among the compound remedies, bdellium with sesame oil is beneficial for hemorrhoids and anal fissures. Likewise, date ointment and rose oil; likewise, blue bdellium and rose oil.

(V.3) The composition of a remedy that should be applied regularly because it shrinks them very much is as follows: Take two ounces from one of the aforementioned oils, one ounce of date ointment, and one ounce of pulverized, sieved blue bdellium. Mix all these ingredients over a low fire, then place the resulting substance in a lead mortar, put a quarter of a *dirham* of ground saffron on it, and pound it with a lead pestle in the burning hot sun for an entire day. He who does the pounding should sit in the shade, and the mortar should be in the sun until the power of the lead emerges into the remedy, and that which is dissolved from the lead becomes mixed with the ingredients, and the entire substance turns black and becomes thick. One should not cease to apply this remedy as a suppository every time one has washed one's bottom, for it is the most appropriate remedy for removing hemorrhoids with the passage of time.

(V.4) Similarly, lead extract alone, if applied regularly as a suppository, makes the hemorrhoids shrink and alleviates their pain. It is prepared by putting one of the aforementioned oils in a lead mortar and by rubbing it with lead in a strong sun for days until it thickens. This is called lead extract. One should always wash one's bottom with sweet water and beware of sitting on marble or of touching the anus with cold water, even in the summertime.

Chapter Six

On that which one should rely upon when this disease flares up

(VI.1) It is well known that all chronic diseases do not remain in one and the same condition, but sometimes are quiescent and at other times flare up, and their danger increases for days and then slowly diminishes. The same is the case with those suffering from hemorrhoids; sometimes the hemorrhoids flare up, become swollen, and are very painful, and it becomes impossible to relieve nature because of the narrowness of the passages due to the swelling. Sometimes part of the hemorrhoids protrudes and swells on the outside and becomes very painful and is followed by fever and distress.

(VI.2) The first thing that one should do is rapidly let blood from the basilic vein, if the strength of the patient can tolerate this. To bleed from the vein in the inner side of the knee is the most beneficial thing that exists. If the strength of the patient does not support this because of his age or the season of the year or because of any other obstacle that prevents bleeding, one should apply cupping glasses between the hips. After the evacuation, one should administer a thinning diet, consisting of thinning foods such as young chicken soup with mallow, or spinach, or beetroot, or safflower seed and sugar.

(VI.3) Thereafter, one should attend to alleviating the pain by means of topical remedies, which should be inserted as a suppository or put as a liniment on the protruding part of the hemorrhoids, and by means of sitting in waters that alleviate the pain and reduce the swelling. This includes sitting in hot waters in which common marshmallow leaves or roots, or melilot, or peeled lentils, or *bābūnaj* (German or Roman camomile), or dill, or common flax have been cooked. Each of these should be cooked—on its own, or all together, or only those that can be easily found—until the power of the remedies emerges in the water; and one should sit therein while it is warm and not leave until one feels it turning cold. Then one should get out of it and heat it again. As for those things that are applied as a liniment or are used to sit upon so that the pain becomes less and the swelling is reduced, the first of these is *ʿasīda* (porridge), made from fine white flour with sesame oil and duck or chicken fat. If one adds some saffron to it, it has an even stronger alleviating effect.

(VI.4) Another liniment: Take one ounce of of apricot kernel oil, dissolve two *dirhams* of liquid styrax in it and two *dirhams* of bdellium, and use it as a salve.

(VI.5) Another liniment: Take rose oil, and yolk, and duck fat—or chicken fat if duck fat is not available—and saffron; dissolve the fat in the rose oil, let it cool, and use it as a liniment after adding to it the yolk and some of the saffron. Then one should pound it and use it.

(VI.6) Another one mentioned by Ibn Wāfid: Take one ounce of fragrant rose oil and three ounces of white wax and put this into a glass vessel. Then put the glass vessel in hot water, and light a fire under the water, and let it boil until the wax melts. When it becomes a wax salve, sprinkle rose water on it, drop by drop, and stir it well with a spoon, and leave it on the fire until nothing of the rose water is left, and then apply it; for it has, as he said, a wonderful alleviating effect immediately. [*Kitāb al-Wisād*].

(VI.7) Another one, mentioned by al-Rāzī: Take two *dirhams* of washed zinc oxide and one *dirham* of Indian lycium juice. Knead this with wax salve prepared from rose oil and white wax.

(VI.8) Another one, mentioned by Ibn Sīnā: Take one part each of melilot, peeled lentils, and common marshmallow; pulverize this and sieve it and combine it with yolk and rose oil; and insert it as a suppository, or use it as an ointment. [*Kitāb al-Qānūn fī al-ṭibb* (*The Canon of Medicine*)]. And the following remedy belongs to that which alleviates the pain and reduces the swelling:

Dissolve duck fat in rose oil and mix this—that is, one ounce of it—with one-eighth of a *dirham* of saffron and one *dirham* of bdellium, pulverized and sieved like a powder, and apply it as a suppository.

(VI.9) One of the strongest compounds in alleviating the pain is that mentioned by Ibn Sīnā. Its composition is: Take two *dirhams* each of sagapenum and bdellium, one *dirham* of liquid styrax, half a *dirham* of opium, and one and a half ounces of apricot kernel oil; dissolve these resinous substances in oil over fire; then throw half a *dirham* of pulverized castoreum onto it; stir this mixture thoroughly; and insert it as a suppository or apply it as an ointment. [*Kitāb al-Qānūn fī al-ṭibb*]. One should apply this remedy only when one has exhausted all other means and the pain does not subside. Lead extract alone alleviates the pain if it is prepared with one of the aforementioned oils or with butter that has been melted and whose froth has been removed. This is the most effective remedy for reducing the swelling and alleviating the pain. It has been said that fat of a skink with rose oil has a wonderful specific property to alleviate the pain of hemorrhoids. One should use one of these topical remedies in the case of pain and swelling only when they are actually hot.

Chapter Seven
On the fumigations that should be prescribed for this illness

(VII.1) The remedies with which hemorrhoids are fumigated, dried, and shrunk and that can be easily found are the following: *sandarūs* (resin from the arar tree), leek seed, snake's skin, colocynth, cotton seed, Syrian rue seed, black henbane seed, long birthwort, and fenugreek root. The physicians say that all these, if used as fumigations singly or compounded, are beneficial for the illness of flatulence.

(VII.2) One of the compound remedies to be used for fumigation is the following: Take one part each of leek seed and of *sandarūs* and half a part of bdellium; knead this with honey and fumigate with it.

(VII.3) The fumigation should be carried out in the following way: Dig a hole in the ground and make a coal fire in it. Cover the hole with an earthen pot by putting it upside down on the hole, and make a hole the size of a walnut in the bottom of the pot. Wrap a garment around the pot and cover it with earth so that nothing of the vapor escapes except through the opening in the pot.

Then throw some of the substance to be used for the fumigation on the fire through the opening in the pot. When the smoke rises, the patient should sit down on the pot, put his garments around him, and lower the round part of the buttocks as far as possible. When he feels that the smoke has finished, he should stand up and throw some more into the pot and then once again sit on the bottom of the pot, as he did initially. One should do so for three consecutive times in one hour and should apply this kind of fumigation once a week. This is the amount of information that your servant thinks is very useful and that can be derived from a book. As for letting blood from those hemorrhoids from which no blood streams, or stopping the blood flow if it is excessive, or excising hemorrhoids, or the ingestion of purgatives, if this becomes necessary in whatever circumstance—all this does not belong to that which should be included in this treatise. Nor would anyone among those who look into any of these matters according to what is stated in the medical handbooks and encyclopedias benefit from it. On the contrary, sometimes someone who proceeds on the basis of books suffers severe harm, for remedies that make the blood flow or that retain it if it is excessive, or purgation of the bowels, or excision of the hemorrhoids should only be performed by an experienced physician who takes into account the temperament of the patient, his age, his strength, the current time of the year, and how far other illnesses and symptoms are associated with this illness. All this should be directed by him in accordance with the situation at hand.

May God—He is exalted—strengthen the health of our master
and relieve him of all this by
His grace, magnanimity, beneficence, favor, and goodness.

BOOK 4

On Rules Regarding the Practical Part of the Medical Art

First published in:

Maimonides
On Rules Regarding the Practical Part of the Medical Art

A Parallel Arabic-English Edition
by Gerrit Bos and Y. Tzvi Langermann.

Provo/UT (Brigham Young University Press) 2014
MWMM 8

(0) He said: My honorable master, the Pillar of Faith—may God protect him—, enjoined me to compose a treatise on rules regarding the practical part of medicine using concise aphorisms. I carried out his command—may God grant him lasting happiness—, and I followed the path whose goal came to fruition in writing it. I had intended, at the time that I wrote the treatise on the illness my master was suffering from (asthma), to put these aphorisms together with what was in the treatise *On Asthma*, but I was prevented from doing so by illness and thus did not carry out my intention at that time. Now, however, I will begin to do so, God willing.

(1) The first thing to consider is the improvement of the air, then the improvement of the water, and then the improvement of foods. Know that one's body is composed of matters that are in a constant state of dissolution and fluidity. For this reason, the body does not remain in exactly the same condition, but in conditions that resemble each other, and this is called health. When the body deviates from the correctly proportioned causes, this is called disease. For this reason, health should be preserved by means of those things that maintain the correct mutual proportion, while illness should be treated by things that oppose the illness until the body returns to a harmonious condition.

 | DOI:10.1163/9789004498884_006

(2) There are three things by which health is maintained:

1. Replacing the innate heat that has dissolved from the body and its organs;
2. evacuating the residues that have accumulated in the body; and
3. taking care that the body is not quickly affected by old age.

These three objectives can be realized if one puts before one's eyes the assessment of the quantities and qualities of the established factors of health to which the physicians pay attention.

(3) Pay attention every day to improving the air that reaches the body through inhalation so that it will be perfectly balanced and free from all that might pollute it. The finer the pneuma is, the more sensitive it is to alterations in the air. The natural pneuma is coarser than the vital pneuma, while the vital pneuma is coarser than the psychical pneuma. Likewise, pay attention to the concoction of the bodily humors in the stomach, vessels, liver, and other organs. Take care to decrease their quantity when it is too large and to increase their quantity when it is too small, to refine the humors that are coarse, and to dilute the humors that are viscous, and to balance these humors. Take care to exchange these unhealthy materials with opposite ones, so that every single one becomes again as it should be.

(4) Pay attention to the preservation of health through exercise, massage, bathing, and other means that strengthen the organs, expel their residues, and preserve their temperament. This holds good especially for the major organs and for those organs that carry out an activity in the body that is of major importance, such as the heart, liver, stomach, and brain. These kinds of organs need more attention than the other ones.

(5) There are two kinds of exercise: The first is the kind that is both exercise and art work, such as agriculture and every art in which the body is put into action. The other is mere exercise, such as running, wrestling, and playing with the small ball.

(6) One should exercise only after the food in the body has been digested and its residues expelled. Digestion in the stomach and intestines is indicated by the evacuation of excrements in a natural way, and in the liver and its vessels, by the evacuation of the urine in a proper way.

(7) Massage, or rubbing, should be applied judiciously; in the beginning it should be done little by little and softly, then increased slowly until one reaches the right quantity. Every massage should be done with the hands moving in

different directions so that not one spot remains without rubbing or massage. The right quantity also entails heating the body and concocting the humors in the organs. Massage should be applied either before exercise, and then it should be soft; or afterward, and then it should be hard. If one rubs the body in order to moisten it, one should do so after bathing in sweet, lukewarm water.

(8) Those whose health is deficient should exercise, bathe, and receive massage and rubbing in air contrary to their bodily condition.

(9) Exercise is not safe for those bodily parts that suffer from a discharge of superfluous matters into them. On the contrary, one should let them rest. Those parts that are opposite to the affected parts—namely, those parts away from which the superfluous matters are diverted—should also rest.

(10) Children need that which strengthens their bodily parts and their functions and which prepares these parts for the function they are intended for when they reach puberty. They also need that which preserves the innate heat in them and expels only the residues. Young people need that which preserves the powers of their bodily parts and which moistens according to the surplus of dryness in them. They also need that which expels the vaporous and other residues from them. The elderly and old people need that which heats and moistens commensurate to their tendency toward cold and dryness. They also need that which strengthens the faculties of their organs and which expels the residues. One ought to do likewise for the seasons of the year, the other temperaments, foods, and so forth, so as to provide for every case that which is fitting for it.

(11) If a body is on the verge of putrefaction, it can endure hunger and thirst more easily than other bodies. One should protect one's body against putrefaction using ingredients that expel the bile and that have a cooling and drying effect. One should also be wary of things that cause putrefaction, such as extreme heat and indigestion. A bilious body cannot endure hunger, thirst, or excessive exercise. Such a body should be protected from becoming ill through moderate exercise and massage; bathing in sweet, lukewarm waters; and foods that produce pleasant vapors, cool, and moisten without viscosity. Such foods are barley broth, well-prepared bread, chickens that lay eggs, the testicles of roosters, the yolk from chicken eggs, soft-boiled eggs, rockfish, and every fish that does not have bones. In general, one should beware of everything that is sharp, that obstructs the smoky vapors from leaving the body, and that closes

the pores. One should also avoid exertion, anger, sleeplessness, bathing in astringent waters, and the like. One should similarly take care of the other types of bodies.

(12) A body that is extremely fat should be made more lean by eating less food; by eating salty things; by drinking thinning beverages; by taking refining drugs, especially diuretics; by promoting perspiration through exercise; by bathing on an empty stomach; by sleeping before taking a meal; and by bathing in salty waters. A body that is extremely lean should be made more fat by eating abundant food; by taking sweet and fat things and thickening beverages; by bathing in sweet waters with a full stomach; and by sleeping after taking a meal. If one intends to increase the size of a fleshy part, one may do according to the story that is told—namely, that a coppersmith irritated part of his body by beating it lightly with branches and then rubbing pitch on it, and that he used to do so once every three or four days, and that, in a short time, he greatly increased the size of that part.

(13) Obese bodies that have a hot and moist temperament and a hot and sweet vapor originating in them can endure the postponement of the consumption of food, because of the small quantity of smoky vapor that they contain. But lean bodies that have a hot and dry temperament and a sharp vapor originating in them cannot endure such a postponement. Bodies most unable to endure fasting are those that are cold and dry, because a dry body is emaciated by abstention from food.

(14) Health should be preserved and increased, while illness should be decreased and abolished. Health is preserved through the soundness of the organs, the pneuma, and the innate heat. This can be achieved through suitable nutrition, a quiet life, the generation of good blood and only few superfluities, and by improving breathing through the inhalation of healthy airs and winds.

(15) To apply oneself in acquiring knowledge of every single part of the body and its peculiarities is doubtlessly useful for therapy. This is so because if, for instance, the liver suffers from a hot tumor, it needs a remedy that opens that tumor and cleanses it without irritating it so that it does not trigger pain. Remedies with these properties are those that are fine of substance and not viscous, such as barley groats—among foods—and filtered *hindibā'* (endive or chicory) juice—among other remedies. But *hindibā'* syrup, although it is fine and not viscous, thickens the liver because of its sweetness, for all sweet things have the property that thickens the liver and spleen. And apple syrup

and pomegranate syrup, even though they are coolants, block the openings of the passages through their astringency and thus increase the obstruction. A remedy does not reach remote organs unless it has been transformed and weakened in strength; this is not the case with organs that are close to where the remedy enters the body. The eye, because of its extreme sensitivity, will tolerate only medications that alleviate pain, such as egg white and mucilage of fenugreek, and so also tolerates only those remedies that are extremely fat. Since this is the case, treatment necessarily differs according to the differences in organs and diseases.

(16) If someone's body contains a remnant of the material of a disease, it should be expelled; the body's temperament should be balanced before reviving its strength. If it is suddenly emaciated through excessive evacuation, its strength can be revived in such a way that it regains its initial condition within one or two days, by replacing that which has departed from the body with a large quantity of suitable foods and agreeable smells. This can happen because the powers of organs of such a body have been preserved intact, without any loss. If someone's body has become emaciated over a long period of time, its treatment will take a long time as well, because the powers of his organs are weak. Therefore, it is necessary to give him well-prepared bread along with chickens, fish, and the like, from among those foods that digest quickly, are absorbed quickly, and produce good humors. One should increase their quantity every day according to his capacity to bear the increase in the amount of food. One should also let him drink watery, astringent wine because it increases the total heat of the body, penetrates into the food, helps its digestion, and breaks up the winds. One should take care that the food does not weigh heavily on the stomach. One should do all one can until the patient's condition is such that he can have kid, after which comes lamb. He should be careful that the food does not float in the stomach as a result of drinking a large quantity of water. If he suffers from severe thirst, let him drink a small amount of water mixed with wine.

(17) Arriving at the best treatment will come from knowing several factors, including:

1. The kind of disease someone is suffering from, its cause, and its symptoms.
2. The temperament of an ill person: If a hot temperament alters in the direction of heat (becomes even hotter), then it will return to its natural state through a small amount of cooling; but if a hot temperament alters in the direction of cold, then it will return only through a large amount of heating.

3. The activities of the organs: The powers of bodily parts with noble activities should be preserved, and one should beware of evacuating these parts forcefully. For this reason, if we want to dissolve and evacuate a residue from these parts, we mix the remedies we use with some aromatic, astringent ingredient that preserves the power of the bodily part, even if it affects the treatment adversely.
4. The disposition or nature of the organs: The stomach is cleansed through both excretion and emesis; the rectum can be cleansed only by excretion, and the liver can be cleansed from its residues by excretion and urination.
5. The location of the parts: External parts can be reached by medicines before their powers are changed, whereas for most of the internal parts, the opposite is the case.
6. The reciprocity of the parts: When the head hurts, the stomach shares in the pain; therefore, both the stomach and the head should be cleansed so that the head is not affected by the matter rushing to it from the stomach.
7. The capacities of the parts: Parts affected by high fever cannot endure hard treatment, nor can weak parts.

The remedies themselves: The dose of strong remedies should be calculated precisely and should be mixed with other ingredients according to the need, and so also for other remedies.

The things that, through their conformity or difference, indicate what sort of treatment is needed.

(18) One should evaluate the cause of the ailment, the ailment itself, and its symptoms, as each one stands in relation to the others; then one should pay attention to the thing that causes the strongest disturbance in the body and weakens its strength most of all. If you come across something that counteracts all these things together or that counteracts that which is most severe but is beneficial for the other things, you should rely on it. But if you do not come across something like that, you should turn to treating that which is most important without neglecting the other things. If the cause of the fever is alarming very dangerous, one should take care to root it out, even if this action increases the heat of the fever. And sometimes the fever itself is so high and severe that one should hasten to cool it and extinguish it, even if this treatment worsens the cause. And in some cases, the fever is accompanied by severe symptoms—such as a collapse of strength, excessive diarrhea, and fainting—and one should quickly attend to the symptom first, so that it disappears, and then start treating the fever.

(19) If a humor flows into the stomach, it should be expelled from it using emesis or purgation. The influx should then be stopped through the evacuation

of that humor from the body, and its cause should be neutralized. The stomach should be strengthened so that it does not absorb the humor anymore. If the stomach has been affected by a bad temperament because of the lengthy influx of the humor, that temperament should be changed into a better one once the stomach has been cleansed. If the humor has entered into the lining of the stomach and adheres to it, the condition should be treated with drastic remedies, such as *hiera picra*. When the humor is viscous, it should be refined and diluted before its evacuation. Those suffering from it should be given such foods that cleanse the humor. One should proceed in this way with every single organ.

(20) The issue of food to be given to someone ill has six aspects:

1. One of these is the strength of the patient: If it is sound, then he can tolerate waiting and a lightening of his diet. The opposite also holds true—if his strength is weak—then he must be given food right away, and his diet should not be lightened.
2. The length of the disease: If the disease lasts for a long time, the patient's strength should be maintained by means of food.
3. The disease itself: The quality of the food given should be opposite to that of the disease. For instance, in the case of fever caused by the putrefaction of thick, viscous humor, the food should thin out the thickness of the humor.
4. The time: The food should be administered at the usual time, both during healthy periods and when the attack abates.
5. The digestive organs: If the stomach or liver is affected by a tumor and food is administered before a fever attack, the nourishment is detrimental for the patient, especially when the body is overfilled. When one of these organs is weak because of a bad temperament or because of the influx of humor but is not affected by a tumor, food is appropriate, even during a fever attack, especially when the body is not congested.
6. The magnitude of overfilling: When the body is overfilled, one should take less food; but when it is deficient, one should take more food, even during a fever attack.

(21) The superfluous matter in the lower parts of the body is drawn upward and evacuated by exercising the upper parts that are opposite to the lower parts. The reverse holds true for the superfluous matter in the upper parts: it is drawn downward by exercising the lower parts. Cupping glasses also have a strong attractive force, upon their application. In keeping with this principle, they should be applied to the opposite side if the goal is to divert the matter to

that other side. But if the goal is to draw the superfluous matter from the afflicted part itself, they should be applied on that part either by using fire or with or without scarification.

(22) Overfilling should be treated by bleeding, sweating, exercise, massage, diet, and remedies that evacuate the residues or that refine the humors. Bad humors should be treated by evacuation and then by bringing the humors back into equilibrium.

(23) If the body contains a very raw humor, do not even consider bleeding, lest the innate heat become too weak to concoct the humor. Likewise, do not think of exercise, purgation, or bathing, lest the fine part of the humor be expelled and the crude part remain and flow to one or more of the noble organs. One should remove the humor only by means of massage, which concocts the humor and which should be applied as follows: Start with the legs and rub them from the joint of the knee to the feet; then rub the thighs from the groin to the knee. Once these parts have been softened through rubbing and the body has become warm, rub the forearms, then the upper arms, followed by the spinal column. Then go back to the legs. Repeat this for the whole day, except for the time in which the patient takes a nap, for sleep is beneficial in this case because it concocts the crude humor. Accordingly, at the moment when the patient is fatigued, let him be rubbed with an oil that has a dissolving effect; then rub this off and let him rest. Once the patient has recovered from his fatigue, one should massage him again. Bodies of a moderate temperament should be massaged with linen cloths of moderate softness or roughness, and those of a dry temperament with rough linen cloths. Those with this bodily condition should live in a house that is only moderately hot and cold, for heat dissolves the humors, and one cannot be free from the fear that they will suddenly stream to a noble organ; and cold increases the thickness of the humors. In cases such as these, one should limit oneself to the ingestion of hydromel. If the patient also suffers from fever, one should administer oxymel instead of hydromel, and these patients should feed themselves with gruel prepared from wheat. If they suffer from diarrhea, one should give them pomegranate seeds or tanner's sumach together with the gruel; if the diarrhea becomes severe, one should moisten these ingredients in astringent, diluted wine. In general, the treatment of these patients should consist of refining, dissolving, and evacuating the crude humors. However, if one of them suffers from a tumor in the liver or stomach, there is no hope that he will be saved.

(24) Those whose humors are extremely thin and fluid and whose bodies are quick to dissolve and putrefy should take food in small amounts and repeatedly. Once the first portion of food has passed through the body, they should take a second. If their organs are weak, they cannot take their food all at once; and if they suffer from a tumor in the stomach or liver, they cannot be saved. Their slenderness results from the wideness of their pores and the weakness of their vigor. It should therefore be counteracted with that which thickens the body and strengthens it, externally or internally, by taking astringent ingredients; the thinness of the humors should be counteracted with that which thickens them, and that which has dissolved from the body should be replaced through nutrition.

(25) If pain arises from a biting humor, its harm should be undone by those purgatives that remove, dissolve, and cleanse that humor. If this is not sufficient, one should use that which benumbs the senses—namely, a narcotic. If the pain comes from a thick, viscous humor, it should be alleviated through dissolving, concocting, and evacuating that humor with thinning remedies that do not heat excessively. If the pain comes from inflating wind, it should be treated with foods, remedies, cataplasms, and fomentations that disperse the winds.

(26) One should protect against fainting (syncope) by preserving the substance of the pneuma, the faculties of the organs, and the innate heat. This can be achieved with foods and sweet, pleasant smells; thickening the body when it is porous and thickening the humors when they are thin; thinning the humors when they are thick and thinning the body when its pores are tight; alleviating pain when it is severe; and, in general, by preventing that which causes fainting.

(27) If someone's stomach has a hot dyscrasia, he should be given cold water to drink and fed with cooled sour milk, fruit that has been cooled in the snow or in the cold air, and cooled barley groats. A poultice containing ingredients of this sort should be applied to his stomach. But if it is a cold dyscrasia, he should be given old, pure wine to drink; he should be fed and given a poultice, both the food and poultice being of moderately hot ingredients; and his belly should be brought into contact with things that heat it moderately until his body becomes well fleshed. If the dyscrasia is moist, he should be given roasted food, and a poultice of drying ingredients should be applied to his stomach; but if the dyscrasia is dry, one should give him moist things. If the dyscrasia is composite, the treatment should be composite as well.

(28) Fever is a hot, dry dyscrasia, and it requires for its cure cold, moist things, unless such treatment would lead to a thick, viscous humor or weakness of a noble organ that cannot bear cooling. It may also result in an affliction worse than the fever, such as fainting. Therefore, that which is more important should have precedence, but the other things should not be neglected.

(29) Regarding every fever, observe the change it makes in the temperament in view of the nature of the fever; then bring the temperament into balance. In general, the cause of every fever should be opposed. For instance, although the cause is no longer active in most cases of ephemeral fever, it is still necessary to oppose it. If someone has fever because of sleeplessness, one should make him sleep; if someone has fever because of anxiety, one should give him pleasure. The other kinds of ephemeral fever should be opposed in the same way.

(30) Cold water is appropriate for fever patients because it extinguishes a flare-up by cooling and moistening. It is also appropriate for severe anxiety and distress. It strengthens the intestines and dissolves bile in them, and it invigorates the body from the weakness caused by heat and dryness and prepares it for the intake of food. But one should not administer cold water when the noble organs are weak because of a tumor or because of a cold or moist dyscrasia. And, by God, certainly not when the tumor is [...], and not before the tumor is ripe, nor during the crisis, in order to allow it to ripen. But if the body is well fleshed, dry heat dominates, the humors are concocted and may already have been evacuated, and there is no longer any weak organ within; then cold water should be given to drink.

(31) Once the ephemeral fever has declined, it should be treated by going to the bathhouse in order to dissolve the smoky vapor that arises in the body. If the fever is caused by bathing in astringent water, plenty of massage should be applied in order to relax the tightness of the skin. If it is caused by anger or anxiety, the massage should be moderate and the rubbing with oil should be extensive. When the fever arises from cold, there is more need for hot air; but if it is accompanied by a catarrh or rheum and has not concocted, bathing should be postponed, and one should make the head sweat by rubbing it with hot oil. Someone who has developed a fever because of the heat of poisons should be immersed in cold water and eat cold fruits before going into the bathing basin and after leaving it. If the fever arises from the frequent getting up because of diarrhea, the patient should be fed before entering the bathhouse. One should pay attention to the stomach, especially if it is affected by a burning sensation. The same holds good for the intestines, especially if they are irrit-

ated. If the fever comes from indigestion, one should inquire whether the food has degenerated into something smoky or sour. Each quality—smoky or sour—should be countered with its opposite. In any case, one should take care that the putrefied food is eliminated before the patient enters the bathhouse; after that, the stomach should be strengthened. If the fever comes from a tumor in soft flesh, that tumor should be dissolved before the patient enters the bathhouse.

(32) Those indigestions that are beneath the ribs should be confined. If the food has descended from the stomach to the intestines, one should give the patient with this condition an enema whose ingredients expel. But if it has not gone down, one should give him that which induces emesis and let him drink a pepper stomachic and the like. One should warm his stomach and apply a strengthening poultice to it. If the food is concocted in it, the stomach should be rubbed with olive oil in which common rue or seeds that expel the winds were cooked. When the food has descended and left the body, the patient should have some fine food immediately and then, about six hours later, enter the bathhouse. Know that if the treatment of ephemeral fever is not successful, it will either last for days or lead to putrefaction.

(33) When a fever occurs, one should examine it. If it is an ephemeral fever, the patient should enter the bathhouse when the fever abates, according to the opinion of all physicians. But I caution against taking him to the bathhouse, because we know little about this nowadays. And although there may be someone who knows about the nature of fevers and about the effect of going to the bathhouse, we do not know about it even if we look into it, let alone knowing the effect. If the patient suffers from blood fever (synochous fever), one should hasten to bleed him. If the fever originates from yellow bile, the humor from which it originates should be evacuated using ingredients that have the property to cleanse and evacuate without heating, such as tamarind, pears, pomegranate juice, oxymel, barley groats, and spinach. If the fever is chronic, one should either, in the beginning, give the patient ingredients that refine the coarseness of the humor that causes that fever, thin its viscosity, and help its concoction; or, in the end, when the humor is concocted, give him ingredients that evacuate it. If the patient suffers from hectic fever, one should take care to cool and moisten his body and to revive his vigor.

(34) Those who suffer from hectic fever benefit from going to the bathhouse because it clears their bodies of smoky vapor and moistens their limbs. If one wants them to enter the bathhouse, one should sprinkle much sweet water that

is moderately hot in it so that the air is saturated with moist, sweet vapor. One should make the second room hotter than the first, and the third hotter than the second, and the fourth hotter than the third; but none should be excessively hot. The patient should be given accommodations very close to the bathhouse. Once that has been done, put him on a piece of cloth and tell him to undress in the middle room. Pour lukewarm oil on him and rub him gently with it. While he is lying on a stretcher, put him into moderately hot water by lowering the stretcher into the bathing basin so that it is immersed in the water; then lift him up and immerse him again, and do this repeatedly until he is close to sweating. When he is close to sweating, immerse him in cold water all at once, lift him up quickly, and rub him off immediately with moist towels so that the water goes away; then dress him and carry him on the stretcher to his accommodations. If he follows this regimen, his limbs will acquire much moisture without any harm.

(35) Someone whose body is very emaciated or dominated by a dry dyscrasia should be given milk to drink. The best milk is that of women—after that, the milk of a donkey, and then the milk of a goat. The younger the animal, the better the milk, especially if it has been well fed and well provided for. The best milk to use is that which is sucked from the breast; and if that is impossible, one should bring the animal close to the patient so that he can drink the milk the moment it is milked, while it is still hot and has not cooled off. If one is afraid that it will curdle in his stomach, give the patient something with it that prevents curdling and that causes the milk to be quickly absorbed into the organs, such as honey and fresh milk. The purer the honey, the better it is, but sugar is even better. The milk should be administered as follows: The patient should drink it, then rest for about four hours, and then go into the bathing basin once the milk has been digested and has gone down from the stomach. And when he has left the bathing basin, he should drink milk for a second time; but if he loathes it this time, then leave him alone (do not force him to drink) and replace it with barley gruel and the like.

(36) When the strength of the body supports it, bleeding is beneficial in two ways for all fevers caused by repletion:

1. The evacuation of the putrefied matter;
2. The extinction of the heat of the fever.

The putrid humor should be expelled from the body through purgation, emesis, or micturition. What remains of it should be improved through nutrition and medication.

(37) When fevers originate from a surplus of blood, one should apply venesection until the patient is on the verge of fainting, if his strength allows it. When fevers originate from a humor mixed with blood, bleeding is also beneficial. For this reason, bleeding is beneficial for all continuous fevers in which the humors are concocted.

(38) When the body of the patient is weak, when he suffers from indigestion, or when his body contains a crude humor that has not concocted, one should not bleed that patient. In the case of indigestion, one should postpone bleeding until the corruption of the food has diminished. Crude, viscous humors do not respond to expulsion through bleeding; and when one bleeds a body with weak organs, it becomes even weaker.

(39) If there is a surplus of blood in the body, it should be evacuated all at once, if possible. But if this is not possible, it should be done in several steps. If the blood is bad in quality, it should be evacuated little by little. Each quantity that is evacuated from the body will be replaced with wholesome blood.

(40) In all kinds of treatment, one should pay attention to the condition of the air, the external condition of the body, and the age of the patient. Thinness and a hot temperament dissolve the body; and a thin body that is affected by much dissolution, such as the body of a child, does not endure bleeding. The same holds good for a body with weak organs, such as the body of an old man, especially since an old man has a cold temperament and a small quantity of blood. If bile is produced in the cardia of the stomach of a body, the person is quick to vomit and to develop headache and syncope.

(41) If you encounter other things that require bleeding, even after the seventh day, do not pay attention to the number of days that have passed. Instead, you should determine the quantity to be bled, keeping in mind the other types of therapy, according to the strength of the patient and the quantity of the humor, in order to find out what should be done first and what later.

(42) If much blood has flowed to one of the organs and the organ has become occluded, the patient should be bled as soon as his strength and the other conditions are conducive. If bleeding is impossible, one should apply cupping glasses. If the organ has become congested, one should employ solvents after attempting to evacuate it.

(43) If there is some hardness in one of the organs and it is dominated by heat, it should be softened with ingredients that are not that hot. If the hardness

and rigidness are less thick, but the heat is very strong, the solvents should be mixed with remedies that have a discutient effect, such as vinegar. If one wants to soften something that lies within a noble organ, one should mix the solvent with strengthening remedies so that its strength is preserved.

(44) When one applies poultices with pure, astringent ingredients for the treatment of the internal organs, one should mix them with softening ingredients so that the strength of the external poultice reaches those organs. In the same way, remedies for the treatment of the remote organs should be mixed with remedies that make them reach those organs speedily.

(45) If there is a tumor in the stomach or liver accompanied by fever, it should be dissolved by means of solvent remedies that strengthen the organs. When the stream of putrid matter has stopped, the dissolving effect should be increased. If there is a tumor in the respiratory organs, the astringent effect of the poultices put on the chest should be less strong, so that the tumor does not rise to the heart or to the lungs. If there is a tumor in the lungs, one should beware of astringent ingredients in general, so that the putrid matter does not rise to the heart. One should mix the softening ingredients with ingredients that have a strong heating effect so that the putrid matter is drawn outward. One should draw out the putrid matter either through the application of cupping glasses or through other means. One should do so only once the body has been emptied so that this kind of treatment does not attract superfluous matters to the chest, especially when the body is replete with those matters.

(46) In the case of a hot tumor, the cooling limit should be determined by the magnitude of the heat of the tumor. If the cooling goes so far that the organ is on the verge of compacting, one should diminish the degree of cooling or stop it altogether so that it does not lead to hardness of the tumor. The limit of dissolving a hot tumor that has reached its climax is that the heating effect be of the magnitude of the superfluous matter evacuated from the affected organ. If the heating effect is such that it attracts other matter, one should diminish the degree of heating. One should turn to solvents only after the body has been emptied and the humors balanced.

(47) A hard tumor should be treated first by a softener, then by a discutient, and finally by a solvent. In general, one should see to it that the fine humors are not expelled and that the coarse humors do not remain, turning hard as stone and no longer reacting to the solvents.

(48) Scrofula affecting flesh that serves as filler—such as the flesh of the neck, the armpits, and the groin—should be treated by solvents alone, whereas scrofula affecting flesh that serves some useful purpose—such as the flesh of the breasts and the flesh that produces sputum—should be treated at first with repelling and strengthening remedies, and then, when they reach their climax, with solvents. In general, all scrofula that do not react to solvents should be left to putrefy and then should be extirpated through surgery. During surgery one should be careful not to injure a nerve, artery, or vein.

(49) Some atheromas contain a very thin and fine honey-like moisture; they should be treated with remedies that are powerful solvents. Others contain a very thick moisture; one should let these putrefy and then make an incision because solvents alone are not sufficient. The correct procedure is to make an incision in the whole skin covering the swelling and to uncover it by lifting the edge of the wound with a probe; then one should remove the whole capsule with the swelling. If it is impossible to take it out completely, one should take out whatever one can and let the rest putrefy.

(50) If a soft swelling occurs incidentally following a disease, like that which occurs in the extremities of the body of those suffering from phthisis and dropsy, those extremities should be treated sometimes with rose oil, sometimes with olive oil and salt, and sometimes with vinegar and salt. If it is a disease originating from a small quantity of phlegm flowing to an organ, one should put a sponge that has been soaked in vinegar mixed with an equal amount of water on the organ; but if it originates from a large quantity of phlegm, one should dissolve green vitriol in water and vinegar, dip the sponge in the mixture, and put it on the swelling. If the soft swelling originates from flatulence, it should be treated with sweet, strong medicines whose parts are fine and that dispel the winds—such as olive oil in which common rue, lye from ashes, and vinegar have been boiled—, as well as with the application of cupping glasses.

(51) In the case of bad tumors, take care to improve the temperament and humors of the body; and in the case of carbuncles, evacuate a large quantity of the patient's blood, as long as there is no hindrance. Then put a moderately dissolving and slightly repelling remedy on the surrounding area, and put on the carbuncles themselves remedies that have a strong drying effect and that have been mixed with wine that is either sweet, astringent, or something similar. Never apply a concocting medicine, so that the carbuncles do not putrefy. That would be very bad because carbuncles putrefy easily.

(52) When treating cancer, avoid remedies that produce black bile. Instead, institute a regimen for the liver using those ingredients that produce healthy blood and a balanced temperament, for this tumor originates from hot, melancholic blood. For the same reason—but also because the liver serves as the entry points of the veins—one should use those remedies that dry but do not burn, such as mineral remedies. If one applies surgery, one should examine the cancer minutely and excise it completely so that no trace of it is left. One should let the blood flow and press and squeeze the surrounding area in order to expel the hot, thick, melancholic blood from it. One should not be quick to stop the flowing of the blood. Afterward, one should treat the wound appropriately.

(53) Scarification should be employed in order to either extract the bad matter that causes the organ to degenerate, but only after the body has been emptied, or facilitate the exit of the matter and its attraction outward, as is done with cupping.

(54) Organs that have begun to putrefy and degenerate must be preserved, along with what surrounds them, by means of poultices and fomentations that preserve the innate heat and pneuma and gain strength for the organs, such as rose oil, saffron, meal of bitter vetch, wine, and the like.

(55) If part of the flesh of a nerve, ligament, or sinew degenerates, but its degeneration stops and it did not liquefy, one should then protect that which lies behind it, but it itself should continue to degenerate. Let it fall off with the help of offshoots of chards that are boiled and pounded with old butter and applied several times for a day and a night. If there is a small joint in that spot, one should rub it and [...]; if it is a bone, one should cut it with a saw, but be careful not to cut a healthy nerve. The degenerated nerve, on the other hand, should be putrefied with melted butter until it falls off.

(56) Cauterization should be applied:

1. to stop putrid matter from flowing, as when one cauterizes the head against the disease called elephantiasis;
2. to prevent cankering and putrefaction, as when one cauterizes that which has become malignant;
3. to dry the putrid matter and strengthen the organs, as when one cauterizes the spleen and the ischias; or
4. to prevent blood from bursting forth, as when one cauterizes an artery.

(57) All ulcers should be made to possess angles after surgical removal. And if one has to hollow them out, one should do so in a form appropriate to this concern, so that nature will have appendages from which she can start to grow flesh. The more angular the ulcer is, the easier it is to heal. Roundness hinders fast formation of flesh for three reasons:

1. The fibers are cut off in their length and breadth crosswise,
2. two double bandages cannot unite the two margins, and
3. nature does not find a spot from where she can start to grow flesh.

(58) The successful treatment of an ulcer is achieved through the observation of seven things:

1. The kind of ulcer: From this, one can learn what to do; for if it is simple, one needs only to close it up. If flesh has been destroyed, there is a need for new flesh to be grown in order to replace the other flesh; then the ulcer needs to be sealed and form a scar. If matter flows toward it, that flow needs to be stopped, and then it needs to form a scar. If ugly flesh grows in it, that flesh needs to be extirpated through surgery and drugs that eat away at it; then the ulcer needs to be sealed and to form a scar. If it is accompanied by a bad temperament, that temperament needs to be eliminated; then the ulcer needs to be sealed and to form a scar. If the ulcer is composed of many things, the treatment should be put together according to all these things and each element applied according to its importance.
2. Its cause: If it is caused by the bite of the poisonous animal, the poison should be countered first of all; it should be drawn outward and its effects moderated. Often one needs to widen the ulcer, as in the case of the bite of a mad dog.
3. The part of the body where the ulcer is: Each organ requires a specific treatment.
4. The temperament, strength, external condition of the body, and habits of the patient. A dry body needs medicines that are more dry, and a moist body needs drugs that are more moist, since the aim of the treatment is the restoration of continuity. And a strong body endures the kind of heavy treatment that a weak body does not endure.
5. The things that, through their conformity or lack thereof, are an indication for the kind of treatment needed. In the case of summer and a hot country, the temperament requires medicines that are less heat-producing.
6. The powers of the medicines and foods, so that one can select from them that which is best suited for reaching the goal one aims at.

7. The comparison of some of these points with others so that, from all of them, one can decide upon the right kind of treatment.

(59) Medicines that make the flesh grow in place of an ulcer are those that preserve its temperament, that clean and dry as much foul matter as originates in that ulcer. If their cleansing effect is too strong, they annihilate the matter from which flesh originates; and if their drying effect is too strong, they make the ulcer form a scar and prevent the growth of flesh. If they are too hot or not hot enough, they produce a bad temperament in that part of the body, which in turn sometimes causes something else. The medicines that cause an ulcer to close are those that dry the temperament of the body and its parts to the second degree, so that the foul matter dries up and becomes hard according to their dryness. Medicines that make an ulcer form a scar are those that dry the temperament of the body to the third degree, so that their intense dryness makes the nature of the flesh hard.

(60) Ulcers may be hard to heal because of a bad temperament of the flesh in which they are found, or because of the bad quantity or quality of the blood that reaches them, or because of the kind of drugs administered, or because of their bad arrangement, or because of a bad treatment. The indications for a bad temperament of the flesh that is hot are the heat of that spot, its red or black appearance, the opacity of the ulcer, the large quantity of thin pus within, and the fact that the patient feels a burning heat in it but finds relief in cool things. The indications for a cold temperament are coldness of the spot; a white, green, livid, or leaden color; its lack of pus; and the fact that the patient feels coldness in it and finds relief in hot things. The indications for a moist temperament are severe flabbiness and much foul matter. The indications for a dry temperament are intense dryness and bad blood.

(61) The difference between a swelling occurring from the dissolution of soft flesh by very hot drugs and the swelling occurring from the flow of matter to a certain organ is that the dissolution of the flesh is accompanied by an increase in heat, redness, and hardness of the lips of the ulcer, and heat of the surrounding area. Another difference is that the foul matter occurring from the dissolution of the flesh is thin and red or tending to lividity, while that occurring from the flow of matter is thick and viscous.

(62) Some remedies for ulcers cleanse and dry at the same time, such as frankincense, sarcocolla, aloe, *ḥuḍaḍ* (Mediterranean or rock buckthorn) juice, opopanax, root of Florentine iris, meal of bitter vetch, birthwort, myrrh, and

resin. Others dry and cool, such as gallnuts, pomegranate peels and blossoms, carob, and Maltese fungus. Yet others dry and make the flesh grow, such as Armenian bole and dragon's blood. Some are minerals, such as cadmia, tutty, ceruse, litharge, and green vitriol. Others are liquid, such as vinegar and rose oil. For every situation, one should select from among these the ones that are most appropriate.

(63) One should select remedies according to the difference in the organs. For ulcers in the digestive organs, it is appropriate to apply heat as well as astringent herbs and what is prepared from them, such as Syrian rhubarb, myrtle, tanner's sumach, pomegranate blossom, meadow salsify, pomegranate peels, gum Arabic, quince, apple, wine, and gallnut. The remedies for ulcers in the respiratory organs should be mixed with mineral substances that alleviate cough, such as gum tragacanth, gum Arabic, and starch (amylum). For tumors in the brain, one should use the different kinds of oil and their compositions. It is clear that Armenian bole and similar ingredients are appropriate for all the other ulcers that are accompanied by inflammation.

(64) Ulcers in the intestines and upper part of the stomach should be treated by taking appropriate medicines and foods. Those in the large intestines should be treated by applying clysters and suppositories. Those in the respiratory organs should be treated by remedies that are kept in the mouth or ingested by drinking or inhalation. Those in the mouth should be treated by gargling. Those in the esophagus and stomach—that is, the cardia of the stomach—require agglutinants that adhere to the spot. Moreover, the stomach needs remedies that stay there for a long time; and the remote organs, such as the lungs and the kidneys, need remedies that quickly get through to them and reach them. One should determine the requirements of each organ. One should also apply all the appropriate strong poultices.

(65) Further examples of what the organs need: Ulcers in the nose need remedies that are more drying than those needed for tumors in the eyes. Ulcers in the ears need remedies that are more drying than those needed for ulcers in the thighs, because the ears are naturally drier. They also need more honey, since more foul matter originates in them. Ulcers in the mouth need juice of unripe, sour grapes; tanner's sumach; or a rob of mulberries or walnuts. If they are accompanied by putrefaction, they need caustic remedies with a strong drying effect. Ulcers in the penis, vagina, and anus always need extremely drying remedies, such as burned papyrus and burned seashells and the like. If they are recent, one should treat them with aloe and *ḥuḍaḍ* (Mediterranean or rock buckthorn) juice and the like.

(66) When foul matter accumulates in ulcers, they often need to be washed. If they are in the external parts and have a cold temperament, they should be washed with hot wine; if they are hot, with vinegar mixed in sweet water and with water in which opium poppy has been cooked; if they are moist, with water in which pomegranate peels and myrtle have been cooked; and if they are dry, with sweet water. If there is an ulcer in the internal parts, it should be washed with sugar water and hydromel and milk.

(67) Ulcers in the lungs are most difficult and hard to cure because medicines reach them only after their potency has been weakened and because the lungs are organs that move constantly. Movement prevents the parts of the ulcer from joining together, and it does not allow the medicine to adhere. For this reason, it is not easy to cure them.

(68) If a dissolution of continuity occurs in the lungs, either because of a torn vein or because of something else, one should immediately begin with treatment by telling the patient to rest, to speak little, and to refrain from coughing as much as possible; by attracting the purulent matter from the lungs through bleeding the basilic vein and bleeding the patient many times; by rubbing his hands and feet; and by extracting blood resulting from astringent, glutinous food on the same day, if the strength of the patient allows it. One should apply a poultice with strong, restraining medicines to the chest, such as rose and quince oil in the summer and spikenard oil in the winter.

(69) Internal ulcers need drying medicines, such as the theriac, amber pills, coral, Armenian bole, *terra sigillata* (sealed earth), spikenard, and saffron. For ulcers in the lungs, one should select the strongest among them, adding some opium in order to alleviate the cough, stop the catarrh, bring about sleep, and increase the drying effect. Foods should be those that are quickly digested and that are astringent and viscous, such as the dish called trotters, barley broth, small fish cooked with quince and apples, and the like. In the same manner, one should select the appropriate foods and medicines for every ulcer.

(70) If an ulcer occurs in the lungs because of a hot defluxion in the head, the defluxion should be stopped. The head should be shaved; and one should put vesicatory remedies on it, such as the mustard remedy, so that the vapor that is congested in the head is dispersed and dissolved. Be careful that no oil or no hot or severely cold ingredient reaches the head. Give the patient remedies that dry the ulcer and stop the catarrh, such as the theriac. If he needs to be taken

to the bathhouse in order to ripen the catarrh, this should be done. Give him a refining treatment so that the catarrh does not increase.

(71) Fundamental for returning the lungs to their normal condition are the following: alleviating the cough; stopping the catarrhs; removing the bad humors in the body; taking beneficial medicines and keeping them in the mouth for a while; lying on one's back; relaxing the muscles of the throat so that the medicines go down to the lungs bit by bit; exerting oneself to purge the body with emollient medicines that expel the superfluities from it; balancing the temperament; and giving the patient soft foods prepared from starch (amylum), broad bean flour, and barley flour.

(72) When blood is discharged from the lungs, one should administer to the patient vinegar mixed with a lot of water, hour after hour, in order to stop the discharge of coagulated blood. If there is an ulcer in the lungs or chest and it is accompanied by a rattling sound in the chest and by difficulty breathing, one should administer to the patient cleansing agents that ease the discharge of the feculent matter, such as honey water, barley gruel, julep, or soup. If the feculent matter is thin, the patient should be given a thickener, such as starch (amylum), so that the subsequent discharge by means of honey becomes easier. If, in the case of ulcers in the lungs, one gives the patient wine to drink, one should mix it with water in which quinces or myrtle seed or other astringent ingredients have been cooked, in order to strengthen the lungs and dry the ulcer.

(73) Diverting surplus matter to the opposite side is accomplished by bleeding from the opposite side, extracting the blood therefrom many times, and applying cupping glasses. In the same manner, if we see a nosebleed that increases, becoming more severe, which cannot be stopped with remedies, we bleed from the veins of the arm that is on the same side as the nostril from which the blood flows, and we apply cupping glasses to the hypochondrium. If the blood flows from the right nostril, we apply cupping glasses to the liver; and if it flows from the left nostril, we apply them to the spleen so that the blood is attracted downward. We also tie the hands and feet tightly with bandages once they have been rubbed.

(74) A hemorrhage is stopped by astringent remedies that are cohesive and agglutinant. The best ones are those that make the flesh grow; the faster it grows, the better it is.

(75) If you want to stop a hemorrhage, you should first of all put a medicine on it that stops the bleeding; then apply a bandage and observe: if it still bleeds a little bit, you should not untie the bandage; but if it bleeds a lot, you should untie the first bandage and repeat this procedure after you let the patient rest for a little while. You should leave on the bandage until the third day, then untie it gently, and if you find the medicine still adhering to the wound, you should add some more medicine to it and put a new bandage on it. And if you find that the wound has healed, you should remove the bandage gently and do the same thing again.

(76) If the blood is not contained with the bandage, one should scrape off the skin and catch the vein on a hook, pull it upward, and bind both edges with a silken thread while the vein is in the middle. When there is a hemorrhage, be careful with cauterization. Although cauterization stops the hemorrhage, it is not safe, because it takes away from the flesh of the spot. The bleeding is indeed contained as long as there is a scab on the spot of the wound, but if the scab falls off, a subsequent bleeding is more difficult to treat. Apply cauterization only when it is necessary. Prefer caustic medicines to cauterization. Cauterization is good when bleeding is associated with putrefaction and when it concerns wounds that putrefy quickly, such as those in the anus and testicles. Caustic medicines that are beneficial for these wounds are arsenic, verdigris, lime, sulfur, green vitriol, and the like.

(77) Wounds are either harmless or dangerous. For instance, wounds that affect the chest cavity or the digestive organs are dangerous. Equally dangerous are wounds that occur to nervous parts such as the diaphragm, the joints, and the nerves because they induce spasms and delirium, and wounds that occur to the blood vessels because they cause bleedings. A wound that occurs in very fleshy areas is more dangerous to those areas. And wounds that occur to the large intestines are easier to heal than those that occur to the small intestine, especially the jejunum. If it is torn, it is almost completely impossible to cure because of its thin substance, which is similar to the nature of the nerves.

(78) If much blood flows from a wound right away, it is less dangerous than a wound from which no blood flows. The reason is that this latter wound is close to being a tumor, from which no blood flows, while the wound from which blood flows is not close to being a tumor. For this reason, a wound from which no blood flows, requires venesection.

(79) If there is a wound to the lower part of the belly and the omentum protrudes and some of it turns green or black, then do not hope to heal that which has turned green. Instead, after you have come to the aid of the healthy part, cut off the diseased part by ligating it with a fine silken thread, so that the cut does not result in a hemorrhage from the blood vessels in the omentum. Let the ends of the thread come out from the wound so that it will be possible to extract it if the wound closes up. If the gut protrudes from a wound and becomes inflated and cold because of the air, place on it a hot compress with astringent, hot wine so that it is warmed and its strength is preserved. If that is not possible, take hot pieces of cloth and put them on the gut in the bathhouse, or put a sponge or piece of wool that has been soaked in hot olive oil or hot water on it so that it returns to its former condition.

(80) If the omentum or intestines protrude, raise the patient by his hands and feet, in hot air and in a manner such that the abdomen is drawn upward and becomes clearly visible, while the organ does not become cold. Then the patient should be softly shaken and gently put to sleep in this position on a flatbed raised at its extremities. Once the patient has been put to sleep and tied up in the middle, one should make efforts to return the omentum or intestine inside the body. Then one should draw the edges of the wound together and cut it carefully. If the patient needs to defecate, give him a clyster with ingredients that expel the feces, and alleviate the pain with astringent black wine or the like.

(81) If one needs to suture the wound, one should bring both edges of the wound together and stitch them, then fasten the thread with a double knot and cut it off. Then skip over a small part of the wound, join the two edges, and stitch them in the same way. Continue to operate in this manner until you reach the end of the wound. The threads should consist of [material] that does not decay quickly.

(82) Puncturing a nerve causes severe pain that attracts matter to the spot. And if this results in a tumor in that spot, one should leave the tear open and widen it if it is narrow. One should do what one can to alleviate the pain through rubbing and plastering with oils and hot, fine ingredients that have a heating effect but are not astringent. One should beware of fomentation and bathing in hot water because it has an excessive moistening effect. Since the substance of the nerves is moist and solid because nerves are by nature cold, the nerve would putrefy quickly if it were moistened and heated.

(83) Remedies appropriate for tumors in the nerves are those that are lukewarm, consist of fine parts, and are neither astringent nor pungent, such as sweet olive oil, turpentine resin, asafetida, opopanax, and resin spurge. Select the weakest of these for patients with moist bodies. When the nerve is exposed, the power of the medicine reaches it easily. And select from the strongest medicines for patients with a dry body. When the nerve lies deep within, the power of the medicine cannot reach it. Tumors of the nerves need medicines that are moderately hot and intensely dry and that have a fine substance. If there is a puncture in the arm, rub the neck and armpits with hot oil; if it is in the leg, rub the groins with this medicine. Medicines for all tumors in the nerves should be calefacient, actually, so that the nerves' coldness does not induce spasms. One should pour oil on an abscess so as not to increase its foulness. If a contusion occurs to a nerve without an abscess, one should pour hot, non-astringent olive oil over it time and again.

(84) The setting of a broken bone is effected through straightening the limb so that the deflected part is brought into one line with the straight part above it. Then it should be put together by gently and carefully bringing in the splintered parts, one upon the other, and the fissure should be mended so that the bone returns to its initial shape. Then it should be bandaged, and splints should be put on it such that it reassumes it original shape. The splints should have the same shape as the broken limb so that they preserve the shape. To stop the bleeding, the bandage should be tighter on the site of the fracture and looser on the area around it; bind it high up on those sides. The broader the bandage, the better it is, for then it occupies a large area.

(85) In the beginning of the treatment of someone suffering from a fracture, nutrition should consist of fine foodstuffs, until the patient is out of danger. Then it should produce good, strong blood. Foodstuffs that produce this kind of blood are those that have good chyme and that are very nutritious, so that the secreted nutrition going to the fracture is glutinous and cohesive and the parts of the bone are linked to one another more firmly. A salve that helps the production of the matter exuding from the wound is that which is viscous and slightly heating.

(86) One should set one's mind on all the things discussed in this treatise, compare them with one another, and then act accordingly. Beware of fear and of not being generous in any matter, whether small or large, and do not be excessive in something that the contemporary physicians consider to be needless. Do not treat evil diseases so that you will not be called a "physician of evil." Do

not deviate from the course pursued by physicians in general, and do not try a medicine that has not been tried before and found to be safe. I have mentioned all the precautions one should take in this regard in the treatise on purgatives.

This is what I intended to write,
praise be to God.

BOOK 5

Medical Aphorisms

First published in:

Maimonides
Medical Aphorisms

A Parallel Arabic-English Edition,
Edited, Translated, and Annotated
by Gerrit Bos.

Treatises I–V
Provo/UT (Brigham Young University Press) 2004
MWMM 2

Treatises VI–IX
Provo/UT (Brigham Young University Press) 2007
MWMM 3

Treatises X–XV
Provo/UT (Brigham Young University Press) 2010
MWMM 6

Treatises XVI–XXI
Provo/UT (Brigham Young University Press) 2015
MWMM 9

Treatises XXII–XXV
Provo/UT (Brigham Young University Press) 2017
MWMM 10

In the name of God,
the Merciful, the Compassionate.
O Lord, make our task easy

 | DOI:10.1163/9789004498884_007

(N) Says Mūsā ibn 'Ubayd Allāh, the Israelite, from Córdoba: People have often composed works in the form of aphorisms on different kinds of sciences. The science most in need of this is the science of medicine, because it has branches of knowledge that are difficult to conceptualize, like most of the exact sciences, and because it has branches of knowledge that are difficult only with respect to remembering what has been written down about them, just like the knowledge of one of the perfect languages. As for the science of medicine, its conceptualization and the understanding of its concepts are not as difficult as in the case of the exact sciences. However, aspiring to master this science is difficult in most cases because it requires retaining a very large amount of memorized material, not merely of general principles but also of particulars, which can almost be compared to the individual details that cannot be encompassed by the knowledge of one individual scholar, as one can demonstrate for himself.

These works composed in the form of aphorisms are undoubtedly easy to retain; they help their reader to understand and retain their objectives. Therefore, the most eminent of the physicians, Hippocrates, has written his famous work in the form of aphorisms. [*Aphorisms*]. Later on, many physicians followed his example and composed aphorisms, such as the aphorisms of the famous al-Rāzī [*Kitāb al-Murshid aw al-fuṣūl*], the aphorisms of al-Sūsī, the aphorisms of Ibn Māsawayh [*Nawādir al-ṭibbiyya*], and others.

It is clear to everyone who pays even the slightest attention that everyone who has composed aphorisms in any field of science did not compose them with the intention that those aphorisms would be sufficient for that science or that they would encompass all its principles. But one who has composed aphorisms according to this method has done so concerning matters he thought should always be retained, or thought to be neglected, or thought would be beneficial for describing that which one needs in most cases. In short, the intention of one who has composed aphorisms has not been to encompass everything that one needs in the field of that science—neither Hippocrates in his *Aphorisms* nor Abū Naṣr al-Fārābī in anything he composed in the way of aphorisms, let alone others.

I have made these preliminary remarks merely as a justification for those aphorisms that I have included in my book. And I do not claim to have authored these aphorisms that I have set down in writing. I would rather say that I have selected them—that is, I have selected them from Galen's words from all his books, both from his original works and from his commentaries to the books of Hippocrates. In these aphorisms I have not adhered to the method that I followed in the *Epitomes* [*from the Works of Galen*], in which I quoted Galen's very words, as I stipulated in the introduction to the *Epitomes* [*from the Works of*

Galen]. Rather, most of the aphorisms that I have selected are in the very words of Galen, or in his words and the words of Hippocrates, because the words of both are mixed in Galen's commentaries to Hippocrates' books; in the case of others, the sense expressed in the aphorism is partly in Galen's words and partly in my own; in the case of yet other aphorisms, my own words express the idea that Galen mentioned. What has prompted me to do so is the fact that the idea of that aphorism becomes clear only after reading from scattered places in Galen's lengthy exposition. I have gathered the sum of the idea of that aphorism and have articulated it in a concise expression. Since I know that there are more people who blindly follow the opinion of someone else than people who investigate for themselves and that there are more deficient people than learned people, I considered it appropriate to refer, at the end of every aphorism I cite, to that section in Galen's exposition in which he has explained that aphorism. So, if someone has doubts about the wording of that aphorism or about the idea expressed in it, he can easily look up that section and find that aphorism—whether he finds it in Galen's very words, or mostly so, or whether he finds that idea without omission or addition in Galen's exposition in that section, even if it is expressed in different words—so that his doubts are dispelled.

No one should protest to me that, while I know that this aphorism is mentioned by Galen in a certain section, its idea is also referred to by him in another section, or that he has repeated it in a number of places; for, if I were to refer the reader to one of these other places, the same objection would still apply. To refer to all the places is superfluous and has no use at all; it is, rather, a multiplication of words. But I preferred to quote his expression of an idea that is often repeated in his exposition in only one of its places and have recorded it in that way. Nor should one protest to me and say: How could you write down an aphorism concerning such and such an idea without adducing aphorisms concerning such and such another idea? For no one who composes aphorisms has—as I have said—the intention to encompass everything. Therefore, if someone would consider one of these aphorisms and make an objection by saying: What is the intention behind recording this aphorism but not that aphorism? If you have recorded it so that it may be retained in the memory, it is an aphorism that is very famous and well known among those practicing this art and does not need to be repeated. Similarly, about another aphorism one might say: That aphorism you consider to be of peculiar interest is not of peculiar interest, in my opinion. And, similarly, one might say about yet another aphorism that I recorded because I thought it to be unknown: There is no physician who does not know it. My answer to these objections would be that no person makes a selection for someone else, but he does so for himself in particular.

I have selected these aphorisms for myself only, so that I would have a ready record of them. Similarly, anyone who is like me or who is less knowledgeable than I am can benefit from them. I have not selected them for the benefit of someone who is at the same level as Galen or close to it. I have no doubt that many of these aphorisms are so much more clear to others than to me, that they do not have to be learned by heart. Similarly, what I consider to be of peculiar interest may be not of peculiar interest for someone else, and what I consider to be mostly unknown may be well known to someone else. And in every case concerning which I think that I have solved a difficulty, either through the accurate account of certain ideas or through clarifying certain meanings, there may be someone else for whom that difficulty does not arise in any respect because of his perfection in the art.

In these aphorisms I have included personal remarks, in which I have included only the most essential additional information. To these I refer in my own name. I have also included aphorisms from some of the later physicians, which I attribute to the one who has presented them. I have divided these aphorisms into a number of treatises so that it will be easy to remember them or to show what one wants to show. I have made twenty-five treatises of them.

The first treatise contains aphorisms which concern the subject of the medical art, by which I mean the form of the organs of the human body and their functions and faculties.
The second treatise contains aphorisms concerning the humors.
The third treatise contains aphorisms that concern the principles of the medical art and general rules.
The fourth treatise contains aphorisms concerning the pulse and the prognostic signs to be derived from it.
The fifth treatise contains aphorisms concerning the prognostic signs to be derived from the urine.
The sixth treatise contains aphorisms concerning the other prognostic signs.
The seventh treatise contains aphorisms concerning the causes of diseases which are often not known or which are discussed in a confused way.
The eighth treatise contains aphorisms concerning the correct regimen for the healing of diseases in general.
The ninth treatise contains aphorisms concerning specific diseases.
The tenth treatise contains aphorisms concerning fevers.
The eleventh treatise contains aphorisms concerning the periods and crisis of a disease.
The twelfth treatise contains aphorisms concerning emptying the body by means of bloodletting.

The thirteenth treatise contains aphorisms concerning evacuations by means of purgatives and enemas.
The fourteenth treatise contains aphorisms concerning vomiting.
The fifteenth treatise contains aphorisms concerning surgery.
The sixteenth treatise contains aphorisms concerning women.
The seventeenth treatise contains aphorisms concerning the regimen of health in general.
The eighteenth treatise contains aphorisms concerning exercise.
The nineteenth treatise contains aphorisms concerning bathing.
The twentieth treatise contains aphorisms concerning foods and beverages and their ingestion.
The twenty-first treatise contains aphorisms concerning natural remedies.
The twenty-second treatise contains aphorisms concerning remedies with specific properties.
The twenty-third treatise contains aphorisms on different diseases and symptoms whose names are well known, and the elucidation of the meanings of those names which are known to the physicians, though sometimes not accurately.
The twenty-fourth treatise contains curiosities related in the medical books, and unusual, rare occurrences.
The twenty-fifth treatise contains doubts that occurred to me in different places due to Galen's words.

∴

The First Treatise

Containing aphorisms concerning the subject of the medical art, by which I mean the form of the organs of the human body and their functions and faculties

(I.1) The nerve which conveys to the muscle the faculty of sensation and movement from the brain and spinal cord is inserted into every muscle either at its head or between its beginning and middle […], so that the middle is the head of that muscle. *De usu partium* VII[.14].

(I.2) The muscle called the diaphragm has its head in its center—namely, the sinewy place of the diaphragm to which the parts and ends of the nerves are attached […]. This is the line which encircles the diaphragm. *De usu partium* XIII[.5].

(I.3) Arteries and veins in the whole body are connected with all the parts that need connection with them. They are near one another and sometimes so close together that the veins are in contact with the arteries. Thus, one always finds the veins directly upon the arteries, with the sole exception of the brain; for the arteries ascend to it from below to facilitate the upward movement of the pneuma, while the veins descend to the brain from the crown of the head to facilitate the transport of food to the brain. *De usu partium* IX[.5].

(I.4) To all the parts of the body come arteries and veins from the places that are nearest. But the testes and breasts are distinguished from all the parts of the body by the fact that the vessels that reach them do not come from nearby vessels, but from vessels that are far away, in order to prolong the time that the blood stays in the vessels so that the sperm and the milk will be completely cocted. *De usu partium* XVI[.10].

(I.5) Veins hidden from the eye reach the bones. One does not find any muscle in the body that is devoid of veins and arteries. Nowhere is there an artery without a vein, but a few veins branch off without arteries; this happens close to the skin in the external parts of the body, in the hands, feet, and neck. *De usu partium* XVI[.14].

(I.6) Branches of the arteries and small branches of nerves are intertwined with one another. Therefore, if the nerves are stretched, the arteries share in the pain. *De* [*causis*] *pulsu*[*um* II.12].

(I.7) Someone who is not knowledgeable in anatomy supposes the round ligaments and tendons to be nerves. I would also have been unable to distinguish between them if I had not occupied myself with anatomical dissection. *De methodo medendi* VI[.4].

(I.8) No part of a nerve is attached to cartilage, ligaments, fat, or bones. The only exceptions among all the bodily parts are the teeth, for soft nerves are attached to their roots. Similarly, no nerves are attached to all glands which serve as a filling and foundation for the division of vessels. But glands needed for the necessary generation of fluids do have a few nerves attached to them in a few rare cases, just as they also have arteries and veins. *De usu partium* XVI[.2].

(I.9) Tendons are softer than ligaments but harder than nerves. The volume of the substance of a tendon is equal to that of a ligament and nerve together. In many places within muscles, one finds the size of a ligament to be ten times that of a nerve that is attached to that muscle at its head. Every nerve is sensitive, but no ligament has sensation. Every tendon has less sensation than a nerve because it is in part a ligament. *De motu musculorum* 1[.2].

(1.10) The body has three structures which are similar in bodily form. One of these is the nerve, another is the ligament, and a third is the tendon. A tendon is one of the two ends of a muscle and resembles a nerve. It is the product of nerve and ligament. Every nerve is exactly round, but not all the tendons are like that; some of them are round and others are somewhat flat. Most of them become so wide that they resemble a membrane. *De placitis Hippocratis et Platonis* 1.9[.1–3].

(1.11) All membranes are extremely thin and soft, but a ligament is mostly hard and thick. Some ligaments are in between the nature of nerves and cartilage. But no membrane or nerve or tendon can approach anywhere near to the hardness of a ligament; similarly, the hardest nerve cannot achieve the hardness of a tendon. [*De placitis Hippocratis et Platonis* 1.9.1–3].

(1.12) These three structures—namely, nerve, tendon, and ligament—are all white, solid, and bloodless. If you dissect them, they separate into lengthwise fibers, except for the very hard ligaments, for these cannot be taken apart into fibers. *De placitis Hippocratis et Platonis* 1[.9.8].

(1.13) A muscle is an instrument for motion only and not for sensation, because every voluntary motion occurs exclusively through a muscle. Everything that is not a muscle has sensation, because everything to which a nerve is attached has sensation, even though it has no voluntary motion. [*De motu musculorum* 1.1].

(1.14) The ligaments with which muscles are attached to bones give rise to membranes that envelop the muscles and from which strands spread into the flesh of the muscles. [*De motu musculorum* 1.1].

(1.15) Every tendon is attached to a bone for the most part, but not every muscle ends in a tendon, for none of the muscles which move the tongue and the lips and the eyes has a tendon, since these muscles do not move a bone. Most of the parts of the face move voluntarily, while the bones are motionless and do not need tendons. [*De motu musculorum* 1.3].

(I.16) If someone rapidly suffers from an obstruction in the liver, it happens because the ends of the vessels in which the food arises from the concave side of the liver to the convex side are narrow. *De alimentorum facultatibus* III[.15].

(I.17) The constitutions of bodies that are extremely susceptible to illness are, in particular, those composed of parts with an opposite temperament. An example of this is the case where the stomach is extremely hot and the brain is cold. Similarly, the lungs and entire chest are often cold while the stomach is hot, and frequently the opposite is the case. Many times, the other parts are cold and the liver is extremely hot. One should suspect the very same thing to be true for the other parts of the body. *De alimentorum facultatibus* III[.16].

(I.18) At every place in the body where a nerve or tendon has to pass through the large protuberance of a bone, one of these three things necessarily occurs: either a groove is made into the bone to receive it, or the bone is pierced through, or the nerve or tendon encircles the bone—but it never extends bare over the convexity of the bone. All the nerves, tendons, and veins which lie in bony grooves are covered and protected by strong membranes. *De usu partium* II[.7].

(I.19) Within arteries and veins are two parts: blood and pneuma, which remain separate except that a little thin, vaporous blood flows in the arteries, while a little mist-like pneuma flows in the veins. Arteries in the whole body communicate with veins and exchange blood and pneuma through certain invisible narrow passages. *De usu partium* VI[.10].

(I.20) In his *De usu pulsuum* [VI.10], Galen said: The arteries return a small amount to the heart during their contraction. The thinnest and lightest substance in the body is pneuma, followed in second place by vapor, followed in third place by thin, completely cocted blood. *De naturalibus facultatibus* [III.14].

(I.21) Organs that are generally considered unpaired in the body are in reality paired, such as the brain, the tongue, the jawbone, the lung, the chest, the womb, and their like; for the number of parts in the right side of each of these organs is equal to that in the left side. These parts are likewise equal in their dimensions, thickness, thinness, and external form, and their whole nature never changes. Similarly, the category of arteries, veins, and nerves that come to one side of these organs is similar to that which come to the other side. *De providentia creatoris*.

(1.22) Although the tongue seems from the outside to be a single organ, in reality it is double, since each half of it lengthwise has its own specific arteries, veins, and nerves attached to it. Similarly, the muscles of one half are different from those of the other half. No muscle, vein, artery, or nerve passes in it from the right side to the left side or from the left side to the right side. *De usu partium* XI[.10].

(1.23) When a small nerve must be conducted over a long distance or when it is responsible for the vigorous movement of a muscle, that small nerve is strengthened and supported by a substance that is thicker than the substance of the nerve, although similar to it. If you look at it, you might think that it has become rounded and that it is attached to the nerve and intertwined with it. But it is not attached to the nerve, nor joined to it. When the nerve thickens with that substance, you will see that the nerve extending from it has a large diameter. *De usu partium* XVI[.5].

(1.24) There are altogether four different kinds of movements of a muscle, namely, these: it is either contracted, or it is extended, or it is twisted, or it remains stretched and tense. The first and the fourth kinds of movement are characteristic functions of all muscles. *De motu musculorum* I[.8].

(1.25) Says Moses: A summary of his words about these four movements is thus: When one's will sends the psychical faculty through a nerve to the muscle with which it wants to flex a specific limb, that muscle contracts toward its origin, so that that limb is flexed. Similarly, when one wants that limb to remain stretched and raised, the will stretches that muscle, together with its antagonistic muscle, so that they both become tense. And when one's will ceases its activity altogether and no longer sends any force to the muscle, the muscle becomes like the other inert things, and because of its natural weight, it falls downward, along with that bone to which it is connected, like a lifeless limb. This movement attributed to the muscle is not caused by the activity of the muscle and is therefore not counted among the voluntary movements. The movement of extension is a voluntary and deliberate movement of the muscle; for when one's will wants to stretch a flexed limb, it stops the psychical faculty in the flexed, contracted muscle and sends it to the antagonistic muscle. The result is that the antagonistic muscle is contracted and the first muscle, which had initially flexed the limb, is stretched, since the power which prevented it from doing so is no longer there. If we want to stretch it as far as possible, we must use the psychical faculty to achieve this.

(I.26) Any muscle stretches a limb only when that limb is flexed. Similarly, any muscle flexes a limb only when it is stretched. A limb is flexed by the internal muscle and stretched by the external muscle. Therefore, if either one of them is severed, both movements are abolished altogether—that is to say, the limb will not be flexed or stretched endlessly anymore but will remain in one position, according to the healthy muscle which effects that position. *De motu musculorum* I[.4–5].

(I.27) When we sleep, the positions of our limbs are always between the extreme position and intermediate position; the activity of the muscles is not abolished at that time. When someone is asleep while he is drunk or very tired or weak, he causes all the limbs of his body to be extremely relaxed; his muscles are in the intermediate position and are completely at rest during sleep. *De motu musculorum* II[.4].

(I.28) The muscles of the anus, the urinary bladder, and the diaphragm are all round. Those around the urinary bladder and around the anus were not created for expelling superfluities, as some people think, but for retaining them; for they retain the superfluities and prevent them from streaming when it is not the proper time. But when one's will lets them go and releases them so that they are no longer retained and restrained, then the superfluities are expelled by the natural expulsive faculties, which receive help from the action of the abdominal muscles and from the stretching of the diaphragm. *De motu musculorum* II[.8].

(I.29) When the diaphragm becomes tense, as all muscles do—that is to say, when it contracts and draws together—the inhalation of air becomes easy. When it extends from this contraction, which occurs when the abdominal muscles contract alone or when the muscles between the ribs contract alone, exhalation becomes easy. *De motu musculorum* II[.9].

(I.30) The diaphragm alone effects inhalation and exhalation easily. Difficult exhalation and inhalation are effected by the muscles between the ribs and the muscles that reach the chest from the shoulders and neck. *De motu musculorum* II[.9].

(I.31) Every individual muscle carries the bone to which it is attached as if it were carrying a stone; and, as long as it is strong, it is capable of doing so. For the most part, then, it does not feel its burden—not even a little bit. But, when a muscle is weak, it feels its burden and it is hard for the muscle to carry it. It is as if the muscle would like to push it away and to transfer it from one position to another. This is the reason why ill people change the position of their limbs every moment and cannot bear one consistent position. *De motu musculorum* I[.10].

(I.32) All the activities of the muscles become weak during sleep. Only the activity of the muscles that move the chest stays the same. *De locis affectis* V[.1].

(I.33) Do not be surprised that most people, when asleep, perform most voluntary activities, such as speaking, screaming, walking, and turning from side to side; for even those who are awake perform their activities in a state of absentmindedness, such that one may be on one's way with the intention of reaching a certain place while one is absentminded and does not know where one is going until the journey is completed. *De motu musculorum* II[.5].

(I.34) Says Moses: These voluntary activities that one who is asleep and one who is absentminded perform have been extensively verified by Galen in this treatise by his description of his observations, but he verifies the phenomenon without giving a reason for it. Neither did he resolve the doubt—although it calls for a solution—raised by the following question: How can the will of someone who is asleep or absentminded be nullified and yet direct him to carry out voluntary movements? Galen himself confirmed his perplexity and doubt about these movements by saying: Although we do not know the reasons for this, we cannot deny what we see with our own eyes. But I will give the reason for this in a summary, and it should be clear after the following introductory remarks.

(I.35) First introductory remark: Voluntary movements sometimes follow from thought and reflection, as in our movement to observe a certain star. At other times they follow from one's imagination, as, for instance, in the erection of someone's penis when he imagines a certain person. At yet other times they follow from nature—in effect, a sensation—as, for instance, in the contraction of someone's leg when a flea bites him.

(I.36) Second introductory remark: All the voluntary movements of the other, nonrational animals follow from imagination or sensation.

(I.37) Third introductory remark: You know that the imaginative faculty is fully and completely active during sleep, as is the imaginative form in the imagination of someone who is absentminded, even if he thinks of something else.

(1.38) Fourth introductory remark: It is well known that sensation is not nullified in living creatures when they are asleep, as Galen explained in this treatise. However, it is diminished and is similar to the strength of someone who is resting and relaxing after great exertion and lassitude.

After these introductory remarks, it may be clear to you that all those activities which Galen mentioned on the part of those who are asleep result either from imagination only or from the nature of the sensation; for someone who is asleep will awaken if a light is brought close to his eyes, or he hears a loud noise, or he is pricked by a needle, or his body is overcome by strong heat or severe cold, or he is hungry or thirsty. Similarly, if he feels pain in one side of his body, he turns to another side. All these are movements resulting from the nature of the sensation. It is not difficult for you to understand that a drunk person or someone who suffered from a stroke does not notice any of these, because they are not healthy, but ill. The activities resulting from sound thinking are totally nullified in the case of someone who is asleep. The walking of someone who is asleep or who is absentminded results from the imaginative form that initially occurred to the sleeper when he was awake and to the absent-minded one when he was attentive.

(1.39) We remember of our own accord the things we do and the words we say intentionally when we are healthy or when we are reminded of them by others. But drunken people and those with a very confused mind do not remember—once they have recovered—anything of the things they have done, even if one tries to remind them of them. *De motu musculorum* II[.6].

(1.40) Says Moses: The reason for this is that the retentive faculty retains only those things deposited in it intentionally and voluntarily by the healthy cogitative faculty. You can find a confirmation for this in the fact that those things that we strongly intend to remember are better fixed in our retentive faculty than those we do not so strongly intend to remember. Those who keep something in their hands while they are asleep provide clear proof that the movement of tension remains in their muscles, for their fingers continue to be clasped around a small object. The fact that healthy people keep their jaws closed during their sleep is also clear proof for the movement of tension during their sleep. Similarly, the muscle surrounding the place where the superfluities leave the body performs its function with great intensity in the case of those who are asleep. *De motu musculorum* II[.4].

(1.41) The brain has a constant movement of contraction and expansion, just like the pulse in the measured movement of the arteries and the heart. This is clear in the case of small children and in the case of someone whose cranial bone is exposed. If a living creature cries out loudly, the entire brain swells and expands. I suppose that the reason for this is that, at the time of the loud cry, superfluous heat increases and superfluous matters are compressed and tend upward. When the brain expands, air is attracted through the nostrils; and when it contracts, the vaporous superfluity and other superfluities that it contains are compressed and expelled from it. But the heat of the brain always remains well preserved there. *De instrumento odoratus.*

(I.42) The thin brain membrane (*pia mater*) adheres to the brain, whereas the thick, hard membrane (*dura mater*) is separated from the thin membrane. The only connections between them are the emerging vessels. The hard membrane is perforated by straight, solid holes, just like a sieve. These holes are constantly cleansed by the two aspects of respiration: inhalation and exhalation. The bone which protects the brain and is close to the face and palate is hollow; the anatomists call it the "sieve." Its openings are not straight, like those of a sieve, but have an irregular structure, as in a sponge, so that the air, when it is extremely cold and then inhaled, will not enter the ventricles of the brain straightway. *De usu partium* VIII[.6–9].

(I.43) Between the bone of the upper palate and the hard brain membrane is a network woven from arteries (*retiform plexus*). This network lies underneath the entire brain, except for a small part thereof. It consists of many layers—as if you were to imagine many fishermen's nets spread one over the other—in order that the blood will stay there for a long time, so that it is cocted and refined before it flows from it into the ventricles of the brain. *De usu partium* IX[.4].

(I.44) The spinal cord—in effect, the soft substance which emerges from the brain and runs down the entire spinal vertebrae—is surrounded by exactly the same two membranes as those surrounding the brain. One membrane adheres to the other, and both are surrounded by a third tunic that is coiled around them from the outside just like a third membrane—strong, hard, and sinewy—to protect the spinal cord because of its intense, vigorous, and strenuous movement. *De usu partium* [VIII.8].

(I.45) The senses of taste and touch in the tongue originate from one and the same nerve—namely, from that nerve that comes from the third pair of nerves of the brain. It often happens that the sense of taste is harmed, while such a harmful disturbance does not occur to the sense of touch of the tongue, for the sense of taste requires a more exact discrimination. *De locis affectis* IV[.3].

(I.46) The higher the position of a part of the spinal cord, the more prominent it is; and the danger of severe damage to the patient is greater than in the case of a part that is lower in position. *De locis affectis* IV[.6].

(I.47) The most important organ of speech is the tongue, while the most important organ of the voice is the larynx, next to the muscle which moves it and the nerve that conducts the power from the brain to that muscle. *De locis affectis* IV[.9].

(I.48) The inner part of the grape-like tunic of the eye has soft and moist hairs so that its manner of touching the crystalline humor is like touching with a soaked sponge. A fine humor—namely, the albuminoid humor—has been made to pour over the crystalline humor in order to form a barrier between the parts of the horn-like tunic that are opposite the perforations of the grape-like tunic and the crystalline and arachnoid tunics. The albuminoid humor is smooth as a mirror as it covers the crystalline humor on the outside above the vitreous humor. *De usu partium* X[.6].

(I.49) If the membranes surrounding the brain were severed—and, similarly, if one were to cut into the brain substance itself—it would not cause any harm to a living creature. But if the cut should reach the ventricles of the brain, a living creature would be deprived immediately of all its voluntary movements. *De anatomia vivorum* 2.

The bodily movements of living creatures that can be grasped by the senses are of two types: voluntary movements, and the movement of the heart and the arteries. There is also a third type of movement—namely, that of the veins, which cannot be grasped by the senses but which I do not need to describe at this point. *De tremore, palpitatione*[*, convulsione, et rigore* 2].

(I.50) Says Moses: The third movement referred to by Galen here is explained by him in the third book of his work *De naturalibus facultatibus* [III.13]—namely, that the veins sometimes move to attract the food and sometimes make the opposite movement to discharge some of the food they contain through exactly the same channel. He has given a lengthy explanation of it in that book.

(I.51) When we find that the uterus, the stomach, and the gallbladder all attract and discharge through one and the same canal, we should not be surprised that nature often discharges bodily superfluities into the stomach through the veins. Still less should we be surprised that the stomach is able to attract food from the liver through the same veins by which the food was carried to the liver—namely, during a long period of fasting. For if the food canal contains much food, the veins between the liver and the other sides of the stomach discharge the food to the liver, and when the food canal is empty and in need of food, it again attracts the food from the liver through the very same veins. *De naturalibus facultatibus* III[.13].

(I.52) Locomotion consists of firm support and movement. The feet are the instrument of firm support while the thighs and hips are the instrument of movement. *De usu partium* III[.5].

(I.53) Of the two ventricles of the heart, the right ventricle was specifically created for the sake of the lung, which is the instrument of respiration and of the voice. Every living creature that does not inhale the air through its nostrils and mouth has neither a lung nor a right heart ventricle. *De usu partium* VI[.9].

(I.54) The shape of the stomach is round and elongated, but where it approaches the spinal column it flattens against it. In a human being, its lower end is broader than its upper end. The liver surrounds the stomach and is closely clasped by its lobes, just like something that is clasped by the fingers. The spleen touches it on the left side. The lower end of the stomach extends to the right side; behind it is the spinal column and the muscles stretched over it. At its front is a membrane of fat (omentum) that totally surrounds the stomach to keep it warm. *De usu partium* IV[.7–8].

(I.55) The membrane of fat is composed of two dense, fine layers, one lying upon the other, and of arteries, veins, and not a small amount of fat. We do not find in the body of a living creature a membrane that is denser and lighter. *De usu partium* IV[.9].

(I.56) There is a membrane over the stomach surrounding its exterior, fleshy layer, and this membrane attaches it to the spinal column. The membrane of fat originates from this membrane; likewise, the membrane that covers the liver binds it to all the inward parts and surrounds it as a protective skin originates from it. From it, too, originate the membranes of the spleen, urinary bladder, kidneys, and intestines. *De usu partium* IV[.10].

The stomach and intestines are nourished by two things: the first thing is the food that passes through them and is digested in them; and the second thing is that which they attract from the liver. *De usu partium* IV[.19].

(I.57) After the stomach is filled with an adequate amount of nourishment, it stores the best part of it up in its own layers, and then it expels as residues the remaining amount, which is too much for its nature. Each of the intestines functions in the same way. *De naturalibus facultatibus* III[.7].

(I.58) Imagine the whole economy of nutrition divided into three periods. Imagine that in the first period, the nutriment remains in the stomach so that it can be cocted and is then passed to the substance of the stomach until it is satiated from the nourishment. Simultaneously, a portion of the cocted nutriment rises to the liver. In the second period, it passes along the intestines and is passed to their layers and to the substance of the liver. In this period, a small part of it is carried all over the body. Imagine that in this period, that which was passed to the substance of the stomach in the first period is now adherent and attached to it. In the third period, imagine that the stomach receives nutriment by assimilating with its substance that which had become adherent to it in the second period. At the same time, in the intestines and the liver, that which was passed to their substance before now becomes adherent and attached to it, while the rest passes to all the other parts of the body and is added to it. *De naturalibus facultatibus* III[.13].

(I.59) The digestion that takes place in the stomach is a kind of alteration. The same holds true for the digestion that takes place in the veins and the digestion that takes place in every single organ. After this third alteration, there is a fourth alteration called assimilation; and, although this name is different from that of nutrition, their meaning is the same. *De symptomat*[*um causis* III.4].

(I.60) The omentum is an organ that is not necessary for life to exist; its usefulness for the body is slight. However, since veins and arteries are woven into it, we have become careful not to cut something away from it. If a hemorrhage appears in it, it should be tied off from above and then one may excise that spot. *De methodo medendi* VI[.4].

(I.61) The parenchyma of the spleen is loose, porous, and light like a sponge. It contains many large arteries in order to heat it, so that it can break up the coarse humor that it attracts, and so that there can be cleansed from it the vaporous superfluity which originates in it because of the bad and coarse humor streaming through it. *De usu partium* IV[.15].

(I.62) The right kidney lies so high that, in some living beings, it reaches up to the liver. The left kidney lies lower, so that the one does not hinder the other in its attraction, as would be the case if they lay on one line. *De usu partium* [V.5, 6.]

(I.63) The urinary bladder and the gallbladder are reached by vessels that nourish them, apart from the two vessels through which they attract the residue—because the residue reaches them both—in an absolutely pure state without any admixture. And, in particular, the neck of the gallbladder is reached by an artery, a vein, and a nerve, while each of these is endlessly divided throughout the entire body of the gallbladder, and even so the urinary bladder has a similar ramification of vessels. *De usu partium* V[.7–8].

(I.64) The uterus has the nature of a nerve and is hard. Women have been created with two uteri that end up in one beginning point—namely, the neck of the uterus. The body of the uterus is covered by an external membrane which joins the two uteri together in one place, connects what is between them, and ties them together. Women have been created with two breasts, each one like a servant for its half of the uterus. One of the marvels of creation is that in a woman the number of uterine cavities is equal to the number of breasts, whereas in other living creatures the number of breasts is equal to the number of offspring. *De usu partium* XIV[.4].

(I.65) The urinary bladder and the uteri are not different with regard to their location. The bladder is harder and more sinewy, however, and therefore, inflammations occurring in it make the pulse harder than uterine inflammations. *De* [*praesagitione ex*] *puls*[*ibus* IV.7].

(I.66) Four organs have two membranes—namely, the esophagus, the stomach, all the intestines, and all the arteries except for those in the lungs. Four organs have only one membrane—namely, the gallbladder, the urinary bladder, the uterus, and all the veins except for the veins in the lungs. *De naturalibus facultatibus* I[.6;] III[.11]; *De usu partium* VI[.11].

(I.67) The penis grows out from the pubic bones, from their upper parts, as the other ligaments. But, unlike the other ligaments, it has been endowed with a cavity so that it can fill rapidly, empty rapidly, become tensed and hard and then become shrunken and relaxed. This hollow nerve—if you wish, you may call it a "nerve" or give it another name; I mean, the penis—is embedded far from the anus, and the channel for the semen extends longitudinally in its lower parts and is centrally located. *De usu partium* XV[.2–3].

(I.68) There are nerves in the membrane of the two kidneys similar to the nerves of the spleen, liver, and gallbladder; for all these organs receive small nerves that are all connected to the membranes covering them from the outside. But the urinary bladder receives large nerves, so that its sensation is finer and more intense. All these organs are covered by membranes originating from the membrane stretched over the stomach. *De usu partium* V[.9–11].

(1.69) The humors that coagulate and form an obstruction in the very solid organs cause a pain stronger than the pain they cause in those organs that are opposite to these organs in solidity. The reason is that these last organs stretch more, and the severity of the pain follows the intensity of the stretching. Therefore, pains in the urinary bladder are stronger than uterine pains, although the nerves found in both these organs are equal. *De* [*praesagitione ex*] *puls*[*ibus* IV.7].

(1.70) When the muscles of the arms, legs, and face stretch, they become convex; because of the hardness of the bones beneath them, they become convex when they contract toward their middle. When they relax and extend, they flatten. But something happens to the muscles of the chest and abdomen which is opposite to that which happens to the muscles of the arms and legs—namely, when they stretch, they flatten, because below them are soft organs that sink when these muscles stretch. Consequently, the swelling of these muscles is hidden in low places, but when these muscles relax, they become convex because then their protrusion becomes more visible. *De motu musculorum* I[.3].

(1.71) The movements of all muscles have one aspect in common—namely, contraction and gathering to their origin. However, movements of various sorts, like those of arms and head, take place through the use of many muscles. Each such movement is accomplished by different muscles. *De motu musculorum* I[.3].

(1.72) The faculty in the sperm and the faculty that forms out of blood—material suitable for making bones and material suitable for making nerves, and similarly the other materials suitable for forming the homogeneous parts—is called the procreative faculty, because it gives birth to and generates material that was not there previously; it is also called the alterative faculty. And the faculty that gives shape to that material so that it can make a certain bone with a certain size and form, and similarly the other homogeneous parts, is called the formative faculty. This faculty has a rational principle, different from the natural principles. The faculty that causes a small bone or nerve to grow, so that it increases in size and bulk, is called the faculty of growth; and the faculty that feeds the organs so that they grow or replaces what has been used up by them, is the nutritive faculty. This faculty accomplishes its function by means of four other faculties—namely, the attractive, retentive, second alterative, and excretory faculties. The second alterative faculty, which is also called the digestive faculty, achieves its end only by means of the powers of adhesion and assimilation. *De naturalibus facultatibus* I[.5, 6–11].

(I.73) The procreative and formative faculties are the dominant ones as long as the fetus is in the uterus, while the nutritive faculty and the faculty of growth are like handmaids to them. After one's birth, the formative faculty ceases its activity and the faculty of growth dominates until the end of adolescence, while the nutritive faculty and the alterative or procreative faculty are like assistants and handmaids to it. After the end of adolescence, the faculty of growth and the alterative faculty cease activity, while the nutritive faculty remains active until the end of one's life. *De naturalibus facultatibus* I[.7].

(I.74) The fibers within each of the intestines are circular and are altogether intertwined in its two layers widthwise, for the intestines merely surround and hold their contents and do not attract anything. As for the stomach, some of its fibers are stretched lengthwise because they attract food, while other fibers are stretched widthwise because they reject food. *De naturalibus facultatibus* III[.11].

∴

In the name of God,
the Merciful, the Compassionate.
O Lord, make our task easy

The Second Treatise

Containing aphorisms concerning the humors

(II.1) Blood is something composed of all the humors according to a natural ratio. It is called "blood" because of its dominance over the other humors. And this is what comes out through venesection and cupping. When we say that the body contains four humors—blood, phlegm, yellow bile, and black bile—by blood we do not mean something composed of all the humors, but something existing, in our conception, unmixed with the other humors. *In Hippocratis Epidemiarum* [*commentarius*] II.4.

(II.2) Just as milk contains a watery fluid that is, as it were, the extraction of the thick part, so, too, all humors contain a fine watery fluid. This fluid differs from the other fluids according to the nature of the humor of which it forms the watery part. The worst of all is the watery fluid of the black bile; less detrimental is the watery fluid of the yellow bile; even less detrimental is the watery fluid of the phlegm; and the warmest and best of all is the watery fluid or juice of the blood (blood serum). *In Hippocratis Epidemiarum* [*commentarius*] VI.[1–8].

(II.3) The yellow bile, whether it is saturated in color or not—and similarly when it is extremely heated until it becomes like yolk—originates from veins and arteries. Sometimes a green bile originates in the belly which has the color of leek or the greenness of verdigris or of finely colored indigo. *De atra bile* [2].

(II.4) The thick and pure red bile is the one some physicians call "yolk-like." Sometimes I have observed that it is more watery and less red; this one in particular is called the "yellow bile." At other times I have observed that it is mixed with fine phlegm or watery fluid. Another type of bile may originate that has the color of leek. This one often originates in the stomach because of foodstuffs that do not accept coction, such as beetroot, onion, and leek. Sometimes it originates in the veins because of unnatural heat and then streams toward the stomach or intestines. *In Hippocratis Prognostica commentarius* II[.38–39].

(II.5) Sometimes red bile with the color of red arsenic is discharged by vomiting and is called "arsenic bile." And sometimes a sediment thereof similar to red arsenic is discharged in the urine. *In Hippocratis Epidemiarum* [*commentarius*] VI.1[–8].

(II.6) We call every cold, moist humor in the body "phlegm." There are many types of this humor. A very cold type of it causes extremely severe pains and looks like melted glass. This glassy type tastes somewhat sour. Another type that people often spit out or vomit contains noticeable sweetness and is not absolutely cold because of the sweetness. A third type of this humor tastes sour when one vomits it and is less cold than the glassy one but colder than the sweet one. There is also a salty type, and this one originates either from putrefaction of the humor or from the salty, watery fluid mixed with it. *De* [*differentiis*] *febrium* II[.6].

(II.7) When food is cocted in the liver, the residual substance resembling the foam that floats on wine is natural yellow bile, while the residual substance settling in a manner similar to the lees of wine is black bile. This is the case when the body functions in a natural way. But when the body deviates from nature, the yellow bile becomes similar to yolk in color and thickness. This happens when, at any time, bile is burned and roasted because of fiery heat. The other types of bile are, as it were, intermediate between these two. *De naturalibus facultatibus* II[.9].

(II.8) When at the end of *De naturalibus facultatibus* II[.9], Galen speaks about the fact that nature has not made an organ for evacuating the natural phlegm from the blood, he says: The superfluity that descends from the head cannot be properly called "phlegm," but should be called "coryza" (mucous discharge from the nostrils). And nature has provided for its evacuation from the body, as I will explain in *De usu partium* [VIII.6]. I will also explain the device provided by nature to rapidly cleanse the phlegm from the stomach and intestines, for it is the opposite to that portion of the phlegm that streams in vessels, because that phlegm is useful to the body and, therefore, nature does not have to evacuate it. [*De usu partium* V.3]. It is proper for you to understand that when I use the term uncocted for the phlegm that is in the vessels and that has been given by nature the proper disposition that blood can be made from it, it has a meaning that is different from the term uncocted used for the phlegm in the stomach and intestines, for this does not at all have the proper disposition that blood be made from it.

(II.9) The spleen and the gallbladder purify the blood and each of the two attracts from the blood an amount of yellow and black bile of such a quantity and quality that if it were to reach the entire body it would be harmful to it. They leave the remainder in it, for the blood that is very thick and earthy and that has entirely escaped alteration in the liver is drawn by the spleen into itself. The remainder of the blood that is moderately thick and cooked passes to the entire body, for the blood in many parts of the body needs a certain thickness. And the same holds true for yellow bile. *De naturalibus facultatibus* II[.9].

(II.10) Just as in the case of the two biles—whereby one part is useful to a living being and is natural, while the other part is unnatural and useless—so, too, is it in the case of phlegm. The sweet part of it is useful to a living being because it is natural; concerning that part of it that is sour or salty, that part of it that is sour does not accept any of the second digestion in the liver, while the salty part is putrefied. And everything that is not digested in the first digestion, which takes place in the stomach, is not a humor. *De naturalibus facultatibus* II[.9].

(II.11) Sometimes a phlegmatic humor or bile accumulates in the stomach. This phlegmatic humor sometimes varies in quality, because some of it can be sour, salty, sweet, or tasteless. Some of it can also be moist and thin, some can be thick or viscous, and some easily dissolved. The same holds true for bile: some is red and some is yellow. Each of the two types can be more or less red or yellow. This is exclusive of the types of bile originating in the bodies of ill people. *De alimentorum facultatibus* I[.1].

(II.12) The nature of yellow bile is hot and dry. The nature of black bile is cold and dry. Blood is hot and moist, while phlegm is cold and moist. Each of these humors often streams into organs while it is pure, unadulterated, and unmixed. Sometimes, however, one of them streams into organs while mixed with another humor. [*De causis morborum* 6].

These humors are usually mixed with one another. We only rarely find one of them pure, not mixed with another. [*De morborum differentiis* 2].

(II.13) When we speak of "phlegmatic humors," we mean by this all the humors in which moisture and cold dominate their temperament. When we speak of "melancholic humors," we mean by this all those humors in which dryness and cold dominate. The phlegmatic and melancholic humors are of diverse categories and types, as are the characteristics that differentiate them from each other. *De locis affectis* III[.9].

(II.14) The difference between black bile and the other melancholic humors, which often leave the body through vomiting and diarrhea, is that one can taste and smell black bile because it is clearly sour or bitter, or both at the same time, so that flies do not go near to it. If some of it happens to fall on the ground, it has the same effect as very acidic vinegar. Its consistency is thick, and it originates especially in the bodies of ill people. The other melancholic humors cannot be tasted, nor do flies shy away from them, nor do they cause the ground to effervesce. Even though we call the black humor that sometimes originates in the bodies of healthy people "black bile," it is not the same as the one which we have described just now. *De atra bile* [3].

(II.15) When the melancholic humor, which is similar to turbid blood with its sediment—and this humor is extremely thick, just like the lees of wine—is burned through an ardent fever, it causes bubbles on the ground. At the same time, it is only very slightly sour or not sour at all. I usually call it "melancholic humor" or "melancholic blood," because it is not proper to call something in this condition "black bile." *De locis affectis* III[.9].

(II.16) Diseases caused by black bile are cancer, elephantiasis, mange, the disease in which the skin peels off (leprosy), quartan fever, delusion, and thickness of the spleen. *De alimentorum facultatibus* III[.1].

(II.17) The juice that is called "crude" is like that which one can see as sediment in the urine of someone who suffers from fever due to a surplus of raw phlegm. It also settles in the urine of healthy people—namely, of someone who is tired and then eats hard foods that are difficult to digest. This juice is similar to pus. The difference between them is that the crude juice does not stink and is not sticky, although it is similar to pus in color and consistency. *De alimentorum facultatibus* I[.2].

(II.18) The stomach of a young child's body cannot completely digest what he needs for growth and nutrition. Therefore, the bodies of young children draw out the food from their stomachs before it has been thoroughly digested, with the result that these children have a large quantity of raw superfluities. *De crisibus* I[.12].

(II.19) The humor consisting of yellow bile has a drying effect just like salt water and sea water. For this reason, the membranes of the arteries of someone suffering from jaundice are drier than normal. Even if he does not have fever, his pulse becomes harder. *De* [*causis*] *pulsu*[*um* IV.26].

(II.20) When the biting humor in the stomach is the type of yellow bile, it rises to the cardia of the stomach because of the lightness of yellow bile. When this biting humor is like leek or sour or salty, it settles in the cavity of the lining of the stomach and does not rise or ascend to its cardia. [*De compositione medicamentorum secundum locos*] II[.1].

(II.21) Sometimes a sharp humor descends in the direction of the buttocks and—since it refuses to be expelled—is by necessity retained by the person. This humor then goes back and rises again, causing a burning pain in the stomach. It fills the head with vapor that it expels upward. In the same way, it often happens that flatulent gas seeking an exit from below if it is blocked returns and reascends. *De symptomat*[*um causis* III.2].

(II.22) If a superfluity streams from a stronger organ to a weaker organ, it putrefies in that place and becomes even worse, and it corrupts the food that was brought to the organ subsequently, although the food was good and useful on its own. *De causis* [*morborum* 6].

(II.23) Whatever superfluities remain in the body for a long time obviously putrefy, some in a shorter and some in a longer time. When they reach this state, they become pungent and harmful to the organs in which they are retained. This does not happen to the gallbladder, because it possesses only a few nerves. But, if the bile becomes a heavy burden to the gallbladder because of its large quantity or because of a change in its quality, it becomes pungent and acrid and desires to be expelled. Sometimes the bile is expelled toward the liver through the neck of the gallbladder itself, by which it is attracted. *De naturalibus facultatibus* III[.12–13].

(II.24) Constant dyspepsias are extremely strong in producing bad humors and diseases, whether these dyspepsias are due to foods with good chymes or to foods with bad chymes. But dyspepsia caused by bad chymes is much worse than the other one. *De probis malisque* [*alimentorum*] *sucis* [14].

(II.25) There are two kinds of foods with bad chymes: thin and thick. The bad chyme that is thin causes acute diseases and malignant fevers; and, when it reaches an organ, it causes erysipelas, shingles, and other pains. The thick bad chyme causes arthritis, gout, pain in the kidneys, asthma, and hardness of the spleen and liver. When the bad chyme is both thick and melancholic, it causes cancers, peeling of the skin (leprosy), itch, quartan fevers, melancholy, a bad complexion, and hemorrhoids. *De probis malisque* [*alimentorum*] *sucis* [14].

(II.26) Sometimes phlegm occurs with body heat because, when the stomach becomes greatly heated, it cannot digest the food it contains, with the result that the phlegm increases in it. *In Hippocratis De mulierum affectibus commentarius*.

(II.27) Chymes which dominate in quantity or quality are five: phlegm, yellow bile, black bile, blood, and its watery part. *In Hippocratis Aphorismos commentarius* I[.2].

(II.28) Among all the humors, only phlegm does not give rise to black bile, even when it is surrounded by exceedingly strong, burning heat. *In Hippocratis De aere*[, *aquis et locis*] *commentarius* II.

(II.29) The superfluity of black bile is the least abundant of all the superfluities, the superfluity of yellow bile is more abundant than the black, and the watery superfluity is many times more abundant than the others. *De usu partium* V[.6].

(II.30) That melancholic humor is natural which does not produce seething and bubbling on the earth when it is poured over it, while that which has taken on this quality is unnatural, because it has assumed a sharpness owing to its burning caused by the unnatural heat. This occurs when the natural melancholic humor putrefies. *De naturalibus facultatibus* II[.9].

This is the end of the second treatise,
by the grace of God,
praise be to Him.

In the name of God,
the Merciful, the Compassionate.
O Lord, make our task easy

The Third Treatise
Containing aphorisms concerning the principles of the art and general rules

(III.1) The age of adolescence is the one in which the temperament is the best and most balanced. *In Hippocratis De natura hominis commentarius* [III.7].

(III.2) The age between fourteen and twenty-five years is that in which the pubic hair grows. *In Hippocratis Aphorismos commentarius* V[.7].

(III.3) The temperament in the age when one is past one's prime and in old age is cold and dry. A clear, defining difference between the age of those who are past their prime and old age is the domination of the moist superfluities in the latter, along with a clear weakening of all bodily functions. *De marcore* [4].

(III.4) The whole body of a man breathes well when it is clean and free of superfluities and pressure. The body of a woman has the opposite characteristic, because the spaces between her vessels are narrow on account of the fat, tender flesh and phlegmatic superfluities, which occupy them; and, since her skin is thick and firm, hardly anything is dissolved through it. *De* [*causis*] *pulsu*[*um* III.2].

(III.5) The quick dissolution of humors through perspiration taking place in the bodies of young people is of great benefit to them and provides quite a few opportunities for the healing of diseases occurring in their bodies, for the improvement of their temperaments when they differ from their normal state, and for the correction of an abundance and thickness of their humors. *De* [*praesagitione ex*] *puls*[*ibus* IV.4].

(III.6) Porous bodies are quickly affected by diseases caused by external factors, while internal diseases caused by superfluous humors originate in them only rarely. In compact bodies, the situation is the reverse. *De optima* [*corporis nostri*] *constitutione* [4].

(III.7) Bodies with a loose texture are weaker, but their health is more lasting, and when they fall ill, they recover quickly. Dense bodies have the opposite characteristics. *In Hippocratis De alimento commentarius* [IV.2].

(III.8) When an organ is weak, one feels heaviness in it, even when only a small amount of superfluities streams toward it. A hot tumor often occurs due to the weakness of an organ, even though the body is not full of superfluities. *De* [*curandi ratione per*] *venae sectione*[*m* 7].

(III.9) When the flesh, fat, and chymes in someone's body become more than the previous quantity, while its strength remains the same as before, the movements of the body necessarily weaken, since the mover remains the same as before, while those things which are moved became more than their previous quantity. *De plenitudine* [10].

(III.10) Most susceptible to spasms are the bodies of children because of the weakness of the body of the nerves in them. Consequently, this affliction occurs to them through the slightest cause, although it is the least dangerous in them. *In Hippocratis Epidemiarum* [*commentarius*] I.2.

(III.11) It is impossible for the strength of an elderly person to be great. Some physicians think that children also do not have great strength, but they are mistaken in their opinion. *De* [*curandi ratione per*] *venae sectione*[*m* 9].

As far as the requirement of temperament is concerned, the longest-living people are those whose temperament is the moistest. They are also more able than others to keep their health, and up until the last stages of senility they have stronger bodies than others who are of the same age. This is only on condition that they take care to expel the superfluities from their bodies through exercise, through bathing before taking a meal, through cleansing themselves from their urine and excrements, through purging themselves at times, and through occasionally purifying their heads by means of gargling and chewing, for superfluities originate in the bodies of people with this temperament and those with a warm and moist temperament. *De sanitate tuenda* VI[.3].

(III.12) The worst of all temperaments is the one that is dry. This is inevitable, since what happens to old people in the course of time is present in them from the very beginning. Sexual intercourse is most harmful for them and is contrary to the health of everyone whose temperament tends to dryness. *De sanitate tuenda* VI[.4].

(III.13) You should know for certain that if a part of the body is full, or has bad humors, or is very sensitive, or if all these attributes occur together, it will undoubtedly form a tumor if an accident should occur to that part, whatever part it is. It is therefore necessary to not seal the place where the wound might occur, but, rather, to put ingredients on it that soften, alleviate, and allay the pain to prevent the formation of a tumor. *De methodo medendi* VI[.2].

(III.14) If the substance of someone's heart dries only a little bit, he quickly becomes decrepit but may under certain circumstances live for some more years. However, if the substance of someone's heart dries out thoroughly, it will lead to rapid wasting, and he will die shortly. After this in order of harm comes the wasting caused by dryness of the liver. Then comes the wasting originating from the stomach when it dries out, and then the wasting originating from other organs. *De methodo medendi* VII[.6].

(III.15) You should know that if the dryness of the elementary parts lasts for a long time, it will inevitably be followed by coldness, because the organs are nourished by a hot humor—namely, blood—and, when the organs dry out, their nourishment is cut off and they become dry; this is followed by coldness. *De methodo medendi* VII[.7].

(III.16) Bodily superfluities are sparse in winter, because the cold congeals them; but in the summer they are plentiful, because the heat melts them. Only a few people combine much food with much drink. *In Hippocratis De aere*[*, aquis et locis*] *commentarius* I[.8.10].

(III.17) Sperm and blood are of one temperament in the winter and of a different temperament in the summer. Therefore, the fetuses in these seasons are different, because the summer heat burns and dries the sperm, while the winter cold makes it cold and moist. *In Hippocratis De aere*[*, aquis et locis*] *commentarius* [IV.5.15].

(III.18) The rising of the Pleiades marks the beginning of summer, and their setting marks the beginning of winter. The rising of Virgo marks the beginning of autumn, and its setting marks the beginning of spring. *In Hippocratis De aere*[, *aquis et locis*] *commentarius* II[.5.3].

(III.19) Some persons have seen vessels generated in large wounds, as we ourselves have also seen veins that were quite important and numerous in the head and other organs. They do not grow in many people, but only in a few individuals, and that rarely. As for arteries and nerves, no one has ever seen them generated, even rarely, in anyone. *De semine* I[.13].

(III.20) The empty spaces between the elementary parts are filled with moisture. This moisture is the nutriment that is especially fit for the homogeneous parts, which they attract from the adjacent parts, but not from the vessels. *De arte parva* [16].

(III.21) When the vertebrae of the back separate from each other, there is a white, sticky moisture in the space between them, similar to the moisture that has been poured around the other joints. And equally, around the spinal medulla a sticky humor has been poured similar to the humor that has been poured around the ligament through which the vertebrae of the back are bound together and around all the joints, tongue, and larynx, as well as all the parts that must move continually. *De usu partium* XIII[.8].

(III.22) The tendon is the principal instrument for motion. The muscle was created to produce tendons from it and also to provide the use of composite flesh. Part of the tendon of the muscles is connected to the members of hands and feet through its fleshy parts. *De usu partium* XII[.2].

The nose is the first and foremost instrument of respiration in order. As for the mouth, whatever protection it may provide to a living being against the disasters and calamities that might befall him and force him to use it for respiration, it is not primarily an instrument of respiration. *De usu partium* XI[.11].

(III.23) There is no other organ in the body with so great an innate property that enables it to stretch and extend and then to return and contract into a small space, as the uterus. Since it is attached by means of ligaments to the spine on both sides, these ligaments must also, of necessity, stretch and return to their original state, together with the uterus; they must follow it in its coming and going so that they will be protected from being broken off and so that the uterus will be safe and sound. *De usu partium* XIV[.14].

(III.24) The temperament of the nervous system is colder than that of any other organ. Therefore, it is quickly affected by the cold and conveys to the brain the harm that the cold has inflicted on it. Because of that, one should not approach the place of a nerve, nor touch it with something cold, and especially not in the case of abscesses. *De methodo medendi* VI[.3].

(III.25) The worst city is that which is sheltered from the east winds and in which hot and cold winds blow. *In Hippocratis De aere*[*, aquis et locis*] *commentarius* I[.10.1].

(III.26) A bad temperament harms the faculties of the body in their specific essential nature. If the temperament is extremely bad, it annihilates any faculty of the body. *De symptomat*[*um causis* III.1.3].

(III.27) A varying bad temperament can occur in the whole body, as in the case of dropsy of the flesh (anasarca) and in the case of all the fevers except for hectic fever. It can also occur in one part of the body, as in the case of a swelling of the flesh—that is, a phlegmatic swelling or a hot swelling. Any swelling of this type contains a varying bad temperament. *De inaequali intemperie* [1].

(III.28) Insomnia is of two types—namely, the one in which a human being is involved in some activity with no obvious harm done to his strength, and the one which occurs without any external cause but which diminishes his strength, appetite, digestion, and the other natural activities. *In Hippocratis Epidemiarum* [*commentarius*] VI.[1–8].

(III.29) Any very bad temperament which occurs in the heart in whatever way, be it primary or due to another internal organ, exhausts the animal faculty and annuls it. In the same way, a very bad temperament of the brain is followed by weakness of the psychical faculty. This faculty is strangulated when the ventricles of the brain are filled with superfluities and when the passages opening into those ventricles are obstructed. *De* [*praesagitione ex*] *puls*[*ibus* IV.11].

(III.30) The question of the strength of the body is a very grave one and the most important about which to be concerned. The permanence and continuance of the substance of this strength depends on a combination of three things: the substance of the pneuma, the substance of the elementary parts, and the substance of the flesh. Each one of these is preserved by that which is congenial to it. The pneuma is preserved by the respiration of the chest and by the perspiration through all the pores of the body when it proceeds according to its nature, and also through the vapor which arises in the body when it is in proper condition. The substance of the elementary parts is preserved by solid and strong food. The flesh is preserved by food intermediate between moist and solid. *De methodo medendi* XI[.3].

(III.31) A good transformation of blood is the nourishment of the parts of the body through it, but a bad transformation means that it putrefies with a stinking putrefaction. A transformation of blood intermediate between good and bad means that it will turn into pus, for pus is formed from a combination of unnatural and innate heat. *In Hippocratis Aphorismos commentarius* II[.47].

(III.32) Although every organ of the body attracts nourishment to itself, not all have the same attractive faculty. Therefore, the emaciation occurring to them in the case of lack of blood is not the same. The attractive faculty of the heart is the strongest, followed by that of the liver. Therefore, the heart never lacks its nourishment without the other organs of the body suffering from an extreme lack of blood. So, for this reason, we should not think, when the body seems to us emaciated due to prolonged illness, that the situation of the heart and liver regarding emaciation is the same as that of the other organs. *De marcore* [V].

(III.33) A natural characteristic common to human beings and other living beings is that the heart is stronger than the liver in attracting what is useful to it and rejecting what is loathsome to it, and that the liver is more effective and stronger than the intestines and stomach, while the arteries are more effective and stronger than the veins. When the liver is full and stretched, while the stomach is empty and craving to attract nutrition, the force of attraction shifts to the stomach, which then attracts nutrition from the liver. *De naturalibus facultatibus* III[.13].

(III.34) The purified food which arrives from the stomach into the liver is boiled and cocted in the body of the liver and turned into blood. There the yellow and black bile superfluities are separated and attracted by the gallbladder and spleen. Then the blood—thin in substance—enters the large vessel that grows from the convex part of the liver and streams toward the upper and lower parts of the body. As long as the blood is in this vessel, it is mixed with a large amount of a thin watery liquid, which it needs to facilitate its passing through the many fine veins in the liver. When the blood reaches the broad vessel that is close to the right side of the heart, this superfluity that is, the watery fluid is separated and absorbed by the kidneys and then poured by them into the urinary bladder. *De usu partium* IV[.4–6].

(III.35) The liver is nourished by thick red blood, the spleen by thin dark blood, and the lung by blood that is completely cocted, bright red, and spirituous (filled with "pneuma"). *De usu partium* IV[.15].

(III.36) The intestines are coiled and surrounded by innumerable vessels. The mouths of these vessels penetrate into the inside of the intestines in order to grasp the good part of the food. The arteries which penetrate into the intestines take a small amount of food. *De usu partium* IV[.17–18].

(III.37) Both kidneys are nourished by attracting the watery part of the blood. The residue is the watery superfluity which they expel to the urinary bladder. The kidneys do not need a third vessel to bring them nutrition, as is the case with the gallbladder and urinary bladder. *De usu partium* V[.6–7].

(III.38) There is no part of the body to which blood comes more completely cocted in arteries and veins than the breasts. This is so because that blood passes through the heart as it goes up and meets the heart again on its way down and is constantly moved by the movement of the chest and is heated during all this coming and going by its long stay there and by the length of the distance it covers. *De usu partium* VII[.22].

(III.39) The organs nourished with pure blood—namely, the organs on the right side—are warmer than the organs on the left side. So, do not be surprised that the right testicles in males are warmer than the left and that the right uterus in females is warmer than the left. Thus, it is not unreasonable to say that the parts on the right side produce males, and those on the left side, females. *De usu partium* XIV[.7].

(III.40) Since the breasts and uteri were created for a single task only, they have been joined by means of arteries and veins. The origins of these joined vessels are different from those of the other vessels. This is because some begin above the diaphragm and descend to the lower parts of the body, while others begin below and pass upward, so that, during pregnancy, all that is contained in these vessels goes to the uterus and afterwards, during nursing, to the breasts. *De usu partium* XIV[.8].

(III.41) There are five movements of the stomach, and they follow each other in proper arrangement and order. The first is evacuation, the second is the natural appetite of the emptied parts, the third is the absorption of the vessels of the stomach, the fourth is the sensation of absorption experienced by the stomach itself, and the fifth and last one is the natural desire of the stomach, which is the same as hunger. *De symptomat*[*um causis* I.7].

(III.42) There are five functions of the voice, which follow each other in proper arrangement and order. These are the exhalation of air through breathing, exsufflation with noise, exsufflation without noise, sound, and speech. When one of these functions is damaged, all the following ones are damaged as well, but not the previous ones. *De locis affectis* IV[.9].

(III.43) Exhalation of air through breathing is effected through the muscles of the chest. A strong exsufflation is effected by the intercostal muscles. Noiseless exsufflation is effected by pharyngeal muscles. Sound is produced by the larynx and its muscles. Speech is accomplished by the tongue, with the assistance of the teeth, lips, nostrils, uvula, and upper palate. *De locis affectis* IV[.9].

(III.44) That which nature cannot turn into food as part of its transformation activity is that which settles in the urine. It does not change and turn into blood, and it is not like pus, which is generated by nature in normal and abnormal circumstances. *In Hippocratis Prognostica commentarius* [II.38, 39].

(III.45) Says Moses: What is evident to me—and this is a necessary logical conclusion—is that the food which nature cannot turn into blood in the liver is the crude chyme that appears in some urines. And that which nature cannot transform into blood reaching the organs and feeding them is the sediment which appears in the urine of ill people and of some healthy people.

(III.46) Not only does the nutrition of the organs come from the blood, but also the protection of the innate heat. Therefore, when the quantity of blood changes because it is greatly increased or diminished, or when the quality of blood changes because it becomes very hot or it loses much of its heat, the innate heat is corrupted. When this happens in the heart, its corruption extends to the whole body. When it happens in an organ far from the heart, that corruption affects the heat of that organ only, unless it extends so much beyond that organ that it reaches the heart. *De* [*curandi ratione per*] *venae sectionem* [5].

(III.47) The veins that reach the brain expel the superfluities they contain into the ventricles of the brain, but retain and keep the blood they contain. *De usu partium* IX[.4].

(III.48) It is a natural condition that the skin is not stretched while there is an empty space between the skin and the flesh. Similarly, the spaces in the flesh itself are all empty, especially those around the arteries to accommodate their expansion (diastole). In the case of hot tumors, all these spaces fill and the skin is stretched. When the tumor is chronic, pus extends to the tunics, membranes, and vessels, down to the bone below the tumor. In general, there is no organ that remains in the same natural condition if it is affected by a hot tumor that has become chronic. *De tumoribus* [*praeter naturam* 2].

(III.49) There are two types of heat in the body. One is innate, and its substance lies in the blood; and the other is biting while it burns. Under this last category of heat falls fever; and this heat is called "strange heat," "unnatural heat," and also "acquired heat." *In Hippocratis Epidemiarum* [*commentarius*] VI.[1–8].

(III.50) The vessels through which food is transported from the stomach to all the organs are precisely the ones through which many superfluities stream from all the organs to the stomach and intestines in a time of purgation through drugs and in times of crises of diseases. In the case of healthy people, it often happens in a time of severe hunger that pure blood streams to the stomach in order to feed it. Sometimes the phlegm originating in the stomach ascends to the liver, together with the food that ascends to it. *De atra bile* [7].

(III.51) Wind sometimes collects beneath the skin, and sometimes beneath the membranes covering the bones or beneath the membrane covering one of the internal organs. *De methodo medendi* [XIV.6].

(III.52) The crystalline, vitreous, and albuminoid humors, and likewise the horn-like tunic, do not contain any vessels at all. The crystalline humor is nourished from the vitreous humor by transudation, and the vitreous humor is nourished from what reaches it from the net-like tunic, which has many arteries and veins. Similarly, the horn-like tunic is nourished by transudation from what reaches it from the grape-like tunic, for the grape-like tunic also has many vessels. *De usu partium* X[.1].

From the exits of the nerves, arteries and veins enter the spine in order to carry out the same task as with the other parts. *De usu partium* XIII[.9].

Soft nerves were joined to the parts that require minute sensation and hard nerves to the parts that require voluntary motion. Hard and soft nerves were joined to the parts needing both things. Many nerves or large nerves have been joined to the part that needs much sensation, while no nerve has been joined to a part that does not need sensation. *De usu partium* XVI[.2, 3].

No separate, special nerve was made to reach the skin, but it is reached by certain fine subdivisions of the nerves from the parts that lie beneath it. These subdivisions go to these parts in order to serve as bonds between the skin and the parts beneath it and to serve as sensory organs for them. *De usu partium* XVI[.2].

(III.53) Just as the skin has sensation—although no special nerves reach it, since it receives only the faculty of sensation from the nerves, but not the faculty of motion, with the result that it does not move—so, too, the membranes, tunics, arteries, veins, uteri, intestines, urinary bladder, stomach, and all the viscera have sensation but no motion, although the nerves have both faculties, while the instrument of motion is the muscle. *De usu partium* XVI[.2].

(III.54) One should not be amazed that, if the skin overlying a muscle loses its sensation, the movement of that muscle is not abolished; this is because the nerve that spreads in that muscle has not been damaged, whereas that part of the nerve that spreads within the skin was damaged. So, if the skin is pulled from the muscle, it is impossible for that muscle to move without having sensation. But it is possible that the muscle has sensation without motion; this occurs when the muscle is so severely damaged that, although the amount of power it receives from the psychical faculty is still enough to allow sensation through being affected, it is not enough for motion, because motion is a form of activity, while sensation is a form of passivity. *De symptomat*[*um causis* I.5].

(III.55) Twitching occurs in all the parts that can stretch but never occurs in bones and cartilages, because bones and cartilages do not stretch in any way. Therefore, twitching occurs frequently in the skin, and sometimes it happens also in the muscles which are beneath it. It also happens in the stomach, the urinary bladder, the uterus, the intestines, the liver, the spleen, the diaphragm, the arteries, and the heart itself. *De symptomat*[*um causis* II.2].

(III.56) In soft flesh and that which is generally called flesh, only the alterative faculty is similar to that in other organs. The remaining three faculties are weaker in the flesh than in the other organs. Therefore, the soft flesh is quicker to receive superfluous matters than the other organs. Second—after the soft flesh—in rapidity of reception of the superfluous matters comes the lung, because of the softness of its substance and because of the weakness of the other three faculties in it. After the lung in rapidity of reception of the superfluous matters comes the spleen. The brain is similar to the spleen in rapidity of reception of the superfluous matters or even more so, but it is superior to it in the quality of its composition—namely, the spaciousness of its ventricles, the large quantity of passages for its superfluities, and the fact that these passages run from top to bottom. *De* [*curandi ratione per*] *venae sectionem* [8].

(III.57) Every strong organ sends its strength to a weaker organ that is near to it. Thus, the weaker organ attains a strength that is comprised of its own specific power and of the power sent to it. *In Hippocratis De alimento commentarius* I.

(III.58) Sometimes the body is at rest and ease when its temperament is bad because of sharp, bad humors. If the rest and ease last for a long time, this causes fever. Sometimes the rest dries the body, because it weakens the organs so that they are not well nourished. And when the body is not well nourished, it becomes dry and arid. *De somno et vigilia.*

(III.59) The matters that develop in all the tumors and humors that form in arteries and veins when there is an obstruction are all of one and the same order. For, when the alterative and ripening faculty in those organs which have a tumor or in those vessels that have a humor becomes stable and strong, it transforms that which is within the tumors into good white pus, balanced in its consistency, and transforms that which is in the vessels into the sediment which settles in the urine. This kind of putrefaction is not merely putrefaction but is mixed with coction. But when the alterative faculty is very weak, there is an absolute putrefaction; and those various fluids are exuded from the tumors and those bad sediments settle in the urine of those suffering from fever. *De* [*differentiis*] *febrium* I[.7].

(III.60) Nature often purges the whole body in the case of illness, in the case of the ingestion of a purgative or emetic, and in the case of cholera, while the superfluities come and go through the very same vessels by which the organs are nourished. Thus, the superfluities pass from one organ to another until they reach the vessels spreading from the intestines and stomach. No wonder, then, that nutriment returns from the outer skin surface to the depths of the body, and that it reaches the stomach as it returns from the liver and spleen through the very same vessels through which it ascended from the stomach initially. *De naturalibus facultatibus* III[.13].

(III.61) If fluids stream into the cavities of organs that have tumors and remain there for a long time, they undergo a great variety of transformations. In the case of abscesses, one often finds substances similar to stones, sand, potsherds, wood, coal, sediment of olive oil, lees of wine, and other substances of different sorts. *Ad Glauconem* [*de medendi methodo*] II[.9].

(III.62) The penis, genitalia, and neck of the uterus are reached by a surplus of nerves because of the extra sensation which they need during sexual intercourse. The other procreative parts, such as the uteri as a whole and the male testicles with their receptacle—that is, the scrotum—are reached only by small nerves like the nerves which reach the other internal parts, such as the liver, spleen, and kidneys. *De usu partium* XIV[.13].

(III.63) When blood streams to empty places and a tumor forms in an organ, if the innate heat of that organ has greatly deviated from its equilibrium, that blood putrefies just as the bodies of the dead do. But, if the innate heat remains in a balanced state and does not deviate too much from it, it prevails over that blood and transforms it into pus. According to the variation in these two circumstances, the conditions of the pus vary in proximity to putrefaction or to coction. *In Hippocratis Prognostica commentarius* I[.42].

(III.64) When the vessels of any muscle fill with so much warm blood that they become obstructed by it, and when their orifices open and that blood streams to those openings that are in the flesh of the muscle and those that are outside the muscle, and when the substance of the flesh of the muscle becomes hot due to what is inside it and due to what is outside it, then the flesh will be of a varying bad temperament and cause a sensation of pain as long as it is affected in this way. When the heat prevails over the muscle as a whole and the heat of the flesh at the inside and outside is equal, the bad temperament of the muscle does not vary anymore but becomes even, and the sensation of pain stops. The same holds true—as you should understand—for all the other parts of the body. *De inaequali intemperie* [3].

(III.65) Sometimes a bad humor resembling a deadly poison collects in the body and has a gradual effect on the organs of the body. When it reaches its maximum malignancy, its effects become visible all at once, and it kills rapidly. Just as the effect of deadly drugs depends on their quality and not on their quantity, in the same way one should imagine that the effect of diseases which cause agitation and kill rapidly is as if someone takes a deadly drug or is bitten by a viper. *In Hippocratis Epidemiarum* [*commentarius*] III.3.

(III.66) The parts that get tired first are those that receive the defluxion descending from the head. When fatigue occurs through the voice, it results in angina; when it occurs through the hand, paralysis occurs; and, when it occurs through riding, pain in the back develops. The same happens with the other parts. *In Hippocratis Epidemiarum* [*commentarius*] VI.[1–8].

(III.67) The most important and most dangerous element in treating diseases is a bad temperament. This is so because the temperament is the most important of the kinds of things existing in nature. *De methodo medendi* VII[.7].

(III.68) The strongest cause in the generation of diseases is the predisposition of the body which is likely to fall ill. Therefore, not all people die during the course of an epidemic, nor do all of them fall ill with the rise of Sirius. *De* [*differentiis*] *febrium* I[.6].

(III.69) An extreme change in weather causing illness, overeating to the point of oppressing one's strength, excessive physical exercise, excessive bathing, and excessive sleep are all counted among the unnatural causes, for an excess in these natural causes makes them unnatural—they become unnatural, although they are a kind of cause which is not unnatural by itself. *De pulsibus libellus* [*ad tirones* 11].

(III.70) Weak powers often decline and suffer defeat from minor causes, while strong powers are overcome and subdued only by major causes. Therefore, strong bodies that remain free from diseases for a long time come within sight of ruin when they fall ill. But weak bodies which constantly fight afflictions escape from diseases and are saved from them in the easiest of ways. *De* [*praesagitione ex*] *puls*[*ibus* II.4].

(III.71) If someone enjoys lasting and constant health, strong causes will not alter his body. But, in the case of old men, convalescents, and all sickly people, the slightest cause produces a great change in their bodies. Similarly, if an old man or convalescent only slightly exceeds the proper bounds in the quantity or quality of food, he suffers great harm therefrom. But young people suffer only slight harm from serious offenses against their health. *De sanitate tuenda* V[.4].

(III.72) Intrinsically, corruption occurs to a living being, first of all, in two ways: either through the being's drying up and growing old, which results in death, or through the constant dissolution of his essence—namely, the innate heat—which also results in death. But corruption also occurs to a living being in another way intrinsically connected to the food and drink he consumes—that is, through the production of superfluities in him. All these things [occur] intrinsically. But corruption also occurs to him through extrinsic means: One of them is inseparable—namely, the air—, and the other is occasional—namely, the other things which change its temperament or dissolve its continuity. *De sanitate tuenda* I[.4].

(III.73) In the case of one whom you find who falls ill only on rare occasions, do not change any of his habits in his entire regimen. But in the case of one who falls ill frequently, you should look for the cause of the illness and eliminate it. There is no doubt that this should be achieved through a change in one or more of his habits. Consider, also, in the case of someone whose habit you want to change, whether or not such a change can be well tolerated by him. *De sanitate tuenda* VI[.5, 6].

(III.74) In the case of one who suffers from one illness after another because of an affliction in his body, the cause of his illness can be one of two things: either overfilling, in which case he should diminish the intake of food and drink into his body, or a bad humor originating in the body, in which case he should avoid things that produce bad humors. One should take care that one's stools are soft in either case. *De sanitate tuenda* VI[.6].

(III.75) The body that has become weak because of a chronic illness, evacuation, or bad humor needs moist, quickly digestible food with a fragrant, pleasant aroma. For a pleasant aroma adds something to the body, balances its bad temperament, and strengthens the innate heat. *In Hippocratis De alimento commentarius* IV[.27].

(III.76) Concerning chronic illnesses such as orthopnea, stones, tumors in the nose, bad ulcers, and the like, most of these afflictions occurring to youngsters and children are cured in forty days or seven months or seven years. Some of them are cured before the pubic hair starts to grow and, in the case of girls, at the time of menstruation. *De signis mortis.*

(III.77) When the temporal muscles suffer a blow or are harmed in any other way, they bring on spasms, fevers, stupor, and delirium more than any of the other muscles because of their proximity to the origin of the nerves. For this reason, this muscle is well protected and buried between two bones. *De usu partium* XI[.3].

(III.78) If the grape-like tunic is severely torn, the albuminoid humor flows out of the grape-like tunic and meets the horn-like tunic, and this results in two afflictions. One of these is that the grape-like tunic falls on the crystalline humor, and the other is that pneuma escapes from that wound. *De symptomat*[*um causis* I.2].

(III.79) Tumors in the noble organs are fatal. Tumors in the other internal organs that are not noble can be fatal because of their size, or because of the diminished strength of the body, or because of an error in the treatment prescribed by the physician. *In Hippocratis Prognostica commentarius* I[.30].

(III.80) Our bodies do not remain constantly in one condition—either quantitatively, because of dissolution, or qualitatively, because of external influences. Therefore, our bodies have been provided with the nutritive faculty to correct the corruption occurring in terms of quantity. For the correction of the corruption occurring in terms of quality, our bodies have been provided with two kinds of respiration: one through the movement of the chest, and the other through the movement of the pulse. *In Hippocratis Epidemiarum* [*commentarius*] VI[.5].

(III.81) It is difficult to preserve one's health when the stomach is hot and cold superfluities descend to it from the head, or when the stomach is cold and hot superfluities descend to it from the head. I have tested and found that, of these two conditions, the most difficult to treat is the case of a hot stomach to which cold, phlegmatic humors descend. But the worst case is when this is combined with a dry abdomen and difficulty in vomiting. *De sanitate tuenda* VI[.10].

(III.82) Excruciating pains caused by dryness are hard to cure or cannot be cured at all. Mostly, this dryness is associated with a fever occurring due to a hot tumor in the brain. *De methodo medendi* XII[.8].

(III.83) I do not know anyone who suffered from spasms due to a hot tumor in the brain who was cured, nor have I heard of such a case. But spasms due to overfilling of the nervous system, or those due to a biting humor which consumes these parts, or those due to severe cold result in something similar to a hardening of the nerves. These three kinds of spasms can often be cured. *De methodo medendi* XII[.8].

(III.84) A severe headache occurs from heat or cold. The headache occurring because of dryness is mild. Moisture is not accompanied by pain at all. A large quantity of humors in the head causes heaviness but no headache unless obstructions occur from it, because the headache is commensurate with the degree of obstruction. [*De compositione medicamentorum secundum locos*] II[.1].

(III.85) In most cases, one should not use curbing and restraining drugs for abscesses occurring in the roots of the ears in the beginning of their appearance, as with other tumors. Rather, we should do the opposite—namely, treat them with attractive drugs. If this does not work, we should apply cupping glasses until the malignant, harmful humor is extracted from the inside of the body to the region of the skin. I never advise application of a restraining treatment, except for a light one when there is no pain and when the body is clean. [*De compositione medicamentorum secundum locos*] III[.2].

(III.86) When abscesses occurring in the roots of the ears begin to disperse by themselves, one should not use anything either to stimulate this process or to attract the humor. In this case, the whole matter should be left to nature. If pus collects, one should either lance the abscesses so that that pus can stream out of the ear or disperse and destroy them by means of drugs. [*De compositione medicamentorum secundum locos*] III[.2].

(III.87) If hot matter runs from the head to the eye, one should start with a general evacuation of the body through phlebotomy or through purgation of the bowels, followed by emptying of the head, especially by gargling and by attracting the matter to the opposite side by means of cupping glasses and the like. Occasionally, we split or cut the arteries close to the ears or on the temples and then treat the eye itself. [*De compositione medicamentorum secundum locos*] IV[.1].

(III.88) A phlegmatic tumor hardly ever occurs in the chest and liver because the chest is too solid, strong, and firm for this kind of matter to reach it. In the case of the liver, this is true as well not only because it is very solid, but also because it changes and transforms the nature of the food. For this reason, viscous phlegm and thick blood never enter the body of the diaphragm, and especially not the nervous part of it, because of its thickness. *De* [*praesagitione ex*] *puls*[*ibus* IV.4].

(III.89) Weakness of either liver or stomach brings those suffering from it to ruin. Therefore, it is necessary to strengthen these organs constantly. When the strength of the other organs fails, it is not dangerous. When the strength of the intestines or chest fails, one is not safe from bad consequences. However, their condition is intermediate because, to the same degree that they fall short of the eminence of liver and stomach, they surpass the other parts of the body. *De methodo medendi* XI[.15].

(III.90) If a tumor appears in the chest or stomach or one of the parts of the neck and head, one should bind the hands and feet. If a tumor appears in the hands, one should bind the feet; and, if a tumor appears in the feet, one should bind the hands. *De methodo medendi* XIII[.5].

(III.91) The liver and the spleen are the quickest and most susceptible of the organs to become hard if someone neglects them through taking viscous foods. Similarly, the kidneys are quickly affected by hardness. Therefore, some renal diseases cannot be cured, while others are hard to cure. *De methodo medendi* XIII[.15].

(III.92) Pay attention and be extremely careful that no hardness occurs to liver, spleen, or kidneys. Mostly, these hard conditions occur to somebody who suffers from a hot tumor in one of these three organs and then takes foods that produce coarse and viscous humors. *De methodo medendi* XIII[.15].

(III.93) When a wound or ulcer occurs in the large intestine, it is easily healed because the large intestine is very fleshy and thick and medications settle and stay there for a long time. The small intestine is very difficult to heal, while the jejunum in particular cannot be healed at all when a wound occurs in it because of the thinness of its body, its extreme sensitivity, its abundance of vessels, and the passing of bile through it. The jejunum is the only organ that is always free of food. *De methodo medendi* VI[.4].

(III.94) It is, above all, the outer layer of the skin in which humors arriving at it are retained and become stuck—namely, those humors which are thick and earth-like. This results in mange, the disease in which the skin peels off (leprosy), and elephantiasis. *De* [*simplicium*] *medicament*[*orum temperamentis ac facultatibus* XI[.1].

(III.95) Marasmus develops gradually from tumors that are not dissolved or that are hidden from perception. *De pulsibus libellus* [*ad tirones* 12].

(III.96) For the most part, the accumulation of pus in hot tumors takes place after the twentieth day and in cold tumors, after the sixtieth day. *In Hippocratis Prognostica commentarius* I[.35].

(III.97) It is in all cases unavoidable that the heart is afflicted when death occurs. Death always results from an extreme bad temperament of the heart. If the bad temperament of the heart is severe and specific for the homogeneous parts, it is not followed by a quick death. But when it is specific for the composite organs, it is followed by sudden death, which is at times preceded by severe syncope. *De locis affectis* V[.2].

(III.98) It is absolutely impossible for the arteries to undergo a change affecting all of them without the heart suffering through sharing the pain with the ailing organ. The organ with which the heart shares the pain in the quickest possible way more than the other organs is the lung; after the lung comes the liver, and after the liver the diaphragm, and after the diaphragm the chest. *De* [*praesagitione ex*] *puls*[*ibus* IV.1, 3–5].

(III.99) If fineness of a humor, looseness of the substance of the organ, heat of the surrounding air, strength of the medicine applied, and abundant strength in the patient combine, the tumor is quickly and sometimes suddenly dissolved. But, if the opposite conditions combine, the opposite is the case. *In Hippocratis Prognostica commentarius* II[.68].

(III.100) The death of ill people occurs in one of four ways: Either,

1. the patient suffers an absolutely bad crisis and dies the very same day; or
2. the strength of the patient is dissipated slowly until he dies (marasmus); or
3. both things occur together—namely, that the condition of the patient becomes very bad all of a sudden, while his strength continues to decline gradually until he dies; or,
4. sometimes, the patient dies suddenly, without any crisis at all. *De crisibus* III[.7].

(III.101) Says Moses: It is well known that this sudden death without a crisis cannot occur when the disease is abating but, rather, occurs during one of the other three stages which precede the abatement of the disease. Galen himself explained in his *De crisibus* III[.9], that, during the abatement of a disease, death does not occur at all unless the patient dies because of an error.

(III.102) Any illness that subsides without a clear evacuation, or with a fairly large abscess, will return in a worse form than before. *De crisibus* III[.11].

(III.103) The death of those who die without a crisis occurs on the day of the paroxysm of the disease. Some of them die in the beginning of fever attacks, others die when the attack reaches its peak, and yet others die when the attack is receding and their strength is eroded. *De crisibus* III[.9].

(III.104) All the secretions discharged from the body are discharged in two ways: sometimes they are discharged because the bodies which contain them remove and expel them, and sometimes they are discharged because these very secretions flow out spontaneously, since the bodies containing them are too weak to keep and retain them. *De locis affectis* VI[.6].

(III.105) Take care not to prescribe laxatives at the beginning of tumors in the anus and surrounding area, and do not prescribe diuretics when a tumor begins to appear in the urinary bladder, penis, or kidneys. Similarly, do not induce menstruation when a tumor first appears in the uterus or vulva. When a tumor first appears in the throat, the upper part of the mouth, the tongue, or anywhere else inside the mouth, be careful not to prescribe a gargle. For, doing so while there are tumors in those places is similar to prescribing purgatives in the case of a tumor in the intestines, or diuretics in the case of a tumor in the urinary bladder, or emetics in the case of a tumor in the stomach or esophagus. *De methodo medendi* XIII[.4, 6].

(III.106) The application of cupping glasses is one of the strong means to attract that which is in the depths of the body and to eliminate tumors which have become hard and solid. This should be done only once the whole body has been evacuated, for, if one applies cupping glasses to a part of the body while the body is full, they attract the superfluous matter to this part. Therefore, one should apply them on the side furthest from the ailing part of the body so that the matter is attracted from that part to the opposite side, as we have established. *De methodo medendi* XIII[.19].

(III.107) The application of cupping glasses to the neck on the occipital protuberance is one of the best means to prevent the superfluous matters from streaming toward the eye. But one should do so only after the whole body has been evacuated. *De methodo medendi* XIII[.19].

(III.108) Remember that if one treats a part of the body with dissolving drugs while the body is full of superfluities, it is more probable and likely that these drugs will attract those superfluities to that part and fill it with them than that they will evacuate them. Therefore, if one treats hot tumors and the like, one should not rely on the application of dissolving drugs until one has evacuated the whole body. *De methodo medendi* XIII[.22].

(III.109) There are physicians who think that the stronger a medicine is in astringency, the more effective it is, when astringency is required. They also think that the more dispersing a medicine is, the more effective and beneficial it is, when dispersion is required. They do not understand that the stronger either of these powers is, the stronger the pain caused by it in the tumorous part of the body. The reason is that a very astringent medicine causes something similar to a contusion and disruption because the substance of the bodily part is severely drawn together and compressed, while hot medicines with a strongly dispersing action cause something similar to a corrosion in the tumorous part of the body. Truly, a medicine with a power intermediate between these two is better than either extreme one. [*De compositione medicamentorum secundum locos*] V[.5].

(III.110) Do not cool nor restrain the tumor of erysipelas until you have evacuated the entire body through purgation of the abdomen with a drug which expels yellow bile. If you first chill and restrain and then evacuate the body, it often happens that the erysipelas is driven from the organ in which it resides to a principal organ—and this is very dangerous. *De methodo medendi* XIV[.3].

(III.111) The following matter is of great importance, and you must keep it in mind—namely, that a remedy composed with a certain goal and aim is often mixed with other ingredients which do not fit that goal, nor the intended use. But this remedy is mixed with other ingredients so that it will not cause any kind of pain or harm. [*De compositione medicamentorum secundum locos*] VII[.2].

(III.112) Says Moses: In this way, mastic—an astringent remedy—is added to purgatives in order to strengthen the cardia of the stomach and to suppress the urge which is caused by purgatives to vomit and throw up. Similarly, gum tragacanth is added to prevent possible harm caused to the intestines by colocynth.

(III.113) If someone's humors are thin and fine, and if he is close to fainting because of the dissolution of the pneuma which necessarily follows from the thinness of the humors, and if he has a tumor in his liver or stomach, then there is absolutely no cure for him nor remedy: his strength has collapsed, and feeding him in order to strengthen him is impossible because of the tumor. *De methodo medendi* XII[.6].

(III.114) It is impossible to compose a single remedy that can cure all ailing bodies; for difference in temperaments of bodies and difference in ages makes a large variety in medicines necessary. For this reason, one should have two medicines ready: One stronger than all the other medicines of the same kind, and the other weaker than all the others. These one should mix according to the need whenever one wishes. [*De compositione medicamentorum per genera*] III[.3].

(III.115) Sweat is something unnatural, because, when the body functions properly and when nature overpowers and overcomes the food, sweat is not emitted. *In Hippocratis Aphorismos commentarius* I[.15].

This is the end of the third treatise,
by the grace of God,
praise be to Him.

In the name of God,
the Merciful, the Compassionate.
O Lord, make our task easy

The Fourth Treatise

Containing aphorisms concerning the pulse and the prognostic signs to be derived from it

(IV.1) The existence of the pulse is vital and useful for two things. One of these, the most important, is the maintenance of the innate heat. The second is the generation of the pneuma. *De* [*praesagitione ex*] *puls*[*ibus* I.1].

(IV.2) The meaning of the concept of rhythm mentioned in the different types of the pulse is the ratio of the time of expansion of the arteries to the time of rest which follows, and also of the time of contraction of the arteries to the time of rest with follows. The proportion between these two times is without any doubt according to what is natural for each of the different ages of man. Sometimes it is according to its nature, and sometimes it is different. *De* [*differentia*] *pulsu*[*um*] I[.6].

(IV.3) Knowledge about the rhythm can be obtained through the strongest possible pulse only. In other types of pulse, the rhythm either cannot be grasped at all or is grasped far from correctly. *De* [*differentia*] *pulsu*[*um*] VII[.3].

(IV.4) A constant, truthful indicator of the strength of the animal faculty is a strong, equal pulse, and, similarly, a great pulse. *De* [*curandi ratione per*] *venae sectionem* [13].

(IV.5) The pulse of a newborn child is extremely rapid and frequent, while the pulse of old people is extremely slow and rare. The pulses normal for other ages fall between these two by gradation. In the prime of adolescence, the pulse is greatest and strongest. Its greatness and strength diminish gradually until, in old age, it is weakest and smallest. From the time of birth until the prime of adolescence, the pulse gradually increases in greatness and strength. *De* [*causis*] *pulsu*[*um*] XI[.5].

(IV.6) When rarity, weakness, or smallness of the pulse are at their absolute extreme, they are very dangerous, and those who have this pulse are in constant fear for their lives. This is not the case when greatness and strength of the pulse are at their maximum. When rapidity of the pulse is at its maximum, it is more safe and secure than when slowness is at its extreme. *De* [*praesagitione ex*] *puls*[*ibus* II.5].

(IV.7) A pulse that has an irregular inequality indicates that the cause of the inequality shifts from organ to organ and is not stable. It may shift to an inferior organ, so that the patient is spared. But it may also shift to a noble organ, leading to the patient's death. Therefore, one cannot use the irregularity of the inequality of the pulse as a genuine prognostic sign. *De* [*praesagitione ex*] *puls*[*ibus* II.13].

(IV.8) A regular unequal pulse that adheres to one pattern indicates that the cause of the inequality is stable and fixed. When it is the opposite of this, it is neither stable nor fixed. *De* [*causis*] *pulsu*[*um* II.14].

(IV.9) All the types of pulse which are unequal in more than one beat are the necessary result either of an irregular temperament of the heart or of an affliction occurring to the organ or to the faculty. *De* [*causis*] *pulsu*[*um* II.1].

(IV.10) When the faculty is weak in itself, it rarely makes a pulse unequal in its beats. But if the faculty is powerful in itself and is then burdened by a large amount of humors, the pulse becomes unequal in its beats. *De* [*causis*] *pulsu*[*um* II.1].

(IV.11) The first and lowest degree of weakness of the faculty makes the pulse smaller and fainter. The next degree of weakness is that in which one's fingers put on the artery are a burden for the faculty. It turns one's pulse into the recurrent one called "mouse tail." When the faculty is wasted and dissolved even more than this, it turns one's pulse into the permanent "mouse tail." *De* [*causis*] *pulsu*[*um* II.3].

(IV.12) A strong pulse always strikes a forceful beat. Similarly, a hard type of pulse strikes a forceful beat just like the vibratory and spasmodic pulses. *De* [*dignoscendis*] *puls*[*ibus* IV.1].

(IV.13) One never finds that the same pulse is very hard and at the same time very great. One also never finds that the same pulse is very great or very strong and at the same time slow. But in most cases one finds that the pulse which is very great is rapid and not slow. *De* [*dignoscendis*] *puls*[*ibus* I.5].

(IV.14) The pulse that is great, very strong, and hard, and, to the same extent, the pulse that combines hardness with extreme greatness, has a contraction that is clearer and more evident than that of any other pulse. The contraction of the faint pulse is unknown. There is no way to detect or perceive it, either in the beginning of the movement of the expansion or in the end of the movement of the contraction. *De* [*dignoscendis*] *puls*[*ibus* I.5, 9].

(IV.15) Every disease that changes the pulse into a spasmodic one, if it lasts and becomes more severe and more difficult, changes the pulse into a vermicular one. Every disease that changes the pulse into a rare one, if it becomes more severe and more serious and lasts for a long time, makes the pulse unequal, and it seems as if the body of the artery has fragmented and broken into separate, small pieces. *De pulsibus libellus* [*ad tirones* 12].

(IV.16) Inequality of the pulse is in most cases accompanied by irregularity; one hardly ever finds a regular unequal pulse. When an affliction is minor, it turns the pulse into a regular unequal one; and, when it is major, it turns the pulse into an irregular unequal one. *De pulsibus libellus* [*ad tirones* 12].

(IV.17) When the faculty is dissolved, it makes the pulse small, weak, and very spasmodic. When it is oppressed and burdened, it turns the pulse into an irregular unequal one. The greater the affliction, the more the different kinds of variation in pulse, especially in its strength and greatness. Inequality is in most cases followed by irregularity of the pulse. *De pulsibus libellus* [*ad tirones* 10–11].

(IV.18) Sometimes the temperament of the heart is warmer than is necessary and the temperament of the arteries colder than is necessary, or the reverse. Similarly, the body of the heart itself is sometimes cooler than its natural temperament, while the substance contained in the two ventricles of the heart is warmer; or the reverse may occur, in which case the pulse is similar to the natural pulse. These kinds of illnesses lead astray even skilled physicians—let alone other physicians—and cause them to commit mistakes. *De* [*praesagitione ex*] *puls*[*ibus* III.3].

(IV.19) A bad humor often collects in the cardia of the stomach and burns it or cools it, so that the pulse becomes small and unequal. The difference between burning and cooling is that the pulse becomes smaller as a result of cooling and it becomes more unequal as a result of burning. *De* [*differentiis*] *febrium* I[.9].

(IV.20) When biting, pain, pressure, vomiting, fainting, or hiccups occur at the cardia of the stomach, the pulse becomes very spasmodic, small, and weak, and sometimes also rapid. When the cardia of the stomach is compressed or squeezed by a large amount of food or by nonbiting humors streaming to it, the pulse becomes rare, slow, small, and weak. *De puls*[*ibus libellus ad tirones* 12].

(IV.21) If a varying bad temperament occurs in an artery, that part of it containing more moisture and heat has a pulse that is greater and more rapid, whereas the part which is either cold or dry has a pulse that is smaller and slower. *De* [*causis*] *pulsu*[*um* II.6].

(IV.22) In the beginning of all the putrefying fevers, the contraction of the artery is more rapid. This is a very reliable diagnostic sign. One should rely on it as a prognostic sign more than on any other sign. A similar thing happens to the pulse when the attacks of these fevers are increasing and intensifying. And, when they reach the state of their culmination, the movements of contraction and expansion of the pulse are less rapid. *De* [*praesagitione ex*] *puls*[*ibus* III.5].

(IV.23) If at any time during the beginning of a fever you find the pulse strong and great but not hard, that fever is not a hectic fever under any circumstances. For, when the pulse is strong and great but not hard, it is a clear sign that it is an ephemeral fever. But, when you find the pulse weak and small and the artery hard, it is a hectic fever. *De* [*praesagitione ex*] *puls*[*ibus* III.7].

(IV.24) If much cold matter reaches the heart during the beginning of a fever attack, the patient is in a state close to death. This state is indicated by a tremendous change of the pulse into rarity, slowness, and smallness. So, when these three conditions are followed by considerable weakness, the patient will die instantly. *De* [*praesagitione ex*] *puls*[*ibus* III.7].

(IV.25) The arteries which are closest to the diseased organ undergo the greatest change into softness or hardness of the pulse. The arteries which are far from the diseased organ do not change unless the heart mediates between them and the diseased organ. *De* [*praesagitione ex*] *puls*[*ibus* IV.9].

(IV.26) When the pulse beat of all the arteries is weak, the animal faculty is weak in itself because of the bad temperament of the body of the heart, as is well known. When it is weak in one organ of the body, that organ alone is the one with a bad temperament. If the same artery sometimes has a weak pulse beat and sometimes a strong one, the animal faculty is not weak in itself but is burdened and strangled by a large amount of superfluous matter. *De* [*praesagitione ex*] *puls*[*ibus* IV.12].

(IV.27) When the body of the heart itself becomes excessively cold or warm or moist or dry, in proportion to a bad temperament occurring to it, it makes the pulse weak and is an affliction affecting the faculty of the heart itself. When the blood and pneuma contained within the heart become hot or cold, or when the body of the pericardium or the body of the lung become hot or cold and that bad temperament passes to the heart but does not lodge in its body, nothing more happens than the necessary change in the pulse. The affliction does not affect the faculty of the heart. *De* [*praesagitione ex*] *puls*[*ibus* I.4].

(IV.28) When the blood or the pneuma enclosed by the body of the heart or the body of the pericardium or the lung change their temperament to dryness or moistness, their pulse does not necessarily change from what it was, because only heat and cold cause a necessary change. *De* [*praesagitione ex*] *puls*[*ibus* I.4].

(IV.29) In most conditions of a crisis of a disease, the arterial pulse is unequal, especially when the crisis goes with severe exhaustion. When the pulse is hard, it indicates vomiting. When the pulse is undulatory, it indicates sweat; when it is great but not undulatory, it indicates a hemorrhage, because it indicates a movement of nature toward the outside of the body through blood streaming from the nose or from other places. A high pulse and a strong pulse during a crisis are both signs of all kinds of evacuation. *De crisibus* III[.11].

(IV.30) When the heat of the body increases, the pulse changes first of all toward greatness. When the heat increases further, the pulse increases in rapidity together with greatness. When the heat increases even more than that, the pulse becomes more rapid and greater and also more spasmodic. When the body cools off, the first thing that can be noticed about the pulse is rarity, followed by slowness, and then, in the third place, by smallness. *De* [*causis*] *pulsu*[*um* I.7].

(IV.31) When the arteries are surrounded by things which press upon them and occupy the places of their expansion, be these things humors or tumors, the pulse beats will be unequal. Similarly, a large amount of blood discharged into the arteries or veins can make the pulse unequal in the same way. In general, where some sort of heavy pressure or of blockage happens to the arteries, the pulse will be unequal in its beat. *De* [*causis*] *pulsu*[*um* II.2].

(IV.32) Softness of an organ causes greatness of the pulse, and the domination of cold over the body causes smallness of the pulse. Sometimes the degree of smallness caused by the cold and the degree of greatness caused by the softness of the organ are similar, so that the pulse stays moderate. Similarly, if each of the two causes which change the pulse are equal in strength, the pulse will be moderate. In the case of someone who is ill and in this condition, one might think that his pulse is still in its natural condition. However, this is not so, because every natural pulse is moderate between two extremes, but not every moderate pulse is natural. *De* [*causis*] *pulsu*[*um* I.9].

(IV.33) As the undulatory pulse, when it becomes small and light and little, is followed by the vermicular one, so the vermicular pulse, when most of its motions stop and only one motion is left, is followed by the ant-like pulse, which is a very small motion similar to the crawling of an ant. It is actually unequal, but because it is so small the senses cannot distinguish its inequality. This pulse is extremely small, weak, and spasmodic; there is no pulse which is smaller, weaker, or more spasmodic. One may think that it is rapid, but it is not rapid in reality. *De* [*differentia*] *pulsu*[*um*] I[.26].

(IV.34) The dissolution of the faculty is in most cases followed first by the vermicular pulse and then by the ant-like pulse. When the faculty is dissolved without fever or with a light fever, it is especially followed by the vermicular pulse, and it remains so for a long time. *De pulsibus libellus* [*ad tirones* 11].

(IV.35) Sometimes the pulse hardens in the case of ephemeral fever, putrefying fever, or hectic fever; this is caused by one of those things which harden the pulse, but not by the fever. For fever itself—in its capacity of fever—does not necessarily accompany a hard pulse under all circumstances. But the pulse is in most cases found to be hard in the case of hectic fever. *De* [*differentiis*] *febrium* I[.9].

One may think that the pulse of those suffering from spasms is strong and great, while in reality it is neither weak, nor strong, nor small, nor great. Its tension may give the impression of strength, and because of its trembling motion one may imagine that it jumps and rises very much. *De puls*[*ibus libellus ad tirones* 11].

(IV.36) Internal rest of the artery can never be known for certain, but it is possible to perceive it by means of firm palpation when the pulse is very strong.

Do not palpate an artery firmly in any kind of pulse, except for the strong pulse only. But also in this case, one should not palpate so firmly that the strength of the artery is overwhelmed. *De* [*dignoscendis*] *puls*[*ibus* I.11].

(IV.37) When the faculty is powerful and the body of the artery is hard and the need is urgent, the pulse will be vibratory. When one of these factors is missing, the pulse will not be vibratory. *De* [*causis*] *pulsu*[*um* II.6].

(IV.38) When the faculty becomes very weak, not only does it make the pulse weak, but also small and, because of its smallness, dense. When the faculty becomes powerful, it makes the pulse strong and great; if the need does not change at all, it also makes it very rare. *De* [*praesagitione ex*] *puls*[*ibus* I.7].

(IV.39) The vermicular pulse is caused by weakness of the faculty. The undulatory pulse is caused by an excess of moisture and sometimes by extreme softness of the organ (arteries). *De* [*causis*] *pulsu*[*um* II.8].

(IV.40) Something that every unequal pulse has in common is that it is caused either by obstructions, or by pressure which occurs to an organ, or by an amount of humors greater than the measure of the faculty, or by an unequal bad temperament of the heart. Inequality in one kind of pulse is more serious and difficult than when it occurs in many kinds of pulses. A weak pulse does not indicate anything other than a bad temperament of the heart. It is only necessarily followed by inequality of the pulse when it is joined by one of the three other causes mentioned previously. *De* [*praesagitione ex*] *puls*[*ibus* II.4].

(IV.41) Ascites is caused by moisture collecting in the abdomen, whereby the vessels widen and cool off. In this case, the pulse tends toward hardness and becomes small and dense, especially when it is accompanied by fever. Dropsy of the flesh (anasarca) makes the pulse undulatory because it moistens all the hard organs (arteries) of the body and soaks them. *De* [*causis*] *pulsu*[*um* IV.24].

(IV.42) I do not know anyone who was saved from pleurisy when his pulse was extremely hard, small, and very dense. *De* [*praesagitione ex*] *puls*[*ibus* IV.5].

(IV.44) Do not imagine the movement of the artery in three dimensions as a movement in a cubic body or a cone or a similar body, but think of it as a singular movement and a singular rotation, as the movement of a sphere; for the movement of the artery as it appears to the senses is that of a perfect rotation. *De* [*dignoscendis*] *puls*[*ibus* III.2].

(IV.45) The pulse is never extremely slow and small as long as the faculty is strong, even if the need for it has become extremely slight. *De* [*causis*] *pulsu*[*um* I.7].

(IV.46) A pulse with a double beat (dicrotic pulse) is sometimes caused by an extremely bad temperament and a slight hardness of an artery, and sometimes by extreme hardness of an artery with weakness of the faculty, or thickness and abundance of the humors. *De* [*causis*] *pulsu*[*um* II.6].

(IV.47) The pulse is natural when the faculty is in a balanced condition and protected from being moved by either an excessive fullness of the organ (arteries) or its obstruction or compression by something else. *De* [*causis*] *pulsu*[*um* II.6].

(IV.48) An unequal bad temperament of the organ (arteries) makes the pulse fragmented. *De* [*causis*] *pulsu*[*um* I.7].

This is the end of the fourth treatise,
by the grace of God,
praise be to Him.

In the name of God,
the Merciful, the Compassionate.
O Lord, make our task easy

The Fifth Treatise

Containing aphorisms concerning the prognostic signs to be derived from the urine

(v.1) In all the fevers, one should above all examine and inspect the urine, because fevers are illnesses in the veins. In the case of pleurisy, one should first of all inspect the sputum and then the urine, because pleurisy does not occur without fever. When there is an illness in the abdomen accompanied by fever, one should first of all inspect the excrements and then the urine; and, if there is no fever, one should examine only the excrements. *De crisibus* I[.7].

(v.2) The best sediment which descends with the urine in the case of putrefying fevers is that which comes from the putrefying humor when it is cocted in the vessel containing it. The resulting sediment which settles in the urine is white, smooth, and even and has a smell which is not unpleasant. *De [differentiis] febrium* I[.8].

(v.3) If the parts of the urine are all even in color and consistency, it indicates the domination and supremacy of nature over the illness. When bubbles of gassy spirit accumulate in the urine, it is caused by a cold humor and therefore indicates that the illness will be prolonged. *In Hippocratis Aphorismos commentarius* [VIII.33, 34].

(v.4) The best urine in ill people is that which is most similar to the urine of healthy people. The urine which has been cocted extremely well and which comes from someone who is extremely healthy is the urine which is even in its thickness and tends toward yellowness with a little bit of redness. It tends more to being completely yellow, as is the case if one were to take water and mix it with some of the watery part of the blood and yellow bile. *De crisibus* I[.12].

(v.5) The best kind of urine is that which has a good color and a cloud which is white, smooth, and even. If the cloud settles to the bottom of a bottle, it is the best; if it is suspended in the middle, it is second best; and if it floats on the urine, it is third best. These are the three kinds which indicate coction. Of all the other kinds of urine which remain, some indicate the opposite of coction, and others indicate death. *De crisibus* I[.12].

(v.6) The evenness of a sediment is subject to two kinds of conditions. The first is that it should not be scattered and dispersed but combined, and the second that it should remain so all the time. For sometimes one finds the urine clear at one time but with a sediment at another time, and a laudable sediment does not appear continuously. This is a sign that the coction was not completed. *De crisibus* I[.12].

(V.7) The best urine of ill people is that which, when excreted, shows a laudable sediment with perfect characteristics, for this indicates that nature has overcome the illness and has begun to expel the humor causing the illness. The second-best urine is that which is turbid when it is excreted but in which, shortly after its excretion, a laudable sediment is deposited, for this indicates that nature has begun its work and will soon complete it. The third-best urine is that which is turbid when it is excreted but then becomes clear, with no sediment deposited in it, for this indicates that the time of the coction is still far away, although nature has begun to desire it. *De crisibus* I[.12].

(V.8) Someone who is afflicted by fever because of ease of life, rest, and overeating unavoidably deposits much sediment in his urine. But as for those who are afflicted by fever because of taking a small amount of food and because of exertion, their illness often terminates without anything settling in their urine. A sufficient indication for coction is the appearance of a white, smooth, even cloud on top of the urine or suspended in its middle. *De crisibus* I[.12].

(V.9) When diseases originate from crude humors, there is much sediment in the urine. When they originate from bilious humors, there is no sediment at all or only a small amount. *In Hippocratis Prognostica commentarius* II[.26].

(V.10) The worst urine for ill people is the one that is thin and clear, that truly resembles water and persists in that resemblance, and is as far as possible from being cocted. Second in bad quality is the urine which is thin and clear when it is excreted but then becomes turbid after a short time, for this indicates that nature, although it has not yet started its work, will soon do so. Third in bad quality is the urine which is excreted turbid and stays like that, for this indicates that nature has begun to desire the coction but has not yet processed anything. *De crisibus* I[.12].

(V.11) Among the kidney ailments is one in which the patient urinates thin, watery fluid similar to the excrement discharged in the beginning of a liver affection. This discharge is a bit more like blood than that first mentioned. *De locis affectis* VI[.3].

(v.12) If the diarrhea is of the type of the bilious humor and is oily, it indicates the melting of the fat through the heat of the fever. If the urine is oily and its color and consistency are like the color and consistency of olive oil, it is an indication of death, because it comes from the melting of the flesh; for the heat which melts the flesh is stronger than the heat which melts the fat. *In Hippocratis Epidemiarum* [*commentarius*] III.3.

(v.13) When urine resembling water is micturated quickly, it is the disease called diabetes. This urine is the worst of the uncocted urines; and it indicates, as it were, the death of two of the natural faculties—namely, the alterative and retentive faculties. *De crisibus* I[.12].

(v.14) A black sediment indicates either fiery heat or extreme cold, which result in a condition similar to the death of the natural faculties. A lead-colored sediment originates from cold alone. *De crisibus* I[.12].

(v.15) Any urine that turns black is so extremely malignant that I do not know anyone who has micturated black urine and survived. But a black sediment indicates a less serious threat of death. If there is a black cloud in the middle of the urine, it indicates a less serious threat of death than a black sediment. And a black cloud floating on top of the urine is a less serious indication of death than that suspended in the middle of the urine. *De crisibus* I[.12].

(v.16) If urine that is as white and fine as water has a cloud floating on top of it, or if it has a black sediment or what appears to be dark sediment, or if it contains particles similar to cereal or flakes, all of these are fatal signs. Similarly, urine with a terrible smell and fatty urine which is called oily are both fatal. These urines indicate that the illness is of a very serious nature. *De totius morbi temporibus* [6].

(v.17) Any color of the urine apart from white, yellow, and red is a sign of death. Similarly, anything which appears in the urine apart from a sediment or a cloud in a suspended or floating state—all three of which are laudable—is either a bad or a fatal sign. *De crisibus* I[.12].

(v.18) If the illness is prolonged and slow to move and the patient passes thin urine for a long time, the crisis usually comes with an abscess. If he passes much urine which is thick and contains a laudable sediment deposited in it, it is most likely that the illness will coct gradually and that there will not be a crisis with an abscess. *De crisibus* III[.11].

(V.19) If there appear in the urine white particles similar to particles of bitter vetch or of lentils, it indicates that they come from the liver. If these particles are similar to flesh, it indicates that they come from the kidneys; and, if they are similar to flakes, it indicates that they come from the urinary bladder. Particles which are similar to cereal in size and hardness and are not white indicate dissolution in the flesh of the organs. Black particles indicate dissolution in the flesh of the spleen. Oily urine indicates dissolution of the fat. Urine similar to that of animals indicates a large amount of crude matter. *In Hippocratis Epidemiarum* [*commentarius*] VI.5.

(V.20) Says Moses: Galen's words in *De crisibus* can be summarized to this effect: The best urine of ill people is the one in which—when micturated—a laudable sediment is seen. This one is called the first because nature has completed its activity and cocted the illness-producing matter. Second best is the urine which is turbid when it is micturated and becomes clear once it is micturated while a laudable sediment settles in it, for this indicates that nature has started its work and will soon finish it. This is the second-best urine. The third-best urine is the one which is turbid when it is micturated and then becomes clear without a sediment settling in it, for this indicates that nature has started its work but has not approached the time of coction. This is the third-best urine. The fourth-best urine is the one which is turbid when it is micturated and then stays turbid, for this one is even further away from coction than the previous urine. This is the fourth-best urine. The fifth-best is the urine which is micturated clear and thin and then becomes turbid, for this indicates that nature has not yet begun its work but will shortly do so. The worst urine is that which is micturated thin and then remains that way, for this indicates a total absence of coction, both in the present condition and in the near future.

This is the end of the fifth treatise,
by the grace of God,
praise be to Him.

In the name of God,
the Merciful, the Compassionate.
O Lord, make our task easy

The Sixth Treatise

Containing aphorisms concerning the other prognostic signs

(VI.1) One can predict whether an apoplexy will be severe and necessarily fatal or weak and curable—though it is difficult—from the condition of the respiration. For when the movement of the respiration is totally missing, so that it cannot be noticed, it is the fastest killing kind of apoplexy there is. When the patient breathes with difficulty and strain, the apoplexy is also severe and deadly, but to a lesser degree than the first. If the patient breathes without strain and difficulty but in an irregular and disordered way, the apoplexy is still severe but less so than the previous example. And when his respiration is to some extent orderly—although irregular—and is unstrained, the apoplexy is weak and can be cured if proper procedure is followed. *In Hippocratis Aphorismos commentarius* II[.42].

(VI.2) Cessation of respiration occurs either from the weakness of the power which moves the chest or from a severe cold that overpowers the brain. *In Hippocratis Aphorismos commentarius* IV[.34].

(VI.3) When mental confusion results from heat but without superfluous matter, it is similar to the mental confusion caused by drinking wine. When it results from yellow bile, it is accompanied by worry and fear. When the yellow bile becomes increasingly burnt, the confusion turns into madness. *In Hippocratis Aphorismos commentarius* VI[.53].

(VI.4) Sneezing in the case of chronic diseases, except for diseases of the chest and lungs, is a good sign because it indicates coction and great strength of the expulsive faculty of the brain. *In Hippocratis Prognostica commentarius* II[.39].

(VI.5) A special symptom for the kind of overfilling that is commensurate to strength is weight, and a special symptom for the kind of overfilling that is commensurate to the vessels is stretching. *De* [*curandi ratione per*] *venae sectione*[*m* 7].

(VI.6) Sometimes the outer vessels are full and stretched while the inner ones are not, as happens when it is hot and when one takes a bath in hot water. At other times the outer vessels are empty while the inner vessels are full, as happens when it is extremely cold. Fullness of the outer vessels, then, is only an indication of an excess of blood when two conditions are fulfilled:

1. The temperatures of the inside and the outside of the body are equal and
2. no unusual heat such as, for instance, ardent fever pervades the body. *De plenitudine* [10].

(VI.7) Four different types of biting chymes occur in our bodies. The type from which itch develops is only slightly biting. A more biting type is the one that produces shivering. The one that is extremely biting causes rigor, and the one that is even more biting causes a sensation of ulceration. *De plenitudine* [8].

(VI.8) Says Moses: Consider how only the different degrees of sharpness of the humor are turned by Galen into that which forms the difference between itch, shivering, and rigor. There is another distinction between these diseases that he makes in his treatise *De tremore, palpitatione, rigore et convulsione*. I do not say that what he said here is contrary to what he said there. Rather, both statements are true, and by combining them one obtains a complete picture of what he means—namely, that the places where the biting chyme affects the body vary according to the strength or weakness of the pungency of the chyme. In his *De tremore, palpitatione,* [*rigore et convulsion* 6], he explains that in the case of shivering, the biting humor is confined to the skin alone, while that which produces rigor is in all the parts beneath the skin, and this is correct. We should also understand from his statement that itch occurs in the upper layers of the skin and not in those that are adjacent to the flesh.

(VI.9) When sweet phlegm increases in a man's body, he sleeps much. When acid phlegm increases, he suffers from hunger. When salty phlegm becomes dominant, he suffers from thirst. When raw phlegm becomes dominant, it stops the thirst. *De plenitudine* [10].

(VI.10) Pus is formed when innate heat overwhelms those humors in order to coct and transform them. At that time an extremely severe pain arises and sometimes even fever. When the fever is already there, it rises. When the pus is expelled, the organ becomes completely healthy again, as it was before. When the innate heat disappears and becomes weak and does not want at all to coct those humors because of its weakness, no pus originates in the organ and no considerable pain nor fever develops. Rather, it becomes putrefied and corrupted to such a degree that one is often forced to cut the corrupted part off completely. So it may occur with someone that the fever dies away once fatal signs appear in him and there is no indication of improvement. *In Hippocratis Epidemiarum* [*commentarius*] III.1.

(VI.11) Sometimes melancholic delusion and phrenitis occur together. An indication of this is that at one time someone suffering from it talks continually, for this is a symptom of phrenitis, while at another time he is continually silent, for this is a symptom of melancholic delusion. *In Hippocratis Epidemiarum* [*commentarius*] III.3.

(VI.12) A surplus of watery moisture is expelled in one of three ways: through diarrhea, through the urine, or through the sweat. It is expelled by nature in whatever way she prefers, to the exclusion of the other two ways. Therefore, when the feces are retained and the urine is withheld while the crisis of the disease is near, the patient is necessarily afflicted by rigor followed by sweating. *In Hippocratis Epidemiarum* [*commentarius*] VI.1.

(VI.13) The secretion that dries up on the eyes from conjunctivitis and the sweat that dries up on the face until it becomes like dust are bad signs. Similarly, darkening of vision in acute diseases indicates that the faculty of vision is perishing. *In Hippocratis Epidemiarum* [*commentarius*] VI.1.

(VI.14) When the signs are very bad—whether symptoms or diseases—but the face is fine, very similar to its natural condition, it is a good sign. When the signs are minor—whether symptoms or diseases—and the face is very different from its natural condition, it is a bad sign. *In Hippocratis Epidemiarum* [*commentarius*] VI.[1–8].

(VI.15) There is no person suffering from melancholy who does not fear something that is not frightening or who does not have an imaginary fear of something that is not frightening. When the affliction is mild, he is only afraid of one thing; but when it is more severe, he is afraid of two or three things. And some are afraid of everything because of the severity of the affliction. *In Hippocratis Epidemiarum* [*commentarius*] VI.[1–8].

(VI.16) In his treatise *Quod animi mores corporis temperatura sequantur*, Galen has mentioned that the word "melancholy" means "fear" in the Greek language.

(VI.17) When a nosebleed occurs while one is in a healthy condition, it is a sign of bad blood. In this case one should provide the body with good blood by means of fattening kinds of food that do not fill the vessels, such as starch (amylum), emmer wheat (*khandarūs*), milk, young cheese, meat of piglets, lambs, and kid. Sometimes a nosebleed occurs when one is healthy because of an excess of blood. *In Hippocratis Epidemiarum* [*commentarius*] VI.3.

(VI.18) The eyes give a most correct and certain indication of the strength of the body, when one opens them and looks at them with regard to its state of health. *In Hippocratis Epidemiarum* [*commentarius*] VI.4.

(VI.19) The colors of the tongue indicate the dominating chyme in the region of the stomach. The colors of the urine indicate the dominating chyme in the vessels in the regions of the liver, kidneys, and urinary bladder. A dry tongue—that is, a tongue dominated by severe dryness, indicates that ardent fever has burnt the blood. *In Hippocratis Epidemiarum* [*commentarius*] VI.5.

(VI.20) Fat and sweet foods are only enjoyable to a healthy person. Sick people enjoy the rest of the foods apart from these two, commensurate with their illness. *In Hippocratis Epidemiarum* [*commentarius*] VI.5.

(VI.21) Perspiration on the forehead, neck, and chest area indicates weakness of the animal faculty. Frequent dyspepsias and the consumption of things that are partly putrefied and of coarse bread produce abdominal worms. *In Hippocratis Epidemiarum* [*commentarius*] VI.7.

(VI.22) Sometimes physicians are mistaken by thinking that the blood has increased in the body, while in reality it has not increased. Rather, because of the heat of the air, or anger, or fever, something happens to it that is similar to the high tide of the sea. Conversely, they sometimes think that the blood has diminished, while in reality it has not diminished. Rather, because of the cold that pushes the blood inwards, something happens to it that is similar to the low tide of the sea. *In Hippocratis De humoribus commentarius* I[.1].

(VI.23) Black bile is a very deadly sign when it appears in the spittle, vomit, urine, or excrements. After it in danger comes yellow bile when it appears pure. The other humors are less dangerous when they appear in a pure form in one of these excretions. *In Hippocratis De humoribus commentarius* II[.1].

(VI.24) If a growth appears on the tongue similar to the black seed of the castor oil plant, the patient will not survive to the second day. If a black tumor similar to the seed of the bitter vetch appears on the fingers of the hands in combination with any fever and severe pain, the patient will die on the fourth day. *De signis mortis*.

(VI.25) Black chymes are often excreted with vomiting or diarrhea, and this can in some cases be a good sign. But when black bile is excreted with vomiting or diarrhea, it indicates death; its development in the body is a fatal sign, since it originates from the burning of the turbid and residual part of the blood. When it originates from the burning of yellow bile, the damage to the organs is even worse because it corrodes them. It is the clearest sign of impending death. *De atra bile* [3].

(VI.26) If someone has long experience with these two chymes, he will easily understand the reason why the excretion of black bile from the body indicates impending death. Someone who is inexperienced will either be amazed, or he will not believe it and say: How can the excretion of something that is extremely harmful have a fatal effect on the body? *De atra bile* [3].

(VI.27) When the disease is stronger than the strength of the patient, he will most certainly die. One can take as an indication the observation of increasing signs of the lack of coction day by day. The more one looks closely into the disease, the more fatal signs will appear. *De morborum temporibus*.

(VI.28) It is impossible at any time that a sign becomes visible that indicates coction but does not indicate something very good. When the flow of blood from a site in the body, perspiration, and tumors occur at the proper time, the body may benefit from it, but otherwise not. *De crisibus* I[.7].

(VI.29) Signs of coction indicate that the patient will recover and do not necessarily indicate that a crisis will befall him, because the illness will dissolve slowly. *De crisibus* I[.7].

(VI.30) The superfluity in each part of the body indicates its condition. When it is cocted, it indicates that it is healthy; and when it is not cocted, it indicates that it is ill. The urine indicates the coction in the vessels, the excrements indicate the coction in the abdomen, and the sputum indicates the coction in the respiratory organs. *De crisibus* I[.7].

(VI.31) To lie on one's back and to open one's mouth, which are the only ways through which snoring takes place, indicate weakness or drunkenness or relaxation. *De motu musculorum* [II.4].

(VI.32) The madness occurring from melancholic humor is not as bad as that arising from the burning of bilious humor. Phlegmatic humor does not cause any madness at all. *In Hippocratis Aphorismos commentarius* VI[.56].

(VI.33) When the substance of the brain is dominated by the humor that results from the burning of yellow bile, delusion and delirium associated with fever arise from it. The delirium that occurs at the climax of ardent fevers is caused by hot vapors arising to the brain. *De locis affectis* III[.9].

(VI.34) If someone is affected by vertigo and dizziness, he blacks out and falls down on minor occasions when he is turned around. If someone is affected by vertigo or dizziness that originates from the cardia of the stomach, it is preceded by palpitation and nausea. *De locis affectis* III[.12].

(VI.35) Some of those who suffer from migraine feel the sensation of the pain on the outside of the skull, while others feel it deep inside the head. The pain of those suffering from migraine ends at the line that separates the two halves of the head. When the pain originates from wind, it comes necessarily with tension; if it originates from bilious superfluities, the patient feels a sharp pain. When it arises from an excess of humors, he has a feeling of heaviness next to the pain. When the feeling of heaviness is combined with a red complexion and heat, then those excessive humors are hot; but when it is not accompanied by redness and heat, those excessive humors are not hot. *De locis affectis* III[.13].

(VI.36) The movement of the tongue comes from the seventh pair of cranial nerves. When an affliction occurs to both the right part and the left part of the brain at the origin of this seventh pair, the patient is in danger of suffering a stroke. When one part of it is afflicted, the patient will suffer from paralysis. This paralysis will harm the movement of one half of the tongue and it may also harm other parts of the body beneath the head at different times. *De locis affectis* IV[.3].

(VI.37) The signs of phrenitis are sixteen: sleeplessness or disturbed sleep, delirium manifesting itself gradually, acute fever which never subsides, short-term memory loss, lack of thirst, very aggressive and insolent behavior shown by the patient, deep and intermittent respiration, a small and hard pulse, picking flocks from garments or straw from walls, roughness of the tongue, pain in the back of the head, a dry discharge from the eyes and an acid tear streaming from one eye, drops of blood dripping from the nose, acoustic hallucinations, loss of the sensation of touch throughout the body even when one is touched with force, and the patient lies prostrate and is unresponsive to questions. All these symptoms can occur simultaneously, but sometimes only a majority thereof. *De locis affectis* V[.4].

(VI.38) If a nosebleed comes from the side opposite to where the illness is, it is a bad sign. But if it comes from the same side as the illness, it is a good sign. *De crisibus* III[.11].

(VI.39) Just as those animals and plants which grow more rapidly have a shorter life span and those which grow more slowly have a longer life span, so too is the situation regarding fevers and tumors and all other occurrences. That which develops faster is of shorter duration. *In Hippocratis Epidemiarum* [*commentarius* I.3].

(VI.40) In some acute diseases, bad humors stream to the lungs in such a small quantity that they do not cause any tumors, and they are excreted with the sputum. Someone with no experience will think that the patient suffers from pleurisy or pneumonia, but this is not the case. *In Hippocratis Epidemiarum* [*commentarius*] III[.3].

(VI.41) A malignant cough is one whose cause is either a catarrh which descends from the head, or an ulcer or an abscess in one of the respiratory organs, or matter collecting in the chest. A benign cough originates either from a bad temperament of the respiratory organs or from roughness of the pharynx or trachea. In the case of fevers, when the benign cough is very strong, it heats the sides of the chest and lungs and increases the strength of the fever and the severity of the thirst. But when the cough is weak and occurs only at long intervals, it stimulates the organs to attract a moderate quantity of fine moisture, which diminishes the thirst and the heat of the fever. *In Hippocratis Epidemiarum* [*commentarius*] VI.2.

(VI.42) It has been clarified that bad respiration associated with the movement of all the muscles of the chest and the intercostal muscles has three causes: either a weakness of the power that moves the muscles of the chest, or a narrowing in the respiratory organs, or heat dominating the heart and the lungs. If the only cause is the domination of heat, the respiration is rapid, strong, and frequent while the air is expelled in puffs of boiling hot air. If the only cause is the weakness of the power which moves the muscles of the chest, the respiration is neither rapid nor frequent, the air is expelled through the mouth without any puffs whatsoever, and during inhalation one can see the two sides of the nostrils which are called "leaves" contract. This is a strong indication of the weakness of the power. If the only cause is the narrowing in the respiratory organs, one can see the chest expand greatly, and during the expansion, the respiration is rapid and frequent, although the air is expelled freely without puffs. *De locis affectis* IV[.7].

(VI.43) When a usual or unusual bad temperament occurs in the lungs, it causes cough. If the regular bad temperament is insignificant, it changes the rhythm of the respiration. But when it is severe and hot, it causes a desire to inhale cold air and to drink something cold. When this lasts for a long time, it causes fever. A cold bad temperament is followed by a desire for hot air and hot drinks as long as it is insignificant. But when it gets worse, the lungs are filled with matter. *De locis affectis* IV[.11].

(VI.44) The indications of the culmination of pleurisy are that the pain is chronic and that it is not assuaged by the application of warm compresses. Indications of a severe and malignant pleurisy are that the sputum increases in viscosity and that it cannot be expelled because it adheres to the diseased organs and is stuck in them. *In Hippocratis De acutorum morborum* [*victu commentarius*] I[.32].

(VI.45) If someone resembles a person suffering from dropsy in his nature, he is quickly affected by this disease. Similarly, if someone resembles a person suffering from phthisis, soon he will suffer from it, and someone who resembles a person suffering from delusion rapidly develops this disease. This type of analogy can be applied to any disease and to respiratory afflictions, as in the case of someone who moves fast and who acts like a fool, for he quickly falls into a delirium. *In Hippocratis Epidemiarum* [*commentarius*] VI.7.

(VI.46) He also said in *In Hippocratis Epidemiarum commentarius* III.3: light-witted, troubled, and foolish people become delirious for the slightest reason. But someone with the opposite nature only suffers from delirium through a major cause.

(VI.47) If someone suffers from a tumor in the liver, his complexion is pale and green. If someone has a tumor in the spleen, his complexion is green and dark. If someone has a tumor in the lungs, his complexion is pale and faded. But this will only be the case if these tumors are not inflamed. *In Hippocratis De humoribus commentarius* III[.25].

(VI.48) If someone has hiccups accompanied by tumors in the liver, or if someone cannot sleep and suffers from tremors, or if someone suffering from dropsy is affected by cough, he will die. But if someone suffering from hiccups is affected by spontaneous strong sneezing, his hiccups will stop. *De signis mortis*.

(VI.49) A bad temperament of the heart occurs in one of two ways: either in the moistures specific to the heart or in its solid substance itself. A bad temperament of the moistures is accompanied by palpitation of the entire heart. A bad temperament of the solid heart substance itself is free from palpitation. *De* [*praesagitione ex*] *puls*[*ibus* III.4].

(VI.50) Marasmus is mostly caused by inflamed tumors in the liver and stomach when not treated properly. *De febri*[*um differentiis*] I[.12].

(VI.51) An ulcer in the lungs called phthisis causes the nails to become curved as a bow. When the tongue becomes black, it indicates ardent fever. The particular discoloration indicating weakness of the liver is different from the particular discoloration caused by a disease of the spleen. *De locis affectis* I[.5].

(VI.52) The indications of hypochondriac melancholia are that the ingestion of food is followed by sour eructations, watery sputum in large quantity, a burning sensation in the hypochondrium and a gurgling sound not occurring until one hour after the ingestion of food. Despondency and sadness also occur while the mind is affected by something similar to melancholic delusion. Some of these patients develop severe abdominal pains, which in a few of them extend to the back. Others vomit their food after some time or the next day. They only find relief through emesis or evacuation of the bowels or a good digestion. *De locis affectis* III[.10].

(VI.53) Contraction of the hypochondrium is a special sign of an inflammation of the diaphragm and appears from the very beginning. Similarly, when phrenitis has been established, the hypochondrium contracts in the very end. During an inflammation of the diaphragm, respiration is variable; sometimes it is shallow and frequent, and at other times it is deep and similar to groaning. *De locis affectis* V[.4].

(VI.54) The symptoms which always accompany pleurisy are five in number:

1. acute fever,
2. goading pain in the side,
3. shallow and frequent respiration,
4. serrated pulse, and
5. cough, mostly accompanied by colored sputum.

A patient suffering from this disease may also cough without sputum. This indicates either imminent death or a prolonged illness. *De locis affectis* V[.3].

(VI.55) There are eight symptoms of an inflammation in the liver:

1. burning fever,
2. severe thirst,
3. a total lack of appetite,
4. a tongue which becomes initially red and then black,
5. vomiting of bile which initially has the color of yolks and then turns verdigris green,
6. a pain in the right side which extends to the collarbone, especially when the hypochondrium is pulled upwards, and occasionally the patient has
7. a mild cough and a sensation of heaviness inherent to the right side, and he often complains of
8. pain in the ribs of the back if the liver is in its natural structure attached to those ribs.

If the liver itself is not weakened by the inflammation, the patient suffers from constipation. *De locis affectis* V[.7].

(VI.56) Everyone I observed as suffering from a painful illness of the esophagus would feel the pain between his shoulders. The reason for this is that the esophagus stretches along the spinal column. *De locis affectis* V[.5].

(VI.57) Sometimes an inflammation begins on the convex side of the liver, whereas at other times it begins on the concave side. When it begins on the convex side, it causes so much pain and provokes so much cough that the patient feels as if his collarbone is pulled down. When the inflammation begins on the concave side of the liver, the lack of appetite, severe thirst, throwing up of bile, and nausea it causes are worse than the problems caused by an inflammation on the convex side. *De locis affectis* V[.7].

(VI.58) When the liver becomes ill because of a cold bad temperament, it often begins without fever at the time when serous, thin blood is excreted with the excrements. When this lasts for a long time, it is followed by fevers because the blood of the liver is corrupted. Someone who is neither familiar with this disease nor experienced in it may think lightly of these fevers or suppose that the patient has no fever at all. *De locis affectis* V[.8].

(VI.59) The disease which causes headache is sometimes in all the parts of the head outside the skull and sometimes in all the parts within the skull. But it may also be in only one of those parts, namely, the pulsatile vessels, or the nonpulsatile vessels, or the nerves, or the membranes, or the skin. It may even be in the brain substance itself. To determine the exact location of the disease is very difficult and only possible for someone who has personally dealt with it and observed it many times. [*De compositione medicamentorum secundum locos*] II[.1].

(VI.60) A stabbing pain is that which begins from its root and then rapidly passes to the area surrounding that root. This happens in those pains which are extremely severe and strong, such as one-sided headache and inveterate headache. Nerve pains stretch lengthwise all the way from the origin to the end of the nerve, and the patient feels the pain deep in his body. When the pain is in the membrane that lies under the skin and can be stripped off with it, it causes a tensive numb pain. *De locis affectis* II[.8].

(VI.61) Pains in the membranes surrounding the bones are felt by someone suffering from them deep inside. It seems to him that the pain is in his very bones. Some people call these pains "bone-piercing." These pains result mostly from physical exercise. *De locis affectis* II[.8].

(VI.62) If someone suffers from pain which only occurs in a pulsatile vessel or non-pulsatile vessel, it seems to him that it is a pain of something that is being stretched, such as a string. But pain of the flesh does not extend over a great distance. *De locis affectis* II[.8].

(VI.63) Cold sweat cannot possibly come from sites with high fevers because, had it come from there, it would be hot because of the fever. Rather, it comes from sites that have cooled off because the innate heat has become weak or nearly extinguished. Therefore, it is a sign of imminent death or of a prolonged illness. But it only indicates a prolonged illness when a large quantity of cold moistures dominates the body. *In Hippocratis Aphorismos commentarius* IV[.37].

(VI.64) A frequent occurrence of rigor during a fever is a fatal sign because it shakes the body so much that the body's strength dwindles, irrespective of whether evacuation follows thereafter or not. *In Hippocratis Aphorismos commentarius* IV[.46].

(VI.65) Sweat tastes salty with healthy people and tastes the same with ill persons. But in the latter case the saltiness undergoes a minor change and tends towards the taste of the dominating humor which caused the disease. *In Hippocratis Epidemiarum* [*commentarius* I.3].

(VI.66) The main thing to do if one wants to make a diagnosis of the diseased spots of the hypochondrium when they are tense is to palpate them so that you will know whether there is an inflamed swelling or a hard swelling or flatulence or pus or much feces. When one has diagnosed the illness in the hypochondrium, one should apply oneself to dissolve it. *In Hippocratis Epidemiarum* [*commentarius* I.3].

(VI.67) Loss of appetite is sometimes caused by too much humor in the cardia of the stomach or by the humor's bad quality or by the loss of strength in the stomach. When the nature of the liver is harmed, the loss of appetite can be so severe that the patient would rather die than taste something. *In Hippocratis Epidemiarum* [*commentarius*] III.1.

(VI.68) The most benign tumors are those that tend mostly to go outwards; then follow the ones which have a pointed head; then the ones with a less pointed head. Also benign are tumors which tend downwards and those that do not have two heads. Those tumors, which are the absolute opposite to these, are all of the worst kind. The most benign suppurating tumors are those which suppurate evenly and are not very hard. *In Hippocratis Epidemiarum* [*commentarius*] VI.1.

(VI.69) In most chronic diseases the fingers turn cold. But in hectic fevers they stay warm. Because of the small quantity of flesh on the fingers, the heat which is firmly established in the elementary parts appears in them. *In Hippocratis Prognostica commentarius* [II.60].

(VI.70) If someone suffers from a spasm as a result of a blow or from the ingestion of a purgative, he will die. If someone has a spasm in the front and back of the body and then has to laugh, he will die on the spot. *De signis mortis.*

(VI.71) If someone with an intestinal ulcer suffers from severe thirst and gets a black pustule resembling a bitter vetch kernel behind the ears, he will die. When chyme streams down to the thighs, it is difficult to cure them. *De signis mortis.*

(VI.72) When one of the intestines develops an ulcer caused by black bile, it cannot be cured. When it develops an ulcer caused by yellow bile, it is difficult to heal. The same holds for the other internal organs. *De atra bile* [5].

(VI.73) When these four signs combine—the stool is soft and cohesive; it is discharged neither before nor after its usual time, and its quantity is commensurate with the food intake—it is an indication that the food is well-digested and that the stool is digested and cocted. Occasionally one of these is lacking but the stool is still digested and cocted. *De crisibus* I[.11].

(VI.74) Sometimes something is well-digested and firmly cocted in the stomach, and yet the stool is dry because the heat around the stomach or intestines has dried its moistures. Sometimes it is softer than normal because of the weakness of the faculty that transports the food to the organs. Sometimes its evacuation is delayed because its passage through the intestines goes very slowly. Sometimes the stool is evacuated before the proper time because of the weakness of the retentive faculty in one of the intestines. If this is accompanied by a sensation of biting, it indicates that some sort of irritation stimulated the expulsive faculty to evacuate it; this was not because of a deficiency which affected its digestion in the stomach. *De crisibus* I[.11].

(VI.75) When a soft, cohesive stool is discharged at the normal time, but in a quantity smaller than appropriate in comparison with the amount of food ingested, it indicates that some of it remains in one of the intestines, and this is bad in any case. *De crisibus* I[.11].

(VI.76) A stool that indicates bad digestion is coarse, not ground up, and of a soft consistency, retaining the quality of the food from which it is a residue. *De crisibus* I[.11].

(VI.77) An initially green color of the stool may eventually turn black, namely, when a malignant disease is accompanied by green sputum or green stool or green urine, each of which will later turn black. *De crisibus* I[.12].

(VI.78) If you see a person with a stool containing a discharge of something like water in which freshly slaughtered meat has been washed, let it be a sure indication for you of a decline in the strength of the liver. If the blood that is discharged is thick like wine sediment, it is a sign indicating that the liver is burning the blood. If the blood is thin and serous, it indicates that the liver is too weak to make blood. *De locis affectis* V[.8].

(VI.79) First thin serous blood is discharged in the stool, then after a long time, thick blood similar to black bile, and eventually the discharge is pure black bile. *De locis affectis* V[.8].

(VI.80) Sometimes the stool has a variety of discharges with a very bad color and smell, and similarly the urine. This is caused by the strength of the liver and organs, which expelled those bad residues which were retained in them. An inexperienced physician can make a mistake in these matters by supposing that the patient is close to death. These kinds of evacuations simply occur after a prolonged disease and after the manifestation of signs of coction. *De locis affectis* V[.8].

(VI.81) Just as a discharge of blood through the anus occurs to someone whose hand or foot has been cut off, or to someone who gives up physical exercise, or to someone whose hemorrhoidal or menstrual blood was retained, so a similar discharge occurs to some people through vomiting. The blood of those who eliminate blood either through vomiting or through diarrhea is pure like that of slaughtered animals. If the blood is eliminated because of ripe abscesses bursting, that blood, whether coming out from above or from below, is turbid like wine sediment. *De locis affectis* V[.8].

(VI.82) Bloody diarrhea due to a liver disease may occur suddenly. But if it comes because of a disease of the intestines, it does not happen suddenly, but rather begins as a bilious diarrhea which is extremely acrid; this is followed by shreds of intestinal tissue, and then with the shreds some blood is excreted. *De locis affectis* VI[.2].

(VI.83) The blood which is excreted from the liver with the stool is sometimes retained for two or three days. It then becomes worse than what it was the first time but is not accompanied by shreds. These two prognostic signs do not occur in any intestinal ulcer. *De locis affectis* VI[.2].

(VI.84) The stool that is deep yellow comes from a large amount of yellow bile that streamed to the abdomen. The stool is green when it is mixed with a large quantity of verdigris green bile. When the stool is black, it indicates that it is mixed with black bile or with blood that was burned there. When it tends to lead gray, it indicates that the cold was so severe in the internal organs that they were close to death. One should know from which food the stool is a residue, because sometimes the color of the stool derives from the nature of the particular kind of food. In this case the color is not a prognostic sign. *De crisibus* I[.11].

(VI.85) When the stool is greasy, it is a sign that fat has melted. When it is viscous, it indicates melting of the solid parts, which is worse than the previous case. An excessively putrid stool indicates severe putrefaction. All this is on the condition that it is not due to the nature of the food. *De crisibus* I[.11].

(VI.86) A foamy stool indicates one of two things: either extreme heat melting the body, whereby foam results from the boiling of the body moistures which were boiled by the extreme heat, or from an anomalous disturbance resulting from the struggle between thick flatulence and moisture. *De crisibus* I[.11].

(VI.87) A stool with different colors indicates that the body suffers from different diseases. Thus, it announces that the disease will be prolonged and malignant, because when diseases multiply, they need more time to coct. Their severity and danger are according to their number. *De crisibus* I[.11].

(VI.88) Sometimes the diseases and symptoms caused by the retentive faculty and the expulsive faculty are mixed with one another. An example of this is hiccups. For in the case of hiccups, the stomach has bad contractions over the food, while at the same time the expulsive faculty is making wrong movements. *De* [*symptomatum*] *causis* [III.2].

(VI.89) Black stool originates either from the domination of burning, from foul putrefaction, or from the streaming of a melancholic humor. *In Hippocratis Aphorismos commentarius* IV[.21].

(VI.90) Sometimes a lack of appetite occurs in the beginning of bloody diarrhea. This is not a bad sign, because choleric humors streaming from the liver to the intestines and abrading them stream from there to the stomach so that appetite diminishes. But if the disease is prolonged and a lack of appetite occurs, it is a bad sign because it indicates death of the powers of the body. *In Hippocratis Aphorismos commentarius* VI[.3].

(VI.91) When blood congeals and coagulates and turns into thick, clotted blood in the urinary bladder and, similarly, when it congeals in the intestines or stomach or chest—and in this case it is worse than in that of the bladder—it causes syncope, pallor, and a small, weak, and frequent pulse. The patient becomes hot and weak. This makes a person wonder how it is possible that blood—although it is most dear to nature—causes these bad and malignant symptoms when it leaves its vessels. Sometimes this is followed—after what we mentioned—by putrefaction and death of the organs. *De locis affectis* VI[.4].

(VI.92) Stones develop only in the kidneys and the urinary bladder, though according to some people also in the intestines called "colon." *De locis affectis* I[.5].

(VI.93) That which in the medical art goes according to supposition and conjecture is in most cases the diagnosis of diseases. However, once these diseases are known, their treatment is not arrived at through supposition, guesswork, and conjecture, but through certain knowledge. [*De compositione medicamentorum secundum locos*] II[.1].

(VI.94) Says Moses: It is well known that the physicians speak about psychical faculties, animal faculties, and natural faculties. Now, according to this convention I want to call all the activities of the human body "corporal activities" and say that the most eminent bodily activity is respiration, followed by the pulse, and after that, sensation. The most eminent sense is seeing, followed by hearing. After sensation comes craving for food and drink, then speech, and then distinction—that is, thought and imagination. Then comes the movement of the other parts of the body, according to their habit. This gradation in eminence is specifically according to the requirements for life, or its proper continuation.

Following this introduction, you should know that the term "nature" is a homonym which has many different meanings. One of all these meanings is the faculty which governs the body of living beings, for the physicians also call this faculty "nature." This faculty always spares the most eminent activities of the body and always strives to maintain the integrity of all its activities. If a disease-producing cause develops, nature opposes it and expels it. If it finds it difficult to do so, it casts it to that bodily part that is least important and gives up the activity that is least important. But if nature has difficulty doing so, it gives up the next most important activity and holds on to the activity that is more important than the former one, etc. According to this sequence one can distinguish between fatal and nonfatal diseases and draw conclusions regarding the degree of severity or weakness of the disease and the degree of strength or weakness of nature. For cessation or disturbance of respiration is fatal without any doubt, and similarly cessation of the pulse, loss or disturbance of vision, loss of appetite, loss or weakness of speech, amentia or disturbance of the mind; all these afflictions are fatal indications, and their degree of severity is according to my arrangement and according to the strength of the particular affliction.

Therefore, a severe stroke is necessarily fatal and a mild one is difficult to heal, as Hippocrates stated. For during this affliction, namely, a stroke, the eminent activities which nature always spares are either abolished or disturbed. These activities are respiration, mental activity, speech, sensation, and pulse. The prerequisite for all that I have mentioned is that the loss or impairment of that activity is due to a weakening of the general faculty that governs the body of living beings, and not just due to a disease of the particular organ performing that activity.

You know that many of those suffering from madness or melancholy live for a long time, as they have strong bodies. The loss of their mental activities is only due to an affliction of the brain, and not due to a weakening of the faculty which governs that which occurs to patients during their agony. Thus, the weakening of vision due to an affliction in the eye and the weakening of hearing due to an affliction in the inner earhole is unlike the weakening of vision or hearing—when one dies—due to the collapse of the general faculty that governs the body. The same conditions apply to loss of speech and the other bodily activities. Similarly, nature acts sparingly with changes in one's complexion. For when the complexion of a patient is close to that which he has when he is healthy, it indicates that nature is strong, and when his complexion is very far from resembling his normal complexion, it indicates that the general strength is weak. Consider this aphorism carefully, for it contains many things relevant to prognosis.

(VI.95) In the medical art we can find many symptoms, which, when they appear in healthy people, indicate diseases, and which, when they appear in sick people, indicate health. One of these is sleep which is longer and deeper than usual. When it occurs to healthy people, it indicates illness, and when it occurs to sick people, it indicates health. And when a strong appetite occurs to healthy people, there is reason for suspicion, as it indicates a disease, and when it occurs to sick people, it is a laudable sign. Similarly, sneezing, for when it happens often to someone whose health is beyond reproach, it indicates that an affliction has reached the head. And when it occurs to someone who is in a bad state of disease, it indicates that his condition will change for the better. We can find many things of this nature in the art of medicine. *In [Platonis] Timaeum commentarius* II.

This is the end of the sixth treatise,
by the grace of God,
praise be to Him.

In the name of God,
the Merciful, the Compassionate.
O Lord, make our task easy

The Seventh Treatise

Containing aphorisms concerning the causes of diseases which are often not known or which are discussed in a confused way

(VII.1) The things which cause a manifest increase in strength are six:

1. moderate wine consumption,
2. moderate food intake,
3. moderate physical exercise,
4. anything that improves a bad temperament of the heart and pulsatile vessels, whether drink or drug,
5. anger and joy, and
6. the coction of the humors so that they start to dissolve or to be evacuated during the crisis. *De* [*praesagitione ex*] *puls*[*ibus* 1].

(VII.2) The things which weaken and diminish one's strength are eight:

1. fasting,
2. sleeplessness,
3. anxiety,
4. excessive evacuation of any type,
5. severe pain in any spot,
6. abdominal pain, especially that followed by fainting,
7. a very bad temperament of whatever type of the humors of the body, and
8. a very bad temperament of whatever type of the organs of the body. *De* [*praesagitione ex*] *puls*[*ibus* 1].

(VII.3) People can also faint because of the strength of the affections of the soul. This happens mostly to the elderly and to weak people, whatever the cause of their weakness. Many of them faint when they are affected by anxiety, joy, or anger. Sometimes this happens to them because their bodies unnecessarily sweat a little bit. *Ad Glauconem* [*de medendi methodo*] 1[.15].

(VII.4) Constant anxiety dissolves the fat and corrupts the moist flesh, while frequent joy corrupts the blood. Similarly, the blood is corrupted by passionate love, lust for money, political leadership, and fame. The corruption of the blood by any of these comes from bad digestion in the stomach and vessels. The dissolution of the fat is caused by sleeplessness and by [constantly] thinking about these things. *In Hippocratis De humoribus commentarius.*

(VII.5) The reason why the organs on the right side have more strength than the organs on the left side is that the liver lies on the right side while the leaning of the heart towards the left side is very small. When this leaning of the heart is slightly greater, the organs on the left become stronger than those on the right, especially if the liver, in such a case, is weak and small. *In Hippocratis Epidemiarum* [*commentarius* I.3].

(VII.6) The causes of pain are a dissolution of continuity or a sudden change that occurs to the organ through coercion and harshness. If the change happens slowly, it cannot hurt. Pain does not occur in senseless organs. *De methodo medendi* XII[.7].

(VII.7) Any cause of pain inflicts harm through which the expulsive faculty is activated and exerts itself to expel the harmful element. Because of its intense activity to expel the harmful cause, the expulsive faculty often produces a tumor by attracting blood and air together to the [affected] organ. *De methodo medendi* XIII[.3].

(VII.8) Says Moses: When Galen speaks about the healing of syncope, he starts by giving its causes; however, he does not describe them as he usually does when he classifies the various kinds of diseases and their causes and the various kinds of symptoms: according to the method applied in the medical art, as in his classification of fevers in their various classes and species. Rather, he describes the causes of syncope in an amazing way, namely, by saying that it can be caused by this and by that, but does not classify these causes into specific categories. And even more amazing than this is that when he discusses the subject in detail, he remarks, the other causes for syncope are four. I wish I knew why only some causes were given a specific number but not all of them. Moreover, after mentioning the four causes he remarks, and if you want, you can add another one to these four—namely, a bad temperament of the organs. In short, he did not give a systematic discussion in that place, although everything he said is undoubtedly correct. However, as we said, it is disordered.

And since this affliction, namely, syncope, is such a serious one and is a partner and associate of death, which it often precedes, a physician should have a comprehensive knowledge of all the causes of syncope and should always keep them in mind. If he has a detailed and exact knowledge of its causes, he knows how to treat it when it occurs, and how to prevent its occurrence, and how to warn against it when its occurrence is unavoidable. Abū Marwān ibn Zuhr and other physicians said that when a patient suffers from syncope without the physician knowing about it until it actually happens and without his having warned against it, then this physician is undoubtedly responsible for the death of the patient.

(VII.9) Says Moses: This is correct, for if he knew all the causes of syncope, his most important and desired goal would be to prevent its occurrence, and whenever something would appear in the condition of the disease which could trigger syncope, he would hasten to fight that which would cause syncope if it were neglected. And if he had to give up his fight against it, he would warn the patient against its occurrence. Therefore, I thought it a good thing to classify the various causes of syncope and to describe its classes and species so that it will be easy to learn them and know them by heart. All that I will say in the following five aphorisms is either a literal quotation from Galen or the intent of his words. But I will express this intent partly in his words and partly in my own words. All this is gleaned from what Galen taught us in *De methodo medendi* XII[.5]. This is the right moment to start with those five aphorisms that I promised.

(VII.10) Syncope is a quick collapse of the faculties of the body. The existence and permanence of the faculties in their essential nature depends on the balance of the pneumata, humors, and organs in their quantity and quality. The cause for the collapse of the faculties—namely, syncope—can be a quantitative or qualitative change of the pneumata, or a quantitative or qualitative change of the humors, or a quantitative or qualitative change of the organs. The causes of syncope can thus be limited to these three classes, and since each class consists of two subclasses—namely, a quantitative change and a qualitative change—we actually have six classes. [*De methodo medendi* XII.5].

(VII.11) A change in the elementary parts that causes syncope is due either to a dissolution in their substance—and this is a decrease in quantity—or to their bad temperament because of an excess in one of the four qualities. The substance of the organs is dissolved either because of prolonged chronic diseases or because of acute diseases or because of wasting fevers. [*De methodo medendi* XII.5].

(VII.12) A change in the pneumata that causes syncope occurs either because the pneuma dissolves, and this is a quantitative loss, or because the substance of the pneuma is corrupted, and this is a qualitative loss. The corruption of the substance of the pneuma is due to a corruption of the air, or to lethal drugs, or to animal poisons. A dissolution of the pneuma is either due to the movements of the soul such as intense joy, which is called "exultation," or intense pleasure or intense fear, and similarly, anxiety and anger. As part of all these movements, Galen also mentioned pain and sleeplessness. But I say that these two should be counted separately because there is nothing stronger for the dissolution of the pneuma than pain, and after that, sleeplessness. Similarly, the pneuma is dissolved when it becomes excessively thin and fine or because its vessels become too thin and porous. The pneuma can also be dissolved because of a lack of food or because of severe diarrhea. These two causes also effect a change in the organs and the humors, but Galen linked them to the pneuma. [*De methodo medendi* XII.5].

(VII.13) A change in the humors that causes syncope occurs either in their quality or in their quantity. Their quality changes when the humors become very thin and fine and dissolve rapidly. Therefore, if one does not take care to properly nourish these humors, syncope occurs rapidly. Similarly, if the quality of the humors becomes so thick and viscous that they become crude and raw, they cause syncope for the following reasons:

1. The body does not receive enough nutrition,
2. the innate heat is suppressed,
3. the balance of the temperament is changed and corrupted, and
4. these humors oppress the strength of the body through their abundance—when they neither oppress nor obstruct it, they cause fainting, not syncope.

It is clear to you that a surplus of humors that causes oppression or obstruction of the strength of the body also causes syncope, and this is a change in quantity. [*De methodo medendi* XII.5].

(VII.14) It is clear from the foregoing that the causes of syncope comprise six classes and twenty-one kinds. The first class—namely, a quantitative change of the organs—consists of three kinds:

1. a chronic disease,
2. an acute disease, or
3. a wasting fever.

The second class—namely, a qualitative change of the organs—consists of four kinds: they become excessively

1. hot or
2. cold or
3. dry or
4. moist.

The third class—namely, a qualitative change of the pneuma—consists of three kinds, which are

1. corruption of the air,
2. ingestion of a poisonous substance, or
3. the bite of a venomous animal.

The fourth class—namely, a quantitative change of the pneuma, meaning that the pneuma dissolves and disappears or greatly diminishes—consists of seven kinds:

1. thinness and fineness of the pneumata, or
2. thinness and porousness of the vessels, or
3. the movements of the soul, or
4. pain, or
5. sleeplessness, or
6. lack of food, or
7. diarrhea, or other similar evacuations.

The fifth class—namely, a qualitative change of the humors—consists of two kinds, which are

1. thinness and fineness of the humors, or
2. thickness and crudeness thereof.

The sixth class—namely, a quantitative change of the humors—consists of two kinds:

1. a surplus that oppresses the strength of the body, or
2. a surplus that causes an obstruction.

These are all the various classes of the causes of syncope as explained from the words of Galen, and they number twenty-one causes. [*De methodo medendi* XII.5].

(VII.15) Says Moses: The most important way to prevent the occurrence of syncope is to devote all one's attention during any disease to the three major organs and the cardia of the stomach because of the close interaction between the latter and the major organs. One should take care of the faculties of these organs—namely, through balancing their temperament by means of that with which one supplies the body and by means of that which one applies to the organ externally. Having concerned oneself with these organs, one should seek to balance the temperament of the other organs. Similarly, one should give priority to balancing the pneumata of these three organs. As for the psychical pneuma, this should be done through the sniffing of aromatic substances. As for the animal pneuma, it should be done through balancing the outside air, and through opening the pores of the skin, and through cleansing the respiratory organs from the thick and viscous humors, and through opening the obstruction caused by them, and through the consumption of that which, in combination with drugs, has the property to purify the blood of the heart and to remove the turbidity from its air. As for the natural pneuma, this should be done by the consumption of food and drink that should be of the best and most balanced quality and the least detrimental. One should be extremely careful not to let a patient take any food or drink that is mixed with the slightest amount of putrefaction because these kinds of food produce poisonous humors, as mentioned by Galen. [*De methodo medendi* XII.3]. Similarly, one should be careful not to give a patient any food that corrupts quickly, such as milk, or those foods that produce a poisonous humor when they corrupt, such as *biṭṭīkh* (common melon or watermelon), cucumber, and *qarʿ* (field pumpkin or winter squash). One should be careful that the patient does not eat any ingredients such as these because we fear that they corrupt or that they are slow to descend and thus cause severe damage. Similarly, one should constantly strengthen the stomach and beware of bad digestion. If one makes these things one's aim, one prevents the occurrence of syncope to the majority of patients under one's care.

(VII.16) Emaciation of the body originating from an enlarged spleen has two causes. First, the food is not adequately digested in the liver so that the organs do not receive sufficient food, since the food that is most proper to them in this case is that which is slightly bad. The second cause is that the blood is turbid, and most of it is attracted by the spleen, thus not allowing the body to be nourished by it. *In Hippocratis De aere*[, *aquis et locis*] *commentarius* II.

(VII.17) If black bile dominates someone's body, he is very fond of sexual intercourse because many thick inflating winds collect in his body in the hypochondrium. *In Hippocratis Epidemiarum* [*commentarius*] VI.[4].

(VII.18) Emaciation of the body occurs either because of weakness of the powers of the flesh or because the pulsatile vessels and non-pulsatile vessels are filled with bad blood. Obesity of the body occurs through the opposite of these two causes—the flesh attracts most of the blood to it, leaving only a small quantity of it in the vessels. *In Hippocratis Epidemiarum* [*commentarius*] VI.[4].

(VII.19) Humors cause pain in one of six ways: either through

1. their overabundance,
2. their thickness,
3. their viscosity,
4. their heat,
5. their coolness, or through
6. their biting and corrosion of an organ. *In Hippocratis De humoribus commentarius* I.

(VII.20) Just as the humors influence one's character, so one's character influences the humors: if someone is dominated by bile, he is irascible, and when someone is very angry, bilious humors originate in him. [*De plenitudine* 8].

(VII.21) Pruritus occurs because of sharp, biting humors that irritate a part of the body and produce a kind of movement that is similar to that which occurs when moving the fingers in the region of the armpit. *In Hippocratis De alimento commentarius* III.

(VII.22) Says Moses: When the biting humor is of a thin consistency and passes through a sensitive organ, one of the four different symptoms that he mentioned in his *De plenitudine* [8] is caused in that organ. We have mentioned that particular text in one of the aphorisms when we discussed these symptoms. When the biting humor is of a thick consistency or the organ is only a little sensitive, it causes the pruritus that he mentioned.

(VII.23) Sometimes a vitreous phlegmatic humor collects in the body but does not putrefy and thus causes rigor lasting for many successive days. As long as a person is at rest and does not move at all, the rigor is also at rest. But if he moves, his motion is immediately followed by rigor proportional to the extent of the motion. The stronger and faster the motion, the stronger the rigor. I have seen this affliction and treated it with drugs that heat and dissolve the thick humors, such as the various kinds of pepper and mint. *De tremore,* [*palpitatione, convulsione et rigore* 7].

(VII.24) There are three causes of thickness of blood and its blackness and coagulation so that the vessels are filled with melancholic humor. These causes can occur either together or separately. One of these is that the liver is prepared to produce that superfluity. The second cause is that the regimen of food and drink and the like has the property to produce thick blood. The third cause is that the condition of the spleen is so weak that it cannot attract all of the superfluity that is produced in the liver. *Ad Glauconem* [*de medendi methodo*] II[.12].

(VII.25) When sharp humors or sharp drugs that make the organs rough are excessively strong, they produce ulcers in the fleshy parts of the body and caries in the bones. *De causis* [*morborum* 7].

(VII.26) Sometimes dementia and forgetfulness occur from extreme old age and senility. This is an indication that the dementia and forgetfulness originate especially from coldness. But all deliria are the result of hot biting humors, particularly yellow bile. Sometimes they occur because of a hot, bad temperament. Not one of these is caused by a cold humor, except for the delirium that is called "melancholic delusion." The delirium that occurs in the last stages of acute fevers is caused by hot biting vapors that rise to the head. *De [symptomatum] causis* [II.7].

(VII.27) Pain in membranes is dissimilar because their sensitivity is dissimilar. Some spots are very sensitive while others are hardly sensitive. But pain in membranes can also be dissimilar for a different reason—namely, that when during the membrane's stretching it touches the bone. *De locis affectis* II[.8].

(VII.28) The reason some inflamed tumors are accompanied by pulsation and others are not is the presence of a sizable pulsatile vessel in the spot of the inflamed tumor. Whenever the inflamed tumor expands, it compresses this vessel and pulsation occurs. *De locis affectis* II[.4].

(VII.29) Just as a thick phlegmatic humor can produce epilepsy, so a melancholic humor can produce epilepsy when it is retained in the channels of the ventricles of the brain. But when it increases and becomes dominant in the very substance of the brain, it causes melancholic delusion. *De locis affectis* III[.9].

(VII.30) The cause for the hardening of a pulsatile vessel is one of three things: either dryness, or congealment due to the cold, or stretching. Dryness occurs in the case of ardent fevers—when they last for a long time and are bad and malignant—and in the case of melancholy and some quartan fevers. Congealment originates from anything that produces a vitreous humor in the body. Stretching occurs in the case of diseases that are of the same type as spasms and in the case of large inflamed tumors and in the case of hardness and rigidness occurring in the substance of the liver or spleen. *De [praesagitione ex] puls[ibus* I.4].

(VII.31) Tapeworms eat anything by which a human being feeds himself and therefore make the body lean. *De theriaca ad Pisonem.*

(VII.32) Sometimes sneezing is an accidental remedy and cure for moistures that are collected in the lungs, in the stomach, and in the cardia of the stomach and from which hiccups originate. It removes and expels them from those places. This is why sneezing also cures hiccups—by cleansing all the superfluities that are above the stomach. *De [symptomatum] causis* II[.6].

(VII.33) The reason the pain following the extraction of a painful tooth is necessarily alleviated is that, at that moment, the nerve that was connected to the root of the tooth relaxes because it is severed from the bone that caused its initial stretching. And space is formed in the tooth through which dissolved liquids that have gathered there can emerge. [*De compositione medicamentorum secundum locos*] V[.4].

(VII.34) The reason for the breaking and corrosion of teeth lies in their softness. Therefore, it is necessary to harden and strengthen them with astringent drugs. In the same way their color turns livid and the like because of bad moistures streaming towards them. Therefore, they should be treated with drugs that moderately dry—not as some physicians think, that the stronger the drying effect, the more beneficial the drug. [*De compositione medicamentorum secundum locos*] V[.4].

(VII.35) If an inflamed tumor occurs in a sinewy part of the body, it is followed by delirium more quickly than in any other part, either because the heat alone ascends to the head through parts connected to that nerve or because it ascends with a vaporous or smoky gas. *De locis affectis* III[.9].

(VII.36) A tremor occurs because of a weakness of the faculty that supports and moves the body and also because of the natural heaviness of a part of the body. For when someone suffering from such a weakness wants to move a part of the body, it falls downward due to the weakness of the force, and because he cannot support this part of the body, trembling occurs. But if he did not have any desire at all to move it, he would not tremble. Similarly, if the motive faculty were totally abolished, no trembling would occur, but relaxation. That impossibility to move may be clarified for you by thinking of someone who has a heavy burden upon himself and wants to lift his feet in order to go but cannot do so because his legs tremble. Similarly, if he wants to lift something heavy, his arms tremble. In the same way, when someone is frightened or alarmed and then wants to go or to lift something heavy, his arms and legs tremble. Alarm and fear undermine one's strength. For this reason, trembling occurs to the elderly and to someone whose body is weakened and emaciated because of a disease. *De tremore*, [*palpitatione, convulsione et rigore* 3].

(VII.37) Spasms occur because of overfilling or because of emptying. When it occurs because of sleeplessness, exertion, worry, anxiety, or dry ardent fever, the cause of that kind of spasm is the dryness and emptying. If someone who is given to rest and ease and to constantly filling his stomach and to permanent leisure and idleness is stricken by a spasm, we should suspect that it is caused by overfilling. Similarly, epilepsy is a spasm due to overfilling, possibly occurring when the origin of each nerve is moistened by that thick and viscous moisture. However, this spasm is not continuous as is that which is from the front or back or from both sides together. *De locis affectis* III[.8, 9, 12].

(VII.38) The cause of palpitation is something of the nature and substance of the air that streams to the organs. In its essence there is a thick type of vapor. The cause of a spasm in the case of inflammatory diseases is overfilling and in the case of very ardent and dry fevers is emptying. *De* [*symptomatum*] *causis* II.2].

(VII.39) A spasm is caused by a stretching of nerves either because of moisture or because of dryness. The muscles at the origins of nerves also stretch and contract involuntarily, thus causing a spasm. *De tremore,* [*palpitatione, convulsione et rigore* 8].

(VII.40) The cause of palpitation is a thick wind that is confined to a narrow spot from which it cannot escape. This wind cannot dissolve because of its thickness, and it cannot escape because of the density of the surrounding bodies. Since it constantly tries to escape, it causes the mentioned palpitation. And since the cause of palpitation is of one kind, its treatment is also of one kind—namely, everything that thins and heats. When applied internally or externally, castoreum is especially good for this affliction because it is a drug that is heating, thinning, and extremely drying. According to this reasoning palpitation is especially caused by something cold. *De tremore,* [*palpitatione, convulsione et rigore* 5].

(VII.41) When someone's body has a bad humor and becomes hot through exertion or something else, he suffers from shivering even when no fever arises. *In Hippocratis Epidemiarum* [*commentarius*] VI.3.

(VII.42) A weakness of the force that is the cause of a tremor does not have one cause but many causes. Sometimes it is caused by malnutrition, as happens in the case of cholera, severe diarrhea, and the frequent loss of blood, and in the case of someone fasting. Sometimes it is caused by the dissolution of the animal faculty, as happens in the case of syncope. Sometimes it is caused by severe cold, which compresses the pores of the nerves so that only weak impulses of that motive faculty get through. Sometimes it is caused by overfilling, which oppresses the force so that it is too weak for motion. Therefore, the remedies that cure tremors are not of one kind. *De tremore,* [*palpitatione, convulsione et rigore* 5].

(VII.43) A rigor is a severe and suddenly concentrated cold whereby the body goes from a natural to an unnatural condition. That it is a cold affliction is obvious and clear. As for its cause—I mean the cause of a rigor—it is a cold humor that moves and passes through the sensitive organs. Sometimes it is a sharp humor that moves and streams through the sensitive organs. In both cases the innate heat is put to flight by the biting substance and returns to its original site so that the outer parts of the body become cold. Then, when on its return it finds the pores constricted and contracted and its passages obstructed, it stops in its course and returns to its original site and then leaves this site once again. This continues either until it gains the upper hand and heats the outer parts of the body or until it is overpowered and extinguished and the patient dies. During that phase of going back and forth and being hindered from passing through, trembling associated with rigor occurs. The difference between a tremor and rigor is that a tremor results from the hindrance between the voluntary strength of the body and its natural weight. If someone wants to abolish the voluntary strength and does not want it to perform any motion, the tremor ceases. But the cessation of a rigor does not depend on one's will—it results from the hindrance between a natural motion—namely, that of the innate heat—and that which obstructs its course and its passages and channels. *De tremore,* [*palpitatione, convulsione et rigore* 6].

(VII.44) If the cold only moves the outer surface of the body with a shivering movement and shakes it at the moment of the onset of a fever attack but does not move the whole body, this is called "shivering." Shivering is an affliction occurring only to the skin. Its significance for the skin is the same as that of rigor for the whole body. *De tremore,* [*palpitatione, convulsione et rigore* 6]. But in *De febribus* II[.7], he said that shivering is something less severe than rigor but more cold.

(VII.45) For the occurrence of a rigor, it is necessary that the body contain a biting substance and that this humor is moved violently, no matter whether the cause of the rigor is a cold or a hot one. Therefore, a rigor starts simultaneously with the attack of tertian or quartan fevers when that humor moves to be expelled. Sometimes a similar thing happens to someone who suffers from indigestion or to someone whose body is full of bad humors and who then exposes himself to the sun or enters the bathhouse or does physical exercise.

For if someone does this, he is immediately affected by shivering or sometimes by rigor. *De tremore,* [*palpitatione, convulsione et rigore* 7].

(VII.46) Many of those who are affected by rigor are thirsty during that time because the heat remains deep inside the body while the sensation of cold is at that moment in the outer parts of the body, not in the inner ones. *De* [*symptomatum*] *causis* [II.5].

(VII.47) The causes for bad respiration that force the patient to move all the muscles of the upper chest together with the intercostal ones are one of the following three: either weakened strength, or narrowness and pressure in the respiratory passages, or burning heat in the heart or lungs. When all these three causes occur together, the patient dies immediately. When two of them occur together, it is difficult for him to escape, but if only one of them occurs, he will eventually either die or escape. *De locis affectis* IV[.7].

(VII.48) Sometimes respiration comes at intervals and in great gasps because of harm that has occurred to the mind. This illness consists therein that the patient is, as it were, so unmindful and forgetful of his deeds that he does not know when he stops nor when he begins. *In Hippocratis Epidemiarum* [*commentarius* I.3].

Because of the connection between the organs of the chest and the reproductive organs, sometimes a chronic cough stops because of a swelling of the testicles. *In Hippocratis Epidemiarum* [*commentarius* I.3].

(VII.49) Thinness and interruption of the voice are only caused by humors that are either abundant or thick or viscous and that obstruct the vessels in the lung. *In Hippocratis Epidemiarum* [*commentarius* I.3].

(VII.50) There are two reasons why a patient brings up a small amount of sputum in spite of much coughing: either the humors are so thick and viscous that they get stuck and their expectoration is difficult, or the humors are too thin. For when they are lifted by the air, they are dispersed and sink again. *De locis affectis* IV[.11].

(VII.51) If someone wishes to raise his voice, he should become accustomed to opening his mouth wide so that he lets in much air, which widens the larynx. Then the voice is loud. Therefore, those whose larynx is narrow and small have thin, small voices without any substance so that they are broken off quickly. But those whose larynx is wide have a full and powerful voice. Children, women, and eunuchs have thin and weak voices because their larynx is small. *De somno et vigilia.*

(VII.52) The digestive activity only takes place in the parts that are beneath the cardia of the stomach. Therefore, this part of the stomach causes indigestion when it is indisposed, provided that the indigestion is not caused by foods. *De locis affectis* V[.6].

(VII.53) The cause of a gassy disease in the stomach is heat that exceeds the normal balance and takes possession of the vessels that receive the food from the stomach so that the blood becomes thick there. An indication that the disturbance lies there is that the food remains undigested in the stomach because of the obstruction of those channels, and those suffering from it vomit their undigested food. An indication for the domination of heat in that spot is that they obtain relief by cold things and also that they suffer from burning fever. Some people say that the cause of this disease lies in the fact that the opening of the stomach that leads to the intestines is swollen due to an inflamed bloody tumor. This blood is extremely thick and is very much like black bile. *De locis affectis* III[.10].

(VII.54) When there is a large or hard inflamed tumor in the liver, the patient feels the pain in the right collarbone. This results from the stretching of the vessel known as vena cava and not from the stretching of the pleural membranes. In the case of pleurisy, the pain in the collarbone is the result of the stretching of the pleural membranes. *De locis affectis* II[.8].

(VII.55) If you take food without suffering from intestinal rumblings or inflation or palpitation or hiccups, but you do have an unusual feeling of discomfort in your stomach—the food weighs heavily on it—and you do wish that it would descend from it or that eructation would occur to it, and sometimes you also suffer from difficulty of breathing, there is no doubt that the stomach has contracted over the food in a trembling way. [*De symptomatum differentiis* 4].

(VII.56) When whiteness dominates in someone's complexion, his liver is weak and does not produce much blood. If red spots dominate, his spleen is weak; these red spots are caused by the mixture of melancholic humor with the blood. *In Hippocratis Epidemiarum* [*commentarius* I.3].

(VII.57) The first cause of a severe thirst without diabetes is a hot or dry bad temperament, or both, occurring in the stomach and especially in the cardia of the stomach; and after the stomach, the second cause is that this bad temperament affects the liver and especially its concave part. A similar cause is the occurrence of this bad temperament in the esophagus or in the lungs, for it is then transferred to the stomach so that thirst becomes severe. *De locis affectis* VI[.3].

(VII.58) Sleep moistens under all circumstances, while sleeplessness dries under all circumstances. Sleep has not the property to heat or to cool, but when it occurs to a body with cold humors, it digests them and cocts them and produces blood from them so that the body is heated. And when sleep occurs to a body that suffers from fever caused by the putrefaction of cold humors, it cools the body by extinguishing the heat of the fever and by increasing the innate heat. When the humors are bilious, it selects them and expels them from the body so that it cools off. *In Hippocratis Epidemiarum* [*commentarius*] VI.4.

(VII.59) When evident causes of an affliction strike a body that is free of superfluities, the harm inflicted on it can be easily repaired and quickly eliminated. But when they strike the body while it has a surplus of humors or bad humors, their effect can be compared to that of a fiery spark on the wood of fatty pine nuts or that of a burning wick on sulfur. *In Hippocratis Epidemiarum* [*commentarius*] VI.8.

(VII.60) Corrosion is caused by biting humors; biting humors are those humors that are sharp, sour, and salty. *In Hippocratis Epidemiarum* [*commentarius*] VI.[1–]8.

(VII.61) It is not surprising that one who indulges frequently in sexual intercourse is weak because his whole body is free from seminal fluid and pneuma because of their evacuation from it. And besides, there is an accession of pleasure that by itself is enough to weaken and extinguish the animal faculty. Some people who had a sudden intense pleasure died as a result. *De semine* [I.16].

(VII.62) The reason for a frequent discharge of feces is one of three: either because of a weakness of the organs due to a bad temperament, as is well known, or because of biting humors that irritate the organ and prompt it to expel the excrements, or because of excessive sensitivity that is either natural or caused by an ulcer. *De* [*symptomatum*] *causis* [III.5].

(VII.63) The causes of biting superfluities that necessarily lead to a frequent discharge of feces are four: either the strength of a medication that is received by the body together with the food or without it, or the corruption of food, or biting superfluities that descend from the body into various places in the abdomen, or biting superfluities that originate in the stomach or abdomen. *De* [*symptomatum*] *causis* [III.5].

(VII.64) The cold of the outer parts of the body always hardens the belly, while the cold of the inner parts always softens the belly and sometimes causes diarrhea. *In Hippocratis Epidemiarum* [*commentarius*] VI.5.

(VII.65) When the part of the intestines called "colon" becomes full, bad afflictions occur and the stomach feels its pain. The reason for this is that when this part of the intestines becomes full, it distends and the pain ascends to the membrane that surrounds the stomach and the intestines. Thus, the stomach feels the pain from there. There is also a muscle that covers both the stomach and the intestines, and when this part of the intestines distends, the stomach feels the pain from that. *De clysteribus* [*et colica*].

(VII.66) Pain with numbness occurs in the legs in the case of kidney diseases because of the connection between the kidneys and the legs through the two vessels that descend along the spinal column. These are the vessels known as the vena cava and the aorta. *In Hippocratis Epidemiarum* [*commentarius*] VI.1.

(VII.67) There are three reasons why a smooth organ becomes rough: either acrid humors pour into it and peel and strip it, or acrid medications have a similar effect on it, or foreign substances adhere to it, such as smoke and dust. The reason why a rough organ becomes smooth is that it is soaked and moistened by a fat, soft, or viscous liquid. [*De causis morborum* 7].

(VII.68) It often happens that symptoms follow each other in a row. The first symptom comes from the disease itself, the second comes from the first, the third comes from the second, and the fourth from the third. [*De symptomatum differentiis* 6].

(VII.69) If the albuminoid humor is larger or smaller in quantity than necessary, it harms vision. When this humor becomes thick, clarity of vision is diminished so that distant objects cannot be seen at all and close objects cannot be seen clearly. When it becomes extremely thick, as happens in the case of a cataract, it makes vision impossible. When a part of the eye near the pupil becomes covered by the thick humor while another part remains clear, one clearly sees any one object through the clear part, but one cannot see many objects at the same time. When only a small amount of thick humor is in the middle of the pupil while the surrounding area remains clear, one sees everything as if one were looking through a window. When the thick substances are spread out and scattered in that spot, it seems to the affected persons as if they see gnats flying outside. Such images often appear to them when they wake up from sleep, and they occur mostly with children and those whose heads are filled with wine or with something else. *De [symptomatum] causis* [I.2].

(VII.70) Just as someone who suffers from a cataract imagines that the things that are inside the eye are outside, so it happens with the tongue: the faculty of taste turns the quality that lies in the tongue itself into a necessary attribute of the things that are outside it. The reason for this is that the foods that one tastes activate the matter residing in the tongue so that one thinks that the foods themselves contain the quality of saltiness and sourness. *De [symptomatum] causis* [I.4].

(VII.71) As for laughter occurring through tickling the armpits on the outside and the soles of the feet, as well as laughter which occurs when seeing or hearing comical things, it is absolutely impossible to find out its cause. *De motibus [manifestis et] obscuris.*

(VII.72) Says Moses: This statement is correct because laughter is a specific characteristic of human beings. It is well known that each specific property belongs to the generic form, regardless of whether it belongs to the species of animals or plants or minerals. There is no way to give a reason for this. Therefore, one should not look for it in any way, neither regarding laughter nor any other specific property.

(VII.73) If someone looks into these things, he will find that nature has certain steps: the first is that wherein it departs a short distance from plants, resulting in an animal that has one sense, namely, that of touch. The second step is that in which it adds to touch the sense of taste. The third step is that in which one finds an animal who has, next to these two, the sense of smell. The fourth step is that in which it adds to these three the sense of hearing, and the fifth step is that in which is added to these four the sense of vision. And sometimes nature molds the eyes and sketches them in a hidden way and forms them without completing their strength, as with the mole. *De semine* II[.1, 5].

This is the end of the seventh treatise,
by the grace of God,
praise be to Him.

In the name of God,
the Merciful, the Compassionate.
O Lord, make our task easy

The Eighth Treatise
Containing aphorisms concerning the correct regimen for the healing of diseases in general

(VIII.1) If someone has bad, thin humors in his body, it requires more nutrition, and if he has humors with the opposite quality, it indicates the opposite. If it is impossible to find out the required amount of food, it is more prudent to change to the consumption of less food rather than more food because one can increase the consumption of food when one's strength dwindles but one cannot decrease the amount of food that has already gone to the stomach. [*In Hippocratis*] *De acutorum morborum* [*victu*] *commentarius* II[.36, 37].

(VIII.2) The things that help to coct the humors are all those that heat moderately; some of these are foods, some are beverages, some are poultices, and some are fomentations. Moderate massage and moderate bathing equally belong to this category. *In Hippocratis Epidemiarum* [*commentarius*] I.2.

(VIII.3) Raw humors are of two kinds: the first of these is thin and watery, and such humors should be evacuated immediately before they become sharp through the heat of the fever and become biting and corrosive. The other kind is thick and viscous and settled in the organs; these humors should be cocted first so that they stream easily. *In Hippocratis De humoribus commentarius* I.

(VIII.4) Sometimes a patient suffers from three diseases at the same time: One of these has already declined, the second is just beginning, and the third is reaching its climax. A patient dies not as a result of the disease that has declined or that is beginning, but because of the disease that is dramatically getting worse. *De totius morbi temporibus* [7].

(VIII.5) The first and most difficult thing we should examine is the condition of the three organs from which the faculties of the body originate—I mean the heart, the brain, and the liver—next to the condition of the parts that branch out from them—I mean the pulsatile vessels, nerves, and veins. Then we should examine the other parts of the body and look into everything as it is. *De totius morbi temporibus* [7].

(VIII.6) All diseases are weaker in their beginning and end and are stronger during their culmination. Between these two stages their condition is intermediate between weakness and strength. During the culmination the dominant treatment should consist of things that alleviate, and in the beginning and end it should consist of things that fight the disease. In the intermediate stages the treatment should be commensurate with that given during the two extremes. *De totius morbi temporibus* [8].

(VIII.7) When a disease is difficult to coct, the benefit of the therapy becomes apparent only after a long time and after the same medication has been taken repeatedly. *In Hippocratis Aphorismos commentarius* II[.19].

(VIII.8) One should be anxious and careful not to aggravate the disease and not to destroy the strength of the patient, who is likely to be afflicted for some time, although it is very difficult to achieve both things. For to the extent that abstinence is good for rapidly cocting the disease, to that extent it is harmful for the strength of the patient, and sometimes it is even more harmful. And to the extent that food aggravates a disease and delays its coction, to that extent it strengthens the patient. Therefore, one should always turn to that aspect which is most in need of support. *Ad Glauconem de medendi methodo* I[.11].

(VIII.9) One should try to determine exactly the proximity and distance of a disease from its culmination. For if one does not know this, one may potentially inflict great harm upon the patient. Similarly, one may sometimes prescribe a bad regimen if one does not know when the disease culminates. *De crisibus* I[.13].

(VIII.10) If a corruption of the humors occurs together with a weakness of bodily strength, there is absolutely no cure for that illness. And if there is something by which it might be healed, it can only be done after a long time, through exertion and strain and the presence of an expert physician. What should be done in this case is that the patient should not be treated with drugs that heal his disease, but one should feed him and revive his strength until his nature is strengthened so much that evacuation does not harm it at all or only slightly so. Then one should turn to treating the disease with drugs. *De methodo medendi* IX[.10].

(VIII.11) One should be extremely careful not to overheat any cold, thick, and viscous humor with blazing hot substances because when these humors dissolve, vapors arise from them that one can neither dissolve nor disperse. The most harmful situation is when these humors are between the two membranes of the intestines. These humors can be treated, however, with cutting, thinning remedies that do not overheat. *De methodo medendi* XII[.8].

(VIII.12) A complete evacuation of the body is effected through bloodletting or laxatives or emetics or frequent massage or any kind of exercise, or through bathing in the bathhouse, especially when it has a dissolving effect, or through sharp remedies when they are rubbed on the body, or through abstention from food. Evacuate the body of a patient through that which is most appropriate for him. *De methodo medendi* XIV[.7].

One should hasten to evacuate the irritating humor either before it weakens the strength of the body, or before it increases the heat of the fever, or before such a humor reaches a major organ. *In Hippocratis Aphorismos commentarius* IV[.10].

(VIII.13) Strong bodies can endure evacuation in one stroke, but in the case of weak bodies, one should evacuate the superfluity many times, for as long as the strength of the body can endure it. When the strength of the body dwindles, one should stop the evacuation even if there is still some superfluity left in the body. *In Hippocratis Aphorismos commentarius* I[.3].

(VIII.14) The coction of diseases only takes place through a change of the humors from an unnatural into a natural condition and only when the elementary parts in which those humors are present are healthy. But when these organs are ill, then the illness has taken possession of the very substance of the body, and the danger is great, and the patient cannot be cured unless the specific strength of these elementary parts returns to them. *In Hippocratis Epidemiarum* [*commentarius*] I.2.

(VIII.15) When a humor should be evacuated and you see that it tends to be evacuated with the urine, but the kidneys and urinary bladder are sick or weak, direct it to the belly. Similarly, if it tends to the belly but the intestines are ill, direct it to the region of the kidneys and bladder or to the region of the uterus.

And what is impossible for you to direct, let it stream to the region it tends to. *In Hippocratis Epidemiarum* [*commentarius*] VI.2.

(VIII.16) When the humors tend to stream to the inside, one should attract them to the outside; when they tend to stream to the outside, one should attract them to the inside; when they tend to stream to the rear, one should attract them to the front; and when they tend to stream to one side, one should attract them to the opposite side. *In Hippocratis De humoribus commentarius* I[.14].

(VIII.17) One of the things that attracts in the opposite direction is the binding of the hands and feet when the humor tends to the chest. Similarly, sharp medicines put on hands and feet attract the superfluities that tend towards the head or viscera. *In Hippocratis De humoribus commentarius* I[.14].

(VIII.18) One should evacuate the malignant humor either at the time that the disease attacks—namely, from above through a nosebleed or through emesis and the like—or at the time that the disease abates—namely, from below through the urine or excrements and the like. *In Hippocratis De humoribus commentarius* [I.14].

(VIII.19) Chronic diseases have to be treated by means of a thinning regimen. Indeed, for many of these diseases, this treatment alone is sufficient for their cure. I have seen how many patients who suffered from pains in the joints and asthma and a minor form of epilepsy were completely cured by this regimen. But someone who suffers from chronic epilepsy also derives no small benefit from this thinning regimen. This regimen consists of the continuous [consumption of] foods from which the thinning chyme originates, and of goal-oriented exercise, and of avoidance of any food containing thickness. *De victu attenuante*.

(VIII.20) If one fixes the time of consumption of the food and its quantity and quality, it is sufficient for nature to heal diseases. *In Hippocratis Epidemiarum* [*commentarius*] VI.5.

(VIII.21) I know many patients whose strength failed and whom I cured from this affliction by ordering them to abstain from food for a long time while I administered liquid drugs. I know others who suffered from syncope after loss of strength. These I treated by ordering abstention from food and frequent massage of arms and legs. I also ordered massage of the whole spine. These patients regained their strength and recovered fully. With other patients I did the opposite; I prevented them from keeping a restricted diet and administered food. *De optimo medico cognoscendo.*

(VIII.22) In the case of many people I behaved daringly in my treatment. With confidence and certainty, I gave some of them cold water all the time they were ill, and I gave it to others from time to time, although other physicians refrained from letting their patients drink cold water. With utmost confidence and trust, I let someone who suffered from pure ardent fever—but had no tumor in any part of his viscera—drink cold water. Likewise, in the case of someone else where I was not so sure and confident, I administered cold water after I had told his relatives, if he does not drink cold water, he will most certainly die, but if he drinks it, I hope that he will recover. And I swear by God, all those who drank cold water and whom I had hoped would recover actually recovered and regained their health. [*De consuetudinibus*].

(VIII.23) The diet of convalescents should hold the middle between that of healthy and ill people. Sleeplessness is the most harmful for them. To abandon one's habit is very dangerous not only in the case of the diet of convalescents and their like but also in the treatment of sick people. *De methodo medendi* VII[.6].

(VIII.24) The quantity of cold water that a fever patient should drink when he suffers from severe thirst should be as much as that which he can swallow without breathing. Cold substances prevent coction, except for oxymel, which does not because of its dissolving strength. *In Hippocratis De acutorum morborum* [*victu*] *commentarius* I[.43].

(VIII.25) Barley groats have the combined beneficial effects of invigorating one's strength and cleansing the respiratory organs of bad humors through cutting and moistening. These beneficial effects cannot be found together in any other substance. If a patient dislikes barley groats, the next best food is rockfish with water, leek, dill, salt, and a moderate amount of olive oil. If rockfish is unavailable, one should give him a fish that comes close to its temperament, but one should first of all give him some oxymel, except in the case that the nerves are affected. *In Hippocratis De acutorum morborum* [*victu*] *commentarius* I[.26].

(VIII.26) The ingestion of oxymel should precede that of barley broth by two hours so that it can purify, open, and pave the way for the excretions. When both are taken at the same time, disturbance occurs to the stomach because they are unequal in strength. *In Hippocratis De acutorum morborum* [*victu*] *commentarius* III[.35].

(VIII.27) Constipation helps the illness to increase and to become more powerful than nature, and sometimes it causes death. Sometimes it also causes various kinds of fevers and various kinds of external and internal tumors. Constipation stirs up every kind of pain coming from thick humors; it weakens the powers of nature and corrupts the psychical activities. Sometimes it causes a heavy torpor and loss of reason. *De clysteribus* [*et colica*].

(VIII.28) When someone after the meal exerts himself and does physical exercise so much that he becomes very tired and drinks abundantly, a bilious superfluity collects in his body because of the exertion and a raw uncocted superfluity collects because of the physical exercise performed at an improper time. Diseases become most severe when a large quantity of these two humors collects in the body. *In Hippocratis Epidemiarum* [*commentarius*] I.[3].

(VIII.29) Sleep is one of the most harmful things for very cold humors. Similarly, it is harmful in the beginning of fever attacks; it harms the viscera that have a tumor because the heat sinks and the blood sinks with it to the inner parts of the body. But if someone's humors are crude or small in quantity or if his strength is weak, sleep is beneficial for him. *In Hippocratis De humoribus commentarius* I[.17].

(VIII.30) Sleep in the beginning of inflamed tumors that cause fever increases the tumors and the fever. *In Hippocratis Epidemiarum* [*commentarius*] VI[.1–8].

(VIII.31) Anxieties are painful affections for the soul. Thoughts and considerations are exercise for the soul. All movements of the soul produce bile. Rest of the soul produces cold phlegmatic humors. In the case of cold humors, do not restrict yourself to movements of the body but add to that the movements of the soul to arouse the innate heat. For the arousal of anger, it is necessary that one recover one's normal complexion and that one's humors flow from the inner parts to the outer parts of the body. Anger is aroused in someone when the heat of his heart that was weak is increased. *In Hippocratis De humoribus commentarius* I[.18].

(VIII.32) Joyful thoughts and expectations rejoice and stimulate the soul, so that the innate heat expands by it. Conversely, sad thoughts and expectations distress the soul and cause the innate heat to contract. *In Hippocratis De humoribus commentarius* II[.31].

(VIII.33) Sleep is of evident benefit in the decline of diseases. It is good against the dryness of the belly, for while the air entering the body with the inhalation dries the belly by means of its heat, sleep moistens it. *De somno et vigilia.*

(VIII.34) Any feebleness caused by a copious evacuation all at once can be cured by wine mixed with cold water, especially when the evacuation is of moistures that stream to the stomach and what is around it. This applies only if there is no inflamed tumor in one of the viscera, no severe headache, no illness that causes a derangement of the mind, no ardent fever, and no illness that has not been cocted yet. In all these cases, drinking wine is so harmful for the patient that it almost cannot be cured. *Ad Glauconem* [*de medendi methodo*] I[.15].

(VIII.35) To alleviate the severe pain of inflamed tumors on the outer parts of the body, it is enough to take concentrated grape juice and rose oil mixed with a little melted wax. With this one should moisten a greasy piece of wool and put it on these tumors. Make it cold in the summer and lukewarm in the winter. In the same way one should apply poultices. *Ad Glauconem* [*de medendi methodo*] II[.2].

(VIII.36) One should examine the individual characteristics of the natures of people, because I know some who, having been busy at the beginning of the night, missed their normal sleeping time and consequently could not sleep for the rest of the night. There are others who, when they taste barley groats, immediately feel sick, and yet others who suffer from heartburn when they take it. *De methodo medendi* VII[.6].

(VIII.37) Pain arising especially from vaporous wind should be treated with a large cupping glass applied with strong heating. You might think that this is a kind of magical treatment regardless of whether the illness is in the intestines or in any other organ of the body, because the very moment that the cupping glass is applied, the pain disappears and the patient regains his health. But if the humor that activated the vapor is still there, the pain will necessarily return. Therefore, apply the cupping glass once again until the pain subsides and then evacuate that humor. *De methodo medendi* [VII.6].

(VIII.38) Compound remedies that alleviate pain—namely, those remedies that are mixed with narcotics and soporifics—should only be taken in cases where the pain is strong and severe, such as severe colic, stones, and severe sleeplessness, which dissolve the strength, or if one wants to quiet a severe cough that is difficult to bear and detrimental for the patient, such as someone who coughs up blood or who suffers from a very severe catarrh descending from his head. As for cases that are less dangerous than the ones I mentioned, it is sufficient to apply remedies that are not narcotic. [*De compositione medicamentorum secundum locos* IX].

(VIII.39) When one compounds remedies with narcotics to alleviate pain, one should consider three things: first, that by means of them one should numb the sensation of pain; second, that their application should not be followed by a lasting harm in the affected organ; and third, that the affected organ should receive great benefit from them either through dissolving, cutting, or refining the humors that caused the disease or through changing and improving the nature of those humors. I think that Philo composed the remedy named after him only after he had looked into these three necessary properties, and it is one of the oldest and most famous remedies. [*De compositione medicamentorum secundum locos*] IX[.4].

(VIII.40) If a symptom is accompanied by severe harm that damages the strength of the body, then in order to save the patient from death, the physician is obliged to abandon the treatment of the disease itself and eliminate the symptom or mitigate its harm, even if this aggravates the disease. Then he turns to the treatment of the harm that occurred because of the treatment of that symptom and the ensuing neglect of the disease. Sometimes that harm is completely eliminated, but in other cases it leaves a permanent weakness in or the loss of one of his bodily functions, and the patient lives for a long time with that chronic illness. This is the most appropriate course of action. *De methodo* [*medendi*] XII[.1].

(VIII.41) Some symptoms are harmful to the strength and should be attended to immediately when they become urgent. In this case one discontinues the treatment of the disease itself and of its cause unless it happens that the remedy used to combat the symptom is also good for repelling the disease and its cause. These symptoms are sleeplessness, pain, and all the various kinds of evacuations. If one of these occurs to excess, it is taken over by syncope. *De methodo* [*medendi*] XII[.1].

(VIII.42) When one draws blood or performs an evacuation or tries to to attract the malignant humor to the opposite side of the body but the pain persists, then the harmful substance has become fixed and settled in the organ and its treatment should consist of dissolving medications. In the same manner one should persistently treat those pains that arise from an inflating wind with refining foods and drinks, enemas, cataplasms, fomentations, and warm compresses. *De methodo* [*medendi*] XII[.8].

(VIII.43) The method one should always apply is to seek the evacuation and dissolution of the unnatural substance in the body. If this is impossible because of the nature of the affected organ or because the illness is incurable, one should let the unnatural substance suppurate and putrefy. If this is unsuccessful, we excise and extirpate it either by operative treatment or by caustic remedies. [*De compositione medicamentorum secundum locos*] XIV[.13].

(VIII.44) Weakness of the stomach, veins, arteries, and muscles and, in general, weakness of all the animal and psychical systems is caused by a bad temperament. [*De morborum differentiis* 5].

(VIII.45) A bad temperament occurring in any part of the body is an illness of that part. It forms an obstruction and obstacle now for one and then another of that part's powers. Because of this, humors stream towards various parts at various times unequally and irregularly. [*De symptomatum differentiis* 5].

(VIII.46) Remedies with a strong heating effect weaken the strength of the body greatly and suddenly. As a result, the body cannot tolerate treatment anymore. Therefore, the powers of the various kinds of food and drink that cut the thickness of the humors should be moderately hot. *De* [*curandi ratione per*] *venae sectione*[*m* 6].

(VIII.47) Concerning the various steps of treatment, logical reasoning indicates and experience verifies that we should begin by cleansing the whole body from superfluities. Then we should be confident to treat the ailing part with a medication that has only a heating effect. If we do not evacuate the body first, superfluous matter is attracted to that part through the hot medication, analogous to the attraction of a cupping glass. *De methodo* [*medendi*] IV[.4].

(VIII.48) When the illness is severe and difficult, one should hasten to evacuate the body through bleeding or relieving the bowels or emesis, even if overfilling is not indicated. The illness is severe and difficult when a major organ is endangered or when the illness itself is strong and severe, or bad and malignant, in quality, although not widespread in the body. *De methodo* [*medendi*] IV[.6].

(VIII.49) Galen said: If you want to prevent the superfluity from increasing, you should attract it to the side opposite to where it tends to stream. And if you want to evacuate it, you should do so from the side where it is or from the side to which it is nearest. *In Hippocratis De natura hominis commentarius* [III.15].

(VIII.50) Those, whose illness starts from many indigestions or from viscous thick foods and those who suffer from stretching or swelling in the hypochondrium, or from an extremely severe heat of the urine, or from an inflamed tumor in one of the viscera, are not ready to be purged. *In Hippocratis Aphorismos commentarius* I[.24].

(VIII.51) Says Moses: When the indigestion has occurred a very long time ago and you have verified that its effects have worn off, and, similarly, when those humors have become fine and thin and you have ascertained that there was a complete coction, and you see that the patient needs evacuation, then you can evacuate him with peace of mind as long as he is free from tumors in the viscera and from afflictions in the hypochondria—but mind what I said here.

(VIII.52) Take care not to apply a warm compress to the site of the illness before the evacuation, because then you attract more blood from the neighboring organs to it than the quantity that you dissolve. *In Hippocratis De acutorum morborum [victu] commentarius* II[.1].

(VIII.53) Sometimes a partial coction occurs that cannot be trusted, such as the coction of an abscess beneath the ears, for one assumes that the patient has recovered, yet he dies because the humors in the vessels were not cocted and they caused the illness. *In Hippocratis Epidemiarum [commentarius]* I.2.

(VIII.54) To apply a cupping glass without scarification is very beneficial for the other pains that arise from a thick, inflating, cold wind that is retained in solid bodies and that cannot escape because of its own thickness and the solidity of those bodies. *In Hippocratis Epidemiarum [commentarius]* II.6.

(VIII.55) When superfluous matter streams to the upper part of the mouth or the palate or the uvula, one should return it to the nostrils with sharp medications that are put in the nose. Similarly, the attraction of superfluous matter from the eyes to the mouth should take place through gargling with sharp medicines. *In Hippocratis De humoribus commentarius* I.

(VIII.56) A loud voice widens the passages and eliminates the moisture in the stomach and the mouth and stimulates expectoration. It expels viscous bad phlegm and heats the body. For those who need their bodies to be warmed, the use of the voice is better than any medication or foodstuff, because it warms their bodies, stimulates their innate heat, and warms the cold parts of their bodies and dries the moist parts. But if someone has a dry and lean body, he should not use his voice to expel superfluous moisture. Similarly, if someone suffers from bad moistures in his stomach or suffers from indigestion, you should warn him about the use of a loud voice because it lets the malignant humor in the stomach pass into the whole body. *De somno et vigilia.*

(VIII.57) If much blood streams to any part of the body, that part stretches and the vessels within it also stretch. This happens in the large vessels and in those small vessels which, initially hidden from the senses, become visible structures because of their overfilling, just as we can see the vessels that often appear in the eyes because of the whiteness of their tunic. Perhaps there are other vessels smaller than those of the eyes that become visible when they stretch because of overfilling, but these are not seen due to their smallness. *De arte parva* [34].

(VIII.58) I know a man who relied upon bathing in waters mixed with salt or borax or sulfur in order to evacuate his body of yellow bile. In the rest of his regimen he equally pursued the evacuation of the bile, but he did not know that every dominating unnatural humoral quality should be opposed by the opposite quality and that this is much better than evacuation. Nor did he listen to those who told him so. As a result, the elementary parts of his body dried so much that he was afflicted by phthisis and marasmus and then died. *Ad Glauconem [de medendi methodo]* I[.10].

(VIII.59) When you treat tumors that are difficult to dissolve, you should mix some softening medications with the medications that have a strong dissolving effect in order to be sure that those tumors will not turn into the hard tumor called *skirros*. *Ad Glauconem [de medendi methodo]* II[.6].

(VIII.60) When one is healthy, one should massage weak parts of the body more than the other parts, using dry massage especially. When applied during the times that the pains have eased, this kind of massage can prevent their occurrence in the weak parts, especially when applied two or three hours before the pains' actual attack. *De sanitate tuenda* V[.3].

(VIII.61) A change of the temperament to heat or cold can be treated most easily and cured most quickly. A change to moisture or dryness is harder to treat and to cure; to moisten what has become dry takes a long time. When the dryness becomes firmly settled, it is not susceptible to treatment, and when it becomes extremely well settled, it cannot be cured anymore. *De methodo* [*medendi*] VII[.5].

An incurable consolidation of dryness means that the very substance of the elementary parts has dried up. The closer the degree of dryness is to this degree of consolidation, the more difficult it is to heal and the more prolonged. Even the lowest degree of dryness is difficult to cure because the moistening process is difficult and hard and requires a long time. *De methodo* [*medendi*] VII[.5].

(VIII.62) There are four degrees of dryness: The first and the easiest to heal is when the dryness occurs in the small vessels that are specific to every part of the body and that provide nourishment to those parts through their openings. The second degree is when the dryness reaches the point where it eliminates that moisture scattered through the parts of the body which is like drizzle. This is the moisture whose property is to stream out of the openings of those thin vessels and adapt itself to a particular part to provide it with food. The third degree is when the dryness reaches the point where it eliminates the moisture in those parts of the body that are of a moist, nearly coagulated, and hardened substance—just like fat and flesh—that then liquefies and dissolves. The fourth degree is when the elementary parts become dry, such as the substance of the heart and the liver and the like. *De methodo* [*medendi*] VII[.5].

(VIII.63) When the temperament deviates from its balance towards cold, you should continue to heat it until it returns to its balance as long as you feel certain and confident about the result. But to cool a warm temperament is not the same matter—it should be done with caution and care and without taking any risk. If the area surrounding that part which one wants to cool is not completely strong, one cannot be sure that it will not suffer great harm from the cooling substances. *De methodo* [*medendi*] VII[.5].

The stomach and liver need astringent substances when superfluities stream into them more than the other organs of the body, for these two organs are extremely eminent and important and each one of them should—also in case of illness—carry out its specific function perfectly. *De methodo* [*medendi*] XI[.15].

(VIII.64) Remedies that are applied to the liver should combine—according to what is needed—astringent ingredients with attenuating ones so that their astringency is like that of aromatic substances. The best is when a remedy for the liver combines these two properties so that it is both astringent and aromatic. *De arte parva* [34].

(VIII.65) Quotidian fever hardly ever occurs without a stomach illness, just as quartan fever hardly ever occurs without an illness in the spleen. *Ad Glauconem* [*de medendi methodo*] I[.5].

(VIII.66) A compound remedy made up of many simple drugs is not more beneficial for every illness than one of the simple drugs it is compounded of; rather, the simple drug alone may be more beneficial for a particular illness. The intention of making a compound remedy is to have one single medication beneficial for many individual illnesses, each of which needs a simple remedy, although the benefits of such a compound drug are limited. [*De compositione medicamentorum secundum locos*] VIII[.3].

(VIII.67) The application of a moist, hot compress is beneficial for tumors arising from bile, and the application of a dry, hot compress is beneficial for tumors arising from fine, watery blood. The application of a hot compress that holds the middle between moisture and dryness, namely, one that comes into contact with a moderately warm body, is beneficial for biting humors. The application of a biting, hot compress is good for thick, viscous humors in that it dilutes and cuts them. *In Hippocratis De acutorum morborum* [*victu*] *commentarius* II[.2].

(VIII.68) It is only very rarely that one will see the illness of diabetes occur, for I have only seen it twice until now. *De locis affectis* VI[.3].

(VIII.69) Says Moses: I too have not seen it in the Maghreb, nor did any one of the elders under whom I studied inform me that he had seen it. However, here in Egypt I have seen more than twenty people affected by this disease in approximately ten years. This is to show you that this disease occurs mostly in hot countries. Perhaps the water of the Nile, because of its sweetness, plays a role in this.

(VIII.70) The time of the morning can be compared to spring and the time that comes after it can be compared to summer. The time of the evening is similar to autumn and the nighttime resembles winter. Just as diseases are most severe and lethal in autumn, so their attacks are most severe in the evening. *In Hippocratis Epidemiarum* [*commentarius* I.2].

(VIII.71) The best wind is the one that blows from the high sea; the next best is the one that blows from the mountains; the worst is the one that blows from marshes or swamps or morasses. Intermediate between these is the wind that blows from other directions. *In Hippocratis De humoribus commentarius* III[.13].

(VIII.72) The eye and the cardia of the stomach: these two parts of the body cannot tolerate anything put on then and burdening them. The eye can tolerate this so much less than the stomach that we see it already irritated by a medication put on it as a salve. *Ad Glauconem* [*de medendi methodo*] II[.4].

(VIII.73) Dissolution and dilution are in most cases a very successful treatment for any chronic disease. *Ad Glauconem* [*de medendi methodo*] II[.5].

(VIII.74) The first thing to take care of in the beginning of treatment is to expel that which dissolves and destroys the strength of the body. *De methodo* [*medendi*] VII[.12].

(VIII.75) When the Greeks were in doubt about a disease, they left it to nature to expel it. They said: Nature knows the temperament of the organs, and sends to every organ the appropriate kind of food and looks after the health of living beings and treats them in the case of disease. *De clysteribus* [*et colica*].

(VIII.76) Ibn Zuhr said: Every substance you want to use for cleansing the body, whether externally or internally, should be lukewarm. Every repelling or restraining substance should be cold, such as spring water. Every substance that opens should be hot and every substance that dissolves should be slightly warmer than that used for cleansing. When you want to alleviate internal or external pain, you should administer the remedy while it is lukewarm. But when you are afraid of syncope, you should give the medication with cold water.

(VIII.77) Ibn Zuhr said: It has been proved by experiment that every astringent substance has some purgative effect, except for myrtle, which has no purgative force at all. And every purgative has some sort of astringent quality.

This is the end of the eighth treatise,
by the grace of God,
praise be to Him.

∵

In the name of God,
the Merciful, the Compassionate.
O Lord, make our task easy

The Ninth Treatise
Containing aphorisms concerning specific diseases

(IX.1) The humors that produce epilepsy are thick, cold, and viscous. Their improvement consists in the transformation of the temperament of the young in age from moisture into dryness, and in exercise, and a drying regimen together with evacuation by means of medications. *In Hippocratis Aphorismos commentarius* II[.45].

(IX.2) In the case of a nosebleed you should not wait for the strength of the body to collapse. Rather, if you see the blood streaming rapidly, you should bleed the vein at the inner side of the arm on the same side as the hemorrhage, then you should tie the extremities with linen bandages, and then you should apply a cupping glass to the hypochondrium on the side opposite to the nostril from which the blood flows. I have done all this and as a result the flowing of the blood stopped. As for the medications that are put into the nose or on the forehead as prescribed by the physicians, we have tried them and found all of them to be weak. *De* [*curandi ratione per*] *venae sectione*[*m* 2].

(IX.3) If someone's superfluities from the brain are usually evacuated through a discharge from the ear and if this suddenly stops and vertigo and dizziness occur to him, we observe that if we stimulate that evacuation and provoke it to the ears through opening medications, such a patient immediately benefits therefrom. *In Hippocratis Epidemiarum* [*commentarius*] VI.2.

(IX.4) People who suffer from severe pains caused by thick blood or internal cold, such as migraine and the like, clearly benefit from drinking pure wine either immediately after the meal or during the meal. Their pains are alleviated by the heating and diluting effect of the wine. Similarly, one should soak bread or *sawīq* (semolina) in the pure wine because, by mixing the pure wine with food, one is protected from a hot vapor arising from it and harming the painful site. Rather, an even heat arises from it in all the parts of the painful organ. This heat then increases in these parts without vapor and dissolves the obstruction through the dilution of the humors that got stuck. A long sleep follows and the parts that surround the painful organ become lighter; their pores widen, and that which causes the pain is dissolved. For it is in the nature of these things to occur as the result of an even heat. *In Hippocratis Epidemiarum* [*commentarius*] VI.6.

(IX.5) If a nosebleed becomes excessive and does not stop with the application of a cupping glass on the hypochondrium, one should put a cupping glass on the nape of the neck and use something to cool the head. *In Hippocratis Epidemiarum* [*commentarius*] VI.7.

(IX.6) If the mucous discharge from the nose is watery and uncocted, we stop it with things with which we foment the head in order to heat the brain, and with those things that are inhaled through the nose, and with those things that are dripped into the ears. *In Hippocratis De humoribus commentarius* I[.18].

(IX.7) All those suffering from defluxions are adversely affected in the beginning of their occurrence by sneezing because at that moment the humors are raw and congested. Also, the heavy movement of sneezing increases the fullness of the head. Especially at that moment, the various parts of the head and chest need rest, tranquility, and moderate heat so that those raw humors are cocted. When a defluxion occurs after such a period of rest, the humors are—because they have been cocted—dissolved and evacuated through sneezing. *In Hippocratis De humoribus commentarius* I[.18].

(IX.8) The sparks that a person sees before his eyes result from humors whose consistency and color are contrary to the albuminoid humor that gathers between the crystalline humor and the horn-like tunic. *In Hippocratis De humoribus commentarius* I[.17].

(IX.9) Headaches are alleviated by bandaging the head when the humors that effect the headache need moderate heating. *In Hippocratis De humoribus commentarius* I[.18].

Sneezing is especially beneficial in the case of watery humors, but it is harmful in the case of bilious humors because it stimulates and increases them. *In Hippocratis De humoribus commentarius* I[.18].

(IX.10) The treatment of sleeplessness consists of binding the hands and legs at the time when he who suffers from it usually goes to sleep, preventing him from sleeping, and making him open his eyes when he closes them until he is languid and tired. Then the ligatures are loosened, the lamp is removed, and all sudden movements and speaking are stopped, for then he will have a wholesome, deep sleep. *In Hippocratis De humoribus commentarius* [III.19].

(IX.11) If a person is overcome by a torpor, one should grasp the tip of the tongue and press it completely down. Then one should look for a receptacle with a narrow opening, and put some moist liquid food into it, and put it into the mouth on the base of the tongue, and pour the contents into the esophagus. *De motibus* [*manifestis et*] *obscuris*.

(IX.12) It sometimes happens to a person that he lies on his back the entire night and that when he arises in the morning he is overtaken by a stroke, torpor, or an epileptic fit, since the ventricles of his brain are filled with those superfluities. *De instrumentu odoratus* [6].

(IX.13) For the treatment of a child suffering from epilepsy, after I cleansed his body, I often contented myself with a potion of vinegar and honey until I had completely healed him. There was no need for anything else but for this potion. *Puero epileptico* [*consilium* 4].

(IX.14) If there is a nosebleed from one of the nostrils and one puts cupping glasses one at a time on the liver or spleen on the same side as the bleeding nostril, the nosebleed stops. If the nosebleed is from both nostrils and is very severe, one should put cupping glasses on both spots at the same time. *Ad Glauconem* [*de medendi methodo*] I[.15].

(IX.15) All the afflictions and diseases that occur to the leading activities but do not include swellings in the corresponding organs originate from a bad temperament of the brain. Such a bad temperament sometimes occurs in the ventricles of the brain and sometimes in the pulsatile and non-pulsatile vessels that are scattered throughout them. Sometimes it occurs in the fluid that diffuses in the substance of the brain itself, or sometimes the temperament of the substance of the brain itself is corrupted. To find out which kind of bad temperament one is dealing with is not an easy job, but it is one for which a physician should love to exert himself. *De locis affectis* III[.6].

(IX.16) Melancholic delusion occurs from the fact that all the blood in the vessels is melancholic, and the harm done to the brain is comparable to the general harm. But the change in the blood can also be in the brain alone, either because a melancholic humor poured into it or because it developed in the brain as a result of the heat there, which roasts and burns the yellow bile or the thick blood. If the melancholic blood is common to the whole body, begin with phlebotomy, and if it is in the brain only, take care of the brain alone. *De locis affectis* III[.10].

(IX.17) The cold brain tumor, namely, lethargy, and the hot one, namely, phrenitis, have in common that in the beginning both should be treated by phlebotomy and by the application of rose oil and vinegar in order to expel the harming humor—whatever humor it is—from the head. This should be done although one disease goes with sleeplessness and the other with torpor. Hereafter one should try to calm the person suffering from sleeplessness and to awaken and stimulate the person who suffers from torpor. *De methodo* [*medendi*] XIII[.21].

(IX.18) When a brain tumor reaches its culmination, one should rub the head of the person whose illness is accompanied by sleeplessness and delirium with a salve prepared from opium poppy, while the corner of the nostrils and face should be rubbed with substances that cool the brain. If someone's illness is accompanied by torpor, one should heat the thick humor. *De methodo* [*medendi*] XIII[.21].

(IX.19) If either of these two diseases, namely, lethargy or phrenitis, become chronic, we apply cupping glasses and castoreum for their treatment, because they coct both illnesses. When both are in a state of decline, their treatment should also be one and the same. *De methodo* [*medendi*] XIII[.21].

(IX.20) When the lethargy stops getting worse, smear strong and sharp medications on the palate and then apply those drugs that stimulate sneezing, and put similar drugs on the head, even mustard. *De methodo* [*medendi*] XIII[.21].

(IX.21) When someone suffers from a headache caused by inebriety, he should try to sleep and rest for the entire day; in the evening he should enter the bathhouse and feed himself with foods that produce good blood and do not heat, such as barley groats. One should let him eat cultivated lettuce, because it produces beneficial blood and has a cooling effect, and cabbage, because it eliminates and dries the vapors. From the pulses he should eat lentils, and for a drink he should take water, and when his stomach becomes lax because of the water he should suck pomegranate and quince and the like. The next day he should enter the bathhouse and pour lots of hot water over his head in order to dissolve the vapors. Just like all the others suffering from a headache, he should abstain from movement until the headache subsides, and then he should move so that the rest of the vapors dissolve. [*De compositione medicamentorum secundum locos*] II[.1].

(IX.22) For eye pain one should apply to the eye a warm compress with a sponge dipped in water in which melilot and fenugreek have been cooked. When the pain is mild, apply the compress once or twice a day, and when the pain is severe, apply it many times, especially during the long summer days. [*De compositione medicamentorum secundum locos*] IV[.3].

(IX.23) Epilepsy and torpor only originate from the brain. A torpor amongst the voluntary activities is comparable to a deep sleep amongst the sensory activities, while an epileptic spasm amongst the voluntary activities is like sleeplessness amongst the sensory activities. *De* [*symptomatum*] *causis* IV[.8].

(IX.24) Says Moses: What he means is that both a torpor and a deep sleep are a lack of activity, while an epileptic spasm and sleeplessness are a disturbance.

(IX.25) A severe headache occurs from heat or cold. The headache caused by dryness is weak. Moisture does not cause any pain at all. A surplus of humors in the head causes heaviness but not a headache, except when an obstruction occurs from it. For then a headache occurs that is proportional to the degree of obstruction. [*De compositione medicamentorum secundum locos*] II[.1].

(IX.26) Every substance used for treating the ears should be moderately lukewarm; for this we use breast milk or egg white on its own. Amongst the medications for alleviating ear pains caused by biting matters are such as we apply for eye pain. [*De compositione medicamentorum secundum locos*] III[.1].

(IX.27) I know from experience that the hole of the ear should not be touched at all with anything at the time of pain. Rather, one should trickle drops into it that are as warm as can be tolerated. One should suspend one's hand in the air until the medicine flows from the end of the probe to the inner hole of the ear. One should do this repeatedly and not stop until the hole of the ear is filled. Then one should wipe off that which streams out of it very gently without touching the ear itself or any of its parts. This is a very important matter one should be very careful about when one treats the ear in the case of pain. [*De compositione medicamentorum secundum locos*] III[.1].

(IX.28) The remedies with which the inside of the nose is treated are rapidly washed out because of the moisture streaming from the nose. Therefore, one should persist in its treatment with these remedies in the same way one persists in treating the eye. [*De compositione medicamentorum secundum locos*] III[.3].

(IX.29) Any warm compress applied to the teeth either outside or inside the mouth should be applied before having a meal, on an empty stomach, or after a long time following a meal. [*De compositione medicamentorum secundum locos*] V[.4].

(IX.30) Al-Tamīmī said: Chinese snow, which is a white, round, lustrous stone, Indian tutty, glass slag, "glass of Pharaoh," excrement of lizards, shells of turtle dove eggs and musk—if one calculates the proper amounts of these remedies and then prepares an eye powder from them, the powder removes the white opacity of the eye (leucoma) extremely well and cleanses it without irritation or harm. [*Kitāb al-murshid fī jawāhir al-aghdhiya waquwā l-mufradāt mina l-adwiya*].

(IX.31) Inhabitants of hot countries often suffer from ophthalmia but are rapidly cured. Inhabitants of cold countries rarely suffer from ophthalmia, but if they suffer from it, it is severe and hard whereby the eyes are ruptured. There is a similar analogy regarding ophthalmia occurring in the winter and that occurring in the summer. *In Hippocratis De aer*[*e, aquis et locis*] *commentarius* I.

(IX.32) Angina is any illness of the throat whereby the patient has a feeling of narrowness during swallowing. The most deadly one of these is where the swelling or redness does not appear in the pharynx, but in the esophagus or larynx or in their muscles only. Sometimes angina originates from cold, viscous, raw humors. *In Hippocratis Epidemiarum* [*commentarius* I].2.

(IX.33) When the swelling in the case of angina is severe, one should not be content with applying internal medications alone but should also use external ones. One should apply cataplasms, pour hot water over it and let the patient enter the bathhouse. However, this should only be done when the illness is abating. Angina patients should be fed with medicinal soups so that, when the liquid passes the swollen places, it has the same effect as a cataplasm. *In Hippocratis Epidemiarum* [*commentarius* I.2].

(IX.34) Speech is a movement only occurring in the respiratory organs. Therefore, if someone is discharging blood from the larynx, the lungs, the chest, or the windpipe, he should not make a sound nor breathe heavily. To move his arms is not bad for him. Most appropriate for such a condition is a movement of the legs moderate enough that the pulse does not become frequent. *In Hippocratis De humoribus commentarius* I[.18].

(IX.35) The plucking of hair attracts the humors from the depth of the body to its outside. Therefore, it is beneficial for someone who suffers from the disease of forgetfulness and torpor, or for someone in whose body a humor that is not sound streams from the outside of the body to one of his joints or ears. *In Hippocratis De humoribus commentarius* I.

(IX.36) Sometimes an irregular bad temperament occurs in the muscles of the chest followed by a mild cough, which is, as it were, a pain that provokes coughing, because the muscle trembles and shakes out of desire to expel the harmful substance. *De [symptomatum] causis* [II.5].

(IX.37) Medications for the spitting of blood are composed of drugs that dry without biting, or drugs that are somewhat agglutinant, or astringent drugs. This is right for stopping the spitting of blood in general. But when the spitting of blood is from the lungs, chest, windpipe, or larynx, I mix these drugs with those that are hot and fine, even if they are maximally contrary to this illness. The objective of this is that they will lead those astringent drugs and bring them—while protecting them—to the affected sites. When the spitting of blood is from the region of the esophagus, stomach, abdomen, or intestines, there is no need to mix in these hot and fine drugs. [*De compositione medicamentorum secundum locos*] VII[.4].

(IX.38) Sometimes the drugs for the spitting of blood should also be mixed with soporific ones in order to let those who suffer from it fall into a lethargic sleep. This is very beneficial for someone who is harmed and shaken by coughing. Moreover, because of their coldness, these drugs stop the blood and prevent it from streaming to the affected vessel. [*De compositione medicamentorum secundum locos*] VII[.4].

(IX.39) The amelioration of bad humors in the case of those who say that their sputum tastes like seawater takes a long time. If someone is afflicted with an ulcer in the lungs because of these bad humors, he cannot be healed at all. For in the long time that it takes for the humors to become better, the ulcer becomes so dried up and hard that it cannot be cured anymore, or it becomes putrefied and then in turn causes putrefaction to the surrounding area until the entire lung has decayed. *De methodo medendi* V[.14].

(IX.40) Sometimes hiccups occur from coldness of the air, for every coldness prevents dissolution of humors, and for this reason an overfilling occurs in the nervous parts, which then causes hiccups. *In Hippocratis Aphorismos commentarius* VI[.13].

(IX.41) Especially in the case of stomach ailments, the amount of food that one takes should be extremely moderate so that it does not become a burden to the stomach. The same holds true for liver ailments. *In Hippocratis Epidemiarum* [*commentarius* I.3].

(IX.42) Distress originates from humors that are not as bad as those that produce syncope. Yawning comes from the relaxation of the muscles that move the jawbones so that the vapor can be dissolved. Wine mixed with an equal amount of water is beneficial for all these cases because it balances the bad humors, heats the stomach, aids digestion, dissolves the cold vapor, and is good for shivering that originates from hot humors. But one should refrain from giving it as a drink in the case of shivering during which there is only a fever or an inflamed tumor. *In Hippocratis Epidemiarum* [*commentarius* I.3].

(IX.43) I observed that people suffered from epileptic spasms that arose from the cardia of their stomachs when they suffered from severe indigestion, or when they drank wine that was too hot, or when they had too much sexual intercourse at the wrong time. I also saw patients with fever suffering from sudden spasms because of a bad humor that streamed to the cardia of the stomach and irritated it. When they vomited, they found immediate relief. Other persons, burdened by bad food they had eaten and then struck by torpor, only found relief when they had vomited all that which oppressed the cardia of their stomach. When the cardia of the stomach is affected, a sudden and rapid syncope may also arise from it. *De locis affectis* V[.6].

(IX.44) A gassy disease makes the patient suffering from it depressed, sad, hopeless, and despairing of good. In short, their condition is like that of those suffering from melancholic delusion because of the connection between the cardia of the stomach and the brain. Their afflictions become even more severe when they suffer from indigestion. Most of these patients suffer from an affection of the spleen, and this is one of the indications that serous moisture is streaming from the spleen to the cardia of the stomach. *De locis affectis* V[.6].

(IX.45) If someone's food often putrefies in his stomach, he benefits from emesis before eating and from drinking sweet wine. He should eat those foods that are not quickly putrefied and should accustom himself to relieving the bowels from time to time with those substances that have a moderately relieving force, such as *hiera picra*. But if one neglects the bad humor, healing is difficult. *De sanitate tuenda* v[.7].

(IX.46) When a hot, bad temperament mixed with either a small amount of moisture or with dryness dominates the stomach but does not affect the substance of the stomach, we treat it with cold water without fear or hesitation, for cold water is not harmful to the organs close to the stomach because they are in a state of balance. *De methodo medendi* VII[.9].

But if bad humors have entered into the substance of the coats of the stomach, the best kind of treatment is their evacuation with aloe or *hiera picra* ingested with water. The composition of *hiera picra* is six *mithqāl*s each of cinnamon, spikenard, saffron, asarabacca, mastic, and balsam wood, and one hundred *mithqāl*s of aloe. The *hiera picra* should be prepared in two ways, with washed aloe and unwashed aloe. The washed type strengthens the stomach more, while the unwashed type is a stronger laxative. *De methodo medendi* VII[.11].

(IX.47) In the case of indigestion associated with diarrhea so severe that it harms one's strength, one should feed oneself with things that are astringent more and more. Often diarrhea goes with loss of appetite. In this case the patient should take a stomachic of quinces and the like. However, if indigestion is associated with constipation and either with a fever arising from the indigestion or without a fever, and if the spoiled food is in the upper parts of the abdomen, one should bring it down with the various kinds of pepper and the like. When the spoiled food has gone down, one should expel it either with a suppository or with an enema of honey, water, and olive oil. If the patient has a strong biting sensation there, administer to him an enema of olive oil in which duck fat has been melted. If duck fat is not available, use chicken fat instead. If this is not available, use goat fat or olive oil and washed wax. If the patient suffers from flatulence, administer to him an enema of olive oil in which common rue was cooked or in which seeds that disperse the winds, such as cumin, caraway, celery seed, and the like, were cooked. *De methodo medendi* VIII[.5].

(IX.48) When the bowels of someone suffering from indigestion are relieved by means of a suppository or enema, feed him immediately thereafter with foods that are not at all astringent. Do the same on the second day and order the patient to go to the bathhouse when he is completely free of indigestion. When he sleeps well during the night following the bathhouse, he is completely healed. And if he suffers thereafter from a minor attack of fever, do not be worried or alarmed about it, but let him go to the bathhouse the next day and then let him eat. *De methodo medendi* VIII[.5].

(IX.49) If someone is struck by syncope caused by yellow bile that streamed to the cardia of his stomach, let him drink cold, fragrant, watery wine. When the syncope is caused by a surplus of crude humors, let him drink warm pale or yellowish wine, if his head is strong. But let anyone struck by syncope drink fragrant wine. *De methodo medendi* XII[.4].

(IX.50) Patients with illnesses occurring in the stomach and abdomen because of bad humors benefit from medications prepared with aloe. But astringent things, whether foods, beverages, or drugs, cause great harm. When the cardia of the stomach is steeped in moist humors that are not bad in quality but are simply harmful because of their quantity, then the use of astringent drugs, foods, and beverages is most beneficial. [*De compositione medicamentorum secundum locos*] VIII[.2].

(IX.51) Strong and difficult emesis occurs when there is drug-like fluid in the stomach that is incompatible with it and that inflicts serious harm upon it. When, in addition, the stomach is weak, the harm is twice as great. The aim of the treatment of someone with this condition is to eliminate that bad fluid and then to strengthen the stomach with fragrant spices and seeds with similar properties. Just as all malodorous spices and seeds upset the soul and cause nausea, all fragrant ones strengthen the stomach, especially when they belong to the comestibles, for these are most suited to benefit a stomach upset because of that fluid. [*De compositione medicamentorum secundum locos*] VIII[.3].

(IX.52) If someone is attacked by hiccups because of overeating or an acrid humor, emesis will cure him. And when he is attacked by it because of cold, heating will cure him. A similar effect is achieved when one transforms the things that are acrid and eliminates and dissolves them through refining and drying remedies; this is most beneficial. [*De compositione medicamentorum secundum locos*] VIII[.3].

(IX.53) If someone is struck by bulimia, either suddenly or gradually, we restore his strength by making him smell vinegar, pennyroyal, ashes, and mint steeped in vinegar, or by letting him smell apples and similar fruits, or a piece of bread, which he should also be compelled to eat. We also give him roasted or cooked pork to smell. In general, one should have him smell every kind of foodstuff that has a fragrant smell. Similarly, all fragrant substances revive bulimic patients and restore their strength. One should tightly bandage their hands and feet, prick their chests, and pull their hair. When they awaken from their syncope, one should feed them bread steeped in wine or something else that restores their strength. [*De compositione medicamentorum secundum locos*] VIII[.4].

(IX.54) A craving for bad and detestable beverages can also occur in the same way as it occurs for bad foods. This is the case when a bad humor, either salty or biliary, is congested in the coats of the stomach. This craving is excessive when this humor is boiling. The variation in the types of things one wants to drink is commensurate with the variation of the types of humors in quality and badness. *De* [*symptomatum*] *causis* [I.7].

(IX.55) It is difficult to treat weakness of the cardia of the stomach and quick nausea associated with constipation because everything that relieves the bowels causes nausea and upsets the soul, while that which strengthens the cardia of the stomach causes constipation. The most beneficial therapy I found for such patients is to eat vegetables spiced with olive oil and *garum*. Then they should take a small amount of pear or quince or pomegranate, according to what they like most. *De sanitate tuenda* VI[.10].

(IX.56) If you want to strengthen the stomach of those suffering from indigestion and the like even if they have ephemeral fever, put strengthening substances upon the stomach—these should actually be extremely hot because anything lukewarm loosens and softens the cardia of the stomach. *De methodo medendi* VIII[.5].

(IX.57) If someone suffers from indigestion and the like and from a burning in the stomach that is so severe that one imagines that there is an inflamed tumor there, he will benefit from a salve prepared with quince oil. It is my practice to heat the oils in a double vessel because their strength is lost if they are heated in any other way. *De methodo medendi* VIII[.5].

(IX.58) In those suffering from dropsy, water accumulates in those places that are between the intestines and the membrane covering them. [*Introductio sive medicus* 13].

(IX.59) In the case of dropsy of the flesh (anasarca), one should apply that which expels the phlegm—first of all through relieving the bowels, then through emesis, and then through gargling, since gargling evacuates the phlegm from the head. When the phlegm is spread through the whole body, we set about to apply all possible methods in order to evacuate it. In this disease we also give the patient medications to drink with cutting and heating properties so that we stimulate diuresis and evacuate the body completely through the dissolution of the phlegm. *In Hippocratis De humoribus commentarius* I[.12].

(IX.60) [...] And we should cleanse the bodies of jaundice patients from the biles they contain in every possible manner so that we evacuate the body from above and below and through the urine and the palate and the nostrils. *In Hippocratis De humoribus commentarius* I[.12].

(IX.61) Sometimes a jaundice patient benefits from looking at yellow colors because this dissolves the yellow bile. A patient with hemoptysis should be forbidden to look at colors that are primarily red, because this will make the blood stream forth. To evacuate any humor, it is proper to look at the colors of that humor; and to repel any humor into the depth of the body, it is proper to look at the colors opposite to the color of that humor. *In Hippocratis De humoribus commentarius* II[.27].

(IX.62) I have often successfully treated a hard tumor in the liver at its inception. But when it existed for a longer time, I was unable to effect a cure, nor have I seen anyone else who achieved this. All those affected by this disease are also afflicted with dropsy and most of them die after a long time. But if one of them has diarrhea, he dies quickly. *Ad Glauconem* [*de medendi methodo*] II[.7].

(IX.63) The treatment of patients suffering from dropsy caused by a hard tumor in the viscera should be directed towards three goals: firstly, to succeed in healing the hard tumor in the viscera; secondly, to apply poultices that dissolve the moisture; and thirdly, to give the patient diuretic medications to drink. *Ad Glauconem* [*de medendi methodo*] II[.12].

(IX.64) Transudation of blood occurs because of the opening of small vessels or because of the evacuation of the watery part of the blood, as it occurs especially in the case of weakness of the liver or kidneys, for a patient suffering from this illness often urinates or defecates the watery part of the blood. *De* [*symptomatum*] *causis* [III.5].

(IX.65) In all the various types of dropsy, the liver itself fails to transform the food that reaches it into blood because of a cold bad temperament that dominates it. Sometimes this cold bad temperament dominates one of the digestive organs or one of the respiratory organs and passes from there on to the neighboring organs until it reaches the substance of the liver through the common vessels. As a result, the illness settles in the substance of the liver and produces dropsy. Similarly, when an excessive loss of blood occurs in whatever way, the liver becomes cold and dropsy results. *De locis affectis* v[.7].

(IX.66) Sometimes the liver is affected by such a dry bad temperament that it cannot transform the food into blood, and dropsy develops. Sometimes this happens because of a hard tumor in the spleen, because most illnesses of the spleen also affect the liver. *De locis affectis* [v.7].

(IX.67) Obstructions of the liver should be treated with opening remedies, and congestion in the head, with walking before meals. Such patients should also walk slowly after meals. Everything that is good for opening obstructions is also appropriate for a slow digestion; the best of these are oxymel and the various kinds of pepper. A thinning regimen is good for a slow digestion and relieves obstructions of the liver. *De sanitate tuenda* VI[.7].

(IX.68) For treating tumors of the liver and stomach, I prefer absinth wormwood. When I think that the liver and stomach are in a bad condition, I immediately boil absinth wormwood with olive oil and pour it over these parts of the body. If it is not at hand, I use quince oil or mastic oil. In case of a light fever, I use spikenard oil. *De methodo* [*medendi*] XI[.16].

(IX.69) When a tumor occurs in the liver, an extremely strict diet is required. No food is more beneficial to it than barley groats because they cleanse without biting, and there is no medication more beneficial for it than oxymel with cold water. But do not try to treat it with pomegranate juice or apples or other astringent things that cause the openings of the vessels to contract and prevent the evacuation of bile. *De methodo* [*medendi*] XIII[.14].

(IX.70) If there is a tumor on the convex side of the liver, it is time to purge it. One should do so by stimulating micturition. When it is on the concave side of the liver, one should purge it through relieving the bowels by mixing safflower seed, Roman nettle seed, and a moderate laxative into the food. When the tumor subsides, one should continue to do these things with confidence and trust. I have occasionally cooked common polypody with barley groats and black hellebore. One may also purge such patients with enemas initially prepared from water, honey, and borax or natron, and when the illness subsides, with something stronger such as mint, pulp of the colocynth, and common centaury. *De methodo* [*medendi*] XIII[.15].

In the case of a weak liver one should first of all take care to open its obstruction through cleansing and moderately dissolving remedies—such as turpentine resin—so that the openings of the pulsatile and non-pulsatile vessels that the liver contains and that pass throughout it remain open without any obstruction, for an obstruction produces putrefaction. A medication prepared for the liver should not be strongly cooling but only moderately so. [*De compositione medicamentorum secundum locos*] VIII[.6].

(IX.71) Cultivated and wild *hindibā'* (endive or chicory) have a temperament dominated by some cold and are also somewhat bitter, and together they have a moderately astringent effect. Because of the presence of these two qualities, they are amongst the best remedies for the treatment of a hot, bad temperament of the liver. They are not as harmful for a cold, bad temperament as are cold, moist remedies without astringency and without bitterness. The reason for this is that they cool the liver moderately, and strengthen it through their astringency, and cleanse it through their bitterness. They are beneficial for the liver against a simple bad temperament and against one combined with serous matter, for when they are mixed with honey, they make those serous moistures and other moistures flow and descend from the body. [*De compositione medicamentorum secundum locos*] VIII[.8].

(IX.72) Of the remedies for hardness of the liver, the softening ones should be very weak, and those remedies that heat and refine should be more predominant than in the case of the treatment of hardness of the other organs. For the substance of the liver is indeed like congealed moisture, and if those remedies soften it greatly, its powers dissolve. [*De compositione medicamentorum secundum locos*] VIII[.8].

(IX.73) Among the remedies that are very effective for cleansing the liver and for opening its narrow passages without visibly warming or cooling it is male fern, which, because of its bitter taste, strongly predominates. [*De compositione medicamentorum secundum locos*] VIII[.8].

(IX.74) The medications for a tumor in the stomach or liver should be mixed with astringent fragrant substances (remedies); one should not limit oneself to using only softening, slackening medications. If one does so, one endangers the patient and puts him on the verge of death. [*De compositione medicamentorum secundum locos*] VIII[.1].

(IX.75) Astringent and biting substances are not as harmful for tumors on the convex side of the liver as they are for tumors on the concave side, because the powers of the substances that a person takes change before they reach the convex side of the liver. Thus, an astringent substance is not as astringent as it was before, and a biting substance is not as biting as it was before, and a viscous substance is less viscous. *De methodo* [*medendi*] XIII[.14].

(IX.76) When a tumor occurs in the spleen and the body contains superfluous melancholic humor, mixing astringent ingredients with the dissolving medications is unavoidable in order to preserve the body's strength—the superfluities are thus attracted and the body can be cleansed from them. When the body is clean, one should not mix anything at all astringent with other medications for its treatment, unless the astringent quality is as weak as possible. *De methodo* [*medendi*] XI[.16].

(IX.77) The best remedy for hardness of the spleen is a poultice prepared from roots of caper, absinth wormwood, vinegar, and honey. Be careful not to apply a poultice with astringent remedies to the chest. *De methodo* [*medendi*] XI[.16].

(IX.78) A constant use of vinegar together with dissolving remedies in the case of illnesses of the spleen and of hard swelling in the fleshy part of any muscle is a safe remedy. Simple gum ammoniac with vinegar is often sufficient for the treatment of tumors and hardness of the spleen. *De methodo* [*medendi*] XIV[.5].

(IX.79) Sometimes the distress of a melancholic delusion results from an illness of the spleen and often arouses a very strong craving for food, especially when a purely acid superfluity streams to the stomach. Often an aversion and dislike of food occurs and the soul (stomach) becomes upset when the craving is spoiled in another way. *De locis affectis* VI[.1].

(IX.80) There is only one way to evacuate the superfluities that collect in the spleen, namely, through relieving the bowels, because it is not in the spleen's nature to expel its contents to the kidneys. Therefore, when a tumor develops in the spleen, we stimulate it through laxatives, so that it expels the superfluities that got stuck in it. *De methodo medendi* XIII[.17].

(IX.81) Pleurisy should be treated through bleeding, the application of a hot compress, and softening of the stool. Be careful not to administer barley groats when the pleurisy reaches its climax so that a crisis is not hindered. [*In Hippocratis*] *De acutorum morborum* [*victu*] *commentarius* I[.32].

(IX.82) If you want to apply a hot compress to someone suffering from pleurisy, you should put soft wool or a folded garment or a small cushion underneath the hot compress so that the contact of the hot compress with the ribs is without pressure and without any harm whatsoever. [*In Hippocratis*] *De acutorum morborum* [*victu*] *commentarius* II[.3].

(IX.83) The inhalation of the vapor of a hot compress is only beneficial when the vapor is moist and when the pleurisy is dry, without any expectoration. [*In Hippocratis*] *De acutorum morborum* [*victu*] *commentarius* II[.4].

(IX.84) One should avoid phlebotomy when pleurisy is caused by a bilious, melancholic, or phlegmatic humor. It should also be avoided in pleurisy caused by a blood-like humor when the time of the year is extremely hot, or when the humor that dominates the body of the patient consists of bile, or when the blood-like humor has changed into bile—that is, when the patient spits up bile after spitting up blood. *In Hippocratis De humoribus commentarius* III[.33].

(IX.85) Everything necessarily resulting from an inflammation of the nervous part of the diaphragm also results from severe inflammations of the membrane covering the ribs on the inside. *De* [*praesagitione ex*] *puls*[*ibus* IV.5].

(IX.86) Drugs prepared with aromatic herbs are very beneficial for abscesses occurring deep inside the body and especially in the intestines, for these drugs dissolve and melt the humors accumulated in them. There are many other similar remedies; the best of these is the great theriac, and less good are the drugs prepared with water mint. *De methodo medendi* [XIII.17].

(IX.87) An appropriate therapy in general for abscesses occurring deep inside the body is to treat them with refining and drying drugs. Also good for these patients is to drink a little bit of thin wine. [*De compositione medicamentorum secundum locos*] VII[.6].

(IX.88) Says Moses: Among the refining and drying remedies are

1. vinegar, which is cold, and
2. maidenhair fern, a drug intermediate between hot and cold.

The other well-known and often-applied remedies are all of them hot and dry. However, since most internal abscesses are followed by fever, it is necessary for a physician to remember those remedies that Galen has specified as attenuating and drying, next to their degrees of heat and dryness.

Of the medications that dry and attenuate and are hot and dry in the first degree, there are four that are commonly used:

1. common agrimony,
2. camel grass,
3. French tamarisk, and
4. pistachio nuts.

Of the medications that are hot and dry in the second degree, there are eight:

1. Roman nettle,
2. balsam of Mecca,
3. birthwort,
4. Florentine iris,
5. squirting cucumber,
6. rhubarb,
7. asphodel, and
8. *khīrī* (wallflower or hoary stock).

Of the medications that are hot and dry in the third degree, there are twenty:

1. savin juniper,
2. great yellow gentian,
3. wild carrot,
4. cinnamon,
5. *hayūfārīqūn* (bearded or perforate St. John's wort),
6. sweet flag,
7. hyssop,
8. black poplar,
9. glossy forest grape (*ḥamāmā*),
10. cubeb,
11. marjoram,
12. *nānakhwāh* (bisnaga or ajowan),
13. peppermint,
14. broad-leaved thyme,
15. common rue,
16. Chinese cinnamon,
17. sagapenum,
18. mint,
19. fennel, and
20. black cumin.

Of the remedies mentioned by later physicians that dry and attenuate and that are hot and dry in the first degree, there are three drugs that are commonly used:

1. silk,
2. Ceylon ironwood, and
3. common cardamom, which is called *hāl.*

Altogether there are thirty-seven drugs; of these, one should use whatever is available as a simple or compound remedy according to what one deems appropriate.

(IX.89) When internal ulcers do not come with an inflammation, they can be healed quickly with astringent remedies. But those that come with an inflammation and fever cannot be healed. Rather, their size increases every day. Watery vesicles occur more rapidly in the membrane surrounding the liver than in the other organs. *In Hippocratis Aphorismos commentarius* VII[.37, 55].

(IX.90) When in the case of malignant intestinal ulcers one of the two membranes is so much eaten away that it disappears completely, the other membrane replaces the first and the person is saved. *De usu partium* V[.12].

(IX.91) The ancient physicians acted correctly in applying poultices and hot compresses for a colic arising from a vitreous humor that settled in the colon. If someone wants to use this therapy, he should apply warm packs and poultices continuously, for then he heals the disease and relieves the patient from the bad symptoms of the colic. But if he applies a warm pack only once or twice, he harms the patient severely because the distension increases. *De clysteribus* [*et colica*].

(IX.92) When intestinal pain occurs with fever, apply a hot compress with millet. If the pain does not subside, take one of the seeds that dissolve the flatulent winds and cook it in olive oil of a fine consistency, strain it, and melt duck fat in it, and apply this as an enema. If there is no duck fat available, use chicken fat that is unsalted and not very old. If the pain still does not subside, melt some castoreum into that oil and apply this as an enema. *De methodo* [*medendi*] XII[.8].

(IX.93) There are three kinds of abdominal worms:

1. The kind similar to vinegar worms, which originate in the region around the anus;
2. the kind resembling *qarʿ* (field pumpkin or winter squash) seeds, which form in the large intestine (tapeworms); and
3. the kind resembling snakes, which form in the small intestine (roundworms).

They produce pain in the stomach when they ascend in its direction. Sometimes abdominal worms originate from a bad, biting humor. *In Hippocratis Epidemiarum* [*commentarius* I.2].

(IX.94) Sometimes the humors dissolve in the non-pulsatile vessels and a watery serum is formed in them. When the kidneys cleanse that serum from the non-pulsatile vessels and transport it to the urinary bladder, it is excreted with the urine. When the kidneys are too weak to attract this watery serum, one of two things happens to it:

1. the non-pulsatile vessels either expel it to the abdomen, or
2. they disperse it and let it flow throughout the entire body, thereby causing dropsy. *De* [*symptomatum*] *causis* [III.8].

(IX.95) If an abscess forms in a kidney and ripens and the patient micturates pus, he will find relief from his pain, but he should be wary of an ulcer in that kidney. Therefore, one should attempt its cicatrization by all means. If it does not form a scar quickly, a cure will be very difficult. *De locis affectis* VI[.3].

(IX.96) Sometimes no urine at all comes to the bladder because the kidneys have stopped functioning; the urinary bladder is empty and nothing at all is retained in it. *De* [*symptomatum*] *causis* [III.8].

(IX.97) The diseases of the anus are difficult to heal because of four reasons: this part of the body is hypersensitive; it is the outlet for biting humors; drugs hardly stay there; and its temperament is warm and moist, so it needs remedies that are cool and dry. However, cooling and drying remedies are mostly astringent, and astringent drugs are biting, and the anus cannot tolerate biting. Therefore, the best medications consist of mineral substances that are not hot when they are washed. [*De compositione medicamentorum secundum locos*] IX[.6].

(IX.98) Among diseases of the skin due to black bile are mange and peeling of the skin. And when the illness occurs in the flesh or in the non-pulsatile vessels, it is called cancer. Elephantiasis starts from melancholic humor. When much time passes, black bile dominates the blood, and those suffering from this illness smell bad, ulcers appear on their bodies, and their complexion changes. *De tumoribus* [*praeter naturam* 13].

(IX.99) The moisture in the joints is mucous. When it increases so much that it makes the flesh around the joints wet, it produces tumors similar to those in patients with dropsy. These tumors have misled some physicians so that they have cut into them, believing that they would find pus in them. But they did not find pus; on the contrary, they found that all the flesh around the joint was full of mucous. *In Hippocratis Epidemiarum* [*commentarius*] VI.[1–]8.

(IX.100) For marasmus occurring from a condition similar to old age, and for marasmus that is called parching, and for marasmus that is accompanied by syncope—for these three conditions—milk, barley gruel, and groats of emmer wheat (*khandarūs*) cooked in vinegar are appropriate. But the groats should be cooked in the same way as the barley gruel so that it can be distributed throughout the organs. Hydromel is only beneficial in cold conditions. *De marcore* [9].

(IX.101) Much flesh and fat are harmful and detrimental and gives the body an ugly appearance and hinders its activities and movements. Therefore, those suffering from it should travel a lot and do much walking in the sun. Travel over sea is especially good because the sea air dissolves the superfluous moistures. One should let them eat foods with little nourishment, such as vegetables, and that which contains heat, such as onions, garlic, and salted fish, and that which strengthens but does not moisten, such as lean roasted meat. One should not let them bathe in any hot water except that of thermal springs. One should keep them a little thirsty and make their bodies firm in any possible manner. *De extenuatione corporum pinguium*.

(IX.102) Do not be frightened of the severity of illnesses when performing surgery; rather, consider whether these illnesses are dangerous and serious or minor. For instance, you should not be frightened of a large hernia and think that it is a serious illness. Rather, consider and know that a hernia in which the membrane that covers the intestines and stomach, namely, the omentum, descends, is a serious and grave illness although the size of the hernia may not be large. A hernia that encloses water (hydrocele) is a minor illness, although it may reach a large size. And a hernia into which a portion of the intestines has descended is very grave and serious. The same applies to the other illnesses. *De examinatione medici* [14].

(IX.103) In order to stop the superfluous matters that stream to their feet, patients suffering from podagra imbibe only the other medications for their illness. But they do not cleanse the superfluous matters that are already present in the painful limbs. And this is even worse for them, for when the humors do not stream to that place, they circulate in the body until they sometimes choke that patient. I have seen this several times. Therefore, I advise anyone who suffers from this pain not to drink those medications but rather to drink theriac. I have seen many patients with this pain who constantly took this electuary and found relief from their illness. *De theriaca ad Pisonem* [15].

(IX.104) All dissolving medications have a hot temperament. One of the effects of such a temperament is biting, and this occurs when the medication is extremely hot. Therefore, be careful with using very hot remedies amongst the remedies for dissolving superfluous matter in the organ, especially when the affected organ is evidently cold. For if one uses such remedies to the extent that one adds biting to the illness of the organ, not a small pain ensues from this, and every pain stimulates and attracts superfluous matter. Therefore, only that remedy which is moderately hot does not produce pain in such organs. When the organ is markedly cold or when it is deep inside the body and a strong dissolution is required, use an extremely hot remedy. *De arte parva* [34].

(IX.105) The kind of shingles that is associated with corrosion should be treated with remedies that are cooling but not moistening, just like the other kinds of shingles. But next to their cooling properties they should have drying properties. One should initially apply grapevine tendrils and offshoots of blackberry and broadleaf plantain. After this, one should mix these same ingredients with lentils and with some fine honey and *sawīq* (semolina) of barley. *Ad Glauconem* [*de medendi methodo*] II[.3].

(IX.106) The following non-corrosive remedies are applied for erysipelas and shingles: cultivated lettuce, common knotgrass, common duckweed, *nīlūfar* (blue Egyptian, European white, or yellow water lily), fleawort seed, common purslane, *hindibāʾ* (endive or chicory), *ḥayy al-ʿālam* (common houseleek or tree aeonium), and similarly, black nightshade. *Ad Glauconem* [*de medendi methodo*] II[.3].

(IX.107) Elephantiasis and a cancerous tumor can be healed at their onset by means of a constant evacuation of the melancholic humor and by prescribing the patient a regimen that produces good blood. The regimen plays a prominent role in this disease: for instance, we find that many people in Alexandria are stricken by elephantiasis because of their bad regimen and the heat of their place. However, we do not find that this disease occurs in the land of Mysia save in an exceptional case. In the land of the Scyths, who feed themselves with milk, we have never seen anyone afflicted by this disease. *Ad Glauconem Glauconem* [*de medendi methodo*] II[.12].

(IX.108) The nutrition of patients with elephantiasis or cancer should consist of barley gruel and whey, both of which should be consumed in abundance. Of the vegetables they should eat mallow, garden orach, purple amaranth, and *qarʿ* (field pumpkin or winter squash). Among the fish they should eat those that can be sighted amongst the rocks (rockfish). They may eat all kinds of birds, except waterfowl. The consumption of viper flesh is a wonderful remedy for patients suffering from elephantiasis, but it should be eaten once the head and tail have been severed, the abdomen cleansed, the skin stripped off, and the flesh boiled in a lot of water with some olive oil, dill, and leek until it is overdone. *Ad Glauconem* [*de medendi methodo*] II[.12].

(IX.109) When someone is bitten by a scorpion and its sting gets fixed in a nerve, or a pulsatile or non-pulsatile vessel, he is seized by very severe symptoms because the sting of the scorpion may penetrate deep into the body and pass through the entire skin. *De locis affectis* III[.11].

(IX.110) I have often seen that the bodies of those who gave up sexual intercourse while they were used to it turned cold and that their movements became burdensome. Others were afflicted by sadness for no evident reason and evil thoughts. The occurrence of this affliction is similar to what happens to those suffering from melancholic delusion. All this occurs following the putrefaction of the retained sperm because it causes bad vapors to ascend. *De locis affectis* VI[.5].

(IX.111) When milk boiled in an iron vessel is mixed with heating substances such as tutty, it is beneficial for cancerous ulcers and alleviates their pain. *De* [*simplicium*] *medicamentorum* [*temperamentis ac facultatibus* X.8].

(IX.112) Amongst the most efficient oils for healing tautness of the skin is fresh dill oil and oil of grape juice. They completely dissolve fatigue and relax the skin even if the fatigue is severe. Similarly, oil of pine nuts is beneficial for severe fatigue. *De sanitate tuenda* III[.10].

(IX.113) We have seen many perfectly healthy people—both young and old—attacked by sudden palpitations. All of them benefited from venesection and a thinning diet. *De locis affectis* V[.2].

(IX.114) I do not at all recommend treating organs from which blood is being emitted with cooling, astringent substances that are applied externally, because these substances push the blood inwards so that the internal vessels are filled. I know people whose chests were cooled because of blood they spat up from the lungs; others, whose stomachs were cooled externally because of blood they vomited; and still others whose heads were cooled because of a nosebleed. All this clearly inflicted harm on them. One should only do this once the blood is tending to another place or is attracted to the opposite side. *De methodo* [*medendi*] V[.6].

(IX.115) When the affliction of a nerve is accompanied by pain, one should treat it with a poultice prepared from broad bean flour, vinegar, honey, and liquid pitch. This should be well cooked and applied while still hot. *De methodo* [*medendi*] VI[.3].

(IX.116) Those who are stricken by syncope because of the emaciation of their bodies and the severe weakening of the pneuma should be nourished with foods that do not decay rapidly, and bread and gruel from emmer wheat (*khandarūs*), and astringent fruits that do not spoil easily, given sometimes alone and sometimes with bread. One should also feed them yolk and testicles of roosters. And finally, one should thicken their humors and make their skin more dense. *De methodo* [*medendi*] XII[.5].

(IX.117) When an ulcer occurs on the side of a large vessel, whether it is pulsatile or not, the glands swell very rapidly, and that vessel becomes completely visible in that part of the body; it is red and tense and painful upon touch. *De methodo* [*medendi*] XIII[.5].

(IX.118) When glands begin to swell, begin from the first day to alleviate the pain and apply wool soaked in hot olive oil on them. When the body is full of superfluities, heating substances attract them. If this is the case, one should first of all use venesection or scarification on a part that is not affected and that is opposite to it. When the illness is in the arm, the leg should be scarified; when it is in the leg, the arm should be scarified. But if one is slow in purging the body, the glands will swell to the point of suppuration. *De methodo* [*medendi*] XIII[.5].

(IX.119) The evacuation of a poison from someone bitten by an animal is effected by means of agents that have a strong attractive force and that transform this poison. Such a transformation is effected by medications that either change the quality of the poison or that dissolve its substance. Agents that have a strong attractive force without heating are cupping glasses and hollow horns. Some people suck and attract the poison out of the bitten limb with their mouth. *De methodo* [*medendi*] XIII[.6].

(IX.120) For the treatment of hard tumors, softening remedies should always be mixed with a discutient agent. Vinegar is good for that; it is the strongest remedy with which tendons and ligaments can be treated. But one should not use it continuously because an excessive use robs the humors from their thin and fine quality and makes that which remains as hard as stone. Moreover, when vinegar is used for a long time, it harms and damages the substance of the nerves. Therefore, it should not be used in the beginning of the disease nor for a prolonged time. *De methodo* [*medendi*] XIV[.5].

When a cancer is in an initial stage, it can be cured especially by washed mineral remedies and by cleansing the body through purgation. But when the cancer becomes large and this becomes evident, we try to prevent it from increasing even further. *De methodo* [*medendi*] XIV[.9].

(IX.121) Gout and pains in the joints should be treated first of all by the evacuation of the harmful chyme. Then one should first treat the hands and feet with detaining and restraining drugs. But in the case of the hip joint, one should be careful not to use restraining and cooling remedies because it is situated at a deep spot and this kind of treatment would increase the overfilling. Rather, following the evacuation, one should first of all alleviate the pain with agents that heat and do not cool, and the heat should not be as strong as the heat of those agents that one should apply in the end after excessive evacuation. [*De compositione medicamentorum secundum locos*] X[.2].

(IX.122) For ischias, emesis is more beneficial than purging the bowels because it attracts the matters that cause the disease. Do this first of all by means of food and then give emetics—begin with the mildest and lightest. But if the humors get stuck there and are difficult to dissolve because of sharp medications that the physicians initially used and that hardened and roasted the superfluous matter, cupping glasses are very beneficial. The same holds good for purging the bowels by means of sharp purgative clysters that contain colocynth and the like. [*De compositione medicamentorum secundum locos*] X[.2].

(IX.123) In his *Kitāb Al-Murshid* [*fī jawāhir al-aghdhiya waquwā l-mufradāt mina l-adwiya*], al-Tamīmī mentions the following way of treating a hernia before it becomes chronic. He said: Take two *mithqāl*s of savin juniper fruit, one *mithqāl* of its leaves, two *dirhams* of fresh asphodel flour, and one *mithqāl* of Senegal gum. Knead these ingredients with dissolved fish glue and spread the compound while it is hot on a linen cloth. At the end of the bathhouse procedures, put it on the hernia on an empty stomach and lying down. On the cloth put padding, bandage it, and let the patient sleep on his back until the compress dries. Leave it bandaged for forty days. Every day let the patient drink a potion prepared from two parts of pulverized and strained savin juniper fruit and one part of pulverized and strained savin juniper leaves. From this potion he should drink two *dirhams* daily with one ounce of myrtle juice and sugar.

He further said: When one cooks extract of apricot leaves and uses this as a gargle, it is beneficial for a swelling of the uvula, throat, and tonsils. It dissolves and eliminates all the inflamed tumors occurring in the mouth, gums, and uvula.

(IX.124) The therapy for a bone fracture should, after necessary surgery, consist of an extremely thinning diet. It is often first of all necessary to purge the bowels with a remedy. While the fracture heals, one should feed the patient with food that has good chymes and that is nutritious and viscous. The external remedies should be those that by their substance cause to adhere, cleave, and stick, and that heat slightly and dry moderately. *De methodo* [*medendi*] VI[.5].

(IX.125) If part of an inflamed tumor remains in an organ after treatment, sharp remedies cause more irritation and swelling than dissolution. When the remaining part of an inflamed tumor has turned hard, use strong remedies with assurance and confidence. *De methodo* [*medendi*] XIII[.5].

(IX.126) Sometimes, for tumors on hands and feet, it is sufficient to put a sponge on them with cold water and a little vinegar or astringent wine. As for tumors of the liver, do not put anything cold upon them; rather, cook quinces in wine and apply this lukewarm as a poultice in the beginning of the tumor. The same benefit is derived from a fomentation with quince oil or myrtle oil or mastic oil or spikenard oil or absinth wormwood. But none of these should be used cold, nor should any oily substance be used for tumors of the eyes or mouth. Sometimes rose oil and vinegar can be used as eardrops. *De methodo* [*medendi*] XIII[.12].

(IX.127) Says Moses: In [*Historia*] *animali*[*um*] IX[.12], Aristotle has written a chapter that is very useful for medical practice. In my opinion, Galen has not brought up the matter that I am going to mention now, nor has he drawn attention to it. It is the following statement of Aristotle. He said: Normally spasms mostly occur to babies, especially to those who are well nourished and who suck much milk that is very fat and whose wet-nurses are well-fleshed. In this case an excess of milk is harmful.

This is the end of the ninth treatise,
by the grace of God,
praise be to Him.

In the name of God,
the Merciful, the Compassionate.
O Lord, make our task easy

The Tenth Treatise
Containing aphorisms concerning fevers

(X.1) When the digestion of the foods in the stomach and liver is not as thorough as it should be, fevers increase and become sharper. Therefore, in the case of all fevers, one should pay the utmost attention to the proper digestion of the food through strengthening the stomach and liver with astringent things. *De methodo* [*medendi*] XI[.15].

(X.2) Do not permit those suffering from fever to drink enough water to quench their thirst until you have thoroughly looked into the matter. When one of the noble organs is afflicted by an inflamed tumor alone, or an inflamed tumor combined with erysipelas, or a soft or hard tumor; or when the body of the patient has an obstruction or a putrefaction of uncocted humors; or when it has an organ with a cold temperament, which is always harmed by cold water—in all these cases, the patient should not be given cold water to drink until there are clear signs that the putrefying humors are being cocted or that the inflamed tumor has become ripe. Someone suffering from a true erysipelas should be treated through the ingestion of cold water under the same conditions. *De methodo* [*medendi*] IX[.5].

(X.3) In the case of putrid fevers, you should consider and look into three things:
1. The strength of the patient, which is the most important;
2. then the cause of the putrefaction; and, finally,
3. the fever itself.

If you find that the agents with which you want to treat the fever are good for all these three things, it is very good. But if you find that one or more than one agent has a contrary effect on one or more than one of these three things, set your mind on that which maintains and supports the strength. Sometimes you should treat only the cause—namely, when the heat of the fever is weak—and attempt to open the obstruction and to combat the putrefaction. But when the fever is flaring up somewhat, attempt to extinguish the heat of the fever, even if you increase the obstruction. For, sometimes, the fever is so exceptionally high that a human being quickly perishes therefrom because he cannot bear or endure it. *De methodo* [*medendi*] x[.1].

(x.4) If we knew the different natures of fevers for certain, we could risk telling many fever sufferers to bathe in cold water at home and not only in the bathhouse, and some might benefit from that. But since we do not have a real and exhaustive knowledge of the different natures of fevers, and since a mistake therein at an inopportune occasion could lead to great harm, we avoid this therapy in the treatment of fever patients. *De methodo* [*medendi*] x[.10].

If a young man who is well-fleshed and corpulent and does not suffer from an inflammation in his viscera takes a bath in cold water and swims therein during the time of the summer heat and the culmination of the fever, he clearly benefits from such treatment, and I recommend this without hesitation. *De methodo* [*medendi*] x[.10].

(x.5) If you find it necessary to bleed a fever patient, or to purge him, or to alleviate the pain he is suffering from with a poultice or a hot compress, you should not give him barley groats or barley gruel before doing the aforementioned. *In Hippocratis De acutorum morborum* [*victu*] *commentarius* I[.32].

(x.6) The factors that determine the length or brevity of a fever attack, even if there is only one kind of fever present, is the condition of that humor that putrefies and bursts forth by itself, and the condition of the expulsive faculty, and the condition of the passages and channels of the organ close to that humor. A surplus or thickness or viscosity of that humor necessarily makes the attack lengthy, while the opposite makes the attack short. Similarly, a weak expulsive faculty makes the attack lengthy, and a strong expulsive faculty makes it short; and narrow passages and channels make it lengthy, and wide passages and channels make it short. Sometimes all the factors determining the lengthiness of the attack coincide, and sometimes all the factors determining the shortness of the attack coincide. *De* [*differentiis*] *febrium* II[.16].

(x.7) A fever arising from the putrefaction of humors has its own specific symptom that always goes with it—namely, a quick contraction of the pulsatile vessels of the wrist. This becomes especially evident during the increase of the fever attack, although it is not imperceptible during its beginning and climax.

At its beginning, the pulse is small; and at its climax, it is great. *De* [*differentiis*] *febrium* I[.9].

(X.8) If someone whose body is full of humors is attacked by fever and then by diarrhea, no other kind of evacuation is needed. This is sufficient for him, even if it is not commensurate with the degree of fullness of his body. If someone attempts to bleed such a person or make his diarrhea more severe, he brings him into immediate danger. *Ad Glauconem* [*de medendi methodo*] I[.15].

(X.9) If someone who has only recently suffered from indigestion is attacked by fever when he has a feeling of biting and pressure in the cardia of his stomach and while his body is full of blood, one should not attempt to bleed him before paying attention to the cardia of his stomach. When its condition has improved, one may evacuate the whole body. I have often seen how physicians evacuated the bodies of patients with this condition without first strengthening the stomach. Some of the patients died, and others became so dangerously ill that they were on the verge of death. *Ad Glauconem* [*de medendi methodo*] I[.15].

(X.10) If putrefaction occurs in the viscera or large vessels, something similar to the vapor of the humors that have putrefied there reaches the two chambers of the heart. However, in the case of swollen glands or of tumors in any soft, fleshy part of the body, only the heat spreads from there to the heart and warms the surrounding region. The heat continues to spread until it reaches the heart and heats it, without any vapor of the putrid humor reaching the heart together with it, because that humor is confined to those places. Therefore, the first case concerns putrid fever; and the second, ephemeral fever. *De* [*differentiis*] *febrium* I[.7].

(X.11) Cold in the extremities, especially during fevers, occurs either because of a large, inflamed tumor in the viscera; or because of a severe pain in the middle part of the body; or because of fainting or syncope; or because of weakness of the innate heat and its near extinction; or because of its drowning and choking effect due to a surplus of superfluous matters. The extremities are the ears, nose, hands, and feet. *In Hippocratis Aphorismos commentarius* VII[.26].

(X.12) When cold occurs in the extremities in the beginning of fever attacks, it is not a fatal sign. However, it indicates that blood and heat first gather inside the body and then spread. *In Hippocratis Prognostica commentarius* II[.4].

(X.13) When cold and pallor of the extremities occur in combination with acute fever, it indicates death and extinction of the innate heat. *In Hippocratis Epidemiarum* [*commentarius*] III.2.

(X.14) When cold sweat occurs together with acute fever, it is a sign of death. *De signis mortis.*

(X.15) Sometimes putrefaction occurs in all the vessels equally, but sometimes it occurs only in the largest and most eminent vessels—namely, those between the groins and the armpits. This putrefaction is necessarily the root of continuous fever. When putrefaction occurs only in one organ with an inflamed tumor—or even without one—the root and source of the fever are in that organ. This putrefaction is to the fever as a blazing fire. *De methodo* [*medendi*] XI[.4].

(X.16) One should know which remedies are good for curing a fever, which are good for treating putrefaction, and which are good for treating the cause of putrefaction—namely, an obstruction. The remedies good for the treatment of these three things are not always compatible. On the contrary, it often occurs that the effect of one of these remedies is contrary to that of the others. One should look for the most severe and harmful of these three things and treat it first. *De methodo* [*medendi*] XI[.9].

(X.17) You should know for certain that differentiation between fever, putrefaction, and its cause—when also present—is abstruse, difficult, and hard. Discerning it requires a subtle mind and a refined intellect. It is even harder to differentiate between these and the strength of the body. *De methodo* [*medendi*] XI[.9].

(X.18) If someone suffers from fever while his body contains a very large quantity of crude superfluities and his stomach has been weakened through indigestions, his body appears swollen. The complexion of some of these patients becomes white or dark or lead-colored, and their pulse becomes small and unequal. These patients should not be phlebotomized under any circumstances, nor can they tolerate purgation of the bowels, even if they need evacuation. If one of these methods is applied to them, they are overcome by syncope. They only benefit from an evacuation by means of strong massage, which brings the patient to near-exhaustion because of the bruising of the flesh through the intensive massage. One should stop massaging these patients during sleep, because sleep cocts the superfluities, whereas wakefulness causes their dissolution. If someone falls ill because of crude humors, he should be treated equally with these two methods. *De methodo* [*medendi*] XII[.3].

(X.19) There are three kinds of intermittent fevers that stop in a perceptible way: tertian fever, quotidian fever, and quartan fever. Tertian fever originates from yellow bile when it putrefies; quotidian fever originates from humors that strongly tend to become like phlegm when they putrefy; and quartan fever originates from melancholic humors when they putrefy. When the humor that produces the fever streams throughout the body, these three kinds of fevers are clearly intermittent. *De* [*differentiis*] *febrium* II[.1, 2].

(X.20) Continuous fevers occur when the putrid humor that produces the fever is confined within the vessels—this humor is one of the three humors. The continuous fever that does not end on the third day but rather becomes worse is similar to tertian fever and is the so-called continuous tertian fever. And the type that does not end nor depart but occurs every day in the same way is the so-called continuous quotidian fever. This fever does not have a clear end. The same applies to continuous quartan fever, which becomes worse on the fourth day, but which only rarely occurs. *De* [*differentiis*] *febrium* II[.1, 7].

(X.21) Even when a continuous fever is difficult to move and stretches up to forty days, it is still counted among the acute diseases. And even when it really passes away and recurs, it is also counted among the chronic diseases. When I said "a continuous fever," understand that I mean a fever that does not really pass away. *De diebus decretoriis* II[.12].

(X.22) One of the most important symptoms for putrid fever is the quality of its heat: it always bites and smarts, just like the effect of smoke on the eyes. Nothing at all is pleasant about it, not even in the beginning of its attacks, when the heat has not yet spread. If you leave your hand for a long time on the body, the heat ascends and, even more, bites and hurts. In its beginning, one never finds cocted urine; rather, it is uncocted or cocted in a very obscure way. One does not find compression of the pulse or of the heat in non-putrid fevers. Nevertheless, their occurrence is not specific for putrid fevers alone. *De* [*differentiis*] *febrium* I[.9].

(X.23) Sometimes the quality of the blood changes when it putrefies: it turns into yellow bile or black bile. In these cases, the fever is either tertian or quartan. The only difference between these cases is that in the first one, the fever is malignant; but when it originates from the transformation of the blood, it is not malignant. For when the heat tends more toward the vaporous type and is less aggressive and harmful when one touches the body, it comes from the transformation of the blood; but when it is biting and smarting when one touches the body, it comes from the putrefaction of one of the two biles. And if one touches the body and does not find sharpness in the beginning, but later, when one leaves one's hand on it for a long time, one has a sensation of biting that slowly increases and is uneven, so that it feels as if it were transmitted through the holes of a filter or a sieve, then heat originates from the putrefaction of the phlegm. This humor cannot be dissolved from the body evenly because of its thickness and viscosity. *De* [*differentiis*] *febrium* II[.11].

(X.24) The cycle of phlegmatic fever (quotidian fever caused by phlegm) is twenty-four hours; the cycle of tertian fever is forty-eight hours; and that of quartan fever, seventy-two hours. This is clear. For, in the case of phlegmatic fever, which attacks every day, there are twenty-four hours from the beginning of the first attack until the beginning of the second attack. The same analogy can be made for tertian and quartan fevers. If, for instance, you find an eight-hour cycle in which the attacks last for six hours and then remit for two hours and then return in the same manner and remit again for two hours, continuously, you know that this is a case of a threefold phlegmatic fever, because the eight hours represent one-third of the cycle of the phlegmatic fever. Similarly, if you find a cycle every sixteen hours, you know that this is a case of a threefold tertian fever, because the sixteen hours are one-third of the cycle of tertian fever. If you find a cycle of eighteen hours, you know that it is a fourfold quartan fever, because eighteen hours are one-fourth of the cycle of quartan fever. *De circuitibus febrium* [4].

(X.25) The pulse does not return to its natural state in any of the other fevers, not even if a very long interval occurs between the first and the second attack, such as the interval that occurs between the attacks in the cases of tertian and quartan fevers. For, in the cases of those fevers, the symptoms of the fever remain in the vessels, except for quotidian fever. In the case of this fever, the symptoms of the fever disappear and vanish when the fever subsides. *Ad Glauconem* [*de medendi methodo*] I[.2].

(X.26) The regularity in the cycles of a fever is disrupted and altered for one of two reasons: either because of an alteration from one nature to another of the humors that produce the fever, or because of an error in the diet. Sometimes one may think that a fever does not have a certain regularity, while in reality it does. This happens because the fever is composed of many cycles, but the physician does not notice its composite character. *De* [*differentiis*] *febrium* II[.18].

(X.27) Sometimes the intervals between every fever attack occurring from the beginning until the end of a disease are the same, whether the attack comes early or late after the preceding one. The physicians call those early ones "early cycles" and the opposite ones "late cycles." The earliness or lateness thereof does not indicate a strengthening of the disease nor its decline. Rather, it should be taken as an indication of the shortness or length of the attack and of the malignity or badness of the symptoms or the disappearance of these symptoms. *De crisibus* I[.3].

(X.28) The indications for pure tertian fever—which can be derived from the observation of the patient himself in the beginning of the attack—are eleven:

1. A severe rigor whereby one has the sensation of needle pricks.
2. Thirst and burning heat that do not last long.
3. An equal pulse, whatever its condition.
4. A quick climax to the attack.
5. Equal distribution of the heat through the entire body.
6. Abundant and sharp heat at the first contact of the hand with the body, then a decline as the heat is overcome by the heat of the hand.
7. The passage of a hot vapor through the pores of the body during the drinking of water.
8. The emesis of bile or the excretion of bile through diarrhea or through urine in which the bile dominates—sometimes all three occur at the same time.
9. Even perspiration over the whole body.
10. Alleviation and complete disappearance of the fever.
11. The longest period for the total fever attack being twelve hours, and the shortest, six hours. *De crisibus* 2[.3].

(X.29) The indications for pure quartan fever that can be derived perfectly well from the fever itself are four:

1. All the indications for pure tertian fever are absent; moreover, most of the indications that one finds for quartan fever are the opposite of those for pure tertian fever.
2. Quartan fever rarely begins first; rather, it mostly occurs after other fevers.
3. The pulse of such patients is transformed in the beginning of the attack and becomes like the pulse of a very old man, unlike the pulse of patients suffering from any other kind of fever.

4. It begins simply, with a mild rigor that becomes stronger with every attack. With every rigor, the patient feels a cold whose severity matches the severity of the rigor, until he feels, when it is severe, as if his bones were being crushed by snow. *De crisibus* II[.3].

(X.30) The indications for quotidian fever that are clear, evident, and easy to obtain are seven:

1. It does not begin with a rigor on the first day, and as time passes, the patient has, in the beginning of the attack, a sensation of cold in the outer part of his body and the extremities, but not a real rigor.
2. Inequality and irregularity of the pulse occur mostly in the beginning of the attack.
3. There is no burning heat; the heat and thirst are so little that the thirst is less than in the other fevers.
4. Its patients hardly perspire during the first days, while their urine is uncocted.
5. It mostly occurs with pain of the cardia of the stomach and of the liver.
6. The hypochondrium swells and increases in the beginning of the occurrence of the fever.
7. The faces of its sufferers are yellowish white, even at the time of the climax of the attack. *De crisibus* II[.5].

(X.31) In every continuous fever, the putrefying matter is inside the non-pulsatile vessels. It is not accompanied by rigor, or perspiration, or emesis. A fever originating from a bloody tumor is a mild and safe one and very similar to ephemeral fever, which originates from a tumor in the soft flesh in the groin and other places. *De crisibus* II[.6, 12].

(X.32) When various causes of fever occur simultaneously, begin treatment with bleeding through phlebotomy, and then start to dilute and thin the humors, and then work to soften the solid matter and to rarefy contracted spots of the skin. *De methodo medendi* XI[.4].

(X.33) Galen said on the general treatment of tertian fever: If signs of coction appear, confidently administer some absinth wormwood to the patient because it has a laudable effect in different respects. Moreover, it is one of the most adequate means for the treatment of diseases developing at the cardia of the stomach from the biting effect of bile. *Ad Glauconem* [*de medendi methodo*] I[.10].

(x.34) At its inception, tertian fever begins with severe rigor. As for quartan fever, I do not know that I ever saw that it started with severe rigor. But, in the case of this fever, the rigor becomes more severe as time passes and mostly originates from what remained from other preceding fevers and from the fever called "the mixed one." *Ad Glauconem* [*de medendi methodo*] I[.5].

(x.35) When pure tertian fever lasts as long as possible, it ends after seven cycles. In spite of this, it is one of the least dangerous fevers. But when it is impure, the situation is the reverse. I know that this fever once started in a young man in the beginning of autumn and did not leave him until spring. *Ad Glauconem* [*de medendi methodo*] I[.9].

(x.36) The reason that, in some fevers, a sensation of heat and cold occurs simultaneously, and that one finds high fever and cold rigor, is that the vitreous phlegm and the yellow bile humor increase so much that together they dominate the body and move through the sensitive parts of the body until every small part affected by the cold has, next to it, another small part affected by the heat. Someone suffering from this, feels heat and cold inside his body at the same time because both the heating and the cooling humors are dispersed throughout the smallest parts of the body. *De* [*inaequali*] *intemperie* [8].

(x.37) There are two kinds of rigor that do not abate until the time of the climax draws near. One of them is that which does not abate until the climax of the fever attack is near. This one is malignant, but not severe, and originates from the putrefaction of the very cold phlegm called "vitreous." The other one is that which does not abate until the climax of the entire illness is near, for quartan fever cannot reach its climax until the rigor lessens. The rigor that begins with great severity and then abates before the time of the climax is that which happens in the case of tertian fever. *In Hippocratis Epidemiarum* [*commentarius*] VI.1.

(x.38) In pure tertian fever, the longest duration of an attack is twelve hours. In an impure tertian fever, it can last for twenty or twenty-four hours. In some cases, this fever has an extremely long attack, lasting about forty hours, whereas its abatement lasts for eight hours. All this goes back to what we mentioned above, about the causes of the length of an attack. *De* [*differentiis*] *febrium* II[.3, 10].

(x.39) If a patient suffers from two tertian fevers and two quintan fevers, the two tertian fevers attack daily, and the two quintan fevers attack on the third day. Therefore, one might think that the two tertian fevers are a single quotidian fever and that the two quintan fevers are a single tertian fever. *De crisibus* II[.2].

(X.40) Ardent fevers hardly ever originate from the congestion of yellow bile, but, rather, from the domination of the heat in the vessels when the yellow bile becomes sharp and inflamed through the condition of the air, physical exercise, hot dishes, or movements of the soul. *In Hippocratis Epidemiarum* [*commentarius*] I.2.

(X.41) One should first examine the nature of the fever—whether its heat is strong, blazing, and ardent. A fever with such a condition has its crisis with evacuation. When a fever is mild and weak, similar to a smoldering fire, it can last for a long time, and its crisis mostly occurs with abscesses. *Ad Glauconem* [*de medendi methodo*] I[.16].

(X.42) The worst ardent fevers are those which occur because of the liver or stomach. They can also occur because of inflamed tumors in the lung or because of bilious humors that putrefy and spread through the entire body and that, because of their putrefaction, become exceedingly hot, similar to a boiling process. *De locis affectis* V[.7].

(X.43) One of the worst indications is when an acute, ardent fever occurs or when a hot, sharp superfluity streams to the stomach but does not incite thirst. For this indicates that the sensatory faculty in the stomach has stopped functioning and has died. *In Hippocratis Epidemiarum* [*commentarius*] I.1.

(X.44) When the humor that causes the fever is sharp and burning, a tumor hardly ever develops in the area of the ears. When the humor is extremely cold and thick, tumors develop in the lower parts of the body. When the humor is in the middle, between these two conditions, tumors develop beneath the ears. *In Hippocratis Epidemiarum* [*commentarius*] II.2.

(X.45) Sometimes ardent fever is accompanied by a diarrhea of raw material. This is caused by the presence of raw humors in the vessels connected to the intestines and in the concave side of the liver. When ardent fever is accompanied by thin urine, it indicates the presence of many uncocted humors in the the convex side of the liver. *In Hippocratis Epidemiarum* [*commentarius*] III.2.

(X.46) There are two accurate indications for ardent fever: constant thirst, which does not stop or abate, and a blazing heat so intense that it can be felt through touching. *In Hippocratis Epidemiarum* [*commentarius*] III.3.

(X.47) When all the three faculties of the body are strong while there is a severe ardent fever and there are clear, evident signs of coction, give the patient cold water to drink with trust and confidence, unless he is a very old man. *De methodo* [*medendi* XI.9].

(X.48) Ardent fever develops from the putrefaction of yellow bile in the stomach and especially in its cardia, or in the concave side of the liver, but not in any other organ. One of the most specific properties of ardent fever is that its crisis comes through a nosebleed, because the blood ascends and rises, whereat the non-pulsatile vessels burst open. *In Hippocratis Epidemiarum* [*commentarius*] I.1.

(X.49) Ardent fevers develop from either yellow bile or salt phlegm. *In Hippocratis De acutorum morborum* [*victu*] *commentarius* III.

(X.50) When a patient craves inhaling cold air because he has the sensation of a severe burning in the inner parts of his body, yet needs many clothes to warm his body from the outside because of the cold he feels, it is a sign that his illness is fatal, unless it occurs in the beginning of the fever attacks. *In Hippocratis Epidemiarum* [*commentarius*] II.3.

(X.51) When the weather is cold, and yet the patient has the sensation of a severe burning, let your hope that he will recover be slim. If there are no clear signs of coction and he does not have much strength, it is impossible that he will escape death. *De methodo* [*medendi*] XI[.9].

(X.52) We apply clysters with olive oil and water only in ardent, burning fevers, in order to break their blazing and burning heat. *De clysteribus* [*et colica*].

(X.53) In phlegmatic fevers the cause of rigor is not the same as the cause of the fever. The cause of the fever is that part of the phlegm that has putrefied, while the cause of the rigor is the remaining part of the phlegm, which has not yet putrefied. But in tertian fever, it is the yellow bile that produces both the rigor and the fever. *De* [*differentiis*] *febrium* II[.6].

(x.54) With any illness that flares up and attacks in cycles, the causes of its flaring up [in cycles] are the conditions of the organs that occur in a certain order, whether it be the expulsion of the superfluities, or their acceptance, or their production and attraction. All this occurs because of a bad temperament of that organ—or of the other organs—that so weakens it that it accepts that which is expelled to it from another organ or attracts or alters that which is within it and produces superfluities. The organ that produces superfluities produces and expels them in cycles. Sometimes those superfluities remain within the organ until they putrefy. *De* [*differentiis*] *febrium* II[.18].

Any illness that does not have cycles, such as continuous fever, is not caused by something specific for an organ of the body. But the humors in all the vessels, pulsatile and non-pulsatile—and especially those humors in the largest and hottest vessels—become burning hot and boil because of putrefaction or for some other reason, as in the case of quotidian fever. This results in the development of one continuous, synochous fever from the beginning of the illness until its end. *De* [*differentiis*] *febrium* II[.18].

(x.55) The decline and abatement of a fever attack refer to the entire time after the climax of the attack until the beginning of the next attack. *De crisibus* I[.3].

(x.56) I have cured many people from quartan fever by administering the theriac, but first I emptied their bodies, then gave them absinth wormwood juice to drink, and then this electuary two hours before the fever. The fever patient would be healed after two or three ingestions. *De theriaca ad Pisonem.*

(x.57) Sometimes, in hectic fevers, the organ that becomes heated first is the heart. It is heated initially by an external cause: sometimes it is the liver, and sometimes the stomach, and after the stomach, the other organs that are capable of heating the heart until the hectic fever occurs. It is very beneficial to apply cooling remedies as soon as one observes signs of hectic fever in the organ that got heated first and that is the hearth of the fever. Similarly, marasmus occurring from hectic fevers should be treated with cooling substances taken internally, as well as applied externally to the painful organ. *De marcore* [7].

(x.58) A specific, inseparable sign for anyone suffering from hectic fever is the following: when he takes food and waits for an hour, the heat of his body becomes inflamed and intense, but without oppression, and his pulse becomes greater and more rapid. Common to all hectic fevers is that the heat is always equally weak and feeble from its very beginning until its very end. One of the most important signs of hectic fevers is that the pulsatile vessels are found to be warmer than what surrounds them. *De febribus* I[.11–13].

(X.59) When the fever is accompanied by a diarrhea of liquified material, it is a pestilential fever, because this is an inseparable symptom of pestilential fever. *In Hippocratis Epidemiarum* [*commentarius*] III.3.

(X.60) We mostly find that hectic and marasmic fevers occur if the affliction first befell the heart, then the liver, and then the stomach. These fevers can also occur because of a hot and dry bad temperament that dominates the lungs, or the chest, or the mesentery. They can also occur because of an affliction befalling one of the intestines, or the uterus, or the kidneys, and then spreading to the substance of the heart. As for an affliction befalling the diaphragm first, I once saw hectic fever developing from an affliction occurring to it. But I do not know that I ever saw marasmic fever developing from the diaphragm, because the patient would die before getting marasmus. *De methodo* [*medendi*] X[.8].

(X.61) If someone has survived an attack of marasmic fever, then the marasmus occurred only in the flesh and similar structures. If the elementary parts dry out, it is impossible that he should recover in any way. *De methodo* [*medendi*] X[.11].

(X.62) All marasmic fevers belong to the type of fevers that cause the body to waste. The difference between the two is that, in the case of marasmic fevers, the material that is wasted from the flesh is always eliminated through the pores, whereas in the case of other fevers that cause the body to waste, this material streams to the abdomen and is excreted in the stool. If this lasts for a long time, as in the case of someone who suffers from wasting fever but does not die, he develops marasmus. *De methodo* [*medendi*] X[.11].

(X.63) The greatest and most effective means for treating continuous fevers are bloodletting—as much as the strength of the patient can tolerate—and the drinking of cold water after the coction of the humors—when the fever is of the type that develops from putrefaction. We have often observed that people who suffered from ardent fever drank cold water after the moderate coction of their humors, and the fever left them as soon as they drank it. *De methodo* [*medendi*] IX[.5].

If someone suffering from synochous fever falls into the hands of an ignorant physician who does not bleed the patient, then, by abstaining from bleeding him, he lets the fever increase and grow. Moreover, he shuts off all other avenues of treatment. For if he cools him down, he destroys him because cooling, although it extinguishes the heat and balances the temperament, retains and keeps the overfilling within the body and prevents it from dissolving. But if he starts to evacuate the body with those things that are used to evacuate the body—and that are, all of them, hot—he will increase the heat of the fever. If someone neglects bloodletting, he will eventually end up in this perplexing situation. *De methodo* [*medendi*] IX[.5].

(x.64) In all types of synochous fevers one should hasten to bleed the median cubital vein even to the point that the patient nearly faints, if his strength permits this. If someone suffering from this fever is not bled from a vein, he falls into the greatest distress and is on the verge of the most extreme danger, unless he is saved from this by a strong nosebleed or profuse sweating. *De methodo* [*medendi*] IX[.4].

(x.65) There are two types of synochous—meaning continuous—fever. One type results from an obstruction occurring in the pores of the body and is not accompanied by putrefaction of the humors. This synochous fever belongs to the genus of ephemeral fevers. Another type is that in which the obstruction is accompanied by the putrefaction of the humors, and it belongs to the genus of putrid fevers. Each one of these two types lasts for many days and constitutes a single attack from the beginning of the illness until its end. In both types, one finds that the fever remains in the same state until the climax, that it increases little by little, and that it diminishes little by little. All of this depends upon the matter that burns up and the matter that dissolves from that which burns up. *De methodo* [*medendi*] IX[.2].

(x.66) The ephemeral fever that originates from an obstruction is sometimes so slow to abate that it seems as if it is not an ephemeral fever. In this case, one should apply venesection and extract blood in a quantity dependent on the strength of the patient and on the lightness or severity of the obstruction. The more severe the obstruction, the stronger and shorter the fever. One should apply venesection even if no signs of overfilling occur together with the fever. For then the gaseous superfluity diminishes through the decrease in humors, and opening the obstruction will be easier afterwards. After the bleeding, treat the patient with oxymel and then with barley gruel. If you see, on the third day, that only a small amount of fever remains and that there are no clear signs of putrefaction, neither in the urine nor in the pulse, let him go to the bathhouse three or four hours prior to the time that you expect another fever attack. *De methodo* [*medendi*] VIII[.4].

(x.67) No fever develops from an indigestion in which the food turns sour. But fever can occur from an indigestion in which the food becomes gaseous. If someone develops a fever from such an indigestion and also suffers from diarrhea, and if you see that the evacuated matter consists only of that which was corrupted, let the patient bathe and feed him during the abatement of the first attack and take care to strengthen his stomach. But if you see that the earlier or later evacuation was so extreme that it wears out the strength of the patient, the best thing to do is to feed him without having him go to the bathhouse. *De methodo* [*medendi*] VIII[.5].

(x.68) Food intake is the worst thing for anyone whose fever is caused by overfilling, or an obstruction, or an inflamed tumor, or putrefaction of the humors. Do not feed them—not even when the fever attack abates. For anyone whose fever is caused by sleeplessness or worry or anxiety or emotions, abstention from food is the worst. One may feed them at any time during the attack of the fever, but especially when it abates. *De methodo* [*medendi*] X[.5].

(x.69) Someone suffering from continuous fever should be nourished at such time that he feels at ease and better, and especially at the time that he was accustomed to eating when he was healthy. *De methodo* [*medendi*] XI[.5].

(x.70) One should evacuate the putrid superfluities from patients with continuous fever by prescribing diuretics and purgatives, by stimulating perspiration, and by inducing emesis when these superfluities spontaneously move toward the stomach. But if they do not move toward the stomach, do not induce emesis; rather, choose those remedies by which such an evacuation can be effected without producing heat at all or producin] only a minor amount of heat. *De methodo* [*medendi*] XI[.8].

(x.71) To feed someone suffering from inflamed tumors in the liver or stomach before a fever attack is one of the most destructive and fatal things for him. When the liver or stomach is weak but without inflamed tumors, to do so is one of the most beneficial things. *De methodo* [*medendi*] XI[.21].

This is the end of the tenth treatise,
by the grace of God,
praise be to Him.

In the name of God,
the Merciful, the Compassionate.
O Lord, make our task easy

The Eleventh Treatise

Containing aphorisms concerning the periods and crisis of a disease

(XI.1) The periods of a disease are four altogether: beginning, increase, culmination and decline. It is only with great toil that one can come to know the actual period of a disease at a certain moment through an exact conjecture. *De crisibus* 1[.2].

(XI.2) We find that in the case of the disease which is extremely grave—namely, apoplexy—its beginning and increase take place in a short time. The same holds true for epilepsy, for it does not occur in the same way as that which happens to those whose head is cut off, although even here the beheading takes a first and a second and a third time. And when we admit that epilepsy and apoplexy occur without taking time, we mean the symptoms that follow these diseases; while the disease itself that causes apoplexy and epilepsy has, without any doubt, the four periods. *De* [*totius*] *morbi temporibus* [4].

(XI.3) The time of the beginning of a disease is measured from its first minute until signs of coction of the corrupt matter begin to appear. When the coction increases and the disease worsens, all this is the time of the increase, until the disease is as severe as possible; and this is the time of the climax. Any crisis comes only during the time of the climax of the disease, and the time of the entire crisis is the time of the climax. After the climax begins the decline, until the patient is cured. *De crisibus* 1[.20].

(XI.4) In some diseases the time of the occurrence of a disease—that is, the time of its beginning—as well as the time of its increase, are hidden from the senses. But the time of the climax can be perceived in all diseases. If a particular patient is likely to be cured from his disease, this time is followed by a perceptible decline. Thus, it is clear that, in a number of diseases, neither the beginning nor the increase is perceptible. [*De totius morbi temporibus* 4].

(XI.5) Sometimes a hard tumor occurs on the concave side of the liver and persists for a long time, while it is hidden from our senses, and the passage of food becomes spoiled, while we do not know at what time this occurs. With the passage of time, dropsy develops, whereby one assumes that the disease is, at that actual moment, in the phase of beginning or increase. I have seen a similar thing occurring to many people. [*De totius morbi temporibus* 4].

(xi.6) Sometimes the first fever attack covers the beginning, increase, and climax of the disease, so that the beginning of the attack is the beginning of the disease, the increase of the disease is the following phase of the attack, and the climax of the disease falls together with the climax of the attack. Then, in the second fever attack, the signs of the decline of the disease become clearly perceptible. *De crisibus* i[.3].

(xi.7) The end of the time of the beginning of a disease—that is, the beginning of the time of its increase—is marked by the appearance of a clear sign indicating coction. A clear sign holds the middle between hidden, weak signs of coction and signs of complete coction. *De crisibus* i[.17].

(xi.8) A sign of complete coction is that a white, even, and smooth sediment appears in the urine. A sign of weak coction is when the color of the urine changes from that of water to pale yellow, or that it changes from a clear condition into a turbid one. Similarly, when the urine has a fine consistency and is bright yellowish red, it is a weak sign. In the case of all these weak signs, the disease is in its beginning. *De crisibus* i[.17].

(xi.9) A sign that clearly indicates that the beginning of the disease has come to an end is the appearance of a white, even, and continuous cloud in the urine, either suspended in its middle or floating upon it. Similarly, a deep red cloud in the urine, or a deep red sediment, or urine that is moderately thick and has a healthy color but no sediment is a clear sign indicating the beginning of the increase of the disease. *De crisibus* i[.17].

(xi.10) The quick end of a disease which comes with great strain and which is called by the special name "crisis" is especially characteristic of fevers that originate from hot chymes. Moreover, it is found in the case of inflamed tumors that are quick to move18 in the major organs. *De crisibus* ii[.11].

(xi.11) If the illness is severe and strong, it inevitably ends with a crisis. But when it is small and weak, its end does not come with a crisis. A crisis always comes on a day of attack of the illness. It only rarely comes on a day that it is quiescent. I have seen such an exceptional case only once. *De crisibus* iii[.4].

(XI.12) Complete coction occurs especially during the climax of a disease. A salutary crisis comes during the climax or shortly before it. The crisis that is closer to the climax is always more salutary than the one that is more distant from it. Once complete coction has become evident, it is impossible that a non-salutary crisis occurs at any time. *De crisibus* III[.4].

(XI.13) There are five signs that indicate that a current crisis is beneficial: The first and the most important is that the coction comes first. I have never seen anyone die as a result of a crisis coming to him after coction. The second sign is that the coction occurs on one of the days of the crisis. The third sign is that the crisis is announced beforehand on a day bordering on the crisis. The fourth sign is that the crisis is light and easy. The fifth sign is that the evacuation is congenial to the nature and way of the disease. *De crisibus* III[.3].

(XI.14) Perspiration is congenial to all fevers, especially those that are severely burning and ardent. A nosebleed is congenial to all inflamed internal tumors, except for an inflamed tumor on the concave side of the liver, because diarrhea, perspiration, or emesis are congenial to its crisis. The same holds good for diseases of the chest and lungs, for expectoration is congenial to their crisis. *De crisibus* III[.3].

(XI.15) In the case of diseases of the head, a certainly safe crisis is sometimes brought about through tumors appearing at the roots of the ears; and in the case of chronic fevers, through tumors and abscesses appearing in other parts of the body. *De crisibus* III[.3].

(XI.16) The signs which indicate that the next crisis will be bad are not reliable and accurate, especially since a crisis may occur that does not necessarily follow from such signs. The signs which indicate that the next crisis is salutary are reliable and accurate and are therefore followed by a salutary crisis, according to their indication. *De crisibus* III[.10].

(XI.17) Many times a person suffers from sleeplessness, heaviness of the head, indolence, lack of energy to move, lack of appetite, weariness, headache, and the like while he carries out his normal activities. But then these symptoms increase so much that they throw him down and he has to lie down. The beginning of his illness should be reckoned from that moment in which he clearly began to suffer from such a high fever that he was forced to lie down. *De diebus decretoriis* I[.6].

(XI.18) The most eminent and powerful critical day is the seventh. The fourth day is mostly announced by a clear change taking place on it, in either the urine, or sputum, or excrements, or appetite, or understanding, or sensation, or other things. The change that occurs on the seventh day always resembles that occurring on the fourth day. If the change on the fourth day is for the better, then the crisis on the seventh day is good; and if it is for the worse, then the crisis on the seventh day is bad. Most of those whose condition changes for the worse on the fourth day die on the sixth day. *De diebus decretoriis* I[.4].

(XI.19) The fourteenth day is closest in its nature to the seventh. Similarly, the ninth, eleventh, and twentieth days are close to the nature of the fourteenth. Next in closeness comes the fourth day, and then the third, fifth, and eighteenth. *De diebus decretoriis* I[.5].

(XI.20) As for the other critical days after the twentieth until the fortieth day, critical movement is weaker in all of them and slowly becomes less. And those that come after the fortieth day are very weak. During these critical days, the end of the illness occurs either through coction or through an abscess or, in rare cases, through evacuation. *De diebus decretoriis* I[.10].

(XI.21) I have never seen anyone to whom a crisis occurred on the twelfth and sixteenth day of the illness. Similarly, the nineteenth day is not a critical day; neither is the first nor the second day. On the sixth day, a crisis indeed occurs to some patients but is accompanied by severe symptoms and grave danger. It is not a true crisis and does not come to an end but leads to worse symptoms. *De diebus decretoriis* I[.2].

(XI.22) If a crisis happens to occur on the eighth or tenth day, it is similar to the crisis that occurs on the sixth day. *De diebus decretoriis* I[.5].

(XI.23) When it is said of a crisis that it does not come to an end, it means a crisis in which the rest of the symptoms of the illness remain until after that crisis. When it is said of a crisis that it is not a true one, it means a crisis after which the illness returns. A dangerous and incomplete crisis is the one which comes with severe symptoms, whereby one has to fear for the life of the patient. An unclear crisis is that in which there is no clear evacuation nor clear abscess. Sometimes a crisis comes suddenly, without previous announcement. *De diebus decretoriis* I[.2].

(XI.24) An acute illness is one that moves fast and is dangerous. An illness that is very acute to the extreme is one that ends on the fourth day. One that is very acute but not to the extreme is one which ends on the seventh. An absolutely acute illness is the one that ends on the fourteenth day, and this is the one that is really acute. An illness that ends after the fourteenth day and before the twentieth day is somehow reckoned among the acute ones but is only called acute in a figurative sense. The illness occurring from a relapse is also called acute. *De diebus decretoriis* [II.12].

(XI.25) From three things, one can draw conclusions as to whether the periods of an illness will be long or short: from the nature of the illness, from the seasons of the year, and from the evacuations from the body. Conclusions can be drawn from the nature of an illness, as is the case in illnesses arising from black bile—such as quartan fever—and from phlegm—such as sciatica and pain in the kidneys and arthritis—, since these have long beginnings and also remote distant culminations. But ardent fever, pleurisy, and pneumonia have short beginnings and near culminations. The nearness of the culmination is according to the acuteness of the illness. One can conclude the duration of periods from the seasons of the year because all illnesses have shorter beginnings and more rapid endings in the summer and lengthier beginnings and slower endings in the winter. One can conclude the duration from the evacuations from the body because the appearance of good sputum, or similar urine or excrements, or perspiration in the beginning of the illness indicates that the beginning will be short and that the climax is near, while a delay in its appearance indicates that the beginning will be prolonged. *De crisibus* I[.4].

(XI.26) In some incomplete crises, such a large quantity of superfluities streams to a small organ that this organ cannot contain it. Then that superfluity returns to its original site or to a major organ, and the patient dies. *In Hippocratis Epidemiarum* [*commentarius*] II.1.

(XI.27) The days of crisis are every fourth day until the twentieth day: namely, the fourth, the seventh, the eleventh, the fourteenth, the seventeenth, and the twentieth. After the twentieth, they are every seventh day until the fortieth day. After the fortieth, they are computed in terms of every twentieth day until the hundred and twentieth day. After the hundred and twentieth day, one computes these days in terms of cycles of months, just like the cycles of days. And after the cycles of months, one computes them in terms of cycles of years. *In Hippocratis Epidemiarum* [*commentarius*] II.[6].

(xi.28) Illnesses that last longer than forty days hardly ever have a crisis through perspiration and definitely do not have a crisis through some other type of evacuation. But their end comes either through gradual coction or through an abscess. *In Hippocratis Aphorismos commentarius* iv[.36].

(xi.29) In the case of continuous fevers, one should count all the successive days for a prognosis of the future crisis; but in the case of intermittent fevers, one should count only the days of their bouts. For the effect of the seventh day in the case of continuous fevers is similar to the effect of the seventh cycle in the case of tertian fevers. Similarly, in the case of pure quartan fever, a crisis comes in seven cycles, that is, on the nineteenth day. *In Hippocratis Prognostica commentarius* iii[.7].

(xi.30) From six things, one can conclude that a crisis is complete and perfect. The first and the most important is that it is preceded by clear coction. The second is that it occurs through evacuation and not through an abscess. The third is that the evacuated matter consists of bad chyme. The fourth is that the evacuation is from the side of the illness. The fifth is that this is done on a critical day. The sixth is that it is followed by alleviation and total relaxation. *In Hippocratis Aphorismos commentarius* [i.20].

This is the end of the eleventh treatise,
by the grace of God,
praise be to Him.

In the name of God,
the Merciful, the Compassionate.
O Lord, make our task easy

The Twelfth Treatise

Containing aphorisms concerning evacuation by means of bloodletting

(xii.1) From the following three things one can determine the necessity of venesection: severity of the current or expected illness; age of the patient—that he is not too old nor too young—and great strength. *De* [*curandi ratione per*] *venae sectione*[*m* 9].

(xii.2) If someone has broad and large non-pulsatile vessels and his body is somewhat lean and his complexion is not white and his flesh is not soft, one should bleed him without caution and care. But if someone's condition is the opposite, one should bleed him with caution and care. *De* [*curandi ratione per*] *venae sectione*[*m* 13].

(XII.3) Do not bleed children below fourteen years, nor anyone older than seventy. Do not consider the number of years only, but also the external condition of the body, because some people are only sixty years old and yet cannot tolerate venesection, while others who are seventy can tolerate it, because they have much blood and their strength is great. But in spite of this, you should only extract a small amount of blood, even if their blood is like that of those who are in the prime of their life. *De* [*curandi ratione per*] *venae sectione*[*m* 13].

(XII.4) It is a general rule, for anyone whom one wants to bleed in the beginning of spring, that one examines and interrogates him. If he has a weak organ and his body is full of superfluous matter, this fullness will tend to that weak organ. Then one should bleed him from the side opposite that weak organ in order to draw the superfluous matters away from it. But if he does not have such an organ, one may bleed him from whatever spot one likes. *De* [*curandi ratione per*] *venae sectione*[*m* 19].

(XII.5) One should not proceed to perform venesection, even if there are clear signs of overfilling, under the following bodily conditions and symptoms: someone suffering from spasms, severe sleeplessness, heavy pain, severe heat, or severe cold; those residing in countries that are extremely hot or cold; someone with a very hot and dry temperament; someone whose flesh is lax, soft and flabby, and dissolves quickly; someone who is extremely fat or extremely lean; someone who is young or old; someone who is faint-hearted; someone who is not used to bleeding; someone whose cardia of the stomach is so painful that he is weakened by indigestions and suffering from burning bad humors; or someone who has diarrhea. But when the body of a patient is very full of blood besides having one of these bodily conditions, bleeding him is unavoidable. But one should only bleed a small amount with caution and care. These questions are elucidated in *Ad Glauconem* [*de medendi methodo*] 1[.15], and all these conditions lead to weakness of the animal faculty.

(XII.6) When the body is full of raw humors, it is very dangerous to apply venesection, because the strength of the patient is so greatly weakened and undermined that it is absolutely impossible for his body to return to its previous condition—and especially so if the patient also has fever. *De* [*curandi ratione per*] *venae sectione*[*m* 6].

(XII.7) If someone's body contains a small amount of good blood and a very large quantity of raw humors, venesection should not be applied, and he should not carry out any activity at all and not enter the bathhouse. For venesection removes the good blood from the body and attracts the bad blood collected in the primary non-pulsatile vessels of the liver and disperses it throughout the body. When one gives a purgative to such a patient, it causes colic, biting pain, and fainting, but it does not evacuate anything in a significant quantity. For the humors precede the matter to be evacuated and obstruct the passages because of their thickness. For this reason, he should not exercise nor enter the bathhouse. But the humors of such patients should be thinned and cut with ingredients that do not heat excessively. *De sanitate tuenda* IV[.5].

(XII.8) When a person is healthy but has signs of overfilling, it does not necessarily mean that we have to bleed him. Rather, for such a person, one should limit oneself and be content with withholding food from him. In the case of someone else, one should limit oneself to diminishing his food intake, and in yet another, one should limit oneself to prescribing laxatives or purgatives, or frequent bathing in the bathhouse, or exercise only, or much massage—each person according to his fullness and habit. One should be content to apply one of these so that one need not apply bleeding. *De methodo* [*medendi*] IV[.6].

(XII.9) Regarding venesection, one should know that in the case of someone who has little blood, one should first of all treat him by improving his humors. Then one can apply venesection to him and feed him subsequently. If necessary, one may bleed him again. This therapy is most appropriate for someone whose blood is turbid or contains a thick sediment. *De methodo* [*medendi*] V[.14].

(XII.10) If, during a venesection, it happens to a person that the mouth of a non-pulsatile vessel bursts open, or that menstruation sets in, or that diarrhea develops, one should consider its quantity and vehemence. For, if this is sufficient for the amount needed to be evacuated, let nature take care of the complete evacuation. But if you see that it is less than what needs to be evacuated, you should empty again through venesection such a quantity as makes both evacuations together enough to get the required amount. *De methodo* [*medendi*] IX[.5].

(XII.11) If bleeding is required but indigestion occurs, one should postpone the bleeding until the food is digested and its superfluities are excreted from the body. If another type of evacuation occurs, it is absolutely necessary to postpone the bleeding. *De methodo* [*medendi*] IX[.5].

(XII.12) If the chymes have increased evenly, evacuate all of them equally. The most proper way to do so is, above all, through venesection, closely followed by the evacuation effected through scarification of the ankle. Next comes that effected through exercise, massage, bathing in the bathhouse, and abstention from food. *In Hippocratis Aphorismos commentarius* II[.17].

(XII.13) When you know that the body contains a surplus of seething blood, you should evacuate it quickly before it streams to one of the major organs. Therefore, you should not refrain from applying venesection when necessary, whether it is day or night. *De [curandi ratione per] venae sectione[m* 12].

(XII.14) It often happens that blood, before it putrefies, suddenly streams to one of the organs because of its surplus and either mortifies it completely, so that its function is annulled, or causes it severe damage, such as occurs in the disease of apoplexy. For this disease originates from a large quantity of blood streaming to the brain. Therefore, when signs of a surplus of blood become evident, along with strength of the faculties—that is, the psychical, animal, and natural ones—carry out venesection without any caution. *De [curandi ratione per] venae sectione[m* 5].

(XII.15) When the body contains a large quantity of blood that has become extremely hot and seething and causes acute fever, one should evacuate a large quantity of blood at one stroke to the point of syncope, after examining the greatness of the strength of the patient. I know that I have personally evacuated about five *raṭl*s immediately or on the second, third, or fourth day since the beginning of the fever. *De [curandi ratione per] venae sectione[m* 12].

(XII.16) If someone whose strength is weak needs the evacuation of a large quantity of blood, the best thing is to do so in many sessions, either in a single day or on a second and third day as well. Feed him after every evacuation with fine food. Be careful not to evacuate a large quantity at one time unless you are forced to do so for a very strong reason. *De [curandi ratione per] venae sectione[m* 12].

(XII.17) If you want to simply evacuate blood, do so on the day of the bleeding. But if you want to draw someone's blood in a contrary direction, it is better to repeat it (to do so) on the second and third day. In all such cases, you should consider the strength of the patient. *De [curandi ratione per] venae sectione[m* 21].

(XII.18) If you perform a venesection and the blood is streaming, pay attention to a change in its color, especially if the patient suffers from an inflamed tumor. You should also pay attention to a reduction in the intensity of the flow of the blood. But above all, pay attention to a change of the pulse. If you see that it changes in either volume or regularity, stop the bleeding. But a change toward weakness is something I do not have to discuss. *De* [*curandi ratione per*] *venae sectione*[*m* 14].

(XII.19) In all diseases, you should, once you have evacuated a moderate amount of blood, attempt to repeat this either on the first day when possible or on the second day, unless you intend to evacuate to the point of syncope. *De* [*curandi ratione per*] *venae sectione*[*m* 16].

(XII.20) When someone is trained and experienced in the medical practice, he should not refrain from bloodletting when the illness is severe and serious and the patient has great strength. He should do so even if there are no signs of overfilling, but only a severe and serious disease. The same applies to the application of purgatives or emetics, either because of a surplus of humors other than blood or because of the severity and seriousness of the illness, in order to draw this surplus to the opposite side and to evacuate it and to support the strength of the patient. *De methodo* [*medendi*] IV[.6].

(XII.21) Bloodletting always needs great strength, equivalent to the amount to be evacuated. Lack of strength is the most dangerous of all things in the case of bloodletting. When, in the case of continuous fever resulting from the impossibility of dissolution, one's strength is great, bloodletting is mostly safe, far from being dangerous. But in other illnesses, bloodletting is dangerous, and a patient may suffer from very severe afflictions because of it. *De methodo* [*medendi*] IX[.10].

(XII.22) You were often in my presence when I ordered bleeding someone who suffered from either podagra or arthritis or epilepsy or melancholy or chronic hemoptysis; or someone whose chest condition was such that he would easily fall victim to such a disease; or someone suffering from obstruction, or frequent angina, or inflammation of the lungs, or pleurisy, or inflammation of the liver, or severe ophthalmia. For venesection is necessary in all these illnesses at their onset. Similarly, in the case of anyone losing blood from the mouths of his vessels and then stopping, bleed him with confidence and trust. Similarly, in the case of a woman whose menstruation stops or of someone who suffers from a nosebleed, hasten to bleed such persons, taking into consideration their strength and age. *De* [*curandi ratione per*] *venae sectione*[*m* 7].

(XII.23) When someone suffers from ulcerous fatigue, blood should be evacuated to the point of fainting, if there is no contraindication. One should examine the patient; and when he finds that the patient feels tension and pricking pain in his chest, back, and loins, he should bleed the basilic vein. But when the patient feels this in the head and neck, he should bleed the cephalic vein. And when the patient feels the fatigue equally throughout the body, he should bleed the median vein. *De sanitate tuenda* IV[.10].

(XII.24) When a nerve tears in its width, the patient is in danger of suffering from spasms when an inflamed tumor develops. Therefore, one should remove blood from this patient without compassion and in a larger quantity than one would in the case of another illness. And one should prescribe him a regimen of the finest possible food and of rest. One should also apply plenty of hot olive oil, from the site of the wound to the roots of that nerve and on the spine up to the neck. *De methodo* [*medendi*] VI[.3].

(XII.25) If someone lets blood because of a fever, he should do so during the decline of the fever attack, day or night. Beware of letting blood while food is still present in the stomach and as long as the humors in the stomach and first non-pulsatile vessels are not completely cocted. But for someone who does not have fever, such as someone who has ophthalmia, the best time for letting blood is when the pain is severe. And if there is no pain, the best time is at daybreak, one hour after waking up. *De* [*curandi ratione per*] *venae sectione*[*m* 20, 21].

(XII.26) When bleeding someone suffering from a fever, do not consider the number of days that have passed since the beginning of the illness, whether it is the fourth or fifth day. Rather, when you find that the patient is fit for bleeding, you should bleed him at that moment, even if it is the twentieth day since the beginning of the illness. You can find out about the patient's fitness from the severity of the illness, the greatness of the strength of the patient, the support of the age of the patient, and the time of the year. *De* [*curandi ratione per*] *venae sectione*[*m* 20].

(XII.27) When someone complains about an illness in the parts below the collarbone, it is most appropriate to bleed him from the basilic-axillary vein. And when someone complains about an illness in the parts above the collarbone, it is most appropriate to bleed him from the humeral vein. *De anatomi*[*cis administrationibus*] 3[.6].

(XII.28) For illnesses in the parts above the liver, bleeding should be done from the vein at the inner side of the arm; and for illnesses of the parts below the liver, from the vein at the inner side of the knee or from the saphenous vein. *In Hippocratis Epidemiarum* [*commentarius*] VI.1.

(XII.29) For an inflamed tumor in the side of the body, lungs, diaphragm, spleen, liver, or stomach, one derives clear benefit by bloodletting from the basilic vein. For the lower parts, such as those which lie next to the hip, the urinary bladder, and uterus, one should bleed from the vein at the inner side of the knee or at the ankle. Since the kidneys lie in the middle between these parts, one is benefitted by bleeding from the vein at the inner side of the arm, provided this is done when the inflammation is recent and when the whole body is filled with blood. But when the inflamed tumor in the kidneys becomes prolonged and old, one should bleed from the vein in the inner side of the knee or alongside the ankle. *De* [*curandi ratione per*] *venae sectione*[*m* 16, 18].

(XII.30) When ischias is caused by a surplus of blood, do not start with any kind of treatment before evacuating the surplus. Do not be content with evacuating the blood from the leg only, but also do so from the inner side of the elbow. [*De compositione medicamentorum secundum locos*] X[.2].

(XII.31) As for bloodletting from the saphenous vein or from the one at the inner side of the knee, I know that the illness called sciatica is cured in one day through the evacuation of blood from the leg, when it is caused by overfilling with blood. But cupping is of no benefit to such patients. *De* [*curandi ratione per*] *venae sectione*[*m* 18].

(XII.32) When you want to stop the bleeding from the mouths of the vessels, you should let blood from the veins in the arms. If you want to stimulate it, you should bleed from the veins in the legs. Similarly, you should always bleed from these veins to induce menstruation. When vessels in the uterus burst—because of an erosion or because of overfilling—and the woman loses blood and you want to stop the bleeding, you should let blood from the veins in the arms, since this is not menstrual blood which we would like to stimulate. *De* [*curandi ratione per*] *venae sectione*[*m* 19].

(XII.33) When an inflamed tumor begins in the liver, chest, or lungs, bleed from the basilic vein in the right arm. If this vein is not clearly visible, do so from the median vein; and if this one is not clearly visible, do so from the cephalic vein. When an inflamed tumor starts to develop in the parts of the mouth, bleed from the cephalic vein. If this one is not clearly visible, do so from the median vein; and if this one is not clearly visible, from the basilic vein. In the case of angina, as a last resort, let blood from the jugular vein under the tongue. *De methodo* [*medendi*] XIII[.11].

(XII.34) When the illness is in the nape of the neck, let blood from the arm or from the forehead. In the case of inflamed tumors in the kidneys or uterus, let blood from the vein that is at the inner side of the knee. If this is not possible, then bleed from the vein alongside the ankle—namely, the saphenous. For illnesses of the spleen, let blood from the left arm. *De methodo* [*medendi*] XIII[.11].

(XII.35) When the spleen is affected, bloodletting from the vein between the little finger and ring finger of the left hand is of great benefit. The same holds good for bloodletting from the basilic vein of the left arm. However, do not evacuate the amount that you wish to remove at one time, but over two days. *De* [*curandi ratione per*] *venae sectione*[*m* 16].

(XII.36) When, in the case of someone suffering from pleurisy, one bleeds from a vein on the same side as the inflammation, it sometimes brings clear benefit. But when one lets blood from the arm opposite to the illness, the benefit is not noticeable or only becomes visible after a long time. The same applies to severe pain in the eyes, for bloodletting from the cephalic vein on the same side alleviates the pain immediately and is of great benefit. *De* [*curandi ratione per*] *venae sectione*[*m* 16].

(XII.37) When you bleed someone suffering from a nosebleed or apply cupping glasses to his forehead and the nosebleed did not stop, you should not hastily cool his head; rather, put cupping glasses on the occipital protuberance on the back of his head, because it attracts the blood to the opposite side. *De methodo* [*medendi*] V[.6].

(XII.38) For chronic illnesses of the head or eyes that are caused by hot, fine matter, one sometimes lets blood from the pulsatile vessels in the temples or behind the ears, especially when these illnesses occur in the membranes. In these illnesses, the patient feels as if he is being pricked, and then this pain spreads out, while the pricking sensation remains in the center of that site. However, bloodletting from pulsatile vessels is very dangerous because sometimes the flow of blood does not stop or an aneurysm develops. For this reason, physicians avoid bleeding from a large pulsatile vessel—and also from a small one—because it is of little benefit. When a pulsatile vessel is cut widthwise, it is not dangerous because every part contracts to its own side. *De* [*curandi ratione per*] *venae sectione*[*m* 22, 23].

(XII.39) If a surplus of thick blood, or blood with another reprehensible quality, collects in the non-pulsatile vessels, you should first of all apply venesection and then, as a second thing, use a purgative that cleanses the thick humorous part within the blood. *In Hippocratis Epidemiarum* [*commentarius*] VI.1.

(XII.40) When, in the case of melancholic delusion and the like, all the indications suggest to you that the blood in all the non-pulsatile vessels is melancholic, you should bleed from the median cubital vein. If the blood that flows out is not melancholic, stop bleeding immediately. If you observe it to be melancholic, withdraw as much as you think the body of the patient can tolerate. This is a most important diagnostic rule. *De locis affectis* III[.10].

(XII.41) You should not first administer any strong remedy to patients with quartan fevers, nor desire to evacuate their bodies, unless you observe a surplus of blood that strongly prevails. When you let blood, examine it, and if you see that it is black and thick, evacuate with assurance and assiduity. But if you see that it is pure red and thin, stop its extraction. *Ad Glauconem* [*de medendi methodo*] I[.12].

(XII.42) In the case of women who develop dropsy because of the retention of their menstruation, as well as in the case of those in whom dropsy occurs because of a retention of the blood that was streaming from the mouths of the veins or through a nosebleed, one should hurry to bleed them before their strength dissolves and collapses. *In Hippocratis Epidemiarum* [*commentarius*] VI.7.

(XII.43) Sometimes, apply cupping glasses to the hollow in the back of the neck to attract the matter which streams to the eyes in the opposite direction and bleed from the frontal vein to attract the matter which is in the posterior part of the head. *In Hippocratis De humoribus commentarius* I.

(XII.44) If someone has a surplus of thick, melancholic blood, it is most appropriate, first of all, to bleed him and then to purge the black bile. When crude humors prevail in someone's body, evacuate his body with care and caution before the illness begins. But if he suffers from fever, do not evacuate at all. *De* [*curandi ratione per*] *venae sectione*[*m* 10].

(XII.45) When you treat hardness of the spleen and the illness remains unchanged, apply cupping glasses after scarifying the site. Especially beneficial for hardness of the liver and spleen is to bleed from the vein above the left ear and then take from the extracted blood and rub it on the diseased spleen. [*De compositione medicamentorum secundum locos*] IX[.2].

(XII.46) When the chest, the brain, or the membranes of the brain suffer from an inflamed tumor, we do not apply cupping glasses in the beginning of the illness until we have stopped superfluous matter from arriving at these sites and have evacuated the entire body. For, then, the application of cupping glasses is very beneficial. But when the body is full, the cupping glasses attract the superfluous matter from the entire body and move it to the brain or the chest or the lungs, depending on where one has applied them. *De methodo* [*medendi*] X[.17, 18].

(XII.47) If stretching pain is caused by a surplus of blood, such as occurs in the case of inflamed organs, one should bleed such a patient immediately. But if he is afraid of bloodletting or his strength is weak, one should draw the blood to the region opposite to that of the pain through diversion. *De methodo* [*medendi*] XII[.8].

This is the end of the twelfth treatise,
by the grace of God,
praise be to Him.

In the name of God,
the Merciful, the Compassionate.
O Lord, make our task easy

The Thirteenth Treatise

Containing aphorisms concerning evacuations by means of purgatives and enemas

(XIII.1) All purgatives are harmful for the stomach and especially for the cardia, since it is very sensitive. Therefore, it is proper to mix purgatives with some fragrant substances. *In Hippocratis De acutorum morborum* [*victu*] *commentarius* II[.11].

(XIII.2) Compound purgatives are bad when one of the ingredients has a purgative effect as soon as the purgative enters the body, while another ingredient has this effect only long after its ingestion. *In Hippocratis De acutorum morborum* [*victu*] *commentarius* II[.11].

(XIII.3) Says Moses: Latex plants and scammony purge as soon as they arrive in the body, whereas purgative resins purge only after a prolonged period. These resins are opopanax, galbanum, sagapenum, asafetida, and gum ammoniac.

(XIII.4) Fragrant seeds undo the harm of purgatives without hindering their action. Rather, they support their action, because they have the strength to cut and dilute the thick humors and to open the passages through which purgation takes place. *In Hippocratis De acutorum morborum* [*victu*] *commentarius* II[.12].

(XIII.5) Sometimes, when a purgative passes through the esophagus and cardia of the stomach, some of it sticks to these organs or settles in the stomach and causes great harm. Therefore, it is necessary to rinse these organs thereafter by taking some barley gruel or barley groats. *In Hippocratis De acutorum morborum* [*victu*] *commentarius* II[.12].

(XIII.6) Says Moses: This rinsing should be done after the effect of the purgative has worn off but before the intake of soup of young chickens, so that the food does not mix with the residue of the purgative in the lining of the stomach. The rinsing should be done with a viscous substance that has a cleansing and moistening effect. For this reason, Hippocrates and Galen chose barley groats; and since they were used to this ingredient, it seemed fine to them to take a small amount of it, sufficient to rinse the stomach after the ingestion of the purgative. But if any of us would do so, he would quickly vomit the entire remedy. Instead of that, it seems good to me to take a sip of hot julep. However, the consumption of barley groats, once the effect of the purgative has worn off, is something unusual in all the countries I have passed through. It causes nausea, because the stomach quickly needs to throw up even after the effect of the purgative has worn off. It seems to me that the best thing to do is to drink warm water in which common marshmallow root or seed has been boiled together with fresh fennel, or anise, or cinnamon, or the like in order to combine viscosity with that which has a cleansing effect and with fragrance and sweetness. This should be strained into sugar. If one adds myrtle seed, it combines viscosity and fragrance. Moreover, it is a remedy which is good for the heart. Once this compound medicine leaves the stomach, eat the soup; and if the myrtle seed causes thirst, take fleawort seed instead.

(XIII.7) In most cases, the evacuation by means of purgatives or emetics is not suitable. It is only necessary for someone with a drastic need for evacuation and should only be applied with long intervals between uses. *In Hippocratis Aphorismos commentarius* III[.15].

(XIII.8) If you want to evacuate the body by means of a purgative or emetic, first dilute the thick humors, and cut the viscous ones, and widen the passages using a thinning regimen. If you want to purge the body, first use a laxative for a number of times; and if you want to apply emesis, first stimulate the body repeatedly. *In Hippocratis Aphorismos commentarius* II[.9].

(XIII.9) Yellow bile can be evacuated with minimal effort. But phlegm—especially that which is very thick and viscous—and, equally, black bile can only be evacuated with difficulty. *De methodo* [*medendi*] XIV[.16].

(XIII.10) All crude humors are slow to move because of their thickness and coldness. And once they move in order to be evacuated, they precede the other superfluities and close all the narrow passages. Therefore, do not use a purgative as long as there are crude, raw humors [in the body]. *De sanitate tuenda* IV[.5].

(XIII.11) Because of its thickness, one needs a stronger drug for the evacuation of black bile than for the evacuation of yellow bile. *In Hippocratis Aphorismos commentarius* IV.

(XIII.12) For some people, it is sufficient to evacuate their body once a year at the beginning of spring. Others need a second evacuation in the fall. When bad humors have accumulated in the body, evacuate with drugs that cleanse the dominating bad humor. But when large quantities of superfluities have accumulated, evacuate them by venesection. *De sanitate tuenda* VI[.13].

(XIII.13) If you want to cleanse the body from the bad humors in it and, at the same time, want to cleanse the head so that no defluction descends from it, the remedy must be compounded from ingredients of varying strength—such as the pill I compounded from aloe, scammony, pulp of the colocynth, agarikon, blue bdellium, and gum Arabic—because it expels many types of superfluities. If, at the end of the treatment, one needs drugs to expel the black bile, use these. *De methodo* [*medendi*] V[.14].

(XIII.14) When one of the humors is completely evacuated from the body, it is necessarily affected by a bad temperament and a weakening of the vessels. The reason for such an evacuation cannot be attributed to a drug alone but to an excessive purgation resulting from three things: one of these is the weakness of the vessels; the second, the wideness of the mouths of these vessels; and the third, the biting effect of the purgative. *De* [*simplicium*] *medicamentorum* [*temperamentis ac facultatibus*] III[.28].

(XIII.15) If you administer a purgative, the first thing it expels is the humor you intended to expel. If the purgation is excessive, the next thing to be expelled is the thinnest humor that remains, then the thickest, and then the blood. The thinnest humor is the yellow bile, followed by the phlegm, while the black bile is the thickest. However, blood comes last only once the drug overpowers nature and weakens its strength. *De* [*simplicium*] *medicamentorum* [*temperamentis ac facultatibus*] III[.27].

(XIII.16) Purgation becomes excessive if much of the strength of the purgative drug remains in the mouths of the vessels leading to the stomach. This then produces a biting in these vessels, and opens them, and constantly incites and stimulates them to expel their contents; it also destroys the strength in the vessels. *De* [*simplicium*] *medicamentorum* [*temperamentis ac facultatibus*] III[.27].

(XIII.17) If a person takes purgatives without any result, some of them have a bad effect, but others turn into food and do not harm his nature. These last-mentioned purgatives acquire strength from the body, through which they attract and increase so much in purgative power that they turn into potential purgatives again. But if they do not realize that potential, they return to food. *De* [*simplicium*] *medicamentorum* [*temperamentis ac facultatibus*] III[.26].

(XIII.18) I know famous physicians who are perplexed, not knowing what to do, when they administer purgatives that did not have any effect. When I am called in to such patients, I order some of them to bathe in the bathhouse, I prescribe venesection or emesis to others, and to yet others I apply astringent remedies. When I do this to them, their bowels become loose. *De* [*optimo*] *medico cognoscendo* [XI.8].

(XIII.19) It is necessary to bathe one, two, or three successive days before taking a cathartic remedy, because bathing melts the humors. When there is a site in the body that has become hard and tense, it becomes softened and loose through the bathing, and the body becomes prepared so that which streams through it does so in an easy way. *In Hippocratis Epidemiarum* [*commentarius*] VI.5.

(XIII.20) Often, a single purgation is sufficient for curing those diseases that arise from yellow bile or phlegm. Those diseases which are more related to black bile, such as cancer and elephantiasis, cannot be cured by a single purgation, but need a second, third, fourth, or fifth treatment. *In Hippocratis De humoribus commentarius* I[.12].

(XIII.21) The best therapy for someone in whom bile dominates is to evacuate him from below successively, on successive days. This should be done both when he is healthy and when he is ill. *In Hippocratis Epidemiarum* [*commentarius*] II.3.

(XIII.22) When someone is disordered in his regimen and addicted to drinking bad wines, you will not help him much by purging or phlebotomizing him, for crude humors quickly accumulate in his body in a large amount because of his bad regimen. One should not undertake the treatment of such a patient at all. *De* [*curandi ratione per*] *venae sectione*[*m* 10].

(XIII.23) When you have a bowel movement, you should not interrupt it before the proper time, and when it stops by itself you should not leave it just like that. Rather, examine and inspect the condition and quantity of the humors in the entire body. For when a small quantity remains, it causes a grave and dangerous illness. *In Hippocratis Epidemiarum* [*commentarius*] II.1.

(XIII.24) If you give a purgative to a patient, examine what is eliminated from him. If you observe that it has changed, know that his body is clean from the humor that you wanted to evacuate and he therefore benefits from this treatment. But this is not the case if the evacuated material consists of shreds, or something blood-like, or black bile, or something stinking, or a pure humor. For the excretion of humors in a pure state results from unnatural heat, and that of stinking material results from putrefaction, while that of black bile which is not quiescent results from the prevailing burning. *In Hippocratis Epidemiarum* [*commentarius*] II.1.

(XIII.25) Some people are hard to purge, while in others, a small quantity of a purgative effects a strong purgation. When the patient does not suffer from high fever and you know his nature, give him a purgative to drink. [*In Hippocratis*] *De acutorum morborum* [*victu*] *commentarius* II[.12].

(XIII.26) The strength of a body that has been purged is weakened through the purgation. Therefore, it cannot tolerate much food nor digest it very well. Therefore, one should minimize a patient's food intake and increase it later on, slowly, and give him those foods which are quick to digest. [*In Hippocratis*] *De acutorum morborum* [*victu*] *commentarius* II[.13].

(XIII.27) If a very high fever develops, be extremely careful not to administer a purgative. Evacuate especially through bloodletting, because evacuation by means of bloodletting does not involve any danger. [*In Hippocratis*] *De acutorum morborum* [*victu*] *commentarius* II[.11].

(XIII.28) When diarrhea is beneficial, one should not interrupt it—not even with food that only has little binding force, and certainly not with binding drugs. For if it is interrupted, the bad humor reascends, and a fever or tumor develops in the liver, usually, or in another organ. *In Hippocratis Epidemiarum* [*commentarius*] II.2.

(XIII.29) When you intend to administer a purgative, be especially careful during fever attacks or critical days. The strength of the purgative is corrupted if the humors tend toward the upper parts of the body or to the side opposite from where the drug evacuates them. *In Hippocratis De humoribus commentarius* II[.13].

(XIII.30) I have cured countless patients who suffered from jaundice by using purgation only. Similarly, I have cured those who suffered from elephantiasis or from a chronic and long-standing pain and from other chronic illnesses by purgation alone. *De* [*optimo*] *medico cognoscendo* [XI.8].

(XIII.31) Many people are quick to find relief and to rejoice at a strong evacuation. But the more they are evacuated on the first day, the more constipated they are on the following days. *De sanitate tuenda* V[.9].

(XIII.32) When we want to purge infants, we give their wet nurses something from a purgative to drink, for the strength of that purgative stays in the milk. That this is so is evident from other living creatures, for the bowels of some people were relieved from drinking the milk of goats that had fed on the branches of scammony or latex plants. Others ate a lot of quails and were affected by tension in the muscles because of the hellebore on which the quails fed. *In Hippocratis Epidemiarum* [*commentarius*] VI.5.

(XIII.33) One should apply an enema only to someone whose strength is great. But in the case of someone whose strength is weak, one should use a suppository. [*In Hippocratis*] *De acutorum morborum* [*victu*] *commentarius* [I.44].

(XIII.34) Some ancient physicians recommend that someone suffering from a colic take a small stone of salt and use it as a suppository, because it expels the excrements in a light and easy way. Natron may have the same effect if used as a suppository. *De* [*clysteribus et*] *colica.*

(XIII.35) If one takes two parts of tar and one part of olive oil and applies it as an enema, it is very beneficial for a colic, when the stomach is strong. But when the stomach of the patient is weak, avoid it. Similarly, other strong medications should be applied as enemas only when the stomach is strong. When the patient has a weak stomach, he should be given only enemas with mild medications, so that the stomach does not weaken even more and the patient does not get one disease after the other. For when strong medications are applied as an enema, the strength of the enema sometimes reaches the stomach and may, from there, even reach up to the tongue. *De* [*clysteribus et*] *colica.*

(XIII.36) If there are biting moistures in the intestines, one should, first of all, apply an enema with something that washes them, such as hydromel or barley gruel. And once they have been expelled from the intestines, one should apply an enema with that whose property it is to alleviate the biting pain and to have an agglutinant and cohesive effect. *In Hippocratis Epidemiarum* [*commentarius*] VI.6.

(XIII.37) We use an enema with salt water in the case of someone who suffers from putrid ulcers in his intestines, so that it washes all that had putrefied and expels a substantial amount of scales. Once the site is clean, we apply an enema with drugs that are good for the putrefaction. *In Hippocratis De humoribus commentarius* I[.12].

(XIII.38) As much as possible, one should be careful and considerate concerning the other types of evacuation in the case of someone whose bodily condition is such that his flesh is soft and slack, lean, and quick to dissolve. Similarly, one should take care in the case of someone who is extremely fat or lean. Such a person should be evacuated by means of a moderate diet, massage, mild enemas, the application of fomentations and poultices and softening suppositories, and bathing. Be careful to apply these means according to the indications provided by the conditions of the patient. *Ad Glauconem* [*de medendi methodo*] I[.15].

(xiii.39) For ulcerous wombs, we often apply enemas with milk boiled with stones or iron. We also provide benefit with this remedy in the case of hemorrhoids and ulcers in the anus. *De* [*simplicium*] *medicamentorum* [*temperamentis ac facultatibus*] x[.8].

(xiii.40) If you need to apply an enema for someone with constipation, be it someone who has a chronic disease or someone on a diet of a convalescent after a lengthy disease, do not use a sharp enema, but one containing olive oil only. *De sanitate tuenda* v[.9].

(xiii.41) One should attempt to relieve the bowels of someone suffering from a continuous putrid fever; and if his bowels cannot be relieved, one should give the patient an enema with hydromel and olive oil. *De methodo* [*medendi*] xi[.15].

(xiii.42) When biting humors incline toward the intestines, evacuate them by administering the patient an enema from below with an appropriate ingredient. The best and most appropriate ingredient is barley gruel. *De methodo* [*medendi*] xii[.8].

(xiii.43) The enemas to be used for intestinal ulcers should be composed from astringent, cleansing, ripening, stupefying, agglutinant, and alleviating ingredients. If you intend to use an enema with one of these effects, or all of them, or whichever is needed, then the base for these medications should be barley gruel and some astringent wine. Use this for an enema. [*De compositione medicamentorum secundum locos*] ix[.5].

(xiii.44) Rules in hortatory form composed by Abū al-ʿAlāʾ ibn Zuhr for his son Abū Marwān concerning the treatment by means of purgatives which every physician should observe—all of them. He said: Be most careful not to administer strong purgatives initially, but begin with cocting the humors, opening the obstructions, washing the passages, and softening the stool. Then you can purge. When it is necessary to purge the bowels during the cold season, one should mix with the purgatives substances that dissolve the humors, such as the different kinds of salt and long pepper. If you are forced to purge during the hot season, you do not need a dissolving substance. In any case, it is necessary to use, in combination with the purgative, a substance that strengthens the stomach, such as mastic, anise, or absinth wormwood; and a substance that hinders the purgative from passing from the intestines into the liver and that protects against its harmful effects, such as almonds and pistachio nuts and their oils, or a rob of licorice, or gum tragacanth, and or the like.

(XIII.45) He further said: The more one washes purgatives, the more one diminishes their purgative effect. The same applies if one boils them. The more one pulverizes them, the more likely they are to be lethal rather than purgative. When they are safe, they induce micturition. But all astringent things act conversely. The more one washes or boils them, the more astringent they become. Similarly, the more one pulverizes them, the more astringent they become, and they also hold back the urine.

(XIII.46) He further said: Any purgative with which you want to purify the head should be administered in the form of large pills and should have a strong effect. When he goes to bed, the patient should take such a purgative with hot water in which raisins have been cooked until they rise. Always add a little garlic to any medication used for purifying the head.

(XIII.47) He further said: Imagine a boy who is stricken by a fever that dissolves his flesh to the degree that it comes out in the diarrhea. The most effective way to stop the diarrhea is to immerse the patient in cold water. Imagine someone with coarse humors who is given a purgative while the weather is cold, for he suffers from distress and disturbance and pains in the stomach and intestines, but does not respond to the medicine. If you let him go to the bathhouse and he goes into a hot bathing basin, in due time his bowels will be relieved and his humors will respond and leave his body, and his pains and distress will be alleviated. And if someone with thin humors who is given a purgative drug while the weather is cold and who, consequently, suffers from severe diarrhea goes into a hot bathing basin in the bathhouse, his diarrhea will stop. In the first case, the heat of the bath dissolves and expels his coarse humors; while in the second case, the heat of the bath attracts the humors to the outside.

(XIII.48) He further said: There are certain purgatives that have no effect on certain individuals, while a medication that is weaker does have a certain therapeutic effect on them. If you give a medication and it does not have any effect, do not give more of the same, but give a different one, even if it is less potent, be it some days after the initial medication or shortly thereafter. Never allow a patient to eat immediately after taking a purgative. Let him take light food before the ingestion of the purgative and afterwards for some days, according to the strength of the drug.

(XIII.49) He further said: It is a mistake to use musk as a part of purgatives, and, similarly, to drink it with wine. Those who compound this remedy and administer it are mistaken, because they want to strengthen the organs and let the medicine rise to the head; but they forget that the effect of these purgatives is carried to the major organs, and sometimes such an organ cannot tolerate this, and the patient is killed.

(XIII.50) Says Moses: This is correct if the purgation is done by poisonous drugs, such as pulp of colocynth or St. Thomas lidpod, because of their poisonous effect; or by strong drugs, such as bay laurel, because of its strength. But safe drugs—and especially agarikon, which is good for poisons—are very beneficial if imbibed in wine. I have done so several times and used such a drug in order to cleanse the head, and I saw that it is very effective and that it cleanses the brain to a degree any other drug is incapable of. Moreover, the patient taking this drug found new energy and dilation of the soul. Therefore, consider the specific properties of the drugs that you administer.

(XIII.51) He further said: In the case of the rind enclosing the pulp of colocynth and pistachio nuts, followed by almond kernels, this has been confirmed by long experience. The same applies to husks of hellebore and *nīlūfar* (blue Egyptian, European white, or yellow water lily) blossoms. And if one adds almond oil thereto, it is a good decision.

(XIII.52) In his *Kitāb Al-Murshid* [*fī jawāhir al-aghdhiya waquwā l-mufradāt mina l-adwiya*], al-Tamīmī states: If one boils milk and adds thereto—when it boils—seeds of garden cress, without pulverizing them, and lets this boil until the mucilage emerges, and then one drinks this milk, it cures the colics resulting from taking purgatives, whether pills or decoctions. One should drink the milk while it is lukewarm, because it has a glutinous effect on the contents of the intestines and at the same time washes the remainder of the purgative from the stomach and the intestines.

(XIII.53) Says Moses: This is correct on the condition that one uses goat's milk. And if the patient who takes the medicine becomes very thirsty and feels burning in the stomach and intestines, [the ingestion of] fleawort seed with cold water and rose syrup is most appropriate.

(XIII.54) In his *Kitāb Al-Murshid* [*fī jawāhir al-aghdhiya waquwā l-mufradāt mina l-adwiya*], al-Tamīmī further states that, because of its specific properties, an onion, when one crushes it and smells it during the ingestion of a purgative, stops the nausea and prevents the purgative from being vomited.

This is the end of the thirteenth treatise,
by the grace of God,
praise be to Him.

In the name of God,
the Merciful, the Compassionate.
O Lord, make our task easy

The Fourteenth Treatise

Containing aphorisms concerning vomiting

(XIV.1) All the phlegm that streams into the intestines or that originates in it is washed by the yellow bile superfluity and excreted in the stool. Sometimes much phlegm also originates in the stomach, and therefore the ancient physicians advised that once every month, one should induce vomiting after taking food. Some of them thought that one should vomit twice a month. All of them advised that the food taken prior to vomiting should have a sharp taste and a cleansing and detergent strength, in order to clean all the phlegm out of the stomach without the body being harmed by a bad condition of the humors originating from such food; because all detergent, biting foods produce yellow bile, and all of them are unwholesome. *De usu partium* V[.4].

(XIV.2) If someone's body contains sharp, biting humors, one should not induce vomiting for fear that some of the external superfluities retreat inward; for one should be cautious not to attract the biting humors to the inside, just as one should be cautious not to drive the raw humors which surround the liver to the outside. *De sanitate tuenda* IV[.6].

(XIV.3) Melancholic humors should always be evacuated from below and not through vomiting at all. Thus, he said in his [*In Hippocratis*] *De humoribus commentarius* I. And in his [*In Hippocratis*] *Aphorismos commentarius* IV[.12], he said that if a sharp, thin humor floats upward, there is no way to evacuate it through vomiting in wintertime.

(XIV.4) If someone is stricken by syncope because of bad humors that irritate the cardia of his stomach, give him hot, pure water to drink, either alone or mixed with some oil. Then tell him to vomit; but if vomiting is too difficult for him, warm his stomach and its adjacent parts and his feet and hands. But if, even in this way, vomiting does not come to him, induce it by entering your finger or a feather into his throat. But if, even then, vomiting does not come to him, give him the best oil that you can dispose of to drink, heated. But in many cases, this oil has the property not to induce vomiting, but to soften the stool. And this is also beneficial for someone suffering from this condition. *Ad Glauconem* [*de medendi methodo*] I[.15].

(XIV.5) When bilious humor tends upward to the stomach, evacuate it through vomiting after exercise but prior to taking food. To apply vomiting is most appropriate in the case of someone whose temperament tends more toward heat and dryness since the beginning of the illness. *De sanitate tuenda* VI[.3].

(XIV.6) If someone's stomach contains viscous phlegm that fills it completely, and if he is one of those who vomit easily, he will come to no harm if he vomits by means of radish with oxymel. If the phlegm is thin and not viscous, barley gruel alone or hydromel alone is sufficient to induce vomiting, when one takes, of either one of these, a dose larger than that which one would take in order to feed oneself with it. *De methodo* [*medendi*] VI[.11].

(XIV.7) If you want to let someone vomit after a meal, feed him brains seasoned with much olive oil after his meal, because this induces vomiting. *De alimentorum* [*facultatibus*] III[.8].

(XIV.8) The bulb of the narcissus is one of the drugs that induces vomiting. Therefore, we add two or three bulbs to the food of someone in whom we want to induce vomiting, for then he will vomit easily, without any harm. *In Hippocratis Epidemiarum* [*commentarius*] II.6.

(XIV.9) If it is easy for someone to vomit, he should do so before taking food, in order to cleanse his body from the superfluities of the previous food he took. If it is difficult for someone to vomit, he should vomit after taking food, in order to cleanse his body from the phlegm as well. *In Hippocratis De mulierum affectibus commentarius*.

(XIV.10) Galen said: Vomiting can often be applied for cleansing a thick, viscous humor which has settled in the stomach. And there is no hindrance in either one of these cases from vomiting on all days, but they should not apply it on two successive days only. *In Hippocratis De natura hominis commentarius* [III.22].

(XIV.11) If someone's stomach contains biting humors that either originate there or pour into it and if he is nearly fainting, let him vomit by giving him lukewarm water to drink. *De methodo* [*medendi*] XII[.8].

(XIV.12) Heavy movement of the body after the imbibition of an emetic helps vomiting, because the movement stimulates the humors upwards, as happens to sailors. *In Hippocratis Aphorismos commentarius* IV[.14].

(XIV.13) Drugs that induce vomiting should not be taken all at once but little by little, so that they stay in the stomach and dissolve and attenuate. Then one should take a larger dose until the moment that all that is in the stomach and in the main adjacent vessels is evacuated. *In Hippocratis De natura hominis commentarius* [III.18].

This is the end of the fourteenth treatise,
by the grace of God,
praise be to Him.

In the name of God,
the Merciful, the Compassionate.
O Lord, make our task easy

The Fifteenth Treatise
Containing aphorisms concerning surgery

(XV.1) Putrid ulcers that spread and expand to the surrounding area require very strong remedies. From time to time, cauterization is needed as part of their treatment. [*De compositione medicamentorum per genera*] V[.14].

(XV.2) Some ulcers are called carbuncles. The site where they occur looks as if it has been burned by fire and is completely surrounded by an inflammation that is so severe that it brings about fever and great danger. One should put a strong, caustic remedy on the burned site and a cataplasm on the surrounding inflammation. This cataplasm should combine medications that repel and prevent the surrounding inflammation from spreading and that have a cooling and dissolving effect on it. [*De compositione medicamentorum per genera*] V[.15].

(xv.3) One should not cauterize a part of the body that has depth or hollowness—all bodily parts have depth or hollowness except the hands, feet, and loins. *In Hippocratis De aer*[*e, aquis et locis*] *commentarius* II.

(xv.4) If pus has collected in the area between the chest and the lungs and one despairs of cleansing it through expectoration, apply cauterization to the chest. *In Hippocratis Aphorismos commentarius* VI[.27].

(xv.5) Says Moses: Consider how he recommends doing so only in the case of despair. Therefore, it does not contradict his previous statement in his commentary on *De aer*[*e, aquis et locis*] II.

(xv.6) Cauterization with a glowing hot iron or with caustic remedies should be applied to those sites that are affected by a severe illness caused by a surplus of humors or by their bad quality, as in the case of malignant ulcers. *In Hippocratis Epidemiarum* [*commentarius*] VI.6.

(xv.7) One should not hasten to puncture the abdomen of a dropsy patient. One is forced to do so only when so much moisture collects in it that it bears heavily upon the patient and weakens him. One should hasten to cauterize the chest of patients with lung ulcers before they are eaten away by corrosion. *In Hippocratis Epidemiarum* [*commentarius*] VI.7.

(xv.8) If you lance a site and evacuate the pus from it, be careful at that moment and thereafter not to use oil or water to wash the wound. When you have to wash the wound, do so with hydromel, or vinegar mixed with water, or wine alone, or wine mixed with honey. *Ad Glauconem* [*de medendi methodo*] II[.2].

(xv.9) Malignant ulcers that putrefy need medications that are so extremely sharp that they are similar to fire, such as vitriol, yellow vitriol, the two types of arsenic, and lime. For the burning of these medications is like the burning of fire; and often we use fire in treating these kinds of ulcers when these medications are overpowered and cannot have any effect on them. But sometimes these medications are beneficial for the disease called carbuncles when they are put on the site of the eschar, because this is the site that putrefies more than any other. They should not be applied to the surrounding area. *Ad Glauconem* [*de medendi methodo*] II[.3].

(xv.10) When a limb dies to the point that one does not feel it when it is pricked, cut off, or burned with fire and inevitably turns black, hasten to cut it off at the point where it touches the connected healthy site. *Ad Glauconem* [*de medendi methodo*] II[.11].

(XV.11) Medications which are beneficial for putrid sites are bitter vetch with vinegar, darnel flour with honey, broad bean flour with oxymel, a dried pastille, or broad bean flour with oxymel and salt. Select from these and the like according to the temperament of the patient. *Ad Glauconem* [*de medendi methodo*] II[.11].

(XV.12) When you amputate a limb that has putrefied or died, be careful and cautious and use those medications that I have described, after examining the nature of the patient and the nature of the limb. Once you have amputated the limb, cauterize its root, as we often do in the case of pudenda. *Ad Glauconem* [*de medendi methodo*] II[.11].

(XV.13) I have treated the illness of cancer at its beginning many times, and it was cured. However, if the illness becomes serious and the tumor greatly enlarged, nobody is capable of curing it except through surgery, in order to excise the tumor and completely uproot it all around until one reaches a healthy spot. But if there are large vessels—especially pulsatile—one cannot be sure but that it may start to bleed immediately; and if the tumor is also close to a vital organ, excision is dangerous, because it is impossible to cauterize the root of the disease because of its proximity to a vital organ. *Ad Glauconem* [*de medendi methodo*] II[.12].

(XV.14) Those suffering from dizziness and vertigo or various types of severe headache, such as migraine or a headache affecting the whole head, sometimes benefit from venesection of the pulsatile vessels behind the ear. But sometimes they do not benefit from it because the vapors that produce these illnesses rise to the brain through other pulsatile vessels that are not visible on the surface of the body and that ascend to the cerebral plexus. *De locis affectis* III[.12].

(XV.15) Someone suffering from any wound at any site of the body—a site that has tendons and nerves or veins and is free from flesh and has many bones—is in danger and on the verge of being afflicted by pain, sleeplessness, spasms, and delirium. *De methodo* [*medendi*] IV[.6].

(XV.16) When a part of the body is sensitive, treat it with a medication that causes minimal pain. But you may treat a part that has little sensitivity with very strong drugs, when the disease requires a strong kind of treatment. *De methodo* [*medendi*] IV[.7].

(XV.17) If someone is pricked directly in a nerve and he suffers unavoidably, because of the great sensitivity of the nerve, from severe pain, exercise your skill to alleviate the pain and to prevent inflammation of the site. This should be done by keeping the site open and by not allowing it to heal up, and by, as a precautionary measure, increasing the tear in the skin. Phlebotomize the patient if he is strong enough to tolerate it; and, when his body contains bad humors, evacuate them by giving him a purgative. Foment the site where he is pricked with extremely thin olive oil—that is, old and heated. Be extremely careful not to do so with hot water, because this putrefies the nerve and the patient will die. *De methodo* [*medendi*] VI[.2].

(XV.18) If you choose to treat a cancer through surgery, begin by evacuating the melancholic humor through purgation. Then excise the entire site until not even the root thereof remains. Let the blood flow, and do not hasten to stop it. Then compress the surrounding vessels and press the thick blood out of them. Treat it in the same way as other ulcers. *De methodo* [*medendi*] XIV[.9].

(XV.19) Scrofula is a hard tumor that arises in the soft flesh. If it arises in the soft flesh that was created for an important function—namely, that which was created for the production of the sputum and the like—and pulsatile and non-pulsatile vessels are connected to it, its therapy should be similar to that of other hard tumors. But the scrofula arising in the soft flesh created to fill up empty space and to support the vessels should be treated through extirpation of the bad organ in its entirety. This can be done either through surgery, as is done in the case of cancer, or by letting it putrefy. *De methodo* [*medendi*] XIV[.9].

(XV.20) The therapy of abscesses which mostly occur on the surface of the body has three common goals: dissolution, putrefaction, or surgery. For honey-like abscesses, one needs only one of these forms of therapy. Those abscesses whose contents resemble meal boiled in water may be either excised or allowed to putrefy. Fat-like abscesses can only be treated through surgery, since they cannot putrefy nor dissolve. *De methodo* [*medendi*] XIV[.12].

(XV.21) Excess flesh in the inner angle of the eye and excrescences on the anus—namely, hemorrhoids—require surgery. *De methodo* [*medendi*] XIV[.13].

(XV.22) If you consider applying surgery to any part of the body, strive for three things: the first is to complete your work in the shortest time possible; the second is that no pain at all should be felt during the surgery; and the third is the question of safety. This latter goal is achieved by observing three things: the first is that you are sure that your goal can be absolutely realized; the second is that, if your goal is not realized, the patient will not come to any harm in another aspect because of that; and the third is that you are sure that the disease will not return. If you observe these three goals, it will be evident to you that sometimes surgery is preferable, but at other times the application of medications is preferable. *De methodo* [*medendi*] XIV[.13].

(XV.23) If vessels in the legs or testicles become thick, they should be excised and extirpated. Similarly, an excrescence in the nose should be excised, together with the covering internal membrane, and, in some cases, together with the entire nose. *De methodo* [*medendi*] XIV[.13].

(XV.24) As long as the pterygium in the eye is small, it can be treated with cleansing medications similar to medications for trachoma. If it increases and hardens, it should be treated by surgery. *De methodo* [*medendi*] XIV[.19].

(XV.25) Hailstone in the eyelid (chalazion) requires excision. The same applies to the pus collected in the eye in the illness called *kumna*. However, in most cases it can be treated with dissolving medications that do not have a strong drying effect, because these evacuate most of the pus and congeal the rest. I have evacuated this pus by lancing the horn-like tunic in the rim. It can also be evacuated by shaking the head until the pus descends. *De methodo* [*medendi*] XIV[.19].

(XV.26) For the treatment of illnesses associated with pain, one should, first of all, use those medicines which are moist and slightly heating. Then use slackening medicines, namely, those which loosen the stretching of the organs. [*De compositione medicamentorum per genera*] VII[.9].

(XV.27) The uvula can be affected by the illness of extreme relaxation without an inflammation, in which case we generally cut it off. But when the uvula is affected by this illness, remedies that heat and that cleanse the phlegm are really beneficial for it, because, at that time, the uvula mostly tends to turn white, as if it were lacking blood. [*De compositione medicamentorum secundum locos*] VI[.8].

(XV.28) The eye is the most sensitive of organs. Therefore, drip medications into it after extremely gently lifting the upper eyelid. The medications should be steeped in a liquid that does not bite. The ancient physicians were very much in the right to use egg white as a base for eyedrops. *De methodo* [*medendi*] XIII[.22].

(XV.29) A moist, liquid medicine stays at its place only when applied in a ligament. Therefore, medicines for lachrymal fistula should be dry, because the ligament has to cover the whole eye, and the eye cannot tolerate being constantly bandaged for so many days that the fistula in it is cured. [*De compositione medicamentorum secundum locos*] V[.2].

(XV.30) When in the case of a cataract operation the moisture has descended from the surface of the pupil, the couching needle should be held for a long time in the place where one wants the moisture to settle, so that it becomes firmly fixed there. [*In Hippocratis*] *De officina* [*medici commentarius*] I[.6].

(XV.31) If you dissect the horn-like tunic, the first thing you find is a fine and thin liquid streaming and pouring out. It is the moisture that you often see flowing out from the opening made in the eye that is being operated on for a cataract. This is followed by the whole eye becoming shriveled, contracted, and hollow. *De usu* [*partium*] X[.5].

(XV.32) The most beneficial and appropriate medication for nerve wounds is that which dries while it is slightly warming, or one in which the heat is not noticeable but which dries just the same. Everything that has the property to attract moistures from the depth of the body to the outside is suitable for nerve wounds. [*De compositione medicamentorum per genera* III.2].

(XV.33) As medications for nerve wounds, I use sulfur that has not been affected by fire, mixed with olive oil until it assumes the consistency of bath sordes. Sometimes, for young people and those of similar constitution, I use turpentine resin alone, or with resin spurge for dry bodies. Similarly, I use honey bee glue alone or with resin spurge kneaded with old olive oil. For very hard bodies, I use sagapenum, sometimes with old olive oil and sometimes with turpentine resin—so, too, opopanax. Sometimes I also mix the olive oil with washed lime. *De methodo* [*medendi*] VI[.2].

(XV.34) If a nerve lies bare and exposed by the wound, use none of the aforementioned strong medications, but use only lime that has been washed very well with thin olive oil; heat this, and then apply it. *De methodo* [*medendi*] VI[.3].

(XV.35) If any organ is affected by a large tumor, it is dangerous to evacuate the pus therefrom all at once, because the patient will immediately suffer from syncope and from a collapse of his strength. This is because the pus obstructs, as it were, the openings of the pulsatile vessels; and if the entire pus is evacuated all at once, a large amount of pneuma is expelled all at once. *In Hippocratis Aphorismos commentarius* VI[.27].

(XV.36) The evacuation of water retained in the abdomen of someone suffering from ascites is effected either through dissolving drugs or through puncturing the peritoneum by surgery. But the fluid collected in the scrotum should be evacuated by a tube inserted into it. Sometimes, a part of the membrane containing the fluid should be excised in the case of hydrocele. Similarly, the uvula should be excised in some cases with the disease itself. Do not hurry to excise it, but wait until much time has passed and it has turned as thin as a thong; then excise it. *De methodo* [*medendi*] XIV[.13].

(XV.37) In abdominal wounds, always take care that the side of the wound is higher than the other side. If the wound is on the right side, turn the patient on his left side; and if the wound is on the left side, turn him on the right side. After suturing the wound, apply bandages as necessary. *De methodo* [*medendi*] VI[.4].

(XV.38) For any fresh ulcer, except abdominal ones, it is appropriate that blood exude from the wound itself, whether little or much; for, if blood flows therefrom, the ulcer and the surrounding area will be less inflamed. *De methodo* [*medendi*] IV[.6].

(XV.39) When an excessive amount of blood is streaming from wounds because the vessels have burst, the flow of the blood can be stopped either by cauterization, or by drugs whose strength is equal to cautery, or by something that closes and agglutinates, or by transferring it to a nearby site, or by attracting it to the opposite side, or by cooling the whole body and especially the part of the body where the wound is. Many times, the bleeding is stopped by drinking cold water, or by the external application of vinegar mixed with water, of astringent acidic wine, or of other substances with cooling and astringent properties. *De methodo* [*medendi*] V[.5].

(XV.40) If the hemorrhage is from a pulsatile vessel, the bleeding can be stopped by one of two things: either by tying a ligature around it; or by cutting and severing it into two halves, so that each part shrinks and contracts to the nearby side and becomes covered with flesh. Sometimes we are forced to do the same for a non-pulsatile vessel, if the vessel is large or if it is situated in a major part where there is great danger. The most prudent practice is to do both things simultaneously, applying a ligature to the root of the vessel close to the heart or liver and cutting it into two halves. *De methodo* [*medendi*] V[.3].

(XV.41) We are forced to cauterize if the hemorrhage is caused by corrosion or putrefaction affecting the organ. Similarly, if we cut off a part because of corrosion or putrefaction that crept into it, we cauterize its root or apply caustic astringent drugs to it, such as vitriol and the like. *De methodo* [*medendi*] V[.4].

(XV.42) In the case of old ulcers, blood should flow from the ulcer, either much or little. If the diseased part has turned livid or black or red, we scarify it, let it bleed, and place a dry sponge on it. Then we treat it with medicines that have a drying effect. If it is necessary to bleed it a second time, we do so again. *De methodo* [*medendi*] IV[.2].

(XV.43) If you see that only the rim of an ulcer has changed in color or become hard, you should cut it out and uproot it until you reach healthy flesh. If that change has spread over a large area, you should either uproot it or treat it with medicines for a long time. *De methodo* [*medendi*] IV[.2].

(XV.44) If some pus has usually streamed from a fistula for a long time but then the flow is stopped, one should open the blockage. *In Hippocratis Epidemiarum* [*commentarius*] VI.2.

(XV.45) Sometimes, a sinuous ulcer, when it is very dirty, can be syringed with lye from ashes, which is called *al-qāṭir*, or with hydromel. The less dirty it is, the less honey should be used. Hereafter, one may also syringe the sinuous ulcer with wine mixed with honey. Hydromel is more effective for cleansing the pus from the sinuous ulcer, while wine is more beneficial for promoting adhesion after the cleansing. Then put a plaster with agglutinant drugs on it, put a new sponge steeped in wine thereon, and bind these onto it. Begin tying it from the bottom of the sinuous ulcer and end at its opening, so that it presses on the ulcer without causing pain. Change the bandage once every three days. Put on another small cloth, applying it in a circular form, with a plaster on the opening of the ulcer. When the bottom of the sinuous ulcer extends downward and the opening upward, and you cannot change this position, make an incision in the bottom part, so that its contents may flow out. *Ad Glauconem* [*de medendi methodo*] II[.10].

(XV.46) When there is a severe hemorrhage from a pulsatile or non-pulsatile vessel, we concern ourselves with the vessel and cut it transversely, because, although it never closes up, we will rescue the patient from the danger he is in. Similarly, if a nerve is affected by an accident or puncture, we are often forced to cut it transversely and to abolish a movement in order to save the patient from the danger of being afflicted by spasms or delirium or both. Similarly, when a major joint suffers from a dislocation in combination with an ulcer, we treat the ulcer first until it is healed, even if it is not possible to treat the dislocation afterwards. For if we try to combine the reduction of the dislocation with the treatment of the ulcer, the patient is usually affected by spasms. Therefore, we should treat the more dangerous condition first. *De methodo* [*medendi*] III[.9].

(XV.47) The following medicine stops a hemorrhage, even from the jugular veins: Take frankincense, or pulverized frankincense and aloe, and mix these with egg white until the medicine assumes the consistency of honey. Smear this upon the hairs of a hare, and apply it to the torn vessel and the entire wound, and bandage it well. But beware of causing pain, because there is nothing in the world that is more effective in provoking a hemorrhage than pain. Then loosen the bandage after three days; and if you find the medicine still firmly adherent to the wound, do not remove it, but put more of the same medicine thereon, moistening, as it were, the hairs of the hare. Then bandage it in the same way as the first time that you bandaged it. If the hairs of the hare fall off, replace them and apply the bandage again. Continue to replace them until the wound heals up. *De methodo* [*medendi*] V[.4].

(XV.48) If you see that the medications are unable to dissolve the entire quantity of pus, but that the pus overpowers them and prevails over them, it is necessary to lance and incise the abscess at its highest and thinnest point. Let the pus flow out, and then put drying medicines on it that do not have a biting effect. But if you find that part of the bodily part has putrefied, excising that which has putrefied is unavoidable. Sometimes you have to excise, from the skin of armpits and groins, something of the shape of a myrtle leaf, because of the slackness of the skin in these places. Take care that the direction of the incision be in the width of the groin, not in its length. After the incision, fill up the site with pulverized frankincense. *De methodo* [*medendi*] XIII[.5].

(XV.49) When humors become entangled in a part of the body that is between the homoeomerous parts and have to be evacuated from that very part, one should first put medicines on that spot which repels that which streams to it, and then one should evacuate them the humors through an incision and dissolving drugs—especially when you suspect that something of those humors is being retained in those spots that are between the homoeomerous parts. *De arte parva* [34].

(XV.50) If you scarify bloody inflammations that occur without an external cause, the one affected by it suffers from a grave affliction, especially if you do so at the outset. But if the illness lasts for a long time, there is no objection to scarification. Similarly, when the inflammation known as *ḥumra* (erysipelas), has reached the condition of lividness, greenness, or blackness, it should be scarified. *Ad Glauconem* [*de medendi methodo*] II[.3].

(XV.51) In the case of the inflammation which is called *ḥumra*, one should, first of all, cool it. When its seething heat subsides, scarification and the application of a poultice made from barley meal and then heat is beneficial. *Ad Glauconem* [*de medendi methodo*] II[.3].

(XV.52) If an inflamed tumor is difficult to suppurate and dissolve, and the humors that got stuck in that part of the body contain a thick and viscous superfluity, one should apply deep scarification. Also good for these tumors is a cataplasm made of figs. For this, one should boil the figs until their moisture attains the consistency of bees' honey. Mix this one time with barley meal and another time with bread from coarse meal. *Ad Glauconem* [*de medendi methodo*] II[.9].

(XV.53) I found that superficial scarification is of little benefit and use in the case of inflamed tumors. But an incision that is deep and extremely long evacuates such a large quantity of superfluities that the patient almost faints. Therefore, such an incision needs its own special treatment. But an incision intermediate between these two is free from these harmful effects. Therefore, I thought it a good thing to always employ this kind of incision except in the case of the inflamed tumor, which is difficult to coct and dissolve. For then, one should resort to making a deep incision. *Ad Glauconem* [*de medendi methodo*] II[.9].

(XV.54) Two kinds of superfluities necessarily develop in bodies: One of them is thin and dissolves in a hidden way, and the other is thick; and the latter is the filth that accumulates on the surface of a body. The thin superfluity in an ulcer is called *ṣadīd*, while the thick superfluity in an ulcer is called *waḍar*. An ulcer becomes moist or dirty because of an excess of the thin or the thick secretion. When an ulcer is moist, it necessarily needs something that dries it up without biting, and when it is dirty, it necessarily needs something that cleanses it. In deep ulcers, the production of these two superfluities never stops, not even for one moment. *De methodo* [*medendi*] III[.3].

(XV.55) When an ulcer is deep, it always needs a drying and cleansing medication. A remedy that makes the flesh grow should be in the first grade of dryness, moderately drying and cleansing in the manner of frankincense, meal of barley, meal of broad beans, meal of bitter vetch, Florentine iris roots, sweet myrrh, tutty, and wine, for these are excellent remedies for all ulcers. *De methodo* [*medendi*] III[.3].

(XV.56) A remedy that closes a wound with flesh should be more drying than a remedy that makes the flesh grow and does not need the same cleansing and purifying action as a remedy that makes the flesh grow. Rather, a remedy that makes the flesh grow should be astringent. A remedy that seals a wound and promotes cicatrization should be more drying than a remedy that closes a wound with flesh, because the former has to dry and harden the surface of the flesh that has been formed in the wound. It has to dry it and to make it replace the skin. Such a remedy is unripe gallnuts, pomegranate peels, fruit of the acacia tree, pomegranate blossom, and the like. *De methodo* [*medendi*] III[.5].

(XV.57) The overgrowth of flesh in an ulcer needs a very drying remedy that also cleanses or eats away the flesh, such as verdigris. *De methodo* [*medendi*] III[.6].

(XV.58) With many of those in whose cases you want to pour a medicine into their nose as a treatment for a cold and lasting catarrh, you should proceed as follows: Take black cumin, pulverize it until it becomes like dust, mix it with old olive oil, and pound it into a very fine substance. Then tell the patient to fill his mouth with water and to tilt his head back as far as possible, and pour this medicine into his nose and tell him to inhale so that he draws in the medicine more strongly. *De instrumento odoratus*.

(XV.59) The story goes about a man who suffered from a persistent ulcer on his thigh which was hard to heal. He went to an eminent physician (Stratonicus), who bled him from his arm and who, when he saw that his blood was black and thick, extracted a small amount of blood on the first day thereafter and similarly on the third and fourth day. He then purged him three times with a medicine that evacuates the black chyme and fed him with nutriments producing good chymes. Then he turned to treating the ulcer itself, and it healed. *De atra bile.*

(xv.60) If you think it proper to make an incision but the patient is fainthearted or it is distressing for his family, make him think that you are going to palpate or rub the spot you want to incise with oil, and then make the incision, so that you take him unawares. [*In Hippocratis*] *De officina* [*medici commentarius*] I[.13].

(xv.61) There is no advantage in evacuating a humor that is going to turn to pus, for it is a better and quicker way to ensure simultaneous change if one leaves it inside until the rest of what is within changes. [*In Hippocratis*] *De officina* [*medici commentarius*] II[.29].

(xv.62) If a broken nasal bone is set, it will heal and grow together within ten days. Broken jaw, collarbone, and ribs heal within twenty days. A broken upper arm heals within thirty days. A broken leg and forearm heal within forty days. A broken thigh heals within fifty days. *In Hippocratis De alimento commentarius* IV[.22].

(xv.63) Broken bones of young people heal sooner than those of children, because children need material for their growth to replace the matter which has been dissolved. This was mentioned by Asklepios in the first treatise of his commentary on Hippocrates' book *On Fractures* and their setting.

(xv.64) Do not attempt to set any broken bone if only four days have passed, lest you cause the patient severe harm. The third treatise of Asklepios' commentary on Hippocrates' book *On Fractures* and their setting.

(xv.65) In the case of broken bones, apply pads immersed in astringent dark wine, especially in the summer. For, if you use olive oil or cerate, putrefaction develops in those parts. *De methodo medendi* VI[.5].

(xv.66) In the case of fractures and ulcers, the patient should feel more pressure of the bandage on the affected spot itself and less on the extremities. But a bandage with which one intends to increase the flesh of an emaciated limb should be as slack as possible on the emaciated limb itself and exert its greatest pressure on the sound parts nearby, so that blood is admitted to the emaciated limb. [*In Hippocratis*] *De officina* [*medici commentarius*] III[.33].

(xv.67) When you set the arm or leg, place it in the position customary for that patient. For there are some people whose legs are stretched during the entire day, while there are others whose legs are flexed. [*In Hippocratis*] *De officina* [*medici commentarius*] III[.21].

(xv.68) Fractures of the leg require a cast, so that the limb is not troubled during moving. You should carefully investigate the injuries which require a cast, for if the harm caused by the cast is greater than its benefit, do not apply it. [*In Hippocratis*] *De officina* [*medici commentarius*] III[.19].

(xv.69) In cases of fracture, first put a bandage under the pads. Begin from the spot of the injury and end higher up to prevent moistures from streaming to that part so that it does not become inflamed. Then apply the pads; and then put a bandage on top of the pads, so that they do not become disordered, beginning with the spot of the injury and ending downward in order to force the putrid blood from the injured limb to its extremity. After this second bandage, apply the trusses which secure and support all that is behind them. Thus, there are four things that surround the limb: the bandage that has contact with the limb, the pads, the bandage on these, and the trusses. [*In Hippocratis*] *De officina* [*medici commentarius*] III[.4, 12].

(xv.70) The pads should be placed on the thinnest part of the limb so as to make it level with the thick part, so that when it is secured by a bandage, the pressure exerted may be even. For if it is not even, the bandage will work loose. The width of the bandage should be three or four thumbs. [*In Hippocratis*] *De officina* [*medici commentarius*] III[.2].

This is the end of the fifteenth treatise,
by the grace of God,
praise be to Him.

In the name of God,
the Merciful, the Compassionate.
O Lord, make our task easy.

The Sixteenth Treatise

Containing aphorisms concerning women

(XVI.1) The harm caused by the retention of menses is seldom evident in the first month. It becomes evident in the second month though it is still somewhat imperceptible. But in the third and following months the afflictions resulting from the retention become severe. Menstrual blood that streams to the uterus in the first month can be contained by it, but when it becomes full, and consequently the blood that streams towards it does not find an empty place, that blood rises, goes back to its former place, and putrefies, and this results in those severe afflictions. *In Hippocratis De mulierum affectibus commentarius.*

(XVI.2) Four or five days before the menstruation the woman should adhere to a thinning diet and then be bled from her legs to stimulate the menstrual blood. Along with this, she should ingest remedies with hydromel, water mint and peppermint. Stronger than these are savin juniper and Cretan dittany, either in the form of a decoction prepared from one of these or its substance only. The best time to take these drugs that stimulate the menstrual blood is when the woman has left the bath and has dried herself. Similarly, the ingestion of *hiera picra* at that time stimulates menstrual flow. *De* [*curandi ratione per*] *venae sectione*[*m* 18].

(XVI.3) A retention of the menstrual blood results from the weakness of the vessels and the uterus so that they cannot attract it, or because of an obstruction there, or because of a contraction of the uterus. *In Hippocratis De mulierum affectibus commentarius.*

(XVI.4) Says Moses: The aforementioned causes for the retention of the menstrual blood mentioned by him only pertain to the organ when the menstrual blood is still present. He did not mention here those causes that are dependent on the blood, namely, when its quantity greatly diminishes, for then blood is no longer present. Therefore, he speaks of the retention of the menstrual blood and not of its cessation.

(XVI.5) Retention of the menses is usually followed by some or all of the possible bad afflictions—namely, heaviness of the body; loss of appetite; shivering; pain in the loins, neck, forehead, head, or roots of the eyes; ardent fevers; a dark, reddish urine; flow of milk from the breasts. When the retention of the menses lasts for a long time, a swelling may occur in the hollow of the groin. But those women who have a normal menstruation do not suffer from any of these afflictions. *De locis affectis* VI[.5].

(XVI.6) When the evacuation of menstrual blood becomes excessive, it is followed by a bad complexion, swelling of the feet and the whole body, and poor digestion. *De locis affectis* VI[.5].

(XVI.7) Sometimes women suffer from the illness called *nazf* (female flux) whereby the whole body is purged. This mostly occurs to those women whose bodies are soft and phlegmatic in constitution. The discharge from the body through this flux sometimes consists of a reddish serum and at other times of a watery or yellowish serum. But if you observe the blood to be like the blood of venesection, investigate it carefully to determine if it comes from an erosion. Most often, such an erosion occurs at the neck of the uterus. *De locis affectis* VI[.5].

(XVI.8) Just as there are men whose nature tends towards that of a woman and whose bodies are tender and soft, similar to the body of a woman, so too there are women whose bodies are dry and hard, similar to the nature of the body of a man. If the nature of a woman tends towards the nature of a man, there is nothing with which she can be treated to strengthen and stimulate her menstrual flow. *In Hippocratis Epidemiarum* [*commentarius*] VI.8, specifically the last part of the book.

(XVI.9) Superfluities accumulate in the bodies of women because of their state of rest, calm, and lack of exertion. Nature expels these superfluities to the vessels that are connected to the uterus; they accumulate over there, for the uterus has the strength to attract these superfluities. *In Hippocratis De mulierum affectibus commentarius.*

(XVI.10) All the pulsatile and non-pulsatile vessels in the entire body of both male and female are the same, not only in number but also in structure, form, and location. However, male and female are different in their reproductive organs. Yet it is clear from anatomy that the reproductive parts of the male and female correspond to each other and resemble each other, but in the male, they protrude whereas in the female they are internal. This is true to such a degree that if the female reproductive organs were reversed so that their internal side would be external, the uterus would, as it were, become the scrotum, and the testicles, which are on the sides of the uterus, would be located inside this pouch, and the neck of the uterus would correspond to the penis. *De semine* II.

(XVI.11) If too much blood is evacuated from the uterus all at once, apply cupping glasses next to the breasts and it will stop rapidly. Similarly, place cupping glasses on the two groins and thighs of a woman whose uterus is drawn and raised upwards or is inclined sidewards. Place something with an extremely repulsive smell near her nostrils and sweet-smelling medicines with slackening and heating properties near her uterus. *Ad Glauconem* [*de medendi methodo*] I[.15].

(XVI.12) Generally apply cupping glasses to the pudenda and groins if you want to promote and stimulate the flow of the menstrual blood. *De methodo* [*medendi*] XIII[.19].

(XVI.13) In the case of inflammations of the uterus, be careful not to perform a venesection from the arm, because this hinders menstruation. Rather, cut the vein above the ankle, but plan to do so three or four days before the time of the woman's menstruation. Then you may also apply cupping glasses to both ankles. *De* [*curandi ratione per*] *venae sectione*[*m* 18].

(XVI.14) When a woman has a normal menstruation and performs light work, she does not desire sexual intercourse because her body is free from those superfluities that tickle and stimulate the uterus to seek sexual intercourse. *In Hippocratis De mulierum affectibus commentarius.*

(XVI.15) When the flow of menstrual blood is excessive, the nerves and muscles on the spinal column stretch because of dryness, and this causes pain. Sometimes the uterus ascends when it suffers from spasms caused by the dryness resulting from the excessive menstrual bleeding. With the stretching of the uterus, the diaphragm and the viscera also stretch and then hysterical suffocation develops. *In Hippocratis De mulierum affectibus commentarius.*

(XVI.16) Hysterical suffocation occurs if the menses are retained and if the uterus and the vessels that lead to the uterus and its ligaments are filled with superfluous matter and stretch, causing the uterus to stretch upwards and press on the diaphragm. Respiration then becomes difficult, and sometimes pressure on the stomach or on the organs lying on the spinal column causes severe pain. *In Hippocratis De mulierum affectibus commentarius.*

(XVI.17) Sometimes the most likely cause of this illness is the retention of the female sperm and its corruption in the uterus. This was explained at length in *De locis affectis* VI[.5].

(XVI.18) I once saw a woman who had been a widow for a long time. Because of the afflictions she suffered from as a result of hysterical suffocation—for her midwife told me that her uterus had been pulled up—I considered it a good thing that she should use those things for a suppository that are regularly used for this illness. But because of the heat of the things used for a suppository and because of the contact of her hand with her genitals during the insertion of the medications, she experienced a spasm together with pain and pleasure, similar to that experienced during sexual intercourse. Immediately after this, thick semen was discharged from her and the woman found relief from all those harmful afflictions. *De locis affectis* [VI.5].

(XVI.19) Menstrual blood that flows from a pregnant woman cannot come from the vessels inside the uterus because the placenta is attached to all their openings. Rather, it originates from the vessels in the neck of the uterus. *In Hippocratis Aphorismos commentarius* [V.60]. Similarly, Galen mentioned in *De locis affectis* VI[.5] that the blood that flows from pregnant women comes from the bursting of a vessel in the neck of the uterus.

(XVI.20) Rapidity of growth in women indicates that their bodies contain a surplus of heat that matches the moisture of their bodies. This is confirmed by the monthly flow of the menstrual blood from their bodies, for when the blood increases the heat increases too. *In Hippocratis De mulierum affectibus commentarius.*

(XVI.21) In many pregnant women the uterus often protrudes and prolapses if the labor pains are extremely severe and the expulsive faculty itself is extremely active. This is especially the case when the ligaments connecting the uterus with the spine are naturally weak. *De naturalibus facultatibus* III[.3].

(XVI.22) The tumor known as cancer mostly occurs in the breasts of women if their bodies are not cleansed by menstruation. If this cleansing process takes place properly, a woman always preserves her health and is not affected by any illness at all. *Ad Glauconem* [*de medendi methodo*] II[.12].

(XVI.23) A craving for bad foods happens to someone who has bad superfluities inside the folds of his stomach. This happens to women who have bad humors during their pregnancy. Often, they crave for anything sour and astringent, and anything acrid or sharp, and clay and charcoal. This happens to most of them until the third month of their pregnancy; then it subsides in the fourth month because those bad humors are partly evacuated through vomiting and partly concocted during this whole period. For the woman hardly eats anything, since she has no appetite, and by then the fetus feeds itself with substantial things. As a result, the body of the woman is less filled with foodstuff and all the bad humors in it are decreased. *De* [*symptomatum*] *causis* [I.7].

(XVI.24) The symptom of craving for bad things, which happens to women, indeed originates from an illness of the cardia of the stomach. All these symptoms that happen to women—a ravenous appetite, or no appetite at all, or only a craving for bad things—all these are symptoms indicating diseases affecting the stomach. *De locis affectis* V[.6].

(XVI.25) Male fetuses are mostly conceived by the woman on the right side of the uterus and female ones on the left side. The reverse of this situation only happens rarely. *De locis affectis* VI[.5].

(XVI.26) When the breasts of a pregnant woman shrink so much that they become emaciated and thin, you should expect that she will miscarry. If she is pregnant with twins and one of her breasts becomes emaciated and thin, one of her fetuses will be aborted. *De locis affectis* VI[.5].

(XVI.27) When a woman conceives and always has a miscarriage after two or three or four months, you should know that this is caused by a phlegmatic moisture which accumulates in the openings of the vessels in the uterus. Depending on the quantity of that moisture, the connection of the pulsatile and non-pulsatile vessels in the uterus with the placenta will be weak so that it cannot carry the burden of the fetus but easily tears free from it. *De locis affectis* VI[.5].

(XVI.28) During pregnancy the pulse is greater and more frequent and faster. But the other conditions of the body remain the same. *De puls*[*ibus libellus ad tirones* 9].

(XVI.29) A sign of the wisdom of Nature is that the *os uteri* (mouth of the uterus) is completely closed as long as the fetus within it is alive, but if the fetus dies, the *os* opens to the extent which is necessary for it to make its exit. The midwives do not make the women get up and sit down on the obstetric chair during labor pains. But after they have palpated the *os uteri* when it is gradually dilating—and if it has dilated enough for the fetus to make its exit—they make them sit down on the obstetric chair and tell them to expel the fetus by squeezing the muscles in the belly. *De naturalibus facultatibus* III[.3].

(xvi.30) A woman may have a miscarriage because of excessive movement or because of taking a bath, for bathing softens the body and the nerves. She may also abort because of excessive anointing of her head because this produces a catarrh. As a result, she coughs, the uterus is shaken, and the fetus is expelled. *In Hippocratis De mulierum affectibus commentarius.*

(xvi.31) During pregnancy the formative and growth-promoting faculty attracts the best blood to the fetus and leaves the worst blood in the vessels. This blood exits after birth, just like the blood that is quantitatively and qualitatively useless exits every month. *De atra bile* [8].

(xvi.32) The time within which the formation of the fetus is completed is thirty-five or forty or forty-five days. The time within which the fetus begins to move is twice that many days. In three times the amount of time within which it moves, the child is born. *In Hippocratis De alimento commentarius* iv[.20].

(xvi.33) If a woman has a difficult childbirth, the blood which streams during the parturition is mostly retained because the organs of the childbirth swell as a result of the pressure put on them during the difficult delivery. *In Hippocratis Epidemiarum* [*commentarius*] ii.2.

(xvi.34) When a woman gives birth, she needs to evacuate all that corrupt blood that has accumulated during the days of the pregnancy. Her main treatment is the evacuation of that blood. She should be given fluid-promoting food to facilitate the outflow of blood. A food both nourishing and moistening is barley gruel, which, in addition, dilutes and attenuates. It is a food that helps the thick blood to flow copiously. *In Hippocratis Epidemiarum* [*commentarius*] ii.6.

(xvi.35) If the milk of the wet nurse is too thick or too thin, it is a warning that an illness will occur. Plenty of good milk in the breasts indicates that the nature of the breasts is balanced and they are capable of carrying out their activities. *In Hippocratis De mulierum affectibus commentarius.*

(xvi.36) If the milk of a pregnant woman flows copiously, the fetus is weak. Because of its weakness it does not attract the blood, which recedes to the breasts, and milk is produced. If the breasts are firmer, the fetus is healthier. *In Hippocratis Epidemiarum* [*commentarius*] ii.6.

(xvi.37) The milk of the mother fits the newborn infant because its substance is nothing else but the substance of the blood from which he was created. If her milk is spoiled, one should choose other suitable milk. *In Hippocratis De alimento commentarius* IV[.18].

(XVI.38) The accumulation of blood in the breasts indicates that insanity will occur. *In Hippocratis Epidemiarum* [*commentarius*] II.6.

This is the end of the sixteenth treatise,
by the help, guidance, and grace of God,
praise be to Him.

In the name of God,
the Merciful, the Compassionate.
O Lord, make our task easy.

The Seventeenth Treatise
Containing aphorisms concerning the regimen of health in general

(XVII.1) Rest is very bad for the maintenance of one's health just as moderate movement is very beneficial. That is, people do not fall ill if they take care that they do not suffer from any bad digestion whatsoever and that they do not strenuously move after eating. Just as exercise before a meal is more beneficial for lasting health than anything else, movement after a meal is more harmful than anything else. *De bonis* [*malisque*] *sucis* [III.3, 4].

(XVII.2) Hippocrates remarks in *Epidemics* VI that lasting health lies in the avoidance of satiation and in giving up laziness for exertion. Galen says in his first commentary to this statement that the avoidance of overfilling with food is beneficial for all ages and for any bodily condition. *In Hippocratis Epidemiarum* [*commentarius*] VI.1.

(XVII.3) Health is something that all people need. But not everyone is able to follow the regimen that would be appropriate for him, because of gluttony and lust for food, or because he is too busy, or because he does not know what is proper for him to do. *De bonis* [*malisque*] *sucis* [IV.39].

(XVII.4) One should not neglect the movement of one's body as the scholars do, who diligently study the entire night and day. The body and all its limbs should be moved evenly, and every limb should carry out its activity so that both the internal and external parts of the body receive benefit therefrom. *De somno et vigilia*.

(XVII.5) To maintain one's health, one should strive after two goals: One, the replacement of that which has dissolved so that it provides the body with something similar and suitable according to its temperament, and the other, the cleansing of the superfluities that unavoidably develop in the body. And the third goal, that one should not age prematurely, is subordinate to the other two goals. *De sanitate tuenda* I[.3].

(XVII.6) One should first of all pay attention to the maintenance of the innate heat, which can be preserved with different kinds of moderate exercise for both the body and the soul. *De sanitate tuenda* I[.8].

(XVII.7) For a healthy regimen one should begin by paying attention to exercise, then food, then drink, then sleep, and then sexual intercourse. Perform each of these five activities to a moderate degree. *In Hippocratis Epidemiarum* [*commentarius*] VI.6.

(XVII.8) Having sexual intercourse is something which falls under the category of the regimen of one's health, meaning that there are intervals between the times in which one has intercourse that one does not feel feeble or weak. Rather than feeling feeble or weak, one should feel that the body is lighter than before having intercourse. At the time that one has intercourse, one's body should not be very full nor very empty nor very cold nor very hot. The same holds true for dryness and moisture. If someone who has intercourse errs in one of these, his error should be as small as possible, that is, having intercourse with a full or a warm or a moist body is less harmful than doing so in conditions that are opposite to the mentioned ones. *De arte parva* [24].

(XVII.9) Just as sexual intercourse always has a drying effect, it always has a cooling effect. It is only beneficial for him whose body contains a vaporous superfluity because a hot dyscrasia prevails in him by nature. Only in his case sexual intercourse is beneficial, because of its drying and cooling effect. *In Hippocratis Epidemiarum* [*commentarius*] VI.5.

(XVII.10) For the preservation of health one should first of all perform physical exercise, this should be followed by paying attention to food and drink, and then sleep. *De sanitate tuenda* II[.2].

(XVII.11) One should eat after bathing or physical exercise, once the disturbance of the body caused by these activities has subsided. Be careful not to take food prior to these activities so that it is not transported to the organs before it is digested. If one takes food in a state of disturbance of the body, it fills the head and mostly overflows the cardia of the stomach. *In Hippocratis De acutorum morborum* [*victu*] *commentarius* III[.55].

(XVII.12) After a person has exercised properly and has bathed in the prescribed manner and eaten beneficial food and then slept, he can have sexual intercourse if it is appropriate for him. *De sanitate tuenda* II[.2].

(XVII.13) Only someone with a hot and moist body or someone with a body in which much sperm is produced by nature is free from the harm caused by sexual intercourse. But the harm it causes to someone whose temperament tends towards dryness or to old people is very severe. *De sanitate tuenda* VI[.4].

(XVII.14) Some bodily constitutions are very bad. That is, in some people much hot, biting sperm is produced, which stimulates them to eject it. If they do so during sexual intercourse, the cardia of their stomach becomes flaccid as does their whole body; they become weak and dry and lean; their complexion changes and their eyes sink in. But if they abstain from sexual intercourse, their head becomes heavy and they suffer from pain in their stomach. Abstaining from sexual intercourse harms them just as much as having sexual intercourse.

As to the regimen of these people, my advice is that they abstain from anything producing sperm, consume foods and medications that suppress its formation, and exercise the upper parts of their body by playing with a small or large ball or by lifting stones. After bathing he should anoint his loins with cooling oils. If he wants to expel the sperm, he should feed himself with good foodstuff during that day, and in the evening, when he wants to go to sleep, he should have sexual intercourse and then go to sleep. When he wakes up on the following day, his body should be massaged with linen cloths until the skin becomes red, and then he should be moderately rubbed with oil. He should wait a little while and then eat solid bread steeped in diluted wine. Then he should go about his affairs. *De sanitate tuenda* VI[.14].

(XVII.15) I advise all people to abstain from all foods that produce bad humors. Even if someone digests them easily and rapidly, he should not be misled by this because undoubtedly a bad humor will accumulate in his vessels even though he does not notice. It will putrefy from the slightest cause, and from this, malignant fevers will arise. *De alimentorum* [*facultatibus*] II[.6.4].

(XVII.16) One acts prudently and securely when one takes care that the passages and channels of the food through the liver are open and clean, not only in the case of sick people but also in the case of healthy people. *De alimentorum* [*facultatibus*] II[.8.5].

(XVII.17) A good regimen is beneficial for the soul and bestows it with excellent ethical qualities, just as it is salutary for the body and provides it with health. This is especially true if a person adheres to a good regimen immediately after being born. *De sanitate tuenda* I[.7].

(XVII.18) One's moral character is impaired by bad habits in food, drink, exercise, sights, and sounds. Bad humors often cause diseases. *De sanitate tuenda* I[.8].

(XVII.19) The first thing to consider regarding anyone's regimen of health is the calculation of the times of nourishment, whether you should let him eat once or twice a day, depending on his temperament. Some bilious persons should eat three times a day. Be extremely careful that one does not suffer from constipation, but that one's stools tend slightly towards softness. *De sanitate tuenda* VI[.7].

(XVII.20) I advise all educated people not to follow the regimen of most people who behave as dumb animals in seeking that which is most pleasurable and nothing else. Rather, every person should test by experience what foods, drinks, and activities are harmful for him and consequently avoid them. Similarly, he should test whether sexual intercourse is harmful and if so, after how much time it is no longer harmful. His regimen in this matter should be thus: He should look and strive for all that is beneficial for him and avoid all that is harmful to him. Anyone who follows such a regimen has little need for a physician, as long as he is healthy. *De sanitate tuenda* VI[.14].

(XVII.21) If someone needs additional nourishment, he should be given moist food in the morning, such as broth and dry food in the evening such as bread and meat. There are three kinds of dry foods: seeds, parts of plants, and parts of animals. *In Hippocratis De alimento commentarius* I.

(XVII.22) Well-prepared barley groats are better than all the other foods for producing good chyme and for the preservation of health. It is no less nourishing than the nourishment of good bread. *De bonis* [*malisque*] *sucis* [VII.1].

(XVII.23) In seeking health, a bad but regular diet of food and drink is more reliable, safer, and farther removed from danger than if a person suddenly replaces his diet with something else that is better. There are things that are by nature peculiar to some people and similar to their nature while other things are not peculiar to them and not similar to their nature. [*De consuetudinibus*].

(XVII.24) I have seen many people who, although the regimen they followed was not at all good in all the other aspects, yet ended up healthy by the ingestion of sea squill vinegar and sea squill wine. *De victu attenuante* [12].

(XVII.25) Rockfish is rapidly digested. Together with its high digestibility, it is extremely good and beneficial in preserving the health of a human body since it produces blood of an intermediate consistency, neither thin and fine nor thick. *De alimentorum* [*facultatibus*] III[.27.2].

(XVII.26) Children should not be allowed to taste wine for a long time, for wine is very harmful to them. It moistens and heats their bodies more than necessary, fills their heads [with vapors], and corrupts the ethical qualities of their souls. *De sanitate tuenda* I[.11].

It is not good for adult persons to drink more than a moderate amount of wine, because it rapidly brings a person to anger, indecency, and obscene language and makes the rational part of his soul confused and his subtle mind sluggish. *De sanitate tuenda* I[.11].

(XVII.27) In general, the regimen of health of the elderly should consist of massage with oil in the morning after sleep, followed by walking or slow riding, bathing in hot sweet water, drinking wine, and the consumption of heating and moistening foods. *De sanitate tuenda* V[.3].

(XVII.28) Just as wine is extremely harmful for children, so for the elderly it is extremely beneficial. The wine that is most salutary for them is warm and thin and has a bright reddish color. It is the one which Hippocrates calls "tawny." *De sanitate tuenda* V[.5].

(XVII.29) Let a weak old person eat three times a day, for when his strength is weak, he should be nourished by small amounts at short intervals. [*De sanitate tuenda* V.4]. And when his strength is great, he should be nourished with large quantities of food at long intervals.

(XVII.30) Bread for the elderly should be perfectly baked. Milk is not beneficial for all old people but only for those who can digest it well and in whom no flatulence develops in the hypochondrium. *De sanitate tuenda* V[.7].

(XVII.31) Let old people eat ripe fresh figs. Prefer these above other fruits. But in the winter give them dried figs. *De sanitate tuenda* V[.8].

(XVII.32) Watery phlegmatic superfluities have the property of accumulating and increasing in the bodies of the elderly; therefore, it is necessary to stimulate micturition daily, not with drugs but with celery, honey, and wines. Their stools should be softened, above all with olive oil, which they should drink before meals. Similarly, one should give them a clyster with olive oil only, and they should take vegetables with olive oil and *garum* before meals, or plums boiled with honey. *De sanitate tuenda* V[.9].

(XVII.33) Of any food or drink, one should first consume things that soften the stools, like sweet wines and softening vegetables prepared with olive oil and *garum*. After the meal one should consume astringent foods to strengthen the cardia of the stomach. *De sanitate tuenda* VI[.7].

(XVII.34) For the elderly and those with weak bodies, slaughter the animal a day and a night before cooking it and then cook it well. But for young people and for those who have strong bodies and for workers and heavy laborers, boil fresh meat, but do let it become well done during the roasting or cooking. *In Hippocratis De alimento commentarius* IV[.19].

(XVII.35) Old age has three stages: The first stage, that is that in which old age has just begun, is one in which a person is still able to carry out his civic affairs. The second stage is that in which the elderly should follow the regimen mentioned before. The third stage, the age of senility, is that in which a person who is in that stage does not tolerate bathing every day, and in which sharp biting superfluities do not accumulate in his body. *De sanitate tuenda* V[.12].

(XVII.36) To avert or prevent old age is something impossible. However, it is possible to prevent it from arriving rapidly, and this can be accomplished with a fitting diet, frequent bathing, sleeping on a soft bed, and avoiding everything that dries or cools. *De marcore* [5].

(XVII.37) We know that some people suffer from regularly recurring nosebleeds, that others evacuate blood from the vessels in the buttocks, and others when emesis or diarrhea happens to them, and that yet others evacuate blood through venesection or by making an incision or by emptying their bodies through purgatives. When their usual manner of evacuation is discontinued, they fall ill because their regimen is a bad one. Therefore, bad humors accumulate in their bodies, which unless they are expelled by the activity of nature—whether spontaneous or provoked—remain in their bodies and make them ill. But when those who use these evacuations change their regimen and eat less food and increase their physical exercise, they are safe from illness, for a change in habit at that time is something that is beneficial for them. [*De consuetudinibus*].

(XVII.38) I do not advise giving the elderly any aloe or *hiera picra*. If they suffer from constipation for two days, it is sufficient to soften their stools with field bindweed, or olive oil, or safflower hearts with barley groats, or with the hearts of dried figs and safflower seed, or with the amount of one or two hazelnuts of turpentine resin. For this remedy softens the stools without harm, purges the intestines, and cleanses what is in the liver, spleen, kidneys, urinary bladder, and lungs. One should use these laxatives variously so that nature does not get used to one particular laxative and consequently become resistant to it. *De sanitate tuenda* V[.9].

(XVII.39) If someone complains of constant headache because of hypersensitivity of the nerves that spread in the cardia of the stomach, its treatment is a matter of the art of the regimen of health. That is, he should hasten to take food every day before the bile flows into the stomach, and he should change his diet to a cooler and moister one. If bile streams into the stomach, it should be evacuated through emesis and through purging the belly downwards. For drugs he should use, at long intervals, absinth wormwood and the *hiera picra* remedy. His stomach should be anointed externally with quince oil and spikenard oil and similar slightly astringent oils. *De sanitate tuenda* VI[.10].

(XVII.40) If food putrefies in the stomach and the putrefied material is passed through the bowels, it is most beneficial for the preservation of health. But if it is not passed, it should be promoted by that which passes it without biting or harm, such as the cumin stomachic, or the remedy prepared with dried figs and safflower hearts, or other remedies prepared with safflower seed and dodder. The patient also benefits from vomiting the putrefied material. *De sanitate tuenda* VI[.7].

(XVII.41) Galen advises that he who takes the theriac to preserve his health should do so once the food has been digested and left the stomach. One should take an amount of it equal to the size of an Egyptian bean in two spoons of water. If one needs an amount equal to a hazelnut, one should dilute it with three spoons of water. Do not take it in the summertime, and no young person nor someone with a hot temperament should consume it. But if one resorts to it in such a case because of an emergency, it should be a small amount. In the case of children, one should be extremely cautious in administering it to them. He mentioned the case of a man who forced a son of his, while still a child, to drink some theriac, and when the boy had taken this medicine, his nature could not transform it. As a result, the theriac dissolved his body and made him suffer from diarrhea, and the boy died that very night. Similarly, he advised that the elderly and old people, if they take it, should dilute it wine, not with water. *De theriaca ad Pisonem* [17].

This is the end of the seventeenth treatise,
by the grace of God,
praise be to Him.

In the name of God,
the Merciful, the Compassionate.
O Lord, make our task easy.

The Eighteenth Treatise

Containing aphorisms concerning physical exercise

(XVIII.1) If someone is able to exercise before meals, he does not have to be very careful about his diet. But if someone's occupations distract him from exercise, a healthy diet alone is only sufficient if it is combined with the ingestion of drugs that promote health. *De* [*bonis malisque*] *sucis* [II.2].

(XVIII.2) The most beneficial of all types of exercise is that which is able not only to exert the body, but also to gladden and delight the soul, such as hunting and ball playing. For the motion of the soul is so powerful that many have been released from their diseases simply by the pleasure that they experienced. And many, on the other hand, were released from diseases caused by harm inflicted on their soul. *De parvae pilae exercitio* [1].

(XVIII.3) One should pay more attention to the motions of the soul than to those of the body, as the soul has eminence over the body. In all kinds of exercise, one should strive after a combination of exertion with joy, pleasure, and gladness. This can be achieved most easily by playing with a small ball that the players throw from hand to hand. *De parvae pilae exercitio* [1].

One aspect in which exercise with the small ball is superior over the other types of exercise is that with this kind of exercise one can move all the parts of the body together, or move some part to the exclusion of another. It can also be practiced quietly and gently or vigorously and strenuously as long as no danger or harm ensues afterward, as is the case with most of the other types of exercise. *De parvae pilae exercitio* [1].

(XVIII.4) The application of physical exercise is more successful than other means of evacuation because it evacuates that which is spread deep in the body, both in the flesh and in the parts that are more solid than flesh. *In Hippocratis Aphorismos commentarius* III[.15].

(XVIII.5) If someone does not perform physical exercise, both thick and thin humors accumulate in his body: the thick ones because of ease of life and restfulness and the thin and watery ones because he misses their evacuation through exercise. *In Hippocratis Epidemiarum* [*commentarius*] III.3.

(XVIII.6) Physical exercise should not be practiced at all after the poor digestion of food. *De sanitate tuenda* III[.12].

(XVIII.7) If someone happens to do physical exercise with a body that is full of phlegm or yellow bile or black bile or blood, it results in either epilepsy or apoplexy or other afflictions because it dissolves the humors and moves them to the outer side of the body. *In Hippocratis Aphorismos commentarius* III[.20].

(XVIII.8) If someone indulges excessively in idleness, two kinds of overfilling develop in his body as a result: that which pertains to the vessels and that which pertains to the strength of the body. *In Hippocratis De natura hominis commentarius* [II.1].

(XVIII.9) Strenuous physical exercise dries the body and makes it hard and slow of sensation and understanding. Therefore, wrestlers and those who carry heavy burdens and stones are ignorant and have little understanding. *De somno et vigilia.*

(XVIII.10) Extremely hot bodies do not need physical exercise at all. For them walking, bathing, and good rubbing with oil is sufficient. Bathing is beneficial to them after having food. *De sanitate tuenda* VI[.3].

(XVIII.11) Old people need to move their bodies because their heat needs to be fanned. But no elderly person should rest and repose completely so that he does not move at all. On the other hand, he does not need brisk exercise, because brisk exercise cools and extinguishes their heat, which is already weak by itself. *De sanitate tuenda* V[.3].

(XVIII.12) The definition of physical exercise is a vigorous movement that changes respiration. When a person makes any movement that forces him to breathe stronger, faster, and more frequently than before, such a movement becomes exercise for that person. *De sanitate tuenda* II[.2].

(XVIII.13) The best time for physical exercise is after the food of the previous day has been completely acted upon and digested in the stomach and vessels and it is time for the next meal. An indication for this is a moderately yellow urine and the expulsion of all the superfluities retained in the bladder and the lower intestines. Thereafter, recommend physical exercise. *De sanitate tuenda* II[.2].

(XVIII.14) Prior to physical exercise you should rub the patient and massage his body. Then he should exercise gently and increase his exertion until he reaches the optimum level of exercise, that is, as long as his color is healthy and you find him moving quickly, while his movements are even and his sweat is flowing. But as soon as any of these conditions change, he should stop exercising. *De sanitate tuenda* II[.2].

(XVIII.15) After the completion of the exercise, you should pour a generous amount of oil over the body and apply moderate massage while the body is moderately moved and rotated; this massage is called "restorative." Then he should take a bath and wash himself, though he should not stay too long in it, and after the bath he should eat. *De sanitate tuenda* III[.3, 4].

(XVIII.16) If a short quartan fever occurs that is not severe, there is no objection if the patient does some of his usual exercises in the days of the abatement of the fever. *Ad Glauconem* [*de medendi methodo* I.12].

This is the end of the eighteenth treatise,
by the grace of God,
praise be to Him.

In the name of God,
the Merciful, the Compassionate.
O Lord, make our task easy.

The Nineteenth Treatise
Containing aphorisms concerning bathing

(XIX.1) Bathing evacuates only that which is near the skin. That which is deep inside the body, spread in the flesh, is not adequately evacuated by bathing. *In Hippocratis Aphorismos commentarius* III[.15].

(XIX.2) Bathing is beneficial for the other types of dryness, whether that dryness comes with cold—as in the case of marasmus—, from old age, or with heat—as in the case of hectic fevers that are free from putrefaction. This characteristic of bathing is wonderful that it is beneficial for both hot and cold dryness, and it likewise makes him thirsty who does not suffer from thirst and quenches the thirst of him who is thirsty. *De marcore* [7].

(XIX.3) Using the baths weakens the faculties of the body if it has been a long time since one has eaten and one is very hungry. This also happens as a result of bathing in the case of all the other bodily conditions. If one bathes before the digestion of the food, it causes the accumulation of the crude chymes in the body. The best time for bathing is after the digestion of the food, since then it helps pass the food into the organs. *De marcore* [9].

(XIX.4) Bathing is one of the most beneficial things for someone who is to be evacuated of superfluities streaming into his stomach. However, nosebleed and other hemorrhages are strongly stimulated by bathing. And if someone develops syncope because of profuse sweating, bathing is one of the most harmful things for him to do. *Ad Glauconem* [*de medendi methodo*] I[.15].

(XIX.5) —

(XIX.6) Bathing in nitrous or sulfurous water and other kinds of water with drying strength dries the body. Frequent bathing in sweet water, especially after eating, moistens the body. *De causis* [*morborum* 4, 5].

(XIX.7) One should bathe in drinkable water of a moderate temperament. The most appropriate thing to do if bathing in cold water is to jump into it all at once so that the water reaches all parts of the body at the same time and he does not shiver. *De sanitate tuenda* III[.4].

(XIX.8) After bathing in cold water one has more appetite, better digestion, less thirst, a stronger body in general, and skin that is in the best possible condition, that is, harder and firmer. *De sanitate tuenda* III[.4].

(XIX.9) Moderate heat combined with moisture, such as the heat of a bath, has the potential to cool, but the waters should be sweet and drinkable, for these waters cool and moisten the body of him who bathes in them. *In Hippocratis Epidemiarum* [*commentarius*] VI.5.

(XIX.10) You should know that there is nothing better than sleep after bathing for concocting that which can be concocted and for dissolving and dispelling the bad humors. *De sanitate tuenda* IV[.4].

(XIX.11) Bathing in sweet water is the best thing for people from whose bodies a vaporous superfluity dissolves while they are healthy. If you prevent these and their like from bathing, they develop a fever. Someone who suffers from fever because of firmness of the skin also needs bathing. Similarly, someone who suffers from fever because of exposure to the sun should first of all be cooled, and once his fever has abated, let him take a bath. *De methodo medendi* VIII[.2].

(XIX.12) Bathing is most harmful for those whose bodies contain many raw, crude humors. The same applies to very hot or cold air, because bathing and very hot air dissolve their humors so that they stream from one organ to another and one cannot be sure that they will not stream to the major organs or other eminent internal organs. Very cold air makes the concoction of these humors difficult; they can be cured, however, by drinking wine with hot water because this helps the concoction of the crude humors. *De methodo medendi* XII[.3].

(XIX.13) One whose body is emaciated benefits from bathing after meals. But someone who bathes after meals cannot be sure that no obstruction will occur in his liver. If this regimen is continued for a long time, it causes stones in his kidneys. If he has a sensation of heaviness in his right side and in his loins, he should immediately eat capers with vinegar and honey at the beginning of his meal and continue to do so until the feeling of heaviness disappears. *De methodo medendi* XIV[.16].

(XIX.14) If someone suffers from biting humors that irritate the cardia of his stomach, one should hasten, after bathing, to feed him with that which produces good blood. If this is only possible before the bath, he should take such a quantity that does not harm him during bathing. [*De compositione medicamentorum secundum locos*] II[.1].

(XIX.15) Bathing in sweet water is beneficial for the organs of the voice and the other organs affected by tiredness. Those who professionally use a high voice frequently enter the bathhouse and have a bath and eat foods that do not bite but instead have a slackening effect. [*De compositione medicamentorum secundum locos*] VII[.1].

(XIX.16) Bathing is most beneficial for those suffering from an ophthalmia if it is thoroughly ripe and the body is clean, for the pain subsides immediately and the flow of moisture that streams towards the eye stops and the humors become balanced and mixed. *De methodo medendi* XIII[.22].

(XIX.17) For those suffering from an affection of the spleen, poultices should be applied to the spleen after two hours of the day have passed until the ninth hour. The patient should enter the bathhouse while the poultice still adheres to him. When it becomes loose and then falls off in the bathhouse, let him go into the bathing basin. [*De compositione medicamentorum secundum locos*] IX[.2].

(XIX.18) It is best for someone who cannot enter the bathhouse after exercise in the beginning of the day to eat bread only in a quantity that his stomach can digest prior to the time that he takes a bath. *De sanitate tuenda* VI[.7].

(XIX.19) If headaches originate from a hot dyscrasia, baths in drinkable water should be administered frequently because that disperses the hot vapors originating in the head and completely changes the temperament of the body for the better. If the head is very warm and burning, the best thing to do in the summer is to rub the head with oil of roses prepared with omphacine oil. *De sanitate tuenda* VI[.9].

(XIX.20) Cold and moist bodies are prone to deterioration; they quickly suffer from diseases originating from the streaming of superfluities. Those who suffer from such a condition benefit from abstention from bathing, from physical exercise, and from adherence to a thinning regimen. *De sanitate tuenda* VI[.4].

(XIX.21) For him in whose body vaporous superfluities originate, bathing is appropriate, even twice a day and especially in the summer. But if someone with a cold and moist temperament abandons bathing, it is not harmful for him. A cold and dry temperament needs bathing, as is the case with the elderly. Superfluities increase in the bodies of those who have a hot and moist temperament; the application of bathing before the evacuation of these superfluities is dangerous, but after the evacuation it is beneficial. *De sanitate tuenda* V[.12].

(XIX.22) Someone whose body is full with raw, crude humors should not take a bath, for bathing prompts those humors to exit and they quickly obstruct the narrow channels. *De sanitate tuenda* IV[.5].

(XIX.23) He says concerning the regimen of those suffering from quartan fever in its initial phase: As for massage, walking, bathing, and their other usual activities, one should not withhold these from them completely. But if they can completely abstain from bathing and be satisfied with massage only, it is most beneficial to them. *Ad Glauconem de* [*medendi methodo*] I[.12].

(XIX.24) A thick humor dissolves and becomes thinner by drinking pure wine and by taking a bath immediately thereafter. *In Hippocratis Aphorismos commentarius* VII[.46].

(XIX.25) Hippocrates says in his [*Regimen*] *on Acute Diseases* III and Galen in his commentary thereon that those who suffer from pleurisy and pneumonia and acute fevers benefit from bathing. *In Hippocratis De acutorum morborum* [*victu*] *commentarius* III[.57].

(XIX.26) Says Moses: That sufferers from fever benefit from bathing after the concoction of their humors is a subject raised in several sections of Galen's books. As for the statement of both Hippocrates and Galen that bathing is beneficial for pleurisy and pneumonia, it seems to me that they are referring to those who suffer from pain in the side or in the lungs because of a dyscrasia or because of thick or biting humors but without inflammation or fever. These are the patients who benefit from bathing.

(XIX.27) Bathing is beneficial for someone suffering from diarrhea because it attracts the superfluous matters to the skin. But someone whose body is full or who is constipated should not take a bath. *In Hippocratis De acutorum morborum [victu] commentarius* III[.58].

(XIX.28) Someone suffering from a nosebleed or nausea or bilious superfluities in his stomach should not take a bath. If he does so, he ruins his strength and brings about syncope. Similarly, someone whose strength is weak should not bathe. *In Hippocratis De acutorum morborum [victu] commentarius* III[.58].

(XIX.29) In the case of fevers, one should bathe after the concoction of the humors so that it helps the completion of the concoction and dissolves the humors. One should be wary of bathing before the concoction and, in general, be very cautious in the case of fevers caused by salty putrid phlegm because the phlegm cannot be dissolved through the skin in the way that bile can be dissolved, nor can its heat be extinguished or suppressed. *In Hippocratis De acutorum morborum [victu] commentarius* III[.61].

(XIX.30) One should thoroughly dry one's head after bathing so that no moisture remains on it, not even a little quantity, because that remaining quantity cools the brain and thus harms it. *In Hippocratis De acutorum morborum [victu] commentarius* III[.52].

(XIX.31) During chymous fevers, taking a bath after the chymes have been concocted has a healing effect. It is appropriate at all times for hectic fever. There is no need to be afraid of bathing in the case of these fevers unless one's strength is very weak or the hectic fever comes with a putrefying fever. But do not let the patient take a bath until the chymes are concocted. *De marcore* [7].

(XIX.32) All patients with ephemeral fever should take a bath, except for those to whom this fever occurred because of firmness of the skin or because of a swelling of the glands in the groin or armpit. But if you tell these patients to stay in the air of the bathhouse for a long time, it will not harm them at all. All other patients affected by this fever, if it occurred to them from causes other than the two mentioned, should stay in the air of the bathhouse for a short time only, but are allowed to stay in the water as long as they wish. *Ad Glauconem [de medendi methodo]* I[.3].

(XIX.33) Those suffering from pure tertian fever are allowed to bathe in sweet, drinkable hot water since it extracts and evacuates some of the bile and is extremely beneficial because of its quality. For bathing in this water moistens, cools, and strengthens the body. Your intention in letting someone suffering from this fever have a bath should be to moisten and wet his body. *Ad Glauconem* [*de medendi methodo*] I[.10].

(XIX.34) People suffering from marasmus and all those in whom dryness prevails do not need the hot air in the bathhouse, but rather the extremely temperate water of the bathing basin. Big bathing basins are better than small ones for this illness. The patient should remain in the water for a very long time. The water should be extremely temperate and pleasant so that it encourages the nature of the patient to spread, open, and expand in every direction to meet with that which gives it pleasure to enjoy. It is sufficient when his body is moderately heated in the bath. Then, after the bathing, you should massage him with oil so that the pores of his skin are closed, the acquired moisture spreads within the body, and he is not harmed by the air. *De methodo* [*medendi*] VII[.6].

(XIX.35) If someone of those who have vaporous superfluities develops a fever from becoming chilled, he should take a bath, unless the fever is accompanied by a catarrh or rheum. But do not let him take a bath when the catarrh or rheum is not ripe. If someone has a fever because he has been burned by the sun, he should take a bath even if he has a rheum or catarrh. After the bath, pour cooled rose oil over his head in the same way as you did before the bath. *De methodo* [*medendi*] VIII[.3].

(XIX.36) For all patients with hectic fever, and especially those suffering from marasmus, taking a cold water bath without first bathing in hot water is dangerous, because prior bathing in hot water warms the body, prepares it, and makes it ready for bathing in cold water. *De methodo* [*medendi*] X[.10].

Once signs of concoction of the humors have appeared, taking a bath is beneficial for someone whose fever is only light and whose faculties are not strong. *De methodo* [*medendi*] XI[.9].

(XIX.37) In the case of all fevers, one should pay attention to three things concerning bathing in the bathhouse: First, that the patient is not affected by a shivering fit when he takes a bath; second, that none of the vital organs is weak; and third, that the primary vessels are not congested by a large quantity of crude humors. *De methodo* [*medendi*] XI[.20].

For all intermittent fevers, the best time to take a bath, if one is allowed to do so, is when the heat of the fever begins to dissolve, for then the bath immediately prepares the body and makes it fit to be nourished. But in the case of these fevers, one should always beware of going into a cold water basin. *De methodo* [*medendi*] XI[.20, 21].

(XIX.38) For some people, it is most appropriate to take some food prior to bathing. But for everyone whose temperament is extremely hot and dry it is fitting to bathe after the meal. *De sanitate tuenda* VI[.3].

(XIX.39) You should look into the matter of everyone who seems to you to be bathing after eating. If you notice someone experiencing any pain or heaviness or tension in the region of the liver, do not let that person with such conditions bathe after meals. If he perceives any such condition, hasten to open the obstruction of his liver and let him always abstain from thick foods. *De sanitate tuenda* VI[.3].

This is the end of the nineteenth treatise,
by the grace of God,
praise be to Him.

In the name of God,
the Merciful, the Compassionate.
O Lord, make our task easy.

The Twentieth Treatise

Containing aphorisms concerning foods, beverages, and their consumption

(XX.1) Our first specific goal in the consumption of foods is that the food will be well digested. Our second goal thereafter is that the chyme produced therefrom will be beneficial, that is, that it fits all the other organs. *De bonis* [*malisque*] *sucis* [X.4].

(XX.2) The knowledge of the powers of the different foods is nearly the most useful kind of knowledge in the field of medicine, since there is a constant and never-ending need for food, both during health and sickness. *De alimentorum facultatibus* I[.1.1].

(XX.3) Helpful to repel the harm caused by bad foodstuff is the following: the consumption of only a small amount of it, habit, bodily activity, and a long sleep after its comsumption. *De alimentorum facultatibus* I[.2.8, 9].

(XX.4) For any individual person, the digestion of the food he eats can be easy or difficult, either through its specific substance and nature, or through the occurrence of a symptom. *De alimentorum facultatibus* II[.6.2].

(XX.5) We as physicians focus especially on the benefit that foods should provide, not on the pleasure to be derived from them. But since some foods are distasteful and their distastefulness hinders their digestion, the physician should make efforts to season such food so that it can be well digested. However, cooks usually season food to such a degree that it contributes to a bad digestion. *De alimentorum facultatibus* II[.51.5].

(XX.6) Soft food is easier and faster to digest in the stomach, to turn into blood in the liver and the vessels, and to be absorbed into every singular organ that is nourished by it. But harder food is more difficult to digest and more slow to undergo all these processes. *De alimentorum facultatibus* III[.32].

(XX.7) When we are hungry, we should not greedily stuff ourselves with food like a dog, and when we are thirsty, we should not enjoy a cold drink to the same degree as someone whose body is inflamed with continuous fever and who consequently finishes the whole cup out of greed. We should restrain ourselves from stretching out our hands to all that is presented to us or to something sweet and the like, of those things that gluttons take. *De propriorum animi cuiuslibet affectuum dignotione* [*et curatione*].

(XX.8) Convalescents and weak people should be given stronger food in the evening. But since they cannot digest the food properly, we should feed them little by little, at various times, and we should let them drink little by little, in such a quantity that their distress is alleviated and their food does not float. *De methodo* [*medendi*] VII[.6].

(XX.9) If you want to feed convalescents and all those who are weak, you should make it your first aim that the quantity of food such a person takes does not overburden him. Your second aim should be that he digests his food rapidly, and your third aim should be that it passes quickly through the bowels. If you feed them meat of cows (beef), slaughter the animal one day before they are to eat it when it is winter, for the meat that sits overnight is more rapidly digested. But when it is summer, it is enough that the meat be from an animal that has been slaughtered in the morning and is consumed after sunset. *De methodo* [*medendi*] VII[.6].

(XX.10) Putrid foods and beverages produce corruption similar to that produced by fatal poisons. *In Hippocratis De* [*aere,*] *aquis* [*et locis*] *commentarius* II.

(XX.11) Food can become beneficial or harmful in its inherent healing powers for our bodies. But regarding the nutritional aspect, it is always beneficial for our bodies in all bodily conditions. *In Hippocratis De alimento commentarius* II.

(XX.12) When its strength is weak, the body it is unable to digest a large quantity of food even when its quality is good. Therefore, you should always measure the quantity of food according to the strength or weakness of the body and choose the quality of the food according to the temperament of the body. *In Hippocratis De alimento commentarius* IV[.25].

(XX.13) Some foods soften the stools and relieve the bowels in that they have medicinal powers mixed with them, similar to the powers of scammony, pulp of colocynth, and hellebore, for these foods have the nature both of food and of medicine. But foods do not fall under the definition of medicines when they do not have any of these influences on the body and do not do anything else but nourish it. There are very few foods of this sort, but those that exist are merely nourishing. *De alimentorum facultatibus* I[.1.25].

(XX.14) It is impossible for the humor originating from the *biṭṭīkh* (common melon or watermelon) to become thick and earth-like, even when it well digested, just as the humor originating from lentils or from beef cannot become watery and moist. Similarly, whenever someone who eats cucumbers does not pay attention to the quantity he eats because he relies on his good digestion, a cold, thick humor collects in his vessels that cannot easily be converted into blood, even if the cucumbers are well digested. This is the main thing for the preservation of health and the healing of diseases. *De alimentorum facultatibus* II[.6.3, 4].

(XX.15) The dough of bran bread only needs a small amount of yeast, light kneading, and a short time in the oven. But for extremely pure bread the opposite is needed. *De alimentorum facultatibus* I[.2.3].

(XX.16) The most beneficial and appropriate bread for someone who does not engage in physical exercise and for the elderly is bread that has been properly baked in an oven and that contains a lot of yeast. But completely unleavened bread is not appropriate for anyone. *De alimentorum facultatibus* I[.2.7].

(XX.17) Starch (amylum) is near in power to washed bread inasmuch as it provides only a little nourishment to the body and does not heat, just as washed bread does not heat, although all the other kinds of bread do heat. *De alimentorum facultatibus* I[.8.2].

(XX.18) Our nature prevails over almost all kinds of meat and changes and transforms them and turns them into beneficial blood. But of radishes and beetroots and the like, only a small part can be changed and transformed, and that only with some trouble and much labor—and furthermore, that small part is not beneficial blood, and the remainder exits with the superfluities. *De naturalibus facultatibus* I[.10].

(XX.19) The best meat of land animals is pork; then comes kid and then veal. Lamb is moist, sticky, and slimy. As for the meat of the other land animals, I recommend that anyone who cares about keeping his humors in a healthy condition avoid eating it. *De bonis malisque sucis* [VI.8, 9].

(XX.20) Because of its lightness, the meat of birds produces a large quantity of bile if it encounters increased heat from the body. *In Hippocratis Epidemiarum* [*commentarius*] VI.6.

(XX.21) Roasted meat strengthens the body more than boiled meat. After this comes braised meat, for braised meat strengthens more than any other form of cooked meat. *In Hippocratis De alimento commentarius* IV.

(XX.22) The nourishment that the body receives from all meat that is roasted or baked is drier, whereas the nourishment of all meat that is boiled in water is more moist. All meat boiled in a pot and seasoned with spices and condiments falls between these. *De alimentorum facultatibus* III[.1.16].

Testicles taste badly and produce bad humors. This statement applies only to the testicles of land animals, for the testicles of fatted cocks are delicious and provide good nourishment. The consumption of any brain is harmful for the stomach. *De alimentorum facultatibus* III[.6.2].

(XX.23) The food provided by wild animals—that is, those that live in the mountains and deserts—does not contain any superfluities. For this reason, the nutrition that the human body receives from the meat of wild animals is necessarily stronger and better than that which it receives from the meat of domestic animals. *De alimentorum facultatibus* III[.13.1, 2].

(xx.24) Wine mixed with an equal amount of water heats the whole body and rapidly moves to all its limbs. It ameliorates and improves the humors of the body by balancing their temperament and by evacuating bad humors. *In Hippocratis Aphorismos commentarius* VII[.56].

(xx.25) Wine that is diluted and watery moistens and weakens the stomach and produces intestinal winds because of the coldness and fluidity of the water. Pure wine causes twitching in the temples, heaviness in the head, and thirst because of its heat. *In Hippocratis De acutorum morborum* [*victu*] *commentarius* II[.34].

(xx.26) In the case of a hangover, the head is filled with vapor. Pure wine concocts these vapors and dissolves them. *In Hippocratis Epidemiarum* [*commentarius*] II.6.

(xx.27) We have nothing more effective and appropriate than the ingestion of wine for the case in which someone's strength has diminished, weakened, and collapsed. The same applies to someone whose entire body has become cold or whose complexion has changed. *In Hippocratis Epidemiarum* [*commentarius*] VI.6.

(xx.28) All sweet black wines fill the vessels with thick, dark blood. Thin white wines cut the thick chymes and cleanse the blood through the urine. Yellow wines are in the middle between these two and produce chymes that are intermediate in their consistency. *De victu attenuante* [12].

(xx.29) Thin wine is beneficial for producing good chyme and helps digestion. Yellow wine and wine that tends towards whiteness are good for stimulating micturition. *De sanitate tuenda* IV[.6].

(xx.30) Anyone whose strength needs to be revived should not drink anything but thin white wine which is pure, only contains a small amount of water, and is slightly astringent, as this is one of the most beneficial things for such a person if he does not have a fever. *De methodo* [*medendi*] VII[.6].

(xx.31) Wine is one of the most appropriate things for someone who suffers from a liver affliction without an inflammation or a hot bad temperament, because it nourishes, concocts, strengthens and fights, and counteracts putrefaction. If his dyscrasia happens to be cold and moist, wine heals him. [*De compositione medicamentorum secundum locos*] VIII[.7].

(XX.32) Drinking cold water before meals is harmful for the liver, and in some people, it is also harmful for the nerves. *In Hippocratis De natura hominis* [*commentarius* III.12].

(XX.33) The worst of all waters are those derived from melted snow and ice because the fine part of rainwater dissolves but the thick, bad part freezes and never regains the excellent quality of rainwater. [*In Hippocratis*] *De aer*[*e, aquis et locis*] *commentarius* II.

(XX.34) All extremely cold water is thick and hard, slow to be digested and to pass. All turbid water strengthens the appetite. The reason for this is that in the summer the turbid water corrupts the humors so that these bite the stomach, while during winter these humors bite the cardia of the stomach because they are confined to that place because of the cold. [*In Hippocratis*] *De aer*[*e, aquis et locis*] *commentarius* II.

(XX.35) Rapid transformation of water indicates its goodness and not its badness. Rainwater, once it is spoiled, does not regain its original goodness. Therefore, one should wait until the bad smell lessens and then mix it with honey or wine; but cooking is of no use whatsoever for it. [*In Hippocratis*] *De aer*[*e, aquis et locis*] *commentarius* II.

(XX.36) When bad water that is turbid or foul-smelling or slow to pass through the stomach or another organ is boiled, this removes its badness and makes it fit for drinking; this process should go quickly for then the water's earthen parts are separated from it and settle. Boil it at the end of the day, leave it over for the entire night, filter it, and then drink it. *In Hippocratis Epidemiarum* [*commentarius*] VI.4.

(XX.37) Rainwater does not change into another kind of putrefying quality. If you do not have rainwater available, be satisfied with spring water, for it is sufficient when this water is clean and pure. [*De compositione medicamentorum secundum locos*] VII[.21].

(XX.38) The best water is that in which no taste nor odor is perceptible. This water is the sweetest and most delicious to drink. Any water that streams towards the east over clean sand and that quickly warms and cools is the best water for anyone whatever his age. *De sanitate tuenda* I[.11].

(XX.39) Milk nourishes an emaciated body and revives it. It hinders the bad humors from causing harm and even improves them. It softens the stools. But cheese settles in the passages of the liver and obstructs them and is therefore very harmful for dropsy patients. *In Hippocratis Epidemiarum* [*commentarius*] II.6.

(XX.40) In his [*In Hippocratis*] *De alimento commentarius* IV, Galen says that milk is more nutritious than wheat. And in *De bonis* [*malisque*] *sucis*, he says that milk is the best thing in producing good chymes.

(XX.41) Watery moisture prevails in the milk of camels and donkeys, cheesy moisture prevails in sheep's milk and fat in milk of a cow. Compared to the milk of other animals, goat's milk is intermediate between these unbalanced conditions. It is also intermediate in its effect on the human body. The milk that produces the best chyme—if one drinks it immediately after milking—comes from an animal that is healthy and in a good condition. One acts prudently if one adds a small amount of honey and salt to be sure that it does not turn into cheese. *De bonis* [*malisque*] *sucis* [IV.4, 8].

(XX.42) As for milk that seems to have curdled—and the most curdled kind of milk is cheese—it is one of the things which is extremely thickening when it is eaten dry. Milk that is greatly dominated by the cheesy part, such as milk of a cow and sheep's milk is the thickest of all kinds of milk. The thinnest milk is that in which the watery part dominates, such as the milk of donkeys, for if it is taken with honey or salt, it does not harm someone who needs a thinning diet. But one should be on one's guard against the other kinds of milk. [*De victu attenuante* 12].

(XX.43) Milk of a cow is the thickest and fattest of all sorts of milk, while that of camels is the moistest of all sorts of milk with the least amount of fat. After camel's milk is mare's milk, and after that is donkey's milk. Goat's milk is intermediate between thick and thin milk, but sheep's milk is thicker than it. *De alimentorum* [*facultatibus*] III[.14.1].

(XX.44) All sorts of milk are good and beneficial for the chest and lungs, but they are not suitable for the head unless the head is extremely strong. Milk is unsuitable for the parts below the cartilage of the ribs since these are easily filled with flatulence. *De alimentorum* [*facultatibus*] III[.14.3].

(XX.45) The best sort of cheese is the fresh one that is made from milk from which the fat has been removed. This cheese is the most delicious of all sorts of cheeses and does not harm the stomach. It is the most rapid sort of cheese to pass and does not provide bad nutrition nor unwholesome blood as all other cheeses do. *De alimentorum* [*facultatibus*] III[.16.3].

(XX.46) The foods that are extremely weak are vegetables and most fruits that are surrounded by a hard shell. These have the property to weaken the body, and if one uses them constantly, one shortens one's life. *In Hippocratis Epidemiarum* [*commentarius*] VI.5.

(XX.47) Vegetables do not have good chymes. Cultivated lettuce is a cooling vegetable that is harmless; turnip is between good and bad, and after it nalta jute, and then garden orach, common purslane, and purple amaranth. *De bonis* [*malisque*] *sucis* [VIII.9].

(XX.48) If cucumber and *biṭṭīkh* (common melon or watermelon) are not quickly passed, they corrupt in the stomach and the chyme resulting from the putrefaction is almost a fatal poison. *De bonis* [*malisque*] *sucis* [VIII.7].

(XX.49) Thinning vegetables are garlic, onion, garden cress, leek, and mustard.

Next in strength after these come parsley, fennel, mountain mint, water mint, oregano, *ḥāshā* (lesser calamint or creeping thyme), *nānakhwāh* (bisnaga or ajowan), and Massilian hartwort, when these are taken fresh.

Next in strength after these come garden rocket, wideleaf waterparsnip (*qurrat al-ʿayn*), that is, "water celery" (*karafs al-māʾ*), wild celery, *baṭrasālinūn* (seed of mountain parsley), sweet basil, radish, cabbage, blackberry, and other types of fragrant and sharp plants. *De victu attenuante* [2].

(XX.50) Opium poppy seeds are much less cooling than the plants, so one can sprinkle them on bread and mix them with many other foods that one prepares without causing any harm. But they do cause heaviness in the head and induce sleep. Sesame seeds produce thick and sticky chymes in the body. *De victu attenuante* [5].

(XX.51) All fruits from trees, with a few exceptions, produce bad chymes. Such an exception is the fruit from the sweet chestnut, because in spite of its thickness, it does not produce any bad chyme if it is well digested. All fresh fruits produce bad chymes, and if they spoil in the stomach, they cause fatal poisoning. Figs and grapes are less bad. Dried figs together with walnuts and almonds have beneficial chymes. *De bonis* [*malisque*] *sucis* [VIII.1–3].

(XX.52) Fresh, ripe figs are among the intermediate foods about which one can say neither that they have a thinning effect on the chymes nor that they have a thickening effect on them. Those apples and pears that are eaten when they are cooked are less harmful than those that are eaten while they are raw. *De victu attenuante* [2].

(XX.53) If mulberries do not pass quickly, they spoil in the stomach in an extraordinary, unusual way that is beyond description, just like *biṭṭīkh* (common melons or watermelons) and *qarʿ* (field pumpkin or winter squash) when they are not passed. For although *qarʿ* are the most harmless of the summer fruits, when they are not passed from the stomach quickly, they cause severe corruption. *De alimentorum* [*facultatibus*] II[.11.4].

(XX.54) All dates are hard to digest and cause headache and a sensation of sharpness and biting at the cardia of the stomach when one eats too many of them. *Busr* (unripe dates) fill the body with crude, raw humors that obstruct the liver and cause shivering and rigor that is difficult to warm. *De alimentorum* [*facultatibus*] II[.26.20].

(XX.55) He says in [*De compositione medicamentorum secundum locos*] II[.1].: Dates have a specific property that causes headache.

(XX.56) Olives strengthen the stomach and whet the appetite. The olives most suited to this task are those that are preserved in vinegar. Walnuts are more rapidly digested than hazelnuts but are less nutritious. They are better for the stomach than hazelnuts, especially when they are eaten together with dried figs. *De alimentorum* [*facultatibus*] II[.27.1; 28.1, 3].

(XX.57) Raisins are hardly susceptible to putrefaction. In general, their substance is similar and conformable to the nature of the liver. They cure its bad temperament, and nourish it, concoct the unconcocted humors, and correct the bad humors and improve their temperament. For this reason, they are extremely valuable for healing these sorts of illnesses. [*De compositione medicamentorum secundum locos*] VIII[.7].

(XX.58) The foods that are most similar to blood are those that are intermediate between thin and thick. These include the good types of bread; the meat of chickens, partridges, pigeons, turtle doves, francolins, and pheasants; all sorts of fish that do not contain stickiness or grease or have a repulsive taste; and gently boiled eggs. *De bonis* [*malisque*] *sucis* [III.1].

The best food that does not have any clear medicinal power nor a very nutritious substance is barley gruel that has been well prepared, and after it, barley groats. After these comes gruel from emmer wheat (*khandarūs*) with a small amount of vinegar, and gruel from emmer wheat (*khandarūs*) with no vinegar at all. Bread baked in an oven is also good foodstuff, and of the fishes all those that live among the rocks. The best kinds of birds are the partridge and mountain sparrows. After these come chickens and francolins. Those animals that are very old or young (just born) should be avoided. *De methodo* [*medendi*] VIII[.2].

(XX.59) Foods that produce thick, sticky chyme are very nutritious. If they are well digested in the stomach and liver, they produce beneficial blood. Only someone who performs strenuous physical exercise before his meals should take these foods. But someone who merely looks after the health of his body and not after its vigor should guard against all foods which produce thick chyme and should avoid thickening foods even if they have beneficial chymes. *De bonis* [*malisque*] *sucis* [II.9; III.2, 4].

(XX.60) Thick, sticky foods include all types of bread whose baking was bad—that is, bread that was not well leavened or was insufficiently salted, kneaded, or baked—also all types of cheese, roasted or hard-boiled eggs, all types of large fish with hard, sticky meat, mushrooms and truffles, large pine nuts and dates. Lentils, cabbage, acorns, and sweet chestnuts are not sticky, although they produce thick chymes. *De bonis* [*malisque*] *sucis* [IV.1, 2, 12, 13, 15, 16, 34, 42].

(XX.61) All people should always avoid foods with bad chymes, except for those who work hard during the summer and need to treat the dryness and heat of their bodies. In such a situation it is appropriate for them to eat mulberries, plums, cherries, cucumbers, *biṭṭīkh* (common melons or watermelons), apricots, or peaches before their meal, and also cooled milk and *qarʿ* (field pumpkin or winter squash). If a person practices moderation in his lifestyle, he can cool and moisten the dryness and heat resulting from his hard work with another kind of regimen, namely, by going to the bathhouse and by feeding himself thereafter with foods that have good chymes and that are seasoned with vinegar and the like. *De bonis* [*malisque*] *sucis* [XIII.1–3].

(XX.62) Food that is hard to dissolve is that consisting of thick, sticky things such as pork and pure bread. If someone who does not exercise were to constantly eat this food, he would soon suffer from the illness of overfilling, just as if someone who practices bodily exercise were to constantly feed himself with vegetables and barley juice, his body would be destroyed and quickly waste away. *De alimentorum* [*facultatibus*] I[.2.11].

(xx.63) Everything that is moister in its consistency provides the body with little nourishment. It dissolves and evaporates rapidly and is easily digested so that the body needs other, new food. But everything that is hard and earth-like provides the body with rich, lasting nourishment that is difficult to dissolve and evaporate and is not easily digested nor converted into blood. *De alimentorum* [*facultatibus*] I[.23.4].

(xx.64) One should bear in mind a factor common to all foods: Whatever is sharp and spicy or bitter provides little nourishment, while whatever is tasteless provides the body with rich nourishment; even more so whatever is sweet, especially when its substance is solid. This is the case whether these flavors are natural or acquired through preparation—that is, through cooking, roasting, frying, macerating in water, and the like. *De alimentorum* [*facultatibus*] II[.62.1, 2].

(xx.65) Things that are greasy and sticky, such as the different kinds of fat, satiate and fill someone who eats them from the outset, as soon as they reach the stomach. And then they diminish and lessen his appetite. A human being cannot bear to eat such food constantly. *De alimentorum* [*facultatibus*] III.

(xx.66) Something that is truly sweet is undoubtedly nutritious. But something bitter is not nutritious, and something with an intermediate flavor is less nutritious than something sweet. The same holds true for the other flavors because they are not nutritious, with the only exception of the sweet flavor. And also, something fatty is of the same kind as something sweet and is nutritious. *De* [*simplicium*] *medicamentorum* [*temperamentis ac facultatibus*] IV[.10, 15].

(xx.67) Says Moses: Abū Marwān ibn Zuhr mentions the benefits of some foods that have been confirmed by testing. These foods work through specific properties. He mentions them in the *Kitāb al-Aghdhiya* (*Book on Foodstuffs*), which he composed for one of the Almoravid kings. Some of these were mentioned by his father in his *Tadhkira*. It seems to me a good thing to write them down in the form of aphorisms, and they are the following:

(xx.68) Boiled chicken soup balances the temperament. It is the best medicine and foodstuff for the beginning of elephantiasis. It fattens the body of the emaciated and convalescents. Young pigeons have the specific property of producing migraine, especially their necks. Turtle doves increase memory, sharpen the intellect, and strengthen the senses. Partridges, when boiled, cause constipation, but if they are boiled in their skins, they relieve the bowels. Similarly, hens and roosters are very effective in relieving the bowels.

(XX.69) Sparrows are beneficial for paralysis, hemiplegia, facial paresis, and the different kinds of dropsy, and also increase sexual potency. Domestic pigeons that live together and fly around freely increase the innate heat. Soup made from larks loosens a colic. The nature of quails is close to that of sparrows; its meat is beneficial for healthy people and convalescents; its substance is fine; it dissolves kidney stones and stimulates micturition.

(XX.70) He says: Kid is virtually different from the meat of all other quadrupeds because it is exceedingly good. The meat of gazelles has the specific property of strengthening the soul, and the juice of its meat revives someone whose strength has collapsed and resuscitates someone who has fainted because of excessive evacuation.

(XX.71) The testicles of roosters provide extremely good nourishment and are the best food one can give to emaciated people and convalescents. All testicles of living creatures are hot and moist and clearly help the sexual potency.

(XX.72) Pigeon eggs improve sexual potency and are beneficial to it. All eggs improve the sexual potency, especially when they are boiled with onion or turnip.

(XX.73) In general, all types of milk relieve the bowels, and camel milk strengthens the stomach and liver. Raisins fatten the liver and are beneficial for it through their specific property. Unripe, sour grapes strengthen the stomach through their specific property and by virtue of their nature balance the temperament of those suffering from heat. They stop [the urge to] vomit in an amazing way when it is caused by yellow bile.

(XX.74) The smell of an apple strengthens the heart and the brain and is beneficial for those suffering from marasmus and delusions. However, as to its actual consumption, he states that it is more harmful than the consumption of any other fruit because its fragrance gives rise to gases in the nerves and in the muscles that can only be dissolved with difficulty.

(XX.75) Pears strengthen the stomach and have the specific property of quenching thirst when eaten after a meal. If one lets their juice stand, it turns into a vinegar that strengthens the stomach in a wonderful way and does not harm the nerves because of the astringency and fragrance that it contains.

(xx.76) When eaten with bread, sweet pomegranates have a wonderful and specific property that prevents the bread from spoiling in the stomach. Similarly, if sour pomegranates are cooked with the food, that food does not get spoiled in the stomach.

(xx.77) Excessive consumption of walnuts causes stuttering; therefore, children should not eat them. Almonds induce a regular sleep. If used for cooking, they provide primarily moisture without any superfluities. Their oil, if trickled into the nose, induces sleep and is good for cooking.

(xx.78) Pistachio nuts are the most salutary of fruits; they strengthen the stomach and the liver by their specific property. Their oil has the same effect if rubbed on the stomach and liver. They are beneficial in many ways. If they are eaten either alone or with raisins and sugar before the meal, during the meal, or after the meal, they are beneficial for all conditions. They are of a moderate heat and dryness.

(xx.79) Dates obstruct the liver and cause an inflammation in the head. They have bad chymes; the fresh ones are much more detrimental than the dried ones and have the specific property of producing hemorrhoids. The hearts (pith) of the date palm produce much sperm and help the sexual potency.

(xx.80) Sesame injures the brain and the spinal cord and fills the head with superfluities. It makes the mouth stink, putrefies the sweat, makes women sterile, fattens the abdomen, and sometimes causes scrotal hernia.

(xx.81) Raw or cooked cabbage purifies the voice and removes hoarseness. Eggplant, as a drug, strengthens, fortifies, and reinforces the stomach and is good against nausea and vomiting. But cabbage and eggplant are the worst of all foods and produce a large quantity of black bile. This is the end of the text quoted from Ibn Zuhr.

(xx.82) Says Moses: This man who was on the Temple Mount and whose name is al-Tamīmī and who composed a book on drugs and called it [*Kitāb*] *Al-Murshid* [*fī jawāhir al-aghdhiya waquwā l-mufradāt mina l-adwiya*], allegedly had much experience. Although most of his statements are taken from others and although sometimes, he wrongly understands the words of others, he still, in general, mentions many properties of various foods and of medications, and therefore I decided to write down those which are good in my opinion, whether foods or medications.

(xx.83) From his statement about the special properties of foods: Eating a handful of sweetened, salted white lupine beans every day together with the skins strengthens one's vision by virtue of their specific property. He further states: Young chickens that are separated from their mother alleviate the heat that occurs in the cardia of the stomach. Soup prepared from old roosters is good for chronic phlegmatic fevers and for asthma. Oregano has a specific property of strengthening vision and is good for weak vision arising from moisture. It is also beneficial for scorpion stings.

(xx.84) Garden orach has a specific property of being good for jaundice caused by obstruction of the liver. Spinach is beneficial for pleurisy and for any tumor that arises from yellow bile or blood. Purple amaranth has the specific property of eliminating thirst caused by yellow bile and is beneficial for the chest and lungs. Common purslane has the specific property of eliminating the craving for clay and cures teeth that are set on edge.

(xx.85) Asparagus increases the sperm and has the specific property of being beneficial for backache caused by phlegm and winds. When turnips are cooked in fatty mutton, they increase the milk of a nursing mother and make it flow abundantly.

(xx.86) Concerning wild taro, al-Tamīmī contradicts the statement by Īsā ibn Māssa that it is hot and dry and that it increases the libido. Al-Tamīmī states that it is hot and dry, produces black bile, and has no good in it. He says that saffron has the specific property of stimulating the libido. Anise has a similar effect; it also cleanses white humors from the uterus. Dill has the specific property of being beneficial for hiccups arising from overfilling.

(xx.87) He says: Peels of cucumber, especially those of the smaller variety, if eaten, putrefy and produce a poisonous humor. Similarly, these small cucumbers themselves produce a poisonous humor if they are difficult to digest. If pregnant women constantly eat quinces, it improves the moral character of their children.

(xx.88) He says: The specific property of bananas is to obstruct the passages of the liver and vessels of the spleen through their viscosity and sweetness. *Utrujj* (citron or lemon) peels have the specific property of being beneficial for sharp pain affecting the cardia of the stomach caused by the predominance and irritation of black bile. Hazelnuts have a specific property to strengthen the jejunum and to avert harm from it.

(XX.89) Hearts of date palms have a specific property to extinguish and alleviate the boiling heat of blood. They are beneficial for bloody plague spots.

This is the end of the twentieth treatise.

In the name of God,
the Merciful, the Compassionate.
O Lord, make our task easy.

The Twenty-First Treatise
Containing aphorisms concerning drugs

(XXI.1) A treatment with nutriments, which have therapeutic powers is better than a treatment with drugs that have alimentary powers. Be careful not to use pure drugs, unless you are forced to do so for some reason. When using drugs, you should aspire to mix them with ingredients with alimentary powers that improve their quality. *In Hippocratis De alimento commentarius* IV.

(XXI.2) Physicians have always used their skill to prepare drugs which promote health, specifically those which have attenuating power, because this power opens the narrow passages, cleanses the viscous chymes that adhere to the vessels, and rarefies the thick moistures. But if a person uses them frequently, they make his blood watery or bilious and, with the passage of time, melancholic because these drugs, but for a few of them, heat and dry excessively. *De bonis* [*malisque*] *sucis* [II.5].

(XXI.3) Astringent wine is beneficial in that it stops all kinds of emptying. The best wine for someone suffering from a hot disease is a watery one—that is, a thin white wine with no perceptible taste or flavor—because this wine does not have the harmful effects of water or wine. *In Hippocratis De acutorum morborum* [*victu*] *commentarius* [III.8].

(XXI.4) Wine has the property of concocting humors whose concoction has not been completed. It stimulates micturition and perspiration and induces sleeping. *De sanitate tuenda* IV[.4].

(XXI.5) The harmful effects of water are related to its coolness because water that is cold stays for a long time in the hypochondrium and causes intestinal rumblings and flatulence and weakens and diminishes the strength of the stomach. This causes diminished digestion. And because of its coldness, it does not aid sizably to the transport of food. *De methodo* [*medendi*] VII[.6].

(XXI.6) The excellent qualities of the different kinds of beneficial wine are opposite to the afflictions arising from water. In addition, such wines produce beneficial blood, balance the temperament, concoct that which is retained in the stomach and vessels, increase the strength of the organs, and dispel the superfluities and expel them with the excrement. *De methodo* [*medendi*] VII[.6].

(XXI.7) Water does not alleviate cough and does not help expectoration; instead, it stimulates thirst, is transformed into bile, and weakens the body when drunk on an empty stomach. It increases the size of the liver and spleen when these are inflamed; it produces intestinal rumblings, floats in the stomach, and does not pass the excrements. It does not stimulate micturition, and its passage through the organs is slow because it is raw and uncooked. Water mixed with oxymel or the like is beneficial, however, because the other ingredient passes the water through the body and as a result moistens it; it also prevents its transformation into bile. *In Hippocratis De acutorum morborum* [*victu*] *commentarius* [III.40].

(XXI.8) Barley gruel has a cleansing power that is so sufficient on its own that it does not need to be mixed with some hyssop. If you want to increase its power, mix it with some black pepper. There is no need to mix it with some honey unless you intend to cleanse the sides of the chest and the lungs. *De victu attenuante* [6].

(XXI.9) I have personally observed that barley has a cooling force, whether prepared as bread, groats, or *sawīq* (semolina). Even if its outer shell is not removed, the gruel prepared from it has a strong cleansing effect and, from another point of view, one does not suffer any harm from it. Because barley groats have an effect opposite to that of lentils, a most excellent dish is produced when both ingredients are mixed together. *De alimentorum* [*facultatibus*] I.

(XXI.10) The constant consumption of milk is harmful for the teeth and the gums and accelerates the occurrence of putrefaction and corrosion therein. Therefore, one should rinse one's mouth with diluted wine and honey thereafter. But sour milk is not harmful for the teeth, unless someone who drinks it has a cold temperament. And if the stomach is warmer than necessary, it is able to digest sour milk well and to derive some benefit from it, even if it has been cooled with snow. *De alimentorum facultatibus* III[.14; 15.1, 2].

(XXI.11) The best kind of milk after women's milk, is from animals whose nature is close to that of human beings, such as pigs, sheep, goats, and horses. Milk can be prepared by making solid, smooth stones glowing hot after they have been washed, then extinguishing them in the milk, then boiling the milk so that most of the moist, watery part disappears. When the milk is then taken from the fire and drunk, it alleviates dysentery and stops the diarrhea of oily things. It is good for any biting tumor or ulcer dripping because of a surplus of sharp moistures. If instead of stones one uses an iron object that is free from rust, it is even better because it is somewhat astringent. *De* [*simplicium*] *medicamentorum* [*temperamentis ac facultatibus*] X[.8].

(XXI.12) Milk has the property of changing and altering very rapidly, just like sperm. Therefore, in the case of milk, the best thing to do, for someone who needs it, is to suck it from the breast. Women's milk is the best of all milks for those suffering from marasmus, and after it comes milk of donkeys. *De methodo* [*medendi*] VII[.6].

(XXI.13) The watery part of milk is a thinning substance, too, as well as stool softener. It is good to use it frequently, at certain intervals. *De victu attenuante* [12].

(XXI.14) The watery part of milk is better than all other things that relieve the bowels. I think that for this reason the ancient physicians used this drink whenever it was necessary to relieve the bowels. One should add enough honey to sweeten its taste so that someone who takes it enjoys it without feeling nauseated. And add so much salt to it as does not harm the sense of taste. If you want to cleanse the bowels in a stronger way, put more salt into it. *De alimentorum facultatibus* III[.14.8].

(XXI.15) The most appropriate substance for expectorating the thick humors is hydromel and, for the viscous humors, oxymel. The second best, after hydromel, is barley gruel, and after barley gruel, sweet wine. *In Hippocratis De acutorum morborum* [*victu*] *commentarius* III[.2].

(XXI.16) Hydromel boiled with absinth wormwood is a remedy for passing the thin humors that are retained in the insides of the stomach. *De methodo* [*medendi*] VIII[.11].

(XXI.17) If milk is added to honey, it is good for pains in the chest and lungs, but it is very harmful for the region of the liver and spleen. *De victu attenuante* [12].

(XXI.18) Butter and honey mixed together are amazingly useful for expectoration from the lungs in patients with pneumonia or pleurisy. Moreover, it concocts the humors. If the butter is licked up alone, its concocting effect is greater but its support to expectoration is less. If butter and honey are mixed with bitter almonds, the mixture's strength is greater in helping expectoration but is less in helping concoction. *De* [*simplicium*] *medicamentorum* [*temperamentis ac facultatibus*] X[.10].

(XXI.19) Vinegar, in addition to the fineness of its parts, has a considerable repelling and hindering force. Therefore, the physicians did the right thing to mix it with rose oil and use it in the beginning of brain diseases. If several days of the illness had already passed, they mixed broad-leaved thyme with these two ingredients so that it would have a heating effect as well as a refining one because this drug weakens on its way through the body and its strength is dissolved because of the bones that hinder it. Therefore, in this case, we also use castoreum, although we do not use it for the other inflamed tumors, even if they are in the final stages of decline. But during the decline of tumors in the region of the brain, this medication is most useful. *De methodo* [*medendi*] XI[.18].

(XXI.20) Vinegar is harmful for the womb and the other nervous organs because it is cold, thin, and sinks into them. *In Hippocratis De acutorum morborum* [*victu*] *commentarius* III[.39].

(XXI.21) Strongly acid oxymel either dries out the superfluous matters and increases their viscosity and stickiness so that it becomes difficult to expectorate them, or thins the thick sticky matters that are retained in the chest and lungs, so that they start to flow suddenly and abundantly and choke the patient so that he dies if his vigor is not strong. Therefore, it should be used only if one has great strength. [*In Hippocratis*] *De acutorum morborum* [*victu*] *commentarius* III[.28].

(XXI.22) Slightly acid oxymel moistens the mouth and palate, helps in the expectoration of sputum, quenches thirst, and opens obstructions occurring in the liver and spleen and cleanses them without harm. It checks the bile resulting from the honey, dissolves the flatulent winds, and stimulates micturition by opening the obstructions. It facilitates the passing of superfluities and bile into the intestines without any harm whatsoever, except that it abrades the intestines if constantly used. [*In Hippocratis*] *De acutorum morborum* [*victu*] *commentarius* III[.30–32].

(XXI.23) The most acidic oxymel beverage has three parts honey and one part vinegar. The sweetest oxymel has seven parts honey and one part vinegar. It should be boiled until the two parts become one. Then the foam should be removed little by little. *Puero epileptico* [*consilium* 6].

(XXI.24) We give oxymel to some patients to drink as a medicine, not as a food. Similarly, we give many patients hydromel and barley gruel as medicine, not as food. *De victus ratione in morbis acutis secundum Hippocratem.*

(XXI.25) Oxymel is the most suitable of sweet things that are used for a thinning diet. In addition, it does not have bad chymes, is not harmful for the stomach, and has nothing at all bad in it. It is the most cutting, not only of foods but also of all medicines. If someone wants an extreme cutting and thinning effect on the thick, sticky, phlegmatic superfluity in the body, he should use sea squill wine and sea squill vinegar. *De victu attenuante* [12].

(XXI.26) Ibn Zuhr states that the ingestion of the oxymel beverage with the juice of boiled field eryngo every day on an empty stomach protects against pleurisy and tumors of all the internal organs, and that constant soft stools also protect against that. He also says that the potion prepared with the different kinds of sandalwood is beneficial during times of epidemic diseases.

(XXI.27) Oxymel, if used excessively, causes abrasion of the intestines, stimulates cough, and is harmful for the nervous organs. *De methodo* [*medendi*] X[.11].

(XXI.28) To find a remedy that consists of thin parts and that is really absolutely cold may be impossible, because vinegar, which is thinner than all other cold things that we know and use as a medication, has some warmth mixed with it, and we find that it has a drying effect. Therefore, we mix enough cold water with it as to make it drinkable, and we use it for the diseases that need cooling and moistening. *De methodo* [*medendi*] X[.9].

(XXI.29) We find a single medication having opposite effects, such as common sorrel, whose leaves relieve the bowels but whose seeds constipate. Similarly, broth of cocks, snails, and cabbage juice relieves the bowels, but the meat of cocks and snails and the leaves of the cabbage constipate. Aloe and copper scales are astringent for moist wounds and strongly relieve the bowels. But cheese constipates the belly, while whey relieves the bowels. *De theriaca ad Pisonem* [4].

(XXI.30) We find that some medications are beneficial for some organs of the body, such as common agrimony, for it is clearly beneficial for the liver, and similarly, Chinese rhubarb. Not every medication is beneficial for every person; rather, for each person there is a medication appropriate for him. *De theriaca ad Pisonem* [4].

(XXI.31) The things that are most beneficial for the stomach are between bitter and astringent, such as the tendrils of the blackberry and those of the grapevine. All astringent things are beneficial for the stomach in most cases. *De victu attenuante* [4].

(XXI.32) The best medicine in each of its different kinds neither thin nor meager. Similarly, that which is thicker and fatter than the average amount is more deficient. Every herb for which the type-specific odor is very strong is the best. The same analogy applies to the taste of herbs. The excellence of compound medicines depends on the excellence of the simple ingredients therein. The difference between the two caused by their different preparation is small. *De antidotis* I[.5].

(XXI.33) We should not use white false hellebore in our times because of the bad physical condition of the people. Their bodies are full with phlegm; hellebore attracts it and the patient suffers from strangulation. Instead, we should use agarikon and the like. This was mentioned by Asklepios in his commentary on Hippocrates' book *On Fractures* and their setting.

(XXI.34) Dried figs, if eaten together with walnuts and common rue before the ingestion of a fatal poison, help and protect against its harm. *De bonis* [*malisque*] *sucis* [VIII.4].

(XXI.35) Milk, garlic, boiled wine, vinegar, and salt are beneficial against poisons or against substances similar to poisons developing in the body. *In Hippocratis Epidemiarum* [*commentarius*] VI.6.

(XXI.36) Says Moses: He means that any of these things or any combination may be beneficial against a poison depending on the individual poison and the individual bodily condition.

(XXI.37) Capers whet a jaded appetite and cleanse that which is in the stomach and belly and excrete it in the stools. They open obstructions in the liver and spleen and clean them, if this fruit is taken with vinegar and honey or with vinegar and oil before the consumption of all other foods. *De alimentorum* [*facultatibus*] II[.34.2].

(XXI.38) Long pepper has the property to dissolve thick, flatulent winds and to expel that which has coagulated in the region of the stomach towards the lower abdomen and helps in the digestion of that which remains therein. This is something common to all sorts of pepper. *De sanitate tuenda* IV[.5].

(XXI.39) Garlic is one of the medicines that dissolve winds more than any other dissolving substance. It does not produce thirst and dissolves flatulence more than any other food. Therefore, I call it the theriac of the villagers. *De methodo* [*medendi*] XII[.8].

(XXI.40) Obstructions and hard tumors in the spleen require strong cutting, refining, and opening drugs. The rhizodermis of caper has the same effect on the spleen as absinth wormwood on the liver, and *sqūlūfandriyūn* (rusty-back or hart's-tongue fern) has the same effect on the spleen as common agrimony on the liver. Caper with vinegar and honey is beneficial for both these organs. *De methodo* [*medendi*] XIII[.17].

(XXI.41) Boiled melilot has a concocting and astringent effect and is thus similar to saffron. [*De compositione medicamentorum secundum locos*] IV[.5].

(XXI.42) Cinnamon is a very fine drug; it opens the passages of the stomach, cleanses and attenuates the humors, and has a contrary effect on all the putrefactive serous discharges by changing and dissolving them. Because of its pleasant aroma, it is beneficial for all diseases originating from bad humors; it is good for any putrefaction and counteracts any putrefactive force and restores it to a healthy state. Similarly, it is good for seropurulent discharges, fatal drugs, and animal poisons. After cinnamon, Chinese cinnamon—when it is first-rate—has this effect, and after Chinese cinnamon, the whole class of spices and aromatic herbs, such as spikenard, camel grass, *qaṣab al-dharīra* (geranium or lemon grass), and spicknel. [*De compositione medicamentorum secundum locos*] VIII[.7].

(XXI.43) Aloe, although moderate, exerts an extremely contrary effect on someone affected by a hot, dry dyscrasia, but not by bad moistures. [*De compositione medicamentorum secundum locos*] VIII[.7].

(XXI.44) Absinth wormwood has the property to cleanse, wash, and pass the bad humors retained in the cardia of the stomach, and to contract, strengthen, and fortify it. [*De compositione medicamentorum secundum locos*] VIII[.3].

(XXI.45) Bdellium softens adequately, concocts, and, moreover, dissolves to a moderate degree. Turpentine resin has a potency similar to bdellium and, moreover, cleanses, purifies, and opens the narrow passages. These properties are needed for a weak liver. [*De compositione medicamentorum secundum locos*] VIII[.7].

(XXI.46) Indian spikenard has a considerable concocting strength for all cold diseases. Celtic spikenard is inferior to it regarding this property.

(XXI.47) Similarly, saffron is a drug well known for concocting unconcocted humors and diseases. [*De compositione medicamentorum secundum locos*] IX[.4].

(XXI.48) All drugs that free the body from poisons are of two kinds. Some of them change and transform the poison or fatal poison, and others attract the poison and expel it from the body. Any fatal poison is indeed evacuated by means of drugs that are applied externally, and these attract the poison either through their heat or through their whole substance. Similarly, the drugs that transform the poison and free the body from it do so either through a contrary quality or through their whole substance. *De* [*simplicium*] *medicamentorum* [*temperamentis ac facultatibus*] V[.18].

(XXI.49) Concerning all drugs that free the body from poisons, one should take an amount that does not harm the body because the dose is too large and that is not weaker than all the fatal drugs because its dose is too small, for then the fatal drugs overpower the antidote. *De* [*simplicium*] *medicamentorum* [*temperamentis ac facultatibus*] V[.18].

(XXI.50) For stings or bites by all kinds of vermin, one should administer a dose from the great theriac that is slightly heavier than a hazelnut, with fifteen ounces of diluted wine, which should be nearly pure. And someone who undertakes long journeys should, prior to having his meal, be administered a dose of one large bean with six ounces of hot water as a protection against the harm caused by the consumption of bad waters. *De antidotis* I.

(XXI.51) To heal the effect of poisons, one should take the theriac in a dose of one hazelnut mixed with three spoonfuls of wine. For other illnesses the dose is different, and the dose of the fluids to be mixed with it is different. Just as this electuary is beneficial for afflictions happening to the body, so too it is beneficial for afflictions of the soul and counteracts black bile itself; it removes its substance just as it removes the malignancy of animal poisons. It may be drunk for the bite of a mad dog, but it may also be dissolved in rose oil so that it becomes like a salve and applied on the wound externally. And then this electuary is sufficient for freeing people from the plague. *De theriaca ad Pisonem* [17].

(XXI.52) A skilled physician informed me that once a fatal pestilential disease occurred in Italy, and he recommended that the people take the theriac because no other drug was beneficial against this disease. And every one of those who suffered from this disease and who took the theriac benefited from it and was cured, but everyone who did not take it perished. And whoever took it before the illness affected him was saved from falling ill from it. This is not surprising since this drug is capable of counteracting poisons. In general, in whatever illness other drugs are ineffective, this drug is amazingly beneficial. *De theriaca ad Pamphilianum.*

(XXI.53) The snakes that are used for the preparation of the theriac are the least harmful types of vipers. But nevertheless, one should cut off the head because it contains the poison and the tail because it contains the wastes of their nourishment. *De theriaca ad Pisonem* [9].

(XXI.54) If those who are bitten by a crocodile put crocodile fat on the site of the bite, it heals immediately. I have seen that with my own eyes. And if in the case of a bite by a weasel, if one takes that animal and rubs the site of the bite with it, it heals immediately. The same applies to the bite of a viper: If one takes the viper, pounds it, and puts it on the site of the bite, it alleviates the pain little by little. *De theriaca ad Pisonem* [10].

(XXI.55) When you cook vipers, be careful to have only a charcoal fire beneath them. Add new salt and fresh dill, not dried, to them. *De theriaca ad Pisonem* [13].

(XXI.56) There are four tastes indicating heat:

1. Sweetness, which is the least warming, then
2. saltiness, then
3. bitterness, and then
4. sharpness, which is the strongest of them.

There are four tastes indicating coldness:

1. Tastelessness, which is the least cooling, then
2. sourness, then
3. astringency, then
4. acridity.

An oily taste indicates an intermediate quality between heat and cold and also indicates fineness of the substance. *De* [*simplicium*] *medicamentorum* [*temperamentis ac facultatibus*] IV.

(XXI.57) An astringent substance cools and dries and therefore draws together, compresses, contracts, pushes inwards, and thickens.

A sour substance cuts, separates, refines, opens, cleanses, cools, and repels.

A sharp substance cuts, separates, refines, opens and cleanses just like a sour substance, but it warms, attracts, dissolves, and burns.

A bitter substance opens and purifies the passages and cleanses, refines, and cuts the thick humors without notable heat.

A tasteless substance has the property to thicken, draw and bring together, mortify, and stupefy.

A salty substance collects, contracts, and dries the moisture without notable heat or cold.

A sweet substance slackens, concocts, softens, and rarefies.

An oily substance moistens, softens, and slackens. *De* [*simplicium*] *medicamentorum* [*temperamentis ac facultatibus*] V[.26].

(XXI.58) Some biting remedies have a heating effect just like the sharp and bitter remedies, and others have a cooling effect just as the sour remedies do. Biting includes these three tastes. Remedies are mostly dissimilar in their mixtures; an individual remedy consists of different ingredients, and therefore we find different flavors when we taste it. *De* [*simplicium*] *medicamentorum* [*temperamentis ac facultatibus*] IV[.7, 17].

(XXI.59) Anything that is clearly sharp and biting, according to its smell or taste or both, is hot and has cutting and refining power. Similarly, anything that has a pleasant smell, or that gives you the impression when you taste it that it is aromatic, has less heat than substances that bite. Anything that has an alkaline or salty taste—most of such ingredients have refining power and soften the stools. Bitter things also have a refining power not less than that of alkaline and salty things. *De victu attenuante* [3].

(XXI.60) All bitter substances not only have heating power, but also drying power. At times, some acrid, sharp substances have much moisture mixed with their heat. Therefore, we eat many things with these properties. *De* [*simplicium*] *medicamentorum* [*temperamentis ac facultatibus*] IV[.19].

(XXI.61) Drugs that cleanse without biting are similar to soup prepared from broad beans, barley gruel, roasted common flax seed, and thickened juice prepared from dried figs. Concentrated grape juice has relieving power and is nourishing. It is one of the least biting substances. Greater than the cleansing power of these substances is that of turpentine resin, frankincense, and skimmed honey. Even more cleansing power is found in meal of bitter vetch, Florentine iris roots, and sweet myrrh roots. [*De compositione medicamentorum secundum locos*] VII[.2].

(XXI.62) Drugs that really alleviate pains, whether the cause is a cold or hot humor or a cold or hot wind and whatever the consistency of the humor, are those drugs whose heat is like the heat of the body or that are hot in the first degree. In addition, their substance is so fine that it rarefies, refines, concocts, and evacuates the concocted material and expels it through the pores. Therefore, these drugs should not have any astringency at all. *De* [*simplicium*] *medicamentorum* [*temperamentis ac facultatibus*] V[.19].

(XXI.63) The temperament of the drug that helps against the development of pus and purulent matter is hot and moist, similar to the temperament of the body in which you want to concoct these matters. The most beneficial fomentation for this is lukewarm water and water mixed with oil. The most beneficial embrocation is lukewarm oil, and the most beneficial poultice is meal of wheat with water and oil. *De* [*simplicium*] *medicamentorum* [*temperamentis ac facultatibus*] V[.9].

(XXI.64) The physicians apply the name "softening remedy" to that which softens hard bodies whose hardness was caused by cold, especially if moisture is retained in these bodies, as in the case of a hard tumor. These remedies do not have a strong heating effect and do not have so much dryness that they dissolve and slowly disperse what has become hard. These kinds of remedies are always more heating than the temperament of the body from which the hardness is to be dissolved. Examples of such remedies are gum ammoniac, bdellium, liquid and solid styrax, and some types of marrow and fat. *De* [*simplicium*] *medicamentorum* [*temperamentis ac facultatibus*] V[.5.8].

(XXI.65) All strong diuretics, such as the seeds of the different types of celery, have a strong heating effect, as well as the seeds of fennel, wild carrot, Massilian hartwort, valerian, wild dill, sweet flag and asarabacca. Stone-crushing remedies should have only a little heat so that they cut the stones by their fineness but do not make them more solid or dry them by their severe heat. Examples of such remedies are root of asparagus, root of blackberry, felty germander, Jews' stone, burned glass, and sea squill vinegar. *De* [*simplicium*] *medicamentorum* [*temperamentis ac facultatibus*] V[.13].

(XXI.66) Drugs that stimulate the development of milk, menstruation, and micturition are all of them hot but differ in the degree of heat and the quality of their dryness because the type of drugs that do not dry and moderately heat stimulate the development of milk. And the type of drugs that have a stronger heating effect but not a strong drying effect stimulate menstruation. Both these types of drugs also stimulate micturition, and the type that has an even stronger heating effect than these and dries as well is also a stronger diuretic but does not stimulate menstruation nor the development of milk. Therefore, this last type alone is called "diuretic." *De* [*simplicium*] *medicamentorum* [*temperamentis ac facultatibus*] V[.22].

(XXI.67) Says Moses: If someone makes himself remember that which is not necessary to remember, it causes a deficient remembrance even of the things that should be remembered. Therefore, I advise remembering only the natures of the drugs that are often used in any place, whose names are well known, and that are employed internally. I rely in all this on the book on drugs composed by Ibn Wāfid [*Kitāb al-Adwiya al-mufrada*] because he is known for his skill and for his correct quotations from Galen and others. For some mineral drugs, I rely upon Ibn Sīnā [*Kitāb al-qānūn fī al-ṭibb*].

(XXI.68) Of the drugs that are intermediate between heat and cold, three of them are dry in the second degree: Namely,

1. *utrujj* (citron or lemon) peel,
2. mace, and
3. lentils.

And three of them are dry in the first degree: Namely,

1. maidenhair fern,
2. asparagus, and
3. olive oil.

And three are moist in the first degree:

1. sebesten (Assyrian plum),
2. manna,
3. purging cassia.

Gold is intermediate between these two opposites and is refining. In total there are ten.

(XXI.69) There are twenty-seven drugs that are hot in the first degree and dry in the first degree and that are commonly used:

1. Rice,
2. sarcocolla,
3. French lavender,
4. melilot,
5. camel grass,
6. *bābūnaj* (German or Roman camomile),
7. lemon balm,
8. silk,
9. French tamarisk,
10. cabbage,
11. cauliflower,
12. coriander,
13. *lablāb* (common ivy or field bindweed),
14. sugar,
15. Mediterranean cypress,
16. resin of the arar tree,
17. senna,
18. pistachio nuts,
19. common madder,
20. black cardamom,
21. white lupine,
22. common marshmallow,
23. dates,
24. common agrimony,
25. agarikon,
26. Jews' stone, and
27. corundum.

(XXI.70) There are eight commonly used drugs that are hot in the first degree and dry in the second degree: Namely,

1. absinth wormwood,
2. bitter vetch,
3. dodder,
4. spikenard,
5. male fern,

6. peony,
7. common fumitory, and
8. bush basil.

(XXI.71) There are seven drugs that are hot in the first degree and intermediate between dryness and moisture or minimally dry: Namely,

1. flax seed,
2. wheat,
3. labdanum,
4. Mahaleb cherry,
5. manna,
6. liquid or solid styrax, and
7. pine nut.

(XXI.72) There are nine commonly used drugs that are hot and moist in the first degree: Namely,

1. chickpeas,
2. black-eyed peas,
3. almonds,
4. borage,
5. bananas,
6. nalta jute,
7. sesame,
8. common jujube, and
9. sekakul parsnip.

(XXI.73) There are thirty-two commonly used drugs that are cold and dry in the first degree and are frequently used: Namely,

1. myrtle,
2. usnea cartilage lichen,
3. Senegal gum,
4. emblic myrobalan,
5. yellow (citrine) myrobalan,
6. Indian and
7. chebulic myrobalan,
8. field eryngo,
9. broad beans,
10. acorn,
11. sweet chestnut,
12. soldier thistle,

13. coral,
14. roses,
15. common medlar,
16. common sorrel, which is the same as wild beetroot,
17. caltrop,
18. pear,
19. meadow salsify,
20. *māsh* (mung bean or black gram),
21. *nabiq* (the fruit of Christ's thorn jujube),
22. blackberry,
23. barley,
24. thistle,
25. mulberry,
26. apple,
27. quince,
28. sour pomegranate,
39. vinegar,
30. carob, and
31. Egyptian willow (*khilāf*), which is identical with
32. *al-ṣafṣāf* (silver willow).

(XXI.74) There are ten drugs that are cold and moist in the first degree: Namely,
1. plum,
2. spinach,
3. violets,
4. *hindibāʾ* (endive or chicory),
5. *nīlūfar* (blue Egyptian, European white, or yellow water lily),
6. cherry,
7. garden orach,
8. beetroot,
9. mallow, and
10. licorice.

Licorice is lukewarm and slightly colder than our bodies; it is also moderately moist; its most beneficial part is the juice from its root.

(XXI.75) There are thirty-four commonly used drugs, which are hot and dry in the second degree: Namely,
1. Roman nettle,
2. *faranjamushk* (possibly sweet or wild basil), which is the same as *al-rayḥān al-qaranfulī*,

3. turpentine tree,
4. balsam of Mecca,
5. nutmeg,
6. felty germander,
7. birthwort,
8. bitter ginger,
9. bitumen of Judea (*kufr al-yahūd*), which is the same as *al-ḥumar*,
10. lac dye,
11. turnip,
12. mastic,
13. musk,
14. ambergris,
15. agarwood,
16. *falanja*,
17. rhubarb,
18. *yāsamīn* (white or Arabian jasmine),
19. dog rose,
20. narcissus,
21. *khīrī* (wallflower or hoary stock),
22. *sqūlūfandriyūn* (rusty-back or hart's-tongue fern), which is the same as *al-ʿuqruhān*,
23. autumn crocus,
24. white horehound,
25. aloe,
26. safflower seed,
27. honey,
28. hazelnut,
29. wild carrot,
30. borax,
31. lapis lazuli,
32. green vitriol,
33. salt, and
34. rennet.

(XXI.76) There are six drugs that are hot in the second degree and dry in the first or in the beginning of the second degree: Namely,

1. the edible nut (walnut),
2. saffron,
3. fenugreek,
4. frankincense,

5. Florentine iris, and
6. dried figs.

(XXI.77) There are six drugs that are cold and dry in the second degree: Namely,
1. behen (white behen or red behen, possibly Mediterranean sea lavender),
2. garden rocket,
3. wild senna seed,
4. fruit of the ash tree,
5. *mughādh* (moghat), which is the same as *mughāth*, and
6. coconut.

(XXI.78) There are twelve drugs that are cold and dry in the second degree: Namely,
1. barberry,
2. pomegranate blossom,
3. gum tragacanth,
4. broadleaf plantain,
5. *māmīthā* (blackspot or yellow hornpoppy),
6. tanner's sumach,
7. boxthorn,
8. gallnut,
9. black nightshade,
10. gum Arabic,
11. Syrian rhubarb, and
12. fleawort seed.

The latter is intermediate between moisture and dryness.

(XXI.79) There are eleven drugs that are cold and moist in the second degree: Namely,
1. purple amaranth,
2. *biṭṭīkh* (common melon or watermelon),
3. cucumber,
4. the smaller variety of cucumber,
5. *dullāʿ* (common melon or watermelon),
6. common duckweed,
7. truffles,
8. apricot,
9. *qarʿ* (field pumpkin or winter squash),
10. cultivated lettuce, and
11. peach.

(XXI.80) There are sixty-two commonly used drugs that are hot and dry in the third degree: Namely,

1. asafetida,
2. opopanax,
3. gum ammoniac,
4. bdellium,
5. sagapenum,
6. scammony,
7. galbanum,
8. anise,
9. Syrian rue,
10. cumin,
11. caraway,
12. fennel,
13. dill,
14. black cumin,
15. mugwort,
16. garlic,
17. oregano,
18. mint,
19. radish,
20. sea squill,
21. common rue,
22. white horehound,
23. capers,
24. celery,
25. amber, which is dry in the first degree and Ibn Sīnā says that it is also hot in the first degree,
26. *nānakhwāh* (bisnaga or ajowan),
27. savin juniper,
28. wild carrot,
29. sweet flag,
30. dodder,
31. common polypody,
32. stavesacre,
33. colocynth,
34. ivy-leaded morning glory,
35. St. Thomas lidpod,
36. hellebore,
37. great yellow gentian,

38. *hayūfārīqūn* (bearded or perforate St. John's wort),
39. myrrh,
40. bay laurel,
41. ben seed,
42. asarabacca,
43. hyssop,
44. globe artichoke,
45. turmeric,
46. greater celandine,
47. common centaury,
48. common cardamom,
49. *mūmiyā* (bitumen),
50. cinnamon,
51. *zarnab*, and some say that it is the same as *al-falanja*,
52. glossy forest grape (*ḥamāmā*),
53. *ḥāshā* (lesser calamint or creeping thyme),
54. Chinese cinnamon,
55. costus,
56. clove,
57. greater galangal,
58. great false leopardbane,
59. cubeb,
60. mint,
61. broad-leaved thyme,
62. and castoreum.

The latter is dry in the second degree.

(XXI.81) There are two drugs that are hot and moist in the third degree: Namely,

1. ginger and
2. large elecampane.

(XXI.82) There are two drugs that are hot in the third degree and moist in the first degree: Namely,

1. earth almonds (*ḥabb al-zalam*), which are also called *fulful al-sudān* (Sudanese pepper),
2. thapsia, which is the same as *al-yantūn*.

(XXI.83) There are nine drugs that are cold and dry in the third degree: Namely,

1. poison hemlock,
2. black henbane,

3. mandrake,
4. camphor,
5. tabasheer (a white substance obtained from the nodal joints of bamboo),
6. betel nut,
7. sandalwood,
8. tamarind, and
9. dragon's blood (*dam al-akhawayn*), which is called *al-qāṭir* and also *al-shayyān*.

(XXI.84) There are four drugs that are cold and moist in the third degree: Namely,

1. common purslane,
2. *ḥayy al-ʿālam* (common houseleek or tree aeonium),
3. fungi,
4. common knotgrass (*ʿaṣā al-rāʿī*), which is called *al-qaḍāb* in Egypt—it has a restraining effect that is good for inflammations and stops bleeding.

(XXI.85) There are fourteen commonly used drugs that are hot and dry in the fourth degree: Namely,

1. pepper and
2. long pepper, which is less dry than pepper,
3. mustard,
4. pellitory,
5. marking nut,
6. *kundus* (sneezewort, gysophila, or soapwort),
7. February daphne,
8. pepperwort,
9. garden cress,
10. caper spurge,
11. cocculus indicus,
12. resin spurge (*farbiyūn*), which is the same as *al-tākūt*,
13. leek, which has varieties, and
14. onion, which has varieties that contain moisture.

(XXI.86) Opium poppy is cold and dry in the fourth degree. The total number of drugs whose degrees should be remembered because of their frequent use is 265.

(XXI.87) Amongst the drugs that are not taken internally but that are commonly used externally, there are four that are intermediate between heat and cold:

1. Wax,
2. litharge,
3. cadmia, and
4. *ḥuḍaḍ* (Mediterranean or rock buckthorn) juice;

except that cadmia and *ḥuḍaḍ* juice are drying in the second degree, litharge only dries slightly, and wax is also intermediate between moisture and dryness.

Some of these drugs (those commonly used externally) are cold in the first degree and dry in the second degree: Namely,

1. antimony,
2. henna, and
3. tutty.

And some of these drugs are cold and dry in the second degree: Namely,

1. ceruse and
2. the different kinds of earth.

Lead is cold and moist in the second degree. The total number of these drugs is ten.

(XXI.88) There are six drugs that are not taken internally and that are hot and dry in the third degree: Namely,

1. pitch,
2. pine tree resin, and
3. vitriol in its different types.

Sometimes they are used internally in a small amount. Further,

4. arsenic with its types,
5. sal ammoniac, and
6. burned copper.

Sometimes these too are used internally in a small amount.

(XXI.89) Four of these drugs that are not taken internally are hot and dry in the fourth degree: Namely,

1. verdigris,
2. sulfur,
3. tar, which is sometimes used internally in a small amount, and
4. animal biles.

The total number of externally used drugs whose degrees should be remembered is twenty.

(XXI.90) The color of natural bile is yellow, and this should be used in medical practice. Green bile is less hot because the cause of its greenness is the dominance of moisture over it. If yellow bile is burned, its color turns black. *De* [*simplicium*] *medicamentorum* [*temperamentis ac facultatibus*] X[.2].

(XXI.91) The bile of a bull is stronger than that of any other land animal. Next in strength is the bile of a bear, and after a bear the bile of a goat, and after a goat the bile of a sheep, and after a sheep the bile of a pig. Therefore, the strength of the pig's bile is extremely weak. *De* [*simplicium*] *medicamentorum* [*temperamentis ac facultatibus*] X[.2].

The biles of all birds are sharp, biting, dry, and strong. The bile of chickens and cocks is stronger and more proper in medical practice. *De* [*simplicium*] *medicamentorum* [*temperamentis ac facultatibus*] X[.2].

(XXI.92) I know from experience that when olive oil is applied to the body while the oil is cold, it adheres to it and obstructs its pores, but when it is applied while it is hot, it dissolves residues from the body. *De methodo* [*medendi*] VI[.2].

(XXI.93) If a wax salve that has been prepared with three parts of rose oil and one part of wax is softened with cold water and a little bit of vinegar and is actually made cold, it cools and moistens the bodily part one wants to cool. If it becomes hot while on the body, it should be replaced by another one. Similarly, if a *dabīqī* cloth is moistened with cold juices that have been mixed with *sawīq* (semolina) of barley and vinegar and placed on the bodily parts, it cools them. *De methodo* [*medendi*] X[.4].

(XXI.94) Pains of the eyes and ears caused by such a thick and cold humor and by flatulent wind during fevers should be soothed by applying a hot compress with millet because it is a very light substance and, moreover, drying, while the vapor developing therefrom is neither biting nor harmful. *De methodo* [*medendi*] XII[.8].

(XXI.95) A poultice prepared from wheat meal and moderately cooked in water and oil promotes a quicker suppuration than a poultice prepared from bread. One prepared from bread that was very well cooked after having been soaked in water and oil is more effective in reducing an inflammation because of the salt and yeast in the bread. Even more effective than the latter in preventing suppuration is a poultice prepared from barley meal cooked in water in which root of common marshmallow had been cooked. Hereafter this water was, together with oil, poured over the barley meal and very well cooked. *Ad Glauconem* [*de medendi methodo*] II[.9].

(XXI.96) Al-Tamīmī says in his *Kitāb Al-Murshid* [*fī jawāhir al-aghdhiya wa-quwā l-mufradāt mina l-adwiya*]: Juice of the large elecampane in bees' honey prepared with spices and musk, which is called "the potion of angels," is beneficial for old people and for those suffering from superfluous moisture. It dissolves their superfluous moistures, it is beneficial for pains in the joints caused by cold, it strengthens the stomach and the heart, whets the appetite, and stimulates the libido. He further remarks there that Chinese cinnamon neutralizes the poison of the scorpion and of snakes and clearly helps against these, and that it strengthens the uterus of women if they apply it as a suppository or if they take a sitz bath with it. He also states there that *ungues odorati* (opercula) are beneficial for hysterical suffocation and epilepsy both as a fumigation and as a drink in a dose of a *mithqāl* mixed with apple juice. Similarly, quince juice mixed with musk is extremely beneficial for hysterical suffocation and for palpitation.

This is the end of the twenty-first treatise,
by the grace of God,
praise be to Him.

In the name of God,
the Merciful, the Compassionate.
O Lord, make our task easy.

The Twenty-Second Treatise

Containing aphorisms concerning the specific properties of remedies

(XXII.1) We find medicines that are effective through their powers, and we find other medicines that are effective through their total substance, as I will describe now. *De theriaca ad Pisonem* [4].

(XXII.2) Mouse heads, burned and kneaded with honey, and rubbed on the spot affected by alopecia, stimulate hair growth. Similarly, mouse excrement, if pulverized in vinegar, is beneficial for alopecia. Viper skin is also good for alopecia, if it is grounded with honey. *De theriaca ad Pisonem* [9].

(XXII.3) If the brain of a camel is dried and imbibed with vinegar, it is beneficial for epilepsy. The brain of a weasel has a similar effect. [*De theriaca ad Pisonem* 9].

(XXII.4) The brain of a bat with honey is beneficial for a cataract. The brain of a sheep has a similar effect. [*De theriaca ad Pisonem* 9].

(XXII.5) The gall of a female hyena, if mixed with honey and applied as an eye salve, is beneficial for a cataract. If a falcon is cooked in Florentine iris oil, it is good for weak vision. [*De theriaca ad Pisonem* 9].

(XXII.6) If one rubs the gums of children with the brain of a sheep, it eases the growth of the teeth without pain. [*De theriaca ad Pisonem* 9].

(XXII.7) If the horn of a stag is burned and pulverized with wine, it is beneficial for pain and weakness of the teeth. The anklebone of a cow, if burned and pulverized with wine, is good for pain and weakness of the teeth. [*De theriaca ad Pisonem* 9].

(XXII.8) If one drinks the filings of the horn of a bull with water, it stops a nosebleed. Its thighbones have a similar effect. [*De theriaca ad Pisonem* 9].

(XXII.9) Shrimp empty the body of tapeworms. Similarly, the anklebone of a cow, if burned and drunk with honey, evacuates tapeworms from the belly. [*De theriaca ad Pisonem* 9].

(XXII.10) Excrements of a mouse crumble bladder stones. Similarly, a scorpion—if eaten with bread—crumbles bladder stones. Earthworms have the same effect. [*De theriaca ad Pisonem* 9].

(XXII.11) If earthworms are pulverized and administered to a jaundice patient, his body will be cleansed immediately. [*De theriaca ad Pisonem* 9].

(XXII.12) If dung beetles are boiled in olive oil and that oil is dripped into the ear, it will alleviate the pain immediately. [*De theriaca ad Pisonem* 9].

(XXII.13) If the anklebone of a cow is burned and imbibed with oxymel, it reduces the swelling of the spleen; it also stimulates the libido. [*De theriaca ad Pisonem* 9].

(XXII.14) If goose fat is melted in rose oil, it is beneficial for inflamed tumors. [*De theriaca ad Pisonem* 9].

(XXII.15) The burned skin of a hippopotamus is beneficial for hard tumors. If a river crab is pulverized and put on a hard tumor, it dispels the tumor. [*De theriaca ad Pisonem* 9].

(XXII.16) Milk of a cow is clearly beneficial for intestinal ulcers. Castoreum is clearly beneficial for shivers. [*De theriaca ad Pisonem* 9].

If crocodile fat is put on the spot of its bite, it heals immediately. Similarly, if one takes a weasel and rubs it on the spot of its bite, it is healed immediately. And if one takes a viper, pulverizes it and puts it on the spot of its bite, this remedy somewhat alleviates the pain. [*De theriaca ad Pisonem* 9].

(XXII.17) If one heats the marcasite stone and sprinkles vinegar on it and then places the limb that has a hard tumor above the vapor that arises from it, you will see it dissolve in an amazing way, as if it is an act of magic. *Ad Glauconem* [*de medendi methodo*] II[.6].

(XXII.18) If peony root is tied with something and hung on the neck of children suffering from epilepsy, it cures them. I have tested and tried this and found a similar effect. [*De simplicium medicamentorum temperamentis ac facultatibus* VI.10].

(XXII.19) Asafetida is beneficial for a swollen uvula in the same way. Similarly, roasted black cumin, if it is tied with a finely woven cloth and then its hot vapor is inhaled, will dry up the rheum of someone suffering from it. Similarly, if one takes some of the threads that were dyed with purple hailing from the purple-fish, and that were used for choking a viper, and wraps them around the neck of someone who suffers from an inflammation of the tonsils or from any other inflammation in the throat, you see that it is beneficial for it in an amazing way. *De* [*simplicium*] *medicamentorum* [*temperamentis ac facultatibus*] VI[.10].

(XXII.20) Excrements of a dog that has been nourished with bones—namely, those excrements that appear white and dry and free from stench—should be dried and pulverized and then given as a drink to patients suffering from angina and inflammation of the throat, together with another medicine beneficial for this disease. It may also be given as a drink to those suffering from dysentery, in milk that was boiled with red hot stones or iron. Inveterate ulcers can also be treated with it if it is mixed with some other medicine that is good for this. It may also be mixed with medications that dissolve tumors. *De* [*simplicium*] *medicamentorum* [*temperamentis ac facultatibus*] X[.2].

(XXII.21) A child suffering from an inflammation of the throat should be treated for three days with a diet of oven bread and white lupine and should be given slightly diluted wine to drink and should beware of indigestions. On the third day one should take his stool, dry it, pulverize it, knead it with honey, and smear it on the throat of the child that suffers from such an inflammation of the throat that it endangers his life. *De* [*simplicium*] *medicamentorum* [*temperamentis ac facultatibus*] X[.2].

(XXII.22) If the excrements of a wolf that is nourished with bones—that is, white excrements—are given as a drink to someone afflicted by the pain of a colic, the pain will subside. Sometimes it prevents a colic before it actually occurs, and it does not occur in someone who is used to taking this remedy or the attack is milder than usual. The excrements may also be hung on the neck of someone suffering from a colic, for this brings clear benefit. *De* [*simplicium*] *medicamentorum* [*temperamentis ac facultatibus*] X[.2].

(XXII.23) The excrements of a goat mixed with barley meal and kneaded with vinegar dissolve hard tumors, tumors of the knee and spleen. Do not use this therapy for those with a soft body, like women, children, and eunuchs.

(XXII.24) If dung of a cow is smeared on dropsy patients, it is of great benefit to them. If it is kneaded with vinegar, it dissolves hard tumors. *De* [*simplicium*] *medicamentorum* [*temperamentis ac facultatibus*] X[.2].

(XXII.25) Sheep excrement, dried and kneaded with vinegar, heals warts, fleshy excrescences, ulcers that develop from burning with fire, and shingles in which one has the sensation of crawling ants. *De* [*simplicium*] *medicamentorum* [*temperamentis ac facultatibus*] X[.2].

(XXII.26) Pigeon dung should be pulverized, filtered, and smeared on chronically painful limbs that one wants to heat. Similarly, it is good as a cataplasm for chronic cold pains, such as podagra, migraine, headache, pain in the back, abdomen, kidneys, and joints. *De* [*simplicium*] *medicamentorum* [*temperamentis ac facultatibus*] X[.2].

(XXII.27) I know someone in our times who treated patients by giving them burned human bones to drink without informing them about this, lest they turn away from taking it. This man used to cure with these burned bones many patients suffering from epilepsy and pain in the joints. *De* [*simplicium*] *medicamentorum* [*temperamentis ac facultatibus* XI.1].

(XXII.28) If chicken dung is pulverized and given as a drink with vinegar to someone who chokes by the consumption of fungi, he will vomit thick, viscous humors and be healed. *De* [*simplicium*] *medicamentorum* [*temperamentis ac facultatibus*] X[.2].

(XXII.29) If one burns river crabs alive in a red copper pot, takes one part of their ashes, half a part of great yellow gentian, and one tenth of frankincense, and from this mixture sprinkles a large spoonful on water and gives it to someone bitten by a dog, it is of amazing benefit. Similarly, the ashes of these river crabs alone are very beneficial for such persons, but not the ashes of sea crabs. *De* [*simplicium*] *medicamentorum* [*temperamentis ac facultatibus* XI.1].

(XXII.30) The lung of a fox, if dried and imbibed, cures asthma. *De* [*simplicium*] *medicamentorum* [*temperamentis ac facultatibus* XI.1].

(XXII.31) If one constantly drinks the broth [prepared] from larks and eats their flesh, it cures a colic. *De* [*simplicium*] *medicamentorum* [*temperamentis ac facultatibus* XI.1].

(XXII.32) If earthworms—that is, the long worms that can be found in the earth when one digs or ploughs in it—are pulverized and put on nerves that have been cut off, they immediately provide an amazing benefit. If one drinks them together with concentrated grape juice, they also stimulate micturition. *De* [*simplicium*] *medicamentorum* [*temperamentis ac facultatibus* XI.1].

(XXII.33) Vinegar has a specific property that distinguishes it from other similar substances, namely, that next to its cutting effect it dissolves and at the same time checks the dissolution process. This is because its nature is partially hot, but only in a small insignificant quantity, while most of its nature is cold and fine. [*De compositione medicamentorum secundum locos*] I[.8].

(XXII.34) The spleen of a wild donkey or the spleen of a wild horse should be dried and pulverized and given as a drink to those suffering from a spleen disease in a dose of six *dirhams* with five ounces of diluted wine. [*De compositione medicamentorum secundum locos*] IX[.2].

(XXII.35) Abū Marwān ibn Zuhr has mentioned many specific properties of remedies that he tested. He was one of the great empiricists. His son told me amazing things about his precision and diligence in matters depending upon experience. Therefore, I thought it a good thing to mention them in his name, although some of them have been mentioned by others before. However, he is the one who verified these experiential matters. All those special properties are mentioned by him in his *Kitāb al-Taysīr* [*fī l-mudāwāt wa-l-tadbīr*] (*Book on the Facilitation of Treatment and Diet*) and in the *Kitāb al-Aghdhiya* (*Book on Foodstuffs*), which he composed for one of the Andalusian kings. His father, Abū l-ʿAlāʾ, mentions some of these remedies in his book entitled *al-Tadhkira*. These are the following:

(XXII.36) The ingestion of nine granules of emerald, pulverized and filtered, in a mouthful of water on an empty stomach stops the diarrhea caused by poisons. If it is hung around the neck of someone suffering from diarrhea or lientery, it cures him. If the emerald is hung around the neck, it strengthens the stomach and is beneficial for epilepsy. If it is kept in the mouth, it strengthens the teeth and the stomach, and if one puts it on as a ring, it strengthens the cardia of the stomach and stops emesis and brings the person around. The criteria for the application of the emerald are the same as those for the theriac. It should not be taken together with food, but there should be an interval of nine hours between them. [*Kitāb al-Taysīr fī l-mudāwāt wa-l-tadbīr*].

(XXII.37) Looking in the eyes of a wild ass gives a lasting healthy vision and is beneficial for the formation of a cataract. He says: This is true without any doubt. [*Kitāb al-Taysīr fī l-mudāwāt wa-l-tadbīr*].

(XXII.38) The consumption of the heads of hares, as much as one is able to eat them, is beneficial for trembling. I found by experience that it is also beneficial for numbness and hemiplegia. The consumption of hare meat crumbles kidney stones. [*Kitāb al-Taysīr fī l-mudāwāt wa-l-tadbīr*].

(XXII.39) I found by experience that the drinking of water in which mastic has been cooked protects against diseases of the liver and stomach, and that the drinking of water in which *biṭṭīkh* (common melon or watermelon) seed has been cooked protects against kidney stones, and that the anointment of the eyelids with gold strengthens vision, and that if one cooks therewith or throws some of it into a cooked dish, it strengthens the body in general. I also found by experience that the application of a poultice of fresh rose blossoms to the eyes protects against ophthalmia. [*Kitāb al-Taysīr fī l-mudāwāt wa-l-tadbīr*].

(XXII.40) The anointment of the eyelids with rose syrup made with sugar strengthens vision. Its permanent use cures dilatation of the palpebral membrane. This has been verified by experience; I have not ceased to use it for strengthening vision. I have found that pulverized and filtered clove, sprinkled every night on the forehead during winter, protects against catarrhs, while mace is of a similar effect in all the seasons of the year. But the different kinds of mint are less beneficial than clove, and similarly *utrujj* (citron or lemon) peel is less beneficial than mace. [*Kitāb al-Taysīr fī l-mudāwāt wa-l-tadbīr*].

(XXII.41) Constant anointing of the spine of the back with sweet almond oil, lukewarm, protects against the bending of the body that occurs to the elderly. It has been verified by experience that the consumption of turnip, boiled, sharpens vision. [*Kitāb al-Taysīr fī l-mudāwāt wa-l-tadbīr*].

(XXII.42) The consumption of the heads of sparrows and especially the male ones, and similarly the consumption of turnips cooked either in meat or alone, and similarly the consumption of wild carrots, and similarly the consumption of young pigeons that are able to fly, and similarly the ingestion of juice of chickpeas—each of these substances on its own is good for strengthening the lust for sexual intercourse, let alone when they are eaten together in one dish. [*Kitāb al-Taysīr fī l-mudāwāt wa-l-tadbīr*].

(XXII.43) The consumption of male domestic pigeons cures hemiplegia, paralysis, numbness, apoplexy, and trembling. The inhalation of the odorous breath of pigeons and the inhalation of that which dissolves from their bodies into the air protects against all these diseases, and washing the bottom after defecation with lukewarm sweet water protects against hemorrhoids. [*Kitāb al-Taysīr fī l-mudāwāt wa-l-tadbīr*].

(XXII.44) The wearing of hare furs strengthens the bodies of old and young people, and the wearing of lambskin strengthens the bodies of children. The proximity to cats causes marasmus and phthisis. [*Kitāb al-Taysīr fī l-mudāwāt wa-l-tadbīr*].

(XXII.45) The consumption of radish and cabbage eliminates hoarseness and the consumption of roasted quince after meals gives energy and joy. The consumption of lemon peel strengthens the heart, and its seeds are beneficial against poisons. Lemon peel is also beneficial against poisons, as are the leaves of its tree. [*Kitāb al-Taysīr fī l-mudāwāt wa-l-tadbīr*].

(XXII.46) The consumption of *al-murrī al-naqīʿ* and vinegar removes the causes for the development of worms in the abdomen. The consumption of peaches, in spite of their harmful effects, is beneficial against vapor [arising] from the stomach. Similarly, field eryngo has about the same effect. [*Kitāb al-Taysīr fī l-mudāwāt wa-l-tadbīr*].

The smelling of peaches brings someone around, and the drinking of the juice of their leaves kills worms. [*Kitāb al-Aghdhiya*].

(XXII.47) If mustard oil is dripped into a deaf ear, hearing returns, and the immersion in lukewarm olive oil is beneficial for all pains of the body. [*Kitāb al-Taysīr fī l-mudāwāt wa-l-tadbīr*].

(XXII.48) If the inner coat of the stomach of the male bustard is dried and mixed with collyria, it has the specific property of being beneficial against a cataract. The coat of the stomach of the ostrich has the specific property, if one takes thereof, of being beneficial for those suffering from a stomach disease and for crumbling kidney stones. [*Kitāb al-Aghdhiya*].

(XXII.49) Young hawks and falcons have a delicious taste and strengthen the soul and have the specific property of being beneficial against hypochondriac melancholy and other corruptions of the mind. [*Kitāb al-Aghdhiya*].

(XXII.50) If the penis is rubbed with hedgehog fat, it gives a strong erection and provides increased pleasure during the sexual intercourse. If the penis of a hedgehog is dried, pulverized, and ingested, it gives a strong erection. The penis of a male deer has a similar effect if dried, pulverized, and ingested by its specific property. [*Kitāb al-Aghdhiya*].

(XXII.51) Common jujube has the specific property of being beneficial for diseases of the lung, esophagus, chest, and urinary bladder; it is moist and tends slightly towards heat. [*Kitāb al-Aghdhiya*].

(XXII.52) The acidic inner part of the *utrujj* (citron or lemon) eliminates thirst, vigorously subdues yellow bile, and strengthens the soul. Chebulic myrobalan has the specific property of being beneficial for the stomach. The drinking of half a *dirham* of balsam of Mecca counteracts all poisons. [*Kitāb al-Aghdhiya*].

(XXII.53) If a carnelian is pulverized and the teeth are rubbed with it, it makes them white and prevents their corrosion. [*Kitāb al-Taysīr fī l-mudāwāt wa-l-tadbīr*].

(XXII.54) Broad beans have the specific property of corrupting the mind. Milk has the specific property of being harmful for the brain. Aloe has the specific property of being harmful for the anus. Colocynth has the specific property of being harmful for the liver. Figs have the specific property of producing lice. The true service tree has the specific property of being beneficial for weakness of the liver. [*Kitāb al-Tadhkira*].

(XXII.55) Almonds have the specific property of preserving the substance of the brain, while their moisture preserves the organs in an amazing way, without producing abnormal moisture. Rose jam has the special property to strengthen the lungs. [*Kitāb al-Tadhkira*].

(XXII.56) Agarwood has the specific property of being beneficial for the stomach and of strengthening it, and it eliminates a bad smell from the mouth. Artichoke perfumes winds and breath from the body. Smelling narcissus eliminates children's epilepsy. [*Kitāb al-Tadhkira*].

Its smell has the same effect as that which Galen attributes to peony. [*De simplicium medicamentorum temperamentis ac facultatibus* VI.2]. This is the end of the words of Ibn Zuhr.

(XXII.57) From the words of al-Tamīmī on the specific properties of drugs: He said: If one drinks a decoction of black chickpeas with bees' honey for three consecutive days, it cures the severe pain caused by gout. Opium poppy prevents a defluxion of superfluous matter, whether warm or cold. Common purslane stops the craving for clay.

(XXII.58) He further said: Hemp oil has the specific property of being beneficial for earaches caused by cold and cures chronic illnesses of the ear and dissolves its obstructions. If beef is boiled with vinegar, it has the specific property of being beneficial for jaundice, of expelling yellow bile, and of stopping diarrhea of bilious matter.

(XXII.59) Hedgehog meat, if dried and imbibed in oxymel, is beneficial for pains in the kidneys, elephantiasis, and dropsy of the flesh (anasarca). If children feed themselves with its flesh, it is beneficial for them against epilepsy and bedwetting.

(XXII.60) He further said: Cowries or tellin shells, if burned and ingested in a dose of two *dirhams* with an astringent beverage, are beneficial for intestinal ulcers and dysentery. They also have a strong effect in reducing anal prolapse, if sprinkled thereon, it recedes.

(XXII.61) He further said: If one cooks an egg in vinegar, removes the yolk therefrom, and then seasons it with gallnuts, tanner's sumach, and a little bit of salt and eats it, it is beneficial for severe diarrhea and intestinal ulcers. If garden rocket seed is pulverized and put into soft-boiled eggs with a little bit of salted skink and then sipped, it increases the sperm and greatly strengthens the erection.

(XXII.62) He further said: If one takes one part of the flour of dried arum root and three parts of white flour and pounds all this with sesame oil and kneads it with yeast and salt and makes a bread from it and dries this bread and pulverizes it and takes ten *dirhams* therefrom every morning with a spiced honey drink, it stops and eliminates hemorrhoids within three days. Its benefit against external and internal winds is clear and manifest.

(XXII.63) He further said: If one takes the resin of the olive tree and of Socotra aloe and kneads this with the juice from peach leaves and makes suppositories from this, it cures chronic fistulas, especially those surrounding the anus.

(XXII.64) He further said: Juice from the leaves of the sour apple tree averts the harm caused by fatal poisons and by the bite and sting of all vermin. If one takes three *dirhams* of the leaves of the sour apple tree—once they have been dried—and drinks it with three ounces of sour apple juice, one is saved from the poison of a viper bite, and is healed therefrom.

(XXII.65) He said: The blossoms of the true service tree arouse women to desire sexual intercourse to a point that what happens to cats happens to them, namely, that they scream with joy, even when only smelling this blossom.

(XXII.66) He further said: Greater galangal has the specific property of being beneficial for internal hemorrhoids, especially if it is imbibed together with *dādhī* (bearded or perforate St. John's wort). Similarly, usnea cartilage lichen is beneficial for palpitation caused by black bile. Women should sit in a decoction prepared therefrom for uterine diseases. Common galingale has the specific property of liquefying, dissolving, and crumbling kidney stones, and it stimulates micturition.

(XXII.67) He further said: Autumn crocus dissolves inflammations from gout when applied as a salve through its specific property. It also has the specific property of being beneficial for hemorrhoids if half a *dirham* of it is kneaded with butter of a cow; if it is applied as a suppository in cotton for two nights, one does not need a third night.

(XXII.68) He further said: If one extinguishes the heat of gold in vinegar for some time and then rinses one's mouth with that vinegar, it removes any fetid odor from the mouth and improves the smell of the breath. It has the same effect if it is kept in the mouth.

(XXII.69) He also said: If kidney and bladder stones are burned and used as an eye powder, it cleanses a leucoma, whether it is old or recent. Sherds of transparent white Chinese earthenware, burned and mixed with one of the cleansing drugs, have the same effect.

(XXII.70) He further said: If quartz is burned, pulverized, washed, and imbibed in a dose of one ounce with two *mithqāls* of the milk of a donkey, it is beneficial for trembling, tremor, and phthisis. If a salve therefrom prepared with water is put on the breast, it makes the milk flow. It also cleanses a leucoma. It has all these effects because of its specific property.

This is the end of the twenty-second treatise,
by the grace of God,
praise be to Him.

In the name of God,
the Merciful, the Compassionate.
O Lord, make our task easy.

The Twenty-Third Treatise

Containing aphorisms concerning the differences between well-known diseases and the elucidation of technical terms that are well known to the physicians but whose exact meanings are sometimes unknown to them

(XXIII.1) Overfilling in relation to the vessels means that the blood is markedly increased in quantity but that its quality is good according to its nature. Overfilling in relation to strength means that the quality of the blood has changed either into sharpness and has become biting or into crude, raw humors; even if its quantity is small but the strength of the surrounding organ is weak, it is burdensome to the strength. This matter is repeated in several books. It also features in Galen's *De* [*curandi ratione per*] *venae sectione*[*m* 4, 6, 7, 8] and in his *De plenitudine* [8, 10, 11].

(XXIII.2) It is impossible that the vessels should always contain absolutely pure blood to the point that it is not mixed with some yellow bile, phlegm, or watery chyme. Therefore, understand that this is what I mean when I speak of a surplus of chymes and of a surplus of blood. [*De plenitudine* 10].

(XXIII.3) The chyme that Galen calls "raw" in his *De multitidune*, and of which he says that dropsy of the flesh (anasarca) develops from this chyme, and that it is this chyme which settles in the urine similar to cooked broad bean groats, is a kind of phlegm that he calls "crude" in several places. [*De plenitudine* 11].

(XXIII.4) Serous blood is thin, watery blood with detrimental, biting, toxic power. What comes from the watery part of the blood is hot, calm, and tranquil. *In Hippocratis Epidemiarum commentarius* VI.2.

(XXIII.5) Chyme is a liquid that is found in the body of living beings, and chyle is that which is found in fruits when they are eaten or squeezed. *In Hippocratis De humoribus commentarius* I.

(XXIII.6) The liquids one finds in plants are of two kinds: The first is expressed through squeezing, and the second is that which spontaneously flows from plants. The liquid expressed by squeezing is also of two kinds and results either from squeezing fruits as is done with grapes, pomegranates, quinces, mulberries, and the like or from pounding the twigs and fresh leaves of a plant and then squeezing them. Each of these two types was called "chyle" by the ancients. The kind of liquid that flows spontaneously from the fruit or from the tree and that has the consistency of water is called "tear" by them. And that liquid whose consistency is thicker than a tear such as that which streams from some twigs if one cuts into them is called "milk." And that which is thicker than milk is called "gum." *In* [*Platonis*] *Timaeum commentarius* II.

(XXIII.7) Wheat of a good quality is that in which the pith dominates; inferior wheat is that in which the bran dominates. *Ad Glauconem* [*de medendi methodo*] II[.9].

(XXIII.8) The difference between perspiration and odor is that perspiration is the fine moisture that exudes from the humors, while the odors which emanate from the body are the vapors dissolving from the humors. *In Hippocratis De humoribus commentarius* II.

(XXIII.9) Food that arrives in the stomach should not be said to have been digested when it has been ground and turned into small pieces, but one should say that it has been digested when it is transformed into a quality which is similar and peculiar to the body which wants to be nurtured by it. [*De consuetudinibus*].

(XXIII.10) It is a habit of physicians that when they speak of "bile" or "biles" in an absolute sense, they mean by it the bile whose color is yellow or red and do not add to this term any further qualification indicating its color. But if they want to speak about any of the other kinds of bile, they add the name of its color to its description. *De alimentorum* [*facultatibus* III.38].

(XXIII.11) One should not say of everything that becomes corrupted of the organs of the body and its humors that it has putrefied. We should only say that it has putrefied if its corruption is accompanied by a foul smell. *De* [*simplicium*] *medicamentorum* [*temperamentis ac facultatibus*] V[.15].

(XXIII.12) Inhalation is the entrance of the air into the larynx and trachea. Respiration is the activity that occurs in the entire body through the dilation and contraction of the pulsatile vessels. [*De symptomatum differentiis* 5].

(XXIII.13) The knowledge of that which happens in the organs as a result of a minor, insignificant dyscrasia escapes many people, and for this reason they call it "weakness". [*De morborum differentiis* 5].

(XXIII.14) The illness that occurs in all joints is called "arthritis;" this very illness is called "ischias" if it occurs in the hip joint only and "podagra" if it occurs in the feet. If podagra becomes chronic and persists for a long time, the illness spreads into all joints. In all these illnesses much chyme develops in the joints and spreads to the nerves surrounding them. The chyme that mostly flows in the case of arthritis is that which is called "crude." [*De compositione medicamentorum secundum locos*] X[.2].

(XXIII.15) The diseases that are called "endemic" are those illnesses that are specific for most people of that city. They occur among them either in a well-known season of the year or often occur among them in every season of the year. These last diseases depend on the air and the water in that city and on the general nutrition of its inhabitants. *In Hippocratis De* [*aere,*] *aquis* [*et locis*] *commentarius* I.

(XXIII.16) The diseases that are called "epidemic" are general diseases that occur to the inhabitants of a certain city in certain years. These diseases are consequential upon a change occurring in the air or in the water or in the usual nutrition, or in all three of these. *In Hippocratis De* [*aere,*] *aquis* [*et locis*] *commentarius* I.

(XXIII.17) Sometimes phthisis is associated with anyone whose body wastes away and becomes lean and meagre to such a degree that he dies, regardless whether it is due to an ulcer in the lung, a dyscrasia or something else. However, the name "phthisis" is especially used for an ulcer of the lung because phthisis mostly develops from such a condition. [*In Hippocratis*] *Epidemiarum commentarius* I.2.

(XXIII.18) The uterus is especially called "nervous" and similarly the vulva and the penis because every single one of these organs resembles a nerve in regard to stretching, dilatation, contraction, whiteness, and lack of blood therein; not because of the fact that their substance actually consist of nerves, ligaments, or tendons. [*In Hippocratis*] *Epidemiarum commentarius* VI.1.

(XXIII.19) The simple kind of marasmus is that which develops from the predominance of heat alone. Sometimes it is thought to occur during the abstention from food, whether intentionally or whether due to actual lack of food. If predominance of heat is associated with predominance of cold, one is dealing with a complex marasmus, and this is the marasmus that occurs to the elderly or to someone who suffers from an illness which resembles old age. If predominance of dryness is associated with heat, one is dealing with marasmus that occurs in the case of fevers that are related to the substance of the organs. Such a temperament unavoidably affects the heart, and in that case real marasmus occurs. *De marcore* [1].

(XXIII.20) The marasmus called "burning" is one that arises from ardent fevers, and the marasmus called "syncopal" occurs to someone who suffered from syncope and then escaped this severe affliction but still retains some of the initial syncopal condition. The cold marasmus, on the other hand, which is a condition similar to old age, results in cases where fevers were not cooled properly, namely, through letting the patient drink cold water in the beginning of the illness. What Galen calls "the hearth of fever" is the organ that initially becomes only mildly hot but then increases in heat so much that hectic fevers arise from its heat. *De marcore* [5].

(XXIII.21) Says Moses: If you consider what Galen mentions in his treatise *De tremore, palpitatione, rigore et convulsione*, it will be clear to you that the terms *riʿda* (tremor) and *riʿsha* are synonyms. However, it has become common practice in the field of medicine, and actually for all physicians, to call *riʿda* a tremor, whose cause is related to weakness of strength, as is the case in someone who carries a heavy load or walks on a high spot or is frightened or is emaciated by the length of his illness. And they use the term *riʿsha* for the case of someone whose tremor is caused by afflictions that subsist in the nerves and that may be caused by various factors.

(XXIII.22) The discontinuation and complete cessation of voluntary activities is called "paralysis," and their diminution is called "torpor" (numbness). A bad execution of these activities is called "convulsion." *De* [*symptomatum*] *causis* [II.2].

In his *De puls*[*ibus libellus ad tirones*], Galen says: Paralysis means loss of sensation and movement.

(XXIII.23) Numbness is something composed of difficulty of sensation and difficulty of movement. It arises from coldness of the air, from compression of the nervous parts of the body, or from the shock caused by contact with a sea creature. The bodily parts first turn numb, then lose their sensation and movement. This kind of harm is called "paralysis." *De* [*symptomatum*] *causis* [I.5].

(XXIII.24) "Throat"—by this I mean the windpipe. When I speak to you of "organs of the voice," understand from me that by this I only mean the windpipe, larynx, pharynx, and the membrane covering the pharynx, larynx, and windpipe from the inside, and this is one continuous, thick membrane. [*De compositione medicamentorum secundum locos*] VII[.1].

(XXIII.25) Says Moses: The commentators to Galen's writings have confused some of the technical terms, and it is necessary to point this out. Namely, the internal membranes of the organs are called by them *ṣifāqāt* in their comment upon *De usu partium*. Thus, they speak of the *ṣifāq* of the stomach and the internal and external *ṣifāq* of the esophagus. They use this terminology frequently in their commentary on that book. Similarly, they call the tunics of the eye *ṣifāqāt* in their commentary on the same book. Some of the coverings (membranes) are also called *ṣifāqāt*; thus, they call the third covering (membrane) of the coverings (membranes) of the spinal cord *ṣifāq*. Do not let this mislead you.

(XXIII.26) "Pulse compression," as it is usually called by the physicians, means that the pulse is extremely weak and unequal in the beginning of a fever attack. "Heat compression" means that the heat flames up and becomes strong and is not uniform throughout the body, after it was preceded by shivering, cold of the extremities, clear indolence, and a tendency to sleep. *De febrium* [*differentiis*] I[.9].

(XXIII.27) If you place your fingers on a pulsatile vessel and then lift your hand and put it back again and find that every time you put the hand thereon the movement of the pulsatile vessel diminishes, this condition is called "disappearance and loss of the pulse." It is as if it is completely inactive when one feels it. If, on the other hand, when you place your fingers on the pulsatile vessel, you distinguish movement and if only after a prolonged application of your fingers you find that the movement diminishes and weakens little by little until it becomes completely still when one feels it, this is called a "finished pulse," and this is the lack of activity. *De* [*causis*] *pulsu*[*um* II.3].

(XXIII.28) A strong pulse is a powerful pulse, and a weak pulse is a faint pulse. If you place your hand on a pulsatile vessel and find the second pulse somewhat smaller than the first, and similarly, the third smaller than the second by the same amount, and even so the fourth, and so continually, this is called a "mouse tail's pulse." Sometimes it remains and stays in the smallness of pulsebeats that it reached, and this is called "permanent mouse tail." If the pulsebeats continue to get smaller until they stop completely, it is called a "finished mouse tail." Sometimes the pulse returns from the smallness which it reached and becomes greater little by little until it reaches a greatness which is similar to the original pulse or not completely similar, and it is called the "recurrent mouse tail." *De* [*differentia*] *pulsu*[*um*] I[.10].

(XXIII.29) The pulse that is found to be thick in the middle of the pulsatile vessel but becomes thinner on both sides is the one which is called "tending and inclining." *De* [*differentia*] *pulsu*[*um*] I[.1].

(XXIII.30) "Continuous" fevers and "perpetual" fevers are synonyms. Similarly, the fever called "synochous" is continuous, as is the continuous burning fever. The term "burning" has only been given to it only because of its severe heat. *De crisibus* II[.6].

(XXIII.31) When Galen stated and explained how two different fevers which form two different types can be combined—namely, phlegmatic and bilious and other ones—and said: If one fever is combined or mixed with another, he clarified this statement as follows: With "combined" I mean that the attacks of these two fevers start at different times, and with "mixed" I mean that the attacks of these two fevers start at the same time. *De febrium* [*differentiis*] II[.7].

(XXIII.32) Inflammations may occur in the muscles of the ribs, after which fever arises and respiration becomes fast and superficial. This illness is similar to pleurisy, which is not accompanied by expectoration. The difference between both is that in this illness the patient does not cough at all, the pulse is not hard, the fever is not as high as the fever of pleurisy, and respiration is easier than in the case of pleurisy. And some patients feel pain, if one presses on the site of the illness from the outside. If that inflammation becomes ripe, either the pus in it is dissolved or it protrudes outside the skin and needs an incision. *De locis affectis* V[.3].

(XXIII.33) The term "hot compress" applies to everything that warms the body externally. There are five kinds of it: moist, dry, biting, intermediate, and moderate. The moist one is that which is prepared with hot water with which one fills a skin or a bladder and the like. The dry one is the one that is prepared with rags heated over a fire or with mugwort or with roasted millet. The biting one is that which is prepared with salt heated in bags or with bitter vetch and the like. The strength of bitter vetch is sufficient for cutting, concocting, and dissolving the thickness of the humors. The moderate hot compress is such that one can touch with it the body of a living being, such as a child or a puppy and the like. The intermediate one is that prepared with barley and bitter vetch; they should be pulverized and boiled with acid vinegar mixed with it to a degree that is stronger than could be drunk. Put this in a bag and apply it as a hot compress to the parts of the body you want to treat. The same should be done with bran. *In Hippocratis De acutorum morborum* [*victu*] *commentarius* II[.5, 6].

Moderate massage is that which one stops to apply when the body becomes hot. *De methodo* [*medendi*] VII[.6].

(XXIII.34) Cities that are facing the east are cities that lie on high mountains because the sun shines down upon them for the entire day. He also said: Cities facing the east are those through which an eastern wind blows and that are protected at the western side while the eastern side is exposed. The opposite is the case with cities facing the west. *In Hippocratis De* [*aere,*] *aquis* [*et locis*] *commentarius* I.

(XXIII.35) Every ulcer that spreads on the skin but does not go any further is called by us *namla* (shingles). Every ulcer that passes beyond the skin and spreads into the flesh next to the skin is called *ākila* (canker). *In Hippocratis Aphorismos commentarius* VI.

(XXIII.36) *ʿAbīṭ* is a congelation of copious blood which is clearly visible. *De tumoribus praeter naturam* [2].

A *nāṣūr* (sinuous ulcer) is a narrow, elongated cavity that can be closely drawn together but whose parts can also separate through the flow of the superfluities through it. *De tumoribus praeter naturam* [4].

(XXIII.37) When the skin is extremely thin and stays like that for a long time and does not adhere to the underlying flesh, this illness is sometimes called *nāṣūr* (sinuous ulcer) and sometimes *makhba* (absconsio). *Ad Glauconem* [*de medendi methodo*] II[.10].

(XXIII.38) A carbuncle is an inflammation, but it is formed if the blood is affected by something similar to boiling to such a degree that the skin is burned and that an eschar is formed with it. The boil is preceded by a blister similar to a blister produced by burning with fire. This is followed by acute fever which rapidly endangers the life of the patient. *De tumoribus* [*praeter naturam* 6].

(XXIII.39) And in *De febrium* [*differentiis*] I, he remarks: Boils that are called *jamr* (carbuncles) arise from blood that is very hot and tends towards blackness.

(XXIII.39a) If humors stream from the openings of the vessels into the spaces that have no flesh or muscles and the bodily part is soaked with those humors just as a sponge is soaked with liquids, this is called "inflammation." If the pus corrodes parts of the flesh and the like and a cavity is formed in that place into which pus accumulates, it is called "abscess." If those corrupt matters inside the abscess are surrounded by a cover similar to a membrane, it is called *dubayla* (cystic abscess). If the humor is only in the skin, it is called "furuncle," and it is very hot. If it is deep in the body, it very malignant, and then it is similar to an abscess. The only difference between it and an abscess lies in its hardness. *De tumoribus* [*praeter naturam*].

(XXIII.40) Galen says in his *In Hippocratis Epidemiarum commentarius* VI.1: The term "swelling" as used by Hippocrates indicates every type of swelling. Similarly, Galen uses the term in a number of places for inflammations, and in a few statements, he uses it for every swelling. Pustules differ from tumors only in the quantity of humor that produces them. Also, in the case of pustules, nature strives after the cleansing of the internal parts of the body. If the humor that produces the pustules has only a little heat, it only produces itching. If it is very hot, it produces biting. If the humor is extremely thick or cold, it produces broad pustules. *In Hippocratis Epidemiarum commentarius* VI.2.

(XXIII.41) If the matter streaming to a part of the body is a superfluity composed of blood and yellow bile, both of which are warmer than they should be, or if that which streams to it is only blood but blood that is boiling hot, of a fine consistency, the illness developing therefrom is called "erysipelas." "Scirrhus" is the name of a hard tumor which develops from a thick, viscous humor that settles in those parts in which the tumor occurs. It is of two types: That which is absolutely insensible and incurable and that which is a little bit sensible and is hard to cure. And the sites where the tumor becomes very large and the blood is congested in it and the respiration becomes so small that one reaches a point that the patient dies are called "gangrenes" as long as they are in a stage of mortification but have not actually died. Their therapy consists of evacuating the blood that became congested in that part of the body by a deep scarification and by making incisions in it in several places until as much blood as possible is extracted. *Ad Glauconem* [*de medendi methodo*] II[.1, 6, 11].

(XXIII.42) When the inflammation known as "erysipelas" becomes cold and hard and difficult to dissolve, it is called "hard erysipelas." Similarly, if it is combined with a soft swelling, it is called "soft erysipelas." *De methodo* [*medendi*] XIV[.3].

(XXIII.43) When we speak of a hard tumor, we mean any tumor that combines hardness with absence of pain. It should not be insensible and at the same time painless, for if this is the case, it cannot be cured at all. *De methodo* [*medendi* XIV.6].

(XXIII.44) Every ulcer whose healing and cicatrization is difficult because of many humors, or of hot humors streaming towards it while the bad temperament of the ulcerous part of the body is not firmly established, is called "difficult to heal." But if the bad temperament of the ulcerous part becomes firmly established and the illness overpowers it to a degree that the bad temperament reaches a state in which it corrupts everything it arrives at, even if it is good, I call it with a special name: "malignant ulcer." And those ulcers that are extremely malignant I call "gangrenous ulcers." [*De compositione medicamentorum per genera*] I[.18;] IV[.1.14].

(XXIII.45) A scirrhous tumor consists of two types: One of these originates from thick phlegm, and the second develops from turbid blood and its sediments. Both have in common that they are large, hard, and painless tumors. The second type has as a special feature that it is of a black color. *De tumoribus* [*praeter naturam* 9].

(XXIII.46) Cancer consists of two types, namely, a tumor that arises from black bile, and when the black bile streams into the flesh and is biting, it corrodes the entire adjacent skin and ulcerates it, and this is the ulcerous cancer. But when the black bile is moderate, it produces a cancer that is not ulcerous. *De tumoribus* [*praeter naturam* 12].

(XXIII.47) All cancerous tumors especially develop from a melancholic superfluity. If that superfluity tends to the lower part of the body and the expulsive faculty in the vessels expels it from the openings of the vessels in the anus or vagina, then the parts from which this evacuation takes place are called "hemorrhoids," and blood flows from them. Sometimes those superfluities are forced to the legs and cause varicose veins, and sometimes they are forced to the skin of the entire body, and from this elephantiasis develops. *Ad Glauconem* [*de medendi methodo*] II[.12].

(XXIII.48) Sometimes because of the severe corruption of an ulcer a malignant humor or black bile or verdigris green bile accumulates in the body and spreads and affects the parts around the diseased part until the healthy part adjacent to this diseased part becomes corroded. This illness is called *ākila* (canker). *De tumoribus* [*praeter naturam* 12, 13].

(XXIII.49) Canker is an ulcerous sore that corrodes the flesh deep inside, while herpes is an ulcerous disease that corrodes on the outside. Lanolin is the wool fat extracted from the wool, not the filthy (greasy) wool itself. *In Hippocratis De humoribus commentarius* III.

(XXIII.50) Anasarca (dropsy of the flesh) is sometimes called "leucophlegmasia." It is also called *al-ḥaban*, while the ascites variety is also called *jamʿ al-māʾ* (accumulation of fluid). *De locis affectis* V[.7].

In his *In Hippocratis Aphorismos commentarius* IV[.11], Galen says that tympanites is the illness that Hippocrates calls "dry dropsy."

(XXIII.51) A swelling occurs when thin phlegm accumulates. The illness called "gangrene" is the beginning of the mortification of the solid parts of the body, except for the bones. If the bones perish as well, the illness is called "sphacelus." *De tumoribus* [*praeter naturam* 9, 11].

(XXIII.52) The difference between an inflation (emphysema) and a soft swelling (edema) is that a soft swelling, if you press upon it, stays in its place and remains depressed, but an inflation, if you press upon it with your hand, does not remain depressed, and if you strike upon it, you hear a noise similar to that of a drum. *De methodo* [*medendi* XIV.7].

(XXIII.53) Alopecia and ophiasis are one and the same disease. Their names are only different because of the form of the site, since the site from which the hair comes off in the case of ophiasis is similar to the form of a snake when it is moving forward. [*De compositione medicamentorum secundum locos*] I[.2].

(XXIII.54) The skin of the head (scalp) is affected by an illness that is a type of swelling that has fine, small openings filled with a thin, viscous liquid. This disease is called *saʿfa* (cradle cap). Another illness occurs on the skin of the head and resembles the former in its appearance, but the openings are larger and wider than the openings of cradle cap, and they are filled with a honey-like moisture, and this illness is called "honeycomb". [*De compositione medicamentorum secundum locos* I.8].

(XXIII.55) Cradle cap is a small ulceration on the skin of the head (scalp) from which a fluid streams which is neither watery nor as thick as honey, as is the case with that which streams from honeycomb-like ulcers. It seems likely that this ulceration develops from salty, nitrous phlegm. *De tumoribus* [*praeter naturam* 15].

(XXIII.56) If inflammations occur in the soft flesh in the groin and armpits, and if these glands harden and become firm, that illness is called "scrofula." *De tumoribus* [*praeter naturam* 15].

(XXIII.57) A hardening of the testicles is called "sarcocele," just as the watery fluid accumulated in the tunics around the testicles is called "hydrocele." Epiplocele and enterocele and the illness consisting of both of these, that is, epiploenterocele, are names invented by more recent physicians, who call all the swellings that occur in the area of the testicles "hernia." *De tumoribus* [*praeter naturam* 15].

(XXIII.58) When humors of a bilious type dominate in the head, sleeplessness and delirium develop from it. When cold, phlegmatic humors dominate in it, stupor and forgetfulness develop from it. When the humors are in the middle between these two conditions, stupor develops next to torpor. A stupor is a mild form of delirium. *In Hippocratis Epidemiarum commentarius* II.2.

(XXIII.58a) In his *In Hippocratis Epidemiarum commentarius* III.1, Galen says that raving is a mild form of delirium. One should not say that a patient suffers from stupor until it becomes difficult for him to wake up. If he sleeps for a long time and it is not difficult for him to wake up if he is prodded, it is only a long sleep but not a stupor. Both, however, are caused by coldness of the brain. *In Hippocratis Aphorismos commentarius* II[.3].

(XXIII.59) If cold dominates the brain and moisture becomes added thereto, lethargy develops therefrom. If dryness is added to the cold, catalepsy develops from it. If the brain only becomes warm qualitatively or in combination with superfluous matter, sleeplessness develops. *In Hippocratis Aphorismos commentarius* II[.3].

(XXIII.60) In *De puls[ibus libellus ad tirones]*, Galen says: The illness called "forgetfulness" arises from a phlegmatic swelling that occurs in the membranes of the brain.

(XXIII.61) Apoplexy occurs when the psychical pneuma cannot pass to the parts below the head whether it is due to an illness of some sort of swelling that occurs in the brain or because the ventricles of the brain have become filled with phlegmatic moisture. The severity and graveness of the illness are according to the severity of the cause effecting this disease. *In Hippocratis Aphorismos commentarius* II[.43].

The ancients used to call epilepsy "the divine illness." Some of them called it thus because they thought that this illness comes from the demons, and others give as reason for this designation the fact that its only cause is the constellation of the moon. Plato gives as reason for this designation the fact that this illness arises in the head and harms the pure, divine part whose seat is the brain. *In [Platonis] Timaeum commentarius* IV.

(XXIII.62) Madness is a chronic mental confusion without fever whereas phrenitis is a chronic mental confusion with fever. *In Hippocratis Epidemiarum commentarius* III.3.

(XXIII.63) The "black bile illness," that is, melancholy, is the same as melancholic delusion. *In Hippocratis* [*Aphorismos*] *commentarius* [III.24; IV.2].

(XXIII.64) The loss of imagination is called "torpor" and "catalepsy." Its bad functioning is called "delirium." Loss of reasoning power is called "amentia," and its bad functioning is also called "mental confusion." [*De symptomatum diferentiis*] 3.

(XXIII.65) There is one type of melancholic delusion that has its origin in the stomach. Some of the ancient physicians call this illness the "hypochondriac illness" and the "flatulent illness." It is also called "hypochondriac" and "flatulent." *De locis affectis* III[.10].

(XXIII.66) The illness that the physicians call *bayḍa* and *khūdha* (helmet) is an illness affecting the entire head; it is a chronic headache that is difficult to eliminate whereby minor causes produce attacks that are so severe that the patient does not tolerate the sound of speaking nor a bright light nor any movement. The thing he likes most is to lie down in darkness because of the severity of the pain. [*De locis affectis*] III[.13].

(XXIII.67) Mental confusion that arises from phrenitis, which is an inflammation that occurs in the brain or its membranes, does not happen all at once, but little by little, and does not subside during the decline of the fever. But mental confusion occurring in the case of ardent fevers and caused by illnesses affecting other organs happens all at once and subsides when those illnesses have passed their climax. An exception is the case when the mental confusion is consequential upon an inflammation of the diaphragm, for then it is closely related to the mental confusion that is consequential upon phrenitis and that does not subside immediately after the illness has reached its climax. *De locis affectis* V[.4].

(XXIII.68) If a phlegmatic, thick, cold humor that has not yet putrefied increases in the brain, it produces different kinds of severe stuporific attacks without fever. They are the kinds which are called "stupor," "torpor," and "catalepsy." If the humor putrefies at some time, these things occur together with fever, and this illness is called "lethargy." *De methodo* [*medendi*] XIII[.21].

(XXIII.69) The cataract that occurs in the eye and that the physicians call "extension" lies between the crystalline humor and the horn-like tunic. *De usu partium* X[.1].

(XXIII.70) If the membrane known as conjunctiva suffers from a bloody inflammation, namely, conjunctivitis, it harms the visual ability and hinders its normal function accidentally. But if it is affected by chemosis or pterygium, the darkening of vision resulting from the covering of the pupil does not occur accidentally. *De* [*symptomatum*] *causis* [I.2].

(XXIII.71) If a site on the horn-like tunic becomes corroded and part of the grape-like tunic protrudes from it, this is called *mūzaraj* (prolapse). The pus that originates behind the horn-like tunic is called *kumna*. The eyelids that become thick and hard and whose color turns red and whose hairs fall off is an illness which is called *sulāq* (ptilosis). If the flesh in the inner angle of the eye disappears, it is an illness which is called *dam'a* (rhyas). [*De compositione medicamentorum secundum locos*] IV[.8].

(XXIII.72) A fistula occurring in the inner angle of the eye is called *gharab* (lacrimal fistula). Callous hardenings on the face are called *naḥīlāt*. [*De compositione medicamentorum secundum locos*] V[.2, 3].

(XXIII.73) Deafness means that a person cannot hear a low voice at all and hears a loud voice with difficulty. This process continues to progress slowly until the patient becomes completely deaf in the course of time. [*De compositione medicamentorum secundum locos*] III[.1].

(XXIII.74) The tumor that forms inside the nose as if it were a fleshy excrescence is called *nāṣūr* and also "polypus." [*De compositione medicamentorum secundum locos*] III[.3].

(XXIII.75) The term "aphthae" applies to ulcers occurring on the outside of the mucous membrane inside the mouth and is accompanied by fiery heat. It mostly occurs to infants because of spoiled milk. The term "aphthae" is used only when the illness does not come with putrefaction. But if the aphthae last for a long time and putrefaction occurs with it, this is what the physicians call "corrosion." [*De compositione medicamentorum secundum locos* VI.9].

(XXIII.76) The windpipe is called *ḥalqūm* (trachea). The term *ḥalqūm* is especially used for the site where the two channels, that is, the larynx and the esophagus, arrive at, below the root of the tongue. In the throat there are muscles that are known as *naghānigh*. It is a plural term, meaning the muscles at both sides of the throat. *De voce* [*et hanelitu*].

(XXIII.77) Angina is a swelling in the throat and consists of four types. The first is that the inside of the throat swells up, that is, its cavity up to the end of the larynx, whereby none of the swelling is visible externally. The second is when the throat swells up at the outside and the patient does not have a sensation of choking; this is the safest of all four types. The third is when the swelling includes both the inside of the throat and the outside, and this is the worst of all. The fourth is when no swelling is visible on the outside, but the patient has the feeling of choking. *De locis affectis* IV[.6].

(XXIII.78) All types of asthma that occur suddenly are called "acute asthma," and the pulse of those suffering from acute asthma is always irregularly unequal. *De* [*causis*] *pulsu*[*um* IV.21].

(XXIII.79) If it happens to someone that he breathes uninterruptedly like someone who has run fast without his suffering from fever, the physicians use to call this affliction "asthma." They also call it "orthopnea" because the patient suffering from this ailment keeps his chest erect during respiration. It is caused by narrowness occurring in the chest either because of inflammations in the organs there or because of viscous humors that flowed between the chest and the lungs or thick, viscous humors in the different parts of the windpipe. [*De compositione medicamentorum secundum locos*] VII[.6].

The illness which is called "dyspnea" in particular is that which is originating from thick, viscous humors that are stuck in the different parts of the windpipe. This term is indeed used for this illness in particular. [*De compositione medicamentorum secundum locos*] VII[.6].

(XXIII.80) If the foods change in the stomach into a quality different from the natural one, it is called "dyspepsia," that is, bad digestion. If the retentive faculty of the stomach becomes inactive, it means that the stomach does not contract at all and does not wrap itself around the foods in a tight and firm manner. This happens to the stomach in the illness called "lientery." [*De symptomatum differentiis* 4].

(XXIII.81) A bad craving for food, if unusually severe, is called "canine appetite." It happens when a detrimental acid humor burns the stomach or when the entire body suffers from excessive dissolution. *De* [*symptomatum*] *causis* [I.7].

(XXIII.82) Just as emesis is preceded by nausea, so too coughing is preceded and induced by distress. And just as someone's soul is upset and he is nauseous but does not vomit, so too he feels distress that may prompt coughing, but he does not cough because the cause is too mild. *De* [*symptomatum*] *causis* [II.3].

(XXIII.83) The stomach employs for the expulsion of a harmful substance the opening towards which that superfluity has the strongest inclination to stream to. If this type of disturbance occurs in the entire stomach, it employs for its expulsion the two openings together and expels it both through vomiting and diarrhea, just as in the case of cholera. *De* [*symptomatum*] *causis* [III.2].

(XXIII.84) Sometimes the cause of indigestion is the irregularity in which foods are taken in terms of what is taken first and what is taken later, or their quantity or their quality. *De locis affectis* V[.6].

(XXIII.85) The illness called "bulimia" is a form of syncope that is caused by excessive cold of the cardia of the stomach. *De puls*[*ibus libellus ad tirones* 12].

(XXIII.86) One calls a "stomach patient" someone who has no tumor in his stomach but whose appetite has disappeared, or someone who feels after taking food a heaviness, pressure, anxiety, or nausea that he can hardly bear. One also calls a "stomach patient" someone who has an upset stomach after having food, especially if it requires them to vomit. [*De compositione medicamentorum secundum locos*] VIII[.2].

(XXIII.87) Part of the stomach ailments is that ailment which is called *inqilāb* (upset stomach), which is a lack of appetite without a tumor, nausea, feeling of sickness, or vomiting. The ailment called "bulimia" which is a devouring hunger associated with a burning pain occurring in the stomach that can become so severe that the patient suffers from syncope. The general treatment of all these ailments consists of astringent medicines, many of which are mixed with heating and drying medicines. [*De compositione medicamentorum secundum locos*] VIII[.1].

(XXIII.88) The illness which the physicians call "liver ailment" and whose patient they call "a patient with a liver illness" is an illness of a bad temperament without a tumor, just as they speak of a "stomach illness" and a "stomach patient" in the case of someone whose stomach is ill without a tumor. It is well known that a bad temperament sometimes occurs in the substance of the liver itself and is peculiar to it, whereas at other times it occurs in the pulsatile and non-pulsatile vessels that the liver contains. At yet other times the bad temperament occurs in the matters which those vessels encompass. [*De compositione medicamentorum secundum locos*] VIII[.6].

(XXIII.89) When speaking of "spleen patients," physicians mean those patients whose spleen is affected by induration and calcification without an inflammation. The illness that is really called "dysentery" is an ulceration of the intestines, and this ulceration is either simple without putrefaction or with putrefaction. The illness that the physicians usually call "spreading ulcer" is a cankerous sore. Lanolin is the wool fat. [*De compositione medicamentorum secundum locos*] IX[.6].

(XXIII.90) Lientery means that the food is discharged quickly and unchanged, and diarrhea means softness of the stools and their continuous discharge. *In Hippocratis Epidemiarum commentarius* I.2.

(XXIII.91) Ulceration of the rectum, which is called "tenesmus," produces a severe pricking pain and an urge to relieve oneself, while only a small amount is discharged from the patient. In the beginning, the discharge is phlegmatic and fatty. As time passes, something like shreds of intestinal tissue is discharged from these patients. *De locis affectis* VI[.2].

(XXIII.92) If the superfluities that are harmful for nature are moist, the expulsive faculty eliminates them by the severe and violent shaking that happens during a rigor or cough, and then they go to all the sites that have the property to receive them. Thus, some of them go to the upper part of the abdomen, namely, the stomach, and arrive there, and others go to the lower part of the abdomen, namely, the intestines, and arrive there. Yet other superfluities go to the outside of the skin. *De* [*symptomatum*] *causis* [II.5].

(XXIII.93) If the small intestine is affected by a hard tumor or by a severe obstruction of feces so that the patient vomits his feces, that illness is called "ileus," and hardly anyone can be saved from it. If all parts of the intestines and the stomach fall ill and cannot retain their contents even for a short time, or if the illness does not come with biting pain, that illness is called "lientery." It is also called "abdominal affections." The patient suffering therefrom is called "abdominal patient". *De locis affectis* VI[.2].

What is really called "dysentery" is the illness caused by an ulceration of the intestines. *De locis affectis* VI[.2].

(XXIII.94) The illness called "polyuria" which is called by some "diabetes" and by others "polydipsia;" a patient with this illness suffers from severe thirst and drinks a lot and rapidly urinates what he drinks. This illness of the kidneys and urinary bladder is comparable to lientery of the stomach and the intestines. *De locis affectis* VI[.3].

(XXIII.95) If the stomach suffers harm from the biting effect of food that is not digested, together with the intestines it expels this food until it is completely discharged. This affliction is called "diarrhea." *De propriorum animi cuiuslibet affectuum dignotione* [*et curatione* 9].

(XXIII.96) The neck of the uterus and the cervix of the uterus are two synonyms for one and the same organ. The side of that cervix that is close to the uterus is called "mouth of the uterus" (*os uteri*), and this is the one which is hermetically closed during pregnancy. The side of the cervix that is close to the vulva and into which the penis penetrates is called the "mouth of the neck of the uterus." *In Hippocratis Aphorismos commentarius* V[.46].

(XXIII.97) The illness called *raḥā* that develops in the uteri of women is the formless flesh that a woman produces. *De methodo medendi* [XIV.13].

The medicines that are taken internally are called "antidotes" by the physicians. [*De antidotis*] I[.1].

(XXIII.98) The remedies that are called "useful for many purposes" are remedies that are beneficial for many illnesses and are, so to say, compounded from medicines that are opposite not only in their quality and first degree of their potency, but also in the second degree of their potency. [*De compositione medicamentorum per genera*] V.

(XXIII.99) "Thinning" and "rarefaction" are synonyms. For every medicine that heats without causing harm and that dries less than it heats and whose substance contains some fineness such as *bābūnaj* (German or Roman camomile) and common marshmallow, that medicine widens the pores and loosens the skin. A medicine that is hot and that has a thick substance is called "opening" because it opens the mouth of the vessels from below such as garlic, onion, European cyclamen, and bile of a bull. *De* [*simplicium*] *medicamentorum* [*temperamentis ac facultatibus*] V[.14].

(XXIII.100) A cleansing and clearing medicine uproots sordidness from the outer layer of the pores and openings, such as honey, white lupine flour, barley, broad beans, bitter vetch, and a number of seeds. A medicine that purifies the pores and openings is any alkaline, fine medicine and is also called "opening." The difference between this medicine and a clearing medicine is only a quantitative one. *De* [*simplicium*] *medicamentorum* [*temperamentis ac facultatibus*] V[.12].

(XXIII.101) Remedies that warm and moisten until they corrupt what they encounter are truly called "putrefying remedies." Similarly, all remedies that are hot and dry and whose substance is thick, if they bite or burn somewhat without causing pain, are called "putrefying" because they dissolve and corrode the flesh. They have the same effect on it as the truly putrefying remedies. These include the two types of arsenic, chrysocolla, stinging or urticating caterpillar of the pinewoods, and aconite. *De* [*simplicium*] *medicamentorum* [*temperamentis ac facultatibus*] V [.15].

(XXIII.102) The king's nut is the edible nut (walnut). The small nut is the *jillawz* (hazelnut), that is, *bunduq*. Sorghum is called *shaylam* (darnel) by the ancients; millet is a type of sorghum. *De bonis* [*malisque*] *sucis* [V, VII].

(XXIII.103) Concentrated grape juice is the must that has been extremely well cooked. *De victu attenuante* [12].

(XXIII.104) The difference between soft fat and suet (hard fat) lies in their moistness and dryness. For soft fat is moist, similar to olive oil that has become thick and dry because of its age. Suet is very dry; therefore, if you melt it and then leave it, it solidifies quickly. *De alimentorum facultatibus* III[.10].

(XXIII.105) Sour milk is the milk from which only the buttery part has been removed and that was then left until it turned sour. An egg that has been boiled for a long time is called "hard boiled;" the one that reaches moderate thickness from boiling is called "moderately boiled" and is the same as a soft-boiled egg. The egg that is only heated by boiling is called "the one that can be supped." *De alimentorum facultatibus* III[.21].

(XXIII.106) The least nourishing of all types of wine is that whose color is white and whose consistency is thin and that is similar to water. Such a kind of wine is similar to water that is suitable and fit for preparing honey water from it, which is called "hydromel." *De alimentorum facultatibus* III[.39].

(XXIII.107) Among the names of different types of milk are the following: If milk is churned and its butter removed, the rest is called "buttermilk." It is also called *dūgh*. If buttermilk is boiled until it becomes thick and some salt is added to it, it is called *kashk*. If it is then placed in the sun until it becomes dry and more sour, it is called *maṣl* (whey). If the milk congeals completely either by rennet or by leaving it standing for days until it becomes thick, it is called *rāʾib* (thick, coagulated). It is also called *al-māst*. If it is left standing for a long time until its sourness increases, it is called *al-ḥāzir*. If the milk called *al-māst* is boiled until it is completely thick and dry, it is called *aqiṭ*. From the *Ikhtiyārāt al-Ḥāwī* by Ibn al-Tilmīdh.

(XXIII.108) If the watery part of milk is boiled and the fatty parts which separate from it through the boiling are taken from it, it is called *al-lawr*. Colostrum is that which is produced by the mother's breasts at the time of the delivery and for some days afterwards as long as it is thick. If salt is added to butter and boiled until the watery part vanishes, it is called "clarified butter." From the *Ikhtiyārāt al-Ḥāwī*.

(XXIII.109) Ancient physicians call the alteration of a substance to another type of a different variety "putrefaction." Examples are the alteration of wine if it changes and turns into vinegar, or the corruption that develops in some types of wood until it crumbles and turn, as it were, into dust and ashes. However, modern physicians and people in general apply the name "putrefaction" to an alteration that destroys a substance completely and that is accompanied by a stench. This develops especially in substances that tend strongly towards fluidity and moisture. *In [Platonis] Timaeum commentarius* II.

This is the end of the twenty-third treatise,
by the grace of God,
praise be to Him.

In the name of God,
the Merciful, the Compassionate.
O Lord, make our task easy.

The Twenty-Fourth Treatise

Containing curiosities, which feature and are related in the medical books, and unusual, rare occurrences

(XXIV.1) In the book *Diseases of Women*, composed by Hippocrates, translated by Ḥunayn and commented upon by Galen, I found an addition which is neither part of Ḥunayn's translation nor of Galen's commentary. In that additional commentary there are strange things, among them that he says: Porphyry has related that there was a great eclipse of the sun in Sicily and that in that year women gave birth to abnormally shaped babies that had two heads, and that some women menstruated from their mouth through vomiting.

(XXIV.2) In that additional commentary it is also stated that the uterus sends the menstrual blood through small vessels to the buttocks and that the vessels there open and that this blood flow is instead of menstruation.

(XXIV.3) A stone at this site grows no less than a plant. When something grows, it necessarily feeds itself. This is the wording of Galen's statement at the end of his treatise *De nominibus medicis*.

(XXIV.4) Galen promised a patient that a crisis would befall him, yet it did not befall him. He examined him and found the house in which the patient was to be cold. He heated the air of the house with fire, the patient began to sweat and the crisis befell him. *De [optimo] medico cognoscendo* [VI.5, 6].

(XXIV.5) A young man once suffered from a wound in his breastbone. Then pus developed there, he was operated upon, but subsequently the bone there got corrupted again. The corrupted bone was removed, and his heart became visible and exposed beneath it. He became completely healed since the chest itself had not been perforated. *De anatomicis administrationibus* VII[.13].

(XXIV.6) I once saw an astonishing thing, namely, that a young man suffered from a perforation in one of the two anterior ventricles of his brain, but God saved him and he escaped unharmed. If both anterior ventricles of his brain had been perforated at the same time, he would not have lived even for an instant. *De usu partium* VIII[.9].

(XXIV.7) The reason that I drew blood from one of the pulsatile veins was that I was twice told in my dream to bleed the pulsatile vein between the index finger and thumb of the right hand. I let the blood flow until it stopped by itself because I was told so in my dream. The quantity that flowed was less than a *raṭl* and immediately the pain that I had felt for a long time in the spot where the liver is connected to the diaphragm was alleviated. I was a young man when this pain occurred. *De* [*curandi ratione per*] *venae sectione*[*m* 23].

(xxiv.8) As for the bodies that come out with the urine resembling bundles of hair, sometimes one of these is longer than a span of the hand. They originate from a thick, viscous humor that is heated and dries up in the vessels in the manner of the Guinea worms that are formed in the thighs in certain places of Tihāma, as they say. The substance of these worms resembles the sort of substance that a nerve has, and their external form is similar to that of intestinal worms in color. *De locis affectis* VI[.3].

(xxiv.9) There are other types of cleansing that are different from these and that are almost unknown, as they occur only exceptionally. An example is what I have seen, namely, how an abscess in the lung was evacuated through the urine and an abscess in the chest through the stools. [*De locis affectis* VI.4].

(xxiv.10) A man once carried a pork liver with him from one village to another. When he had to relieve himself, he placed the liver on some herbs until he came back to take it with him again. When he came back, he found that blood serum of the liver had dripped on the herbs. He then took from those herbs and gave it to some people to ingest. Whosoever took it did not stop suffering from bloody diarrhea until he died. With these herbs he killed many people. Then the ruler of that country had him captured and severely tortured until he told him who had informed him about the effect of that herb and from whom he had this information. He told him that he had not heard this from anyone and that he had not passed this information on to someone else, but told the story of what happened to him with the pork liver. He told him that it is a very common herb that grows anywhere. Then the ruler ordered to blindfold his eyes so that he would not be able to point that herb out to someone else so that this person would know about it. Subsequently, he had him executed. *De purgantium medicamentorum* [*facultate* 4].

(xxiv.11) If abscesses are cut open, one finds different types of things in it. Sometimes one finds things similar to mud, urine, clots of blood, a honey-like mucous nasal discharge, stones, nails, and flesh. And sometimes one finds living creatures in it, similar to the living creatures that originate from putrefaction. *De tumoribus* [*praeter naturam* 4].

(XXIV.12) Sometimes a superfluity descends from the head to the lungs and from the lungs to the testicles because of the natural connection between the organs in the chest and the reproductive organs. *In Hippocratis Epidemiarum commentarius* I.1.

(XXIV.13) Galen said in his [*In Hippocratis*] *Epidemiarum commentarius* II.4: If blood flows outside the vessels beneath the skin, that site takes on the color of eggplant.

(XXIV.14) Ibn Riḍwān drew the attention to this statement and said: This proves that the eggplant was known to Galen, but he only mentioned it in this place.

(XXIV.15) Says Moses: It is my most firm opinion that Galen did not know the eggplant and that is why he did not mention it. Perhaps he described a similar plant whose color was between black and red and the translator identified it with the eggplant.

(XXIV.16) Only in a few cases do those suffering from tremor or dropsy or similar ailments benefit from bleeding; in most cases it is harmful to them. It is especially beneficial for someone whose illness started from a congestion of blood streaming from the openings of the vessels in the buttocks and for a woman whose illness started from a congestion of menstrual blood and for someone in whose body such a large quantity of blood has accumulated for whatever reason that there is no guarantee against the extinction of the innate heat. *In Hippocratis Epidemiarum commentarius* II.4.

(XXIV.17) There are bodies that are extremely emaciated and yet have much blood, and there are other bodies that are obese and fat and yet have little blood. Galen reports the case of a woman whose menstruation was retained for eight months and who was extremely emaciated. When he saw that the blood was flowing copiously in her vessels but that it had a livid color, he bled her and extracted on the first day a quantity of one and a half *raṭl* of dark blood resembling liquid tar. On the second day he extracted one *raṭl* and on the third day eight ounces. And he said that she was cured and her body returned to its normal condition in a short time. *In Hippocratis Epidemiarum commentarius* VI.3.

(XXIV.18) Examine a male at the time he reaches puberty. If his right testicle is larger than the left, he will beget male offspring, but if the left testicle is larger than the right one, he will beget female offspring. The same applies to the breasts of a girl at the time of her puberty. *In Hippocratis Epidemiarum commentarius* VI.4.

(XXIV.19) Itches, cough, hiccups, sneezing, and the like sometimes subside when a person endures and tolerates them, especially if they are few and weak. *In Hippocratis De humoribus commentarius* I[.18].

(XXIV.20) If someone sees someone else suffering from ophthalmia and he is not used to seeing such a thing, his eyes will initially fill with moisture, and if he looks for a long time, he will also suffer from ophthalmia. Similarly, sometimes a person sees someone else urinating or defecating or yawning or stretching oneself and this prompts him to do exactly the same thing. *De motibus* [*manifestis et obscuris* VIII.16].

(XXIV.21) Some people often fall asleep while sitting and walk while asleep. I used to hear this but did not believe it until I was obliged to walk while asleep throughout the whole night. I learned the truth by experience and had to believe it. I walked nearly a sixth of a mile and absorbed in a dream, did not wake up until I stumbled upon a stone. *De motu musculorum* II[.4].

(XXIV.22) A man once was delirious for thirteen days and thought that he was in the city of Athens while in reality he was in the city of Rome. He thought that he had just arrived from a long journey and wanted to go to the bathhouse to be treated. He knew very well all he had said and done except for the illusion of his arrival from a journey at Athens. After thirteen days had passed, a severe nosebleed overtook him, and then a sweat suddenly broke out and he recovered. But after his recovery he did not remember anything of what had happened to him. *De motu musculorum* II[.6].

(XXIV.23) A servant once became angry and threw himself on the ground. He held his breath for a long time, and then he convulsed and died. Galen says: Someone stayed silent for a year or more than a year by his own free will. *De motu musculorum* II[.6].

(XXIV.24) A woman who was pregnant for some months at first saw blood, then thin, fetid blood serum. With the passing of time, she miscarried. After this, every day part of the placenta was extruded because it had putrefied internally. When the remains of the placenta stopped coming out, the midwives and all the attending physicians except me thought that she was completely cleansed. When I felt her pulse, I realized from its beat that something remained in her uterus that should be expelled. I informed the woman and her husband about it and that she needed to expel that which remained in the womb. On the sixteenth day after her miscarriage, another putrid fetus was aborted. *De* [*optico*] *medico cognoscendo* [13].

(XXIV.25) A woman suffered from an illness that was so harmful for her stomach that she lost her appetite and was close to death because of her extreme weakness and little intake of food. Physicians famous for their medical practice treated her but without success. I told them to prepare absinth wormwood wine for her. Immediately after she had imbibed it, her stomach strengthened and she wanted to eat immediately. *De theriaca ad Pisonem* [2].

(XXIV.26) A boy suffered from an abscess that was ready to be incised, but he was very fearful of an incision. His father took some theriac, made a salve from it, and put it on the abscess. It perforated the skin more rapidly than surgery and extracted the pus it contained. *De theriaca ad Pisonem* [2].

(XXIV.26a) It is related that the queen of Egypt killed herself by letting a viper free on her breast. The viper bit her and she died immediately. The reason she did so was because another king had defeated her and usurped the land that was in her possession. Says Galen: I saw with my own eyes in Alexandria how fast this viper kills someone. For when the judge in that city sentences a prominent person to death, they bring this viper and let her bite him in the chest and he dies immediately. *De theriaca ad Pisonem* [8].

(XXIV.26b) I was informed about an ancient physician that he wished to have a fair son born to him and that he painted a portrait on the wall of a boy as handsome as possible. When he had sexual intercourse with his wife, he ordered her to look at that portrait constantly and not to look away from it even for a short moment. She got a son who was as beautiful as that portrait but did not resemble his father. [*De theriaca ad Pisonem* 11].

If vipers eat bread, the bread obstructs the passages of the teeth so that they bite without causing any damage. Someone who sees this is amazed, not knowing the wickedness and cunning of their hunters. [*De theriaca ad Pisonem* 12].

(XXIV.27) Once a plague erupted from the borders of Ethiopia to Greece. Hippocrates acted skillfully against the plague and saved the inhabitants of his city by instructing them to ignite a fire around the city and to put onto it large quantities of wood and other things, namely, blossoms and leaves of plants and fragrant trees. He also told them to put on the firebrand many spices and odiferous oils. When they did so, they were saved from the death they were so close to. [*De theriaca ad Pisonem* 16].

(XXIV.28) Who is not amazed over the work of nature and what it does in the case of the female bear? It gives birth to an animal that is similar to a piece of meat in which none of its parts nor the shape of an animal is recognizable. But when she has given birth to it, she does not stop to lick it with her tongue until all the parts of this animal become apparent. [*De theriaca ad Pisonem* 11].

(XXIV.29) If you excise the testicles (ovaries) of a female animal, she does not have sexual desire and does not admit the male to copulate with her and she loses her femininity. Thus, female pigs are castrated by our countrymen in Athens but also by other nations. Then their bodies become fat and corpulent and their flesh becomes sweeter than that which is eaten of other female pigs. If someone wants to castrate a female pig, he is forced to cut around both the flanks. For this reason, the castration of the female is much more risky than that of males. *De semine* I[.16].

(XXIV.30) A female secretes sperm without a man approaching her, and this occurs during nocturnal pollution, which happens to her while she is asleep just as it happens to men. It also occurs during the accumulation of sperm as I described in the case of that woman who was a widow. *De semine* II[.1]. The woman he referred to there is the same whose story he related in the last book of *De locis affectis* [VI.5].

(XXIV.31) He says in *De alimentorum* [*facultatibus* II.38.4]: In the past, people used to live only on acorns because it nourishes the body similar to many seeds and grains from which bread is prepared.

(XXIV.32) I know a man who ate lots of mushrooms that had not been properly cooked. As a result, he felt pressure and heaviness in the cardia of his stomach, his respiration was difficult, he fainted, and his sweat was cold. He was barely saved and rescued from death by taking remedies which disperse thick juices such as oxymel with a decoction of thinning roots. *De alimentorum* [*facultatibus*] II[.67.2].

(XXIV.33) He says: I know a small child whose first wet nurse died and was then nursed by another who had bad humors. As a result, his body was covered all over with many ulcers. This second wet nurse used to feed herself in the springtime with vegetables of poor quality because of a famine that had befallen the inhabitants of her land. Her body, too, became completely covered with ulcers, similar to the ulcers that covered the small child. *De alimentorum* [*facultatibus*] III[.14.10].

(XXIV.34) The intestines have been provided with two tunics, and both are alike to strengthen their expulsive faculty and to minimize the occurrence of injuries. I have frequently seen in many persons such putrefaction of a large part of the intestines that in some of them the inner tunic of their intestines was completely destroyed, and yet they were saved and lived. If there had not been a second tunic to the intestines, besides the one that had putrefied and been destroyed, they could not have lived. *De usu partium* IV[.17].

(XXIV.35) I have seen something amazing and unusual, namely, that a boy was hit on the pupil with the end of a sharp iron instrument. Watery moisture flowed from the opening and his pupil became smaller and the horn-like tunic contracted completely. When he had been treated, he saw well again because that moisture that had suddenly flowed reaccumulated slowly. This is something that occurs only rarely. *De* [*symptomatum*] *causis* [I.2].

(XXIV.36) Someone who was stung by a scorpion recently said that he thought that he was pelted and hit by hailstones. His entire body was cold, and he broke out in a cold sweat. He was barely saved after he was treated with remedies that are used for scorpion stings. *De locis affectis* III[.11].

(XXIV.37) He says: There are illnesses which I have only rarely seen. For instance, that a person suffered from a sudden cough and expectorated a moisture resembling thin bile and that he continued to expectorate this moisture, daily and constantly. Later on, he expectorated sputum and after some months some blood. Then his body wasted away and his strength waned and he died. *De locis affectis* IV[.11].

I have seen someone cough and expectorate pieces of putrefied lung. I have also seen someone who had been coughing for a long time expectorate small pieces of matter. Then he expectorated something resembling small hailstones and continued to expectorate them until his life span was completed. [*De locis affectis* IV.11].

(XXIV.38) One day a person famous for his medical practice met with me. I felt his pulse and noticed therein all kinds of irregularities but without fever and without feeling anything at all during respiration. I told him that in my opinion this irregularity arose from a pressure and stenosis of the pulsatile vessels in his lungs and that this was caused either through an obstruction of thick, sticky humors or through the development of an abscess that was not ripe. He said to me: Then I should be suffering from an asthmatic orthopnea. I then said to him that orthopnea arises from the accumulation of a thick, viscous humor in the subdivisions of the trachea (bronchial tubes) but not from their accumulation in the pulsatile vessels. [*De locis affectis* IV.11].

(XXIV.39) Polyuria, also called "diabetes" or "severe thirst," is an illness that is only rarely found and that I until now have only observed twice. These are Galen's very words. [*De locis affectis* VI.3].

(XXIV.40) Says Moses: This illness has never passed by me in the Maghreb, nor did any one of my elders tell me about it. But here in the land of Egypt, in a period of twenty years I have seen about twenty men and three women suffering from this illness. This prompts me to say: This illness only rarely occurs in cold countries but often in hot ones because it is caused by excessive heat prevailing over the kidneys, as can be deduced from what Galen says in *De locis affectis* VI[.3].

(XXIV.41) I have seen several times that the movement of the pulsatile vessels subsided and abated, and then the patient recovered, regained his strength, lived and was saved, especially a patient who was of the age of the elderly. *De* [*praesagitione ex*] *puls*[*ibus* II.4].

(XXIV.42) I once saw a man on one of my travels who had a vessel filled with honey and who stood before two men who were physicians in a shop and offered it to them for sale. He allowed them to lick some of the honey to try how good it was. They did so and started to bargain with him. He then said to them that he would not sell it to them for the price they offered and left them. Both men died shortly after his departure from them. For this reason and similar ones, no one should not rely on whomever one happens to meet. *De* [*simplicium*] *medicamentorum* [*temperamentis ac facultatibus*] X[.1].

(XXIV.43) Pork resembles human meat. I have seen many innkeepers who are visited by travelers who sell human meat, once it had been cooked together with some pork. Some honest persons told me that they had been eating in some inns what they were sure was pork until they found human fingers in their food. When the Ruler was informed that they slaughter human beings and cook their meat, he had them executed. *De* [*simplicium*] *medicamentorum* [*temperamentis ac facultatibus*] X[.1].

(XXIV.44) Among all the medical works in our possession there is a treatise which bears the title: *A Treatise by Galen on the Prohibition of the Burial [of the Dead] within Twenty-four Hours*, translated by al-Biṭrīq. The authorship of this treatise is without doubt only for someone who is not familiar with the language of Galen. It seems to me that it refers to a man, a physician who was also a Greek and whose name was also Galen, but that he lived later than Galen the eminent physician, famous for his works. When this treatise fell into the hands of al-Biṭrīq he translated it into Arabic and thought that it was composed by the famous Galen because he—I mean al-Biṭrīq—was of a much lower level than Ḥunayn in his capacity of a translator. But to put it briefly, since this treatise belongs to that which has been composed in the field of medicine, I thought it a good thing to mention some unusual aphorisms from it.

(XXIV.45) He says in this treatise: A torpor may happen to a person which lasts for six or seven days, during which he does not use the faculty of reason, and does not eat and does not drink, and his vessels are dry and his respiration is irregular. Then he mentions unusual kinds of treating apoplexy patients.

(XXIV.46) He further says in this treatise: Sometimes black bile increases in the heart and the blood thickens and so much wind is emitted into the vessels that life disappears. It can also happen that all the signs of life disappear from such a patient, except for his complexion and the horripilation of the hair on his fingers. However, this indicates only that he is still alive, nothing else.

(XXIV.47) He further says in this treatise: Sometimes an overfilling occurs that is such that the pulse ceases in the entire body and that the heart does not move and that the person to whom this occurs is as dead. But his large vessels are full and replete and of good appearance and warm to the touch. If you see this, whatever vessel you see replete, whether it is tortuous or not tortuous, hasten to make an incision lengthwise and let the blood flow out because then the pneuma will stream through the vessels and the person will be revived immediately.

(XXIV.48) He further says in this treatise: It sometimes happens because of a fall from a high place or because of a very loud cry or because of a prolonged immersion in water that a person loses consciousness for forty-eight hours and becomes quasi-dead in that he assumes an ashy and dust-colored appearance and his nails become dust-colored as well. He then mentions indications of this person being still alive and gives information about how, in his opinion, one should treat him.

(XXIV.49) He also says therein that if one buries a deceased person who died without fever and without a chronic illness within seventy-two hours following his death, one might kill him because it is possible that one buries him while he is still alive. He then gives indications of this person being still alive and gives information about the treatment of such a person.

(XXIV.50) He also says therein: If someone has not eaten bread for a long time and then suddenly eats it, or if someone has not had intercourse for a long time and has intercourse, or if he stayed for a long time in a dark subterranean place and then suddenly emerges to the light of the sun, he may suffer from a condition similar to death and may really die. He then mentions the indications of this person being still alive and his therapy.

(XXIV.51) He also says therein: Sometimes a condition similar to death occurs because of the consumption of poisons or stings or bites by vermin or by putting on a liniment of soporific ingredients. The same may occur because of immoderate consumption of moistening foods and drinks followed by a sleep on the left side in which he is completely immersed so that one thinks that he is dead. Then he mentions the indications of this person being still alive and his therapy.

(XXIV.52) When Galen mentioned the ignorance of the physicians of his time and that he did not debate with them nor teach them anything when he met them at the bedside of the sick because they made themselves important and swelled over incorrect opinions, he expressed himself in the following words: Teaching the followers of Moses and Christ is easier and faster than teaching these physicians and philosophers who are deluded by heretic tendencies. *De* [*differentia*] *pulsu*[*m*] III[.3].

(XXIV.53) Says Moses: It is known to you without any doubt that the Christian religion had appeared and had become well known and spread before Galen. However, it had not spread to Greece at the time of Galen.

(XXIV.54) He says: A deep wound that occurs in the lobes of the liver can be cured. Similarly, if one of the lobes of the liver is cut off. Sometimes we see that the neck of the bladder is healed from a cut made to extract a stone because the neck of the bladder is fleshy. But all these things happen only rarely. Some say that the wound occurring in the stomach can be cured. I have seen a man who suffered from a large deep wound in the brain and was cured, although such a thing happens only rarely. *In Hippocratis Aphorismos commentarius* VI[.18].

(XXIV.55) In *De placitis Hippocratis et Platonis* I[.6], Galen says: I once told someone who was with me during surgery to hold the heart with a smith's tongs since it jumped and slipped from his fingers when he tried to hold it. During this pressure on his heart, the animal did not lose anything of its sensibility or voluntary movements, but screamed, moved, and breathed. It was not lacking anything except for the movement of the pulsation of the vessels.

On another occasion, when I wanted to excise the broken fragments of a bone of the cranium, I was forced to insert underneath that bone the instrument called "protector of the dura mater" as a precautionary measure. If we increase the contact and pressure on the brain with that instrument only a little bit, the patient's sensation and all voluntary movements are immediately abolished.

(XXIV.56) In *De placitis Hippocratis et Platonis* III[.3], he says: With the Slavs and non-Arabs and barbarians, anger is stronger than reason, but among us, the community of the Greeks, we find a similar matter only in the case of youngsters and those who have neither training nor education.

(XXIV.57) At the end of *De placitis Hippocratis et Platonis* VI[.8], Galen states: People in their generation used to inflict punishment on that bodily part with which that crime was committed. They scarified and beat the legs of a runaway and did the same with the hands of a thief, and, similarly, they scarified and beat the belly and stomach of him in whom gluttony and gormandize became apparent. They did the same with the tongue of prattlers. Therefore, their poet (Homer) says: So-and-so who had shown his passion to the wife of so-and-so and committed adultery with her, two kites ate his liver, which is the source and origin of lust.

(XXIV.58) He states in *In Platonis Timaeum commentarius* [II]: I have seen how many people whose body was naturally strong but whose soul was weak hardly moved or did not carry out any activity at all. They were then afflicted by illnesses that were of the same type as sleeplessness, apoplexy, or paralysis, and illnesses like epilepsy. Women with a similar constitution were affected by hysterical suffocation, and after hysterical suffocation paralysis quickly ensued. But of people whose soul was naturally strong and the body weak, I have only seen a few. One of these was Aristides who was from the people of Mysia. He was one of the best orators, and this happened to him because during his whole lifetime he was so fond of conversation and talking that his body wasted away entirely.

(XXIV.59) In *De simplicium medicamentorum* [*temperamentis ac facultatibus* III], in the translation by al-Biṭrīq, Galen says: If someone takes resin spurge slowly and little by little, it does not harm him. We know this from an old woman who lived in the land of Italy and who, as is related by all the ancients as well, used to take resin spurge and it did not harm her at all. The reason for this was that the first time she only took a small dose thereof. And when she continued to take it in larger doses, it did not harm her at all. For when she continued to take it and got used to it, it became part of her nature.

(XXIV.60) And in [*De simplicium medicamentorum temperamentis ac facultatibus* IX], in the translation by al-Biṭrīq, he says: There is nothing more suitable for the concoction of food by the stomach than to bring the body of another person nearby and to attach oneself to it. Some people approach young children for this purpose and put them on their abdomen during the night and derive great benefit therefrom because their heat is more suitable, better and more intense than the heat derived from a hot compress. There are other people who put a puppy on their abdomen if they want to sleep and find great relaxation in this.

This is the end of the twenty-fourth treatise,
by the grace of God,
praise be to Him.

In the name of God,
the Merciful, the Compassionate.
O Lord, make our task easy.

The Twenty-fifth Treatise

Containing some doubts that befell me concerning Galen's words

(XXV.1) Says Moses: With these doubts that I raise in this treatise, I do not have the same intention as al-Rāzī, as will be clear to the attentive reader, because al-Rāzī did not cast doubt on Galen in medical matters but immediately started to refute him in matters that have no relationship at all to the medical art. Even the matters that pertain to the medical art are only dubious for him in the arguments that Galen adduces for them and of which he seeks to establish that they are not logical arguments. Thus, al-Rāzī tries, as it were, to establish Galen's deficiency in the art of logic. Moreover, al-Rāzī often blames Galen and ascribes to him conclusions derived from the abstract and absolute sense of those words in question, without regard to the sense in which he uses them in that context. Ibn Zuhr and Ibn Riḍwān have already tried to resolve those doubts. I have not set my mind to say anything in this regard, and I am also not going to say anything about those things that al-Rāzī pretends to be doubts or to be solutions of doubts, for all this is, in my opinion, a useless waste of time. It is, even more, a waste of time for the worse because every obstinacy means in most cases to follow preconceived ideas, and every following of preconceived ideas is a mere evil. But I will mention those doubts that befell me concerning Galen's words in matters related to the medical art, since he is the master of this art. It is in this field alone that he should be followed; his words should not be heeded in any other field. That these doubts befell me can only be from one of three causes: It may either come from a mistake that befell the ones who translated Galen's works into Arabic, or it may come from unmindfulness that happened to Galen, as nobody is free from these things except for exalted human beings, or the cause may be my bad understanding. In any case, it is certainly useful to present in a combined form both contradictory statements, so that the point of doubt may become evident and the attentive reader may direct his interest to that matter, and that the truth on which he can rely may become manifest to him and his notions may not be deranged and he may not become confused, if a similar doubt presents itself to him.

(XXV.2) In *De usu partium* V[.10], he says: Only one extremely weak nerve is distributed through the whole liver because it does not need much sensation. These are his words in that place. Similarly, he explained in this treatise that the spleen, gallbladder, and kidneys have little sensation. In [*De usu partium*] VI[.18], he says and these are his words: As for nerves, we do not find any distributed and spread through the heart substance, just as we do not find this in the liver, kidneys, and spleen. But a small nerve reaches the membrane, which surrounds the heart (pericardium). But in those animals that have large bodies, something of a nerve that is perceptible sometimes attaches to the heart. These are his words. If he meant to say that the small nerve that he says that is distributed in the liver, spleen, and gallbladder is nothing else but the nerve that is distributed through the membrane of each of these organs, then that should have been clear from his words, as it is in the case of the heart.

(XXV.3) In *De naturalibus facultatibus* II.[9], he says that the sour phlegm does not undergo any concoction in the liver. In *De locis affectis* V[.7], he says that a cold dyscrasia of the liver makes the humor that ascends to it phlegmatic, crude, and semi-concocted. According to him, then, the crude humor is easier concocted than the sour phlegm because the crude humor undergoes some concoction in the liver, while the sour phlegm undergoes some concoction only in the stomach. This ought to be contemplated.

(xxv.4) In [*De causis pulsuum* I.12], he says that there are three causes that alter the pulse, namely, need, strength, and the constitution of the organs themselves. In *De sanitate tuenda* II.[11], he says that there are four causes for the alteration of the pulse and mentions the three that he also mentions in *De* [*causis*] *pulsu*[*um*] and adds the quantitative dissolution of the psychical pneuma. It is possible that this fourth cause belongs to all that which falls under the category of need. This ought to be contemplated.

(xxv.5) The putrid humor that produces fever within the vessels—I found Galen's discussion of this confused from my own point of view, for from his discourse in *De febrium differentiis* [I.7], it sometimes seems to me that this humor flows throughout the entire body. At other times it seems to me that that putrid humor is confined to one place. Similarly, it is clear from his discussion in *De causis* [*morborum* 2] that it is confined to one place. This is the correct opinion. Were it not so, it would not follow that there could be two or three continuous fevers in the body at the same time. This ought to be contemplated.

(xxv.6) In his *De temperamentis* [II.2], he says that the body heat of children and of adolescents is the same. Yet in *De sanitate tuenda* I[.2], he says that moisture and body heat diminish from the time of birth of a living being until the end of his life. This ought to be contemplated.

(xxv.7) In *De methodo medendi* VII[.5, 10], he says that a transformation to heat or cold is easier to treat and more rapid to cure, whereas a transformation to moisture and dryness is harder to treat and harder to cure. These are his words there. After this, in the very same book, when speaking about the stomach he says: A moist dyscrasia is easier to treat and faster to cure than the other types of dyscrasia. This holds true whether it is only moisture or it is mixed with heat or cold. These are his words as well. One might excuse this contradiction by saying that the first statement is meant in general, while the last one is meant specifically for the stomach, and this seems to be the case. But if the matter really is like this, then the first statement is not a general one, and this is the point of doubt. This ought to be contemplated.

(xxv.8) He says in *De compositione medicamentorum secundum locos* IV[.1]: The thin part of egg white washes and cleanses the moistures from the eye, and through its agglutinant quality it makes the roughness occurring in the eye soft and smooth. These are his words, and later in the same book he says: Egg white has no cleansing quality. This ought to be contemplated.

(XXV.9) In *De alimentorum* [*facultatibus* III.14], he regards the milk of camels as more excellent than that of donkeys. Yet in *De sanitate tuenda* V[.7], he regards donkey's milk as more excellent and gives it preference over all other kinds of milk.

(XXV.10) In his *De bonis malisque sucis* [IV.25; VI.8, 9]., he holds that pork excels any other kind of praiseworthy food. After that in excellence comes kid and after that veal and after that lamb.

(XXV.11) In a number of places, Galen explains to us that superfluous matters in the beginning of their streaming, and also when inflammations get worse or reach their climax, should be attracted to the opposite side. But if they have passed their climax and the humor is retained and settles in an organ and turns old or hard, the matter should be attracted from the filled organ itself, if possible, or from the organ that is closest to it. This is a fundamental rule that is repeatedly mentioned in the writings of Galen and Hippocrates. It is a correct rule and fixed according to analogical reasoning. The entire medical practice is based upon it, and its success is evident from experience. And because of this very beneficial fundamental rule, Galen instructs us to bleed the cephalic vein in the case of severe illnesses of the eye, and angina and the like. If the illness becomes prolonged and the inflammations become hard or adhere to an organ and become settled in it, then he tells us to bleed for illnesses of the eye the vein alongside the inner angle of the eye or a vein in the forehead or the veins behind the ears. And for inflammations of the throat and uvula, he tells us to bleed the veins under the tongue. [*De curandi ratione per venae sectionem* 19]. This is all correct and clear, and one should observe to draw the matter to the opposite side. In his *In Hippocratis Aphorismos commentarius* [VI.36], he remarks: In the case of illnesses above the liver, one should bleed from the arms; and if the illnesses are below the liver, one should bleed from the legs. This rule is repeated several times. However, in his *De* [*curandi ratione per*] *venae sectione*[*m* 16], he says: If someone suffers from epilepsy, vertigo, or dizziness, we should bleed him especially from the leg.

Says Moses: This rule is the opposite of the rule established by him in his previous statement and the opposite of that demanded by analogical reasoning. I do not know any explanation of this inconsistency, but it may be that the last-mentioned activity of bleeding from the leg has special conditions that have been omitted during the translation.

(XXV.12) In his *In Hippocratis Epidemiarum commentarius* I.1, he states that ardent fever does not originate from the burning of yellow bile in whatever organ this occurs. Rather, it develops if the yellow bile in the stomach has putrefied and especially in the cardia of the stomach or the concave side of the liver. Then he says in his *In Hippocratis Epidemiarum commentarius* I.2, that ardent fevers occur if the yellow bile in the vessels—and especially in the vessels close to the liver, stomach, or lungs—putrefies. This ought to be contemplated.

(XXV.13) In his treatise *De clysteribus* [*et colica*], he says: And detrimental foods such as cabbage and the like are among the cold and dry vegetables. And in *De simplicium medicamentorum* [*temperamentis ac facultatibus*] VII[.48], he says that cabbage has no evident sharpness or acridity and that its taste contains bitterness. He also says that its strength heals ulcers that have indurated. Everything that he mentions concerning its activity indicates that it contains some heat, although not strong. In this manner, Ibn Wāfid and others considered it as hot in the first degree.

(XXV.14) In his *De bonis malisque sucis* [XI.23], Galen says: One cannot find any type of cabbage that has a cooling effect, nor any type of onion, garlic, or leek with such an effect. Concerning a solution of the doubt raised by these contradictory passages, it seems to me that it is the moisture in the cabbage that contains heat but that its very substance, if that moisture separates from it, is cold. But Galen should have elucidated this, just as he elucidated such a matter in other cases. And in *De febrium* [*differentiis*] I[.4], he says: Hot foods, such as onion, garlic, leek, garden cress, cabbage and sweet basil.

(XXV.15) If a hot humor ascends to the upper parts of the body, ulcers develop in the head by themselves. Then it is necessary to expel it from the nearest site through emesis and not through bleeding. Says Moses: Galen mentions this matter in his *In Hippocratis Epidemiarum commentarius* II.6. I have very grave doubts concerning this statement, since it is contradictory to what is well known from the medical rules.

(XXV.16) In [*De symptomatum causis* I.5], he makes the following statement and these are his words: Any damage that occurs to any of the senses happens only because of an illness affecting the nerves by which the senses are well supplied when the nerves are healthy.

(XXV.17) Says Moses: I wish I knew whether a cataract and a deep ulceration of the horn-like tunic, if they are opposite the pupil and are joined together, are harmful for the sense of vision or not, and from what kind of damage the nerve through which the sense of vision is active suffers in these illnesses and similar ones. In the beginning of this treatise, Galen has informed us that a sense becomes impaired either on account of the principal organ through which it functions, or on account of the faculty that impels this principal organ, or on account of the parts that were created for the benefit of this principal organ. [*De symptomatum causis* I.1]. All this is correct. If one were to reverse this proposition (state the converse) and say that if the nerve of any sense whatsoever is harmed when the harm to this sense is imparted to the nerve, then this proposition would be correct according to what we have just learned. This ought to be contemplated.

(XXV.18) In his *In Hippocratis De aere, aquis et locis commentarius* II, he says: No part of the body should be cauterized except for the hands, feet, and loins. And in his *In Hippocratis Epidemiarum commentarius* VI.7, he says: In the case of those who suffer from an ulcer in the lung, one should hurry to cauterize their chest. These are his words and this statement annuls the previous one. This ought to be contemplated.

(XXV.19) In *De locis affectis* II[.8], he says the following, and these are his words: Pulsation does not follow an inflammation in all parts of the body, as we said, but only in that part in which there are sensitive pulsatile vessels, if that part itself has sensory perception and the inflammation called "phlegmon" is of noticeable size. For if these things occur together in that bodily part, the patient feels a pulsatile pain, even if the affected part does not have a sensitive pulsatile vessel. These are his words.

(XXV.20) Says Moses: If you consider this statement, it becomes clear to you that it is deficient since he mentions four conditions for pulsatile pain, namely, that there is an inflammation, that it is of a large size, that it is in a sensible part, and that that part has sensitive pulsatile vessels. Then he says that when these conditions occur together, the patient feels pulsatile pain. Then he says that this is the case even if the affected part has no sensitive pulsatile vessel. With this last statement he canceled the specific condition necessary for pulsation which he mentioned before, namely, the existence of a sensitive pulsatile vessel. The most probable solution of this inconsistency, in my opinion, is that during the translation of this book from one language into another some words were omitted so that the meaning of this text was corrupted. I also think that the intention of Galen's statement is that the joined occurrence of these four conditions in the inflamed part necessarily leads to a pulsatile sensation, even if that sensitive pulsatile vessel is not in the inflamed part itself but in a part close to it. This ought to be contemplated.

(XXV.21) Others than us and many physicians have contemplated Galen's words on the causes of pain. We found that in a number of places he gives only one cause for it, namely, a dissolution of continuity. He says about a hot cause of pain that it is comes with a loosening of a tight structure, and about a cold cause of pain that it comes with contraction and thickening. It goes beyond doubt that if some parts of an organ become more tight, other parts become more loose. All of it goes back to a dissolution of continuity. On this fundamental principle he bases his statement in [*De symptomatum causis* I.2] in a number of places. Then he explains in his *De inaequali intemperie* [6] that a varying kind of dyscrasia is one of the causes of pain. This is correct, and therefore every pain may have one of two causes: either a varying kind of dyscrasia or a dissolution of continuity. It is on this that he bases his assertion. There is no doubt that initially he had the first opinion and that then it became clear to him that the matter is as he mentions it eventually, namely, that there are two causes of pain. [*De locis affectis* II.5].

(XXV.22) In his *Puero epileptico consilium* [4], he allows an epileptic boy the consumption of some common vegetables and some fruits because he is still young and is not capable to abstain from food like a philosopher. Then he mentions all the vegetables that he allows him and says, and these are his words: Also, from these he should only take a moderate quantity. Similarly, leek, celery, and mountain parsley. These are his very words. But when he continued his statement and started to speak about the things that he should abstain from entirely he said the following, and these are his words: And amongst those things that are similar to those which I mentioned to abstain from entirely are all the things that ascend to the head through their heat and sharpness and fill it with vapors, such as wine, mustard, celery, garlic, and onions. These are his words. It is dubious to me that first he permits two species of celery and then forbids it absolutely. Also dubious to me is that he permits leek, but forbids onion and garlic while all three of them equally fill the brain with vapors, just as Galen treats them as equal in his *De alimentorum* [*facultatibus* II.69].

(XXV.23) Says Moses: We do not know the causes of everything whose existence has been ascertained. The fevers that arise from the putrefaction of the humors belong to this class of things. That is, when Galen wanted to furnish the cause why some of them abate and others do not, and why some of the abating and attacking ones adhere to one pattern and one cycle, while others of the abating and attacking ones follow no pattern, he started to present the causes of each of these four things whose existence is manifest. He said whatever he said in his book *De febrium* [*differentiis*]. He explained the difficulty of furnishing the cause for the regularity of the cycles. Moreover, he explained that he had shifted from one opinion to another but that later on he became confirmed in his final opinion. His explanation was quite lengthy. He claimed to have removed any difficulties and that what he stated was the most appropriate thing to be said about it. But when I contemplated his words thoroughly, I saw that there was some confusion in them. They became ever more dubious for me. The matter was not at all clear to me. I shall here quote his very words, and then I shall explain to you that which I found difficult. In *De febrium* [*differentiis* 1], he stated the following and these are his words:

As for the humors that putrefy in the viscera and in the major vessels—because these humors are always flowing, they cause to putrefy whatever they encounter. For their putrefaction and the heat that originates from them are joined together and result in a putrefying heat that affects one thing after another over a longer period. In sum, the determining factor of these things that happen inside the body is similar to the determining factor of that which happens at the outside to all the bodies that suffer from an unnatural heat, for whatever reason. For if that which becomes hot belongs to those things that do not putrefy, such as a stone or a piece of wood and other similar things, it keeps its warmth for some time until it starts to cool off slowly. But if it is one of those things that can putrefy, its heat spreads continuously from that part that is heated first to the part that is joined to it, like that which I once saw happening in some village to the dung of some animals and doves that had been collected in one place. One part of it became so heated by a very hot sun that a very large quantity of hot vapor started to arise from it, similar to smoke that has a strong biting effect and that is harmful for the eyes and nose of whoever gets close to it. Moreover, the heat of the dung was so strong when one touches it that if one put one's hand or foot into it and kept it there very well, it burned it. However, this symptom did not last forever, for the next day all the dung that had reached the highest degree of boiling heat on the previous day cooled off. And that part of the dung that was joined to the first part and that gradually absorbed the heat during the time that that first part was boiling hot started to become boiling hot as well when the heat of the first part began to diminish.

Shortly afterwards the second part became extremely hot, while the first part had cooled off. Then the heat of that second part also began to diminish, and the part that was joined to it was gradually becoming hotter. And it did not take long before that third part became blazingly and extremely hot, while the second part of the dung cooled off. This cycle took about a day and a night so that it is an example of what is particular for quotidian fever. If this cycle would take two days and two nights, it would be an example of tertian fever. If it would take three days, it would be an example of quartan fever, and if it would take five days, it would be an example of quintan fever, if there would be a fever that would attack on the fifth day. But I have not really seen such a cycle nor another one beyond the cycle of quartan fever. This is his first formulation, in accordance with his first opinion. [*De febrium differentiis* I.7].

Then, in [*De febrium differentiis* II.2], he said, and these are his words: Intermittent fevers, that is, those that have a sensible abatement, occur only when the humor that produces the fever moves and flows throughout the entire body. But continuous fevers occur only when the humor that produces the fever is confined within the cavity of the vessels. This is the text of his second statement. He then said something else in this book, namely, the statement in which he retracted his original opinion. These are his words: If you examine the matter closely, you will find that with some fevers, paroxysms occur in cycles even more wondrous than these.

For the example of the dung that putrefies part after part and that I gave above, it is almost impossible that that would happen in the body of a living being, because it does not take long before the humors that putrefy get mixed with other humors that did not putrefy since the humors stream from every site in the body to every other site. If this is the case, then it is impossible that there is putrefaction in one part of the body but not in another and only at a certain moment but not at another, except when there is an inflamed tumor in some part that has bound the putrefied humor and retained it inside. If our words turned out to be opposite to the ones stated before and it is evidently more difficult to find the cause for fevers that attack in cycles than for continuous fevers, then we should attempt to discuss the situation with regard to both of them together. This is the formulation of his third statement. [*De febrium differentiis* II.13].

Later on in the same book, after he became confirmed in the second opinion, he said, when giving a cause for the cycles, that the organ expels its superfluities from one set time to the next and that it is those expelled superfluities that putrefy. He gave the cause for the length or brevity of the paroxysm in accordance with his last opinion. Then he said the following, and these are his words: Moreover, according to this reasoning it will not be difficult for you to know the cause whereby some bouts of fever abate, while others do not abate. The former are doubtless of such brevity that they terminate before the next bout begins. The putrefying humor flows and moves through the entire body. Thus, the entire period between the end of the first bout and the beginning of the second is a period of abatement and freedom from fever. However, when the second bout comes earlier, and it occurs before the first bout really ends, then no time at all remains between them during which the body is free from fever. This is his fourth formulation. [*De febrium differentiis* II.17].

(XXV.24) Says Moses: The gist of his first statement is that the humor that putrefies gradually is within the vessels, and the period of abatement is that period between the putrefaction of a part of that thing and of that part that lies next to it, as he illustrated with the example of the dunghill. The fever attacks and the humor putrefies within the vessels, as he said. But the gist of his second statement is that there is no sensible abatement unless the putrefying humor is outside the vessels and moves and flows throughout the entire body. And this is most astonishing, how it can be outside the vessels in one place, without any doubt, but also streaming and moving throughout the entire body. And the gist of his third statement—the one in which he became confirmed—is that the organ expels its superfluities outside of itself, and it then putrefies there, until that which is consumed is consumed and that which burns into ashes burns into ashes. This is a bout of fever. Later on, it abates until it expels another superfluity to that place. The gist of his fourth statement is that continuous fever is the result of one paroxysm immediately following upon another. This ought to be contemplated.

(XXV.25) What I am going to say in this aphorism is not to express doubt over Galen but is something that those engaged in speculation should consider and contemplate, namely, to which extremes the following of one's passion ultimately leads and how it blinds the perceptive faculties of the mind. For this Galen was an earnest seeker of the truth, had a predilection for syllogistic demonstrations, composed a book entitled *De demonstratione*, and questioned Aristotle's sayings about natural or supernatural matters when Aristotle did not demonstrate them logically, by using, for instance, mathematical demonstrations. But although Galen had reached such a high level in seeking logical proof for everything, when he found out about the usefulness of the testicles and it became evident to him and he held it for the truth, while Aristotle had paid no attention to that usefulness and ignored it, he was very pleased with himself and, in a lengthy discussion, killed Aristotle off as an animal that is weakened by hunger kills its prey when it has found it. He then began to exalt the usefulness of the testicles and to magnify their importance until he made them more eminent than the heart with his analogical reasoning. These are his words in *De semine* I[.15].

(xxv.26) He says: Only the heart is the origin and root of living, but the testicles are the root and cause of living well. By as much as living well is better than plain living, by so much, among animals, are the testicles better than the heart. These are the very words of this eminent, truth-seeking man, and this is his reasoning.

Consider then, ye who possess insight, whether this is correct, because if the heart would be excised from a living being, could he remain alive to live a good life? That is, could he have sexual intercourse and show his male sexual potency and not lack any vital function? But if his testicles are cut off, he remains alive as we see in the case of eunuchs. Are then the testicles more eminent than the heart? In short, this statement is so deficient that one does not have to refute it.

(xxv.27) In [*De symptomatum causis* II.7], he makes the following statement and these are his very words: The afflictions that occur in the case of epilepsy are, in my opinion, caused by a surplus of phlegmatic superfluity that collects in the ventricles of the brain. Therefore, they appear suddenly and terminate suddenly. And this is something that can in no wise happen because of cold of the body. These are his words over there.

(xxv.28) And in *De locis affectis* III[.11], he says: There are three types of epilepsy. One of these is that the illness originates in the brain itself, the second is that it originates from the cardia of the stomach and ascends to the brain, and the third that the illness ascends from any organ until it reaches the brain. About the third type he states the following, and these are his words: That which arises is similar to a cold breeze. This cannot be anything else but a quality that arises and is guided from organ to organ, or some vaporous substance which comes with this quality, just as is the case with poison. These are his words. The point of doubt is clear: How can epilepsy be merely a dyscrasia without any substance whatsoever that happens in the brain? He himself has rejected this and said that it is not all possible. This ought to be contemplated.

(xxv.29) In a number of places he says that males are warmer and drier than females, and in accordance to this statement, he devised the fundamental principles of the entire medical art. He adduced proof for this question and gave a lengthy explanation of it in *De semine* II[.4]. In his commentary on Hippocrates' book *Diseases of Women*, he says that the rapid growth of women indicates that they have extra heat that is matched by the moisture of their bodies. This is confirmed by the menstrual flow from their bodies every month, because where there is much blood, there is much heat. These are his words.

If he means with this that the principal organs of a woman are colder and moister than those of men and that blood is more abundant in women, this is also problematic, because the vessels of men are wider. In addition, that first judgment of his in which he compares the female of every species with the male has a general character. Moreover, how can one conclude from a surplus of superfluities in a woman that there is necessarily a surplus of blood? It seems to me that Galen found this statement with another, earlier author, either with Hippocrates or with one of the commentators of his books, and that he copied it once he found that commentary. He must have thought that it was correct, either because at that time he did not know about Aristotle's statement concerning this matter or because he had seen it but did not remember it when he commented upon this book [*Diseases of Women*].

Listen to the wording of Aristotle's statement concerning this matter in *De* [*generatione*] *animali*[*um* IV]. He says: The heat found in female living beings is weak. However, some people assume the opposite, that is, that the blood in a female living being is more abundant than in a male one, and for this reason they think that a female living being is warmer than a male one, and this is so according to them because of the emission of menstrual blood—for blood is hot, and therefore that living being that has more blood has more heat. They imagine that this accident (menstruation) occurs only because of an excessive surplus of blood and heat. They also believe that all the blood can appear in this form (menstruation) and content themselves in this respect with the conclusion that the menstrual blood is moist and that it has the color of blood. They do not know that pure blood that consists of good juices forms only a small part of the menstrual blood, for menstrual blood, taken as a whole, is not pure. This is the wording of Aristotle's statement there, and it is correct, and Galen expresses himself in the same way in all his compositions.

(XXV.30) Whenever he mentions milk, in every place where he refers to it, he says that it consists of three substances: the watery part, the cheesy part, and the fatty part. In *De bonis* [*malisque*] *sucis* [IV.4.8], he makes the following statement, and these are his words: Watery moisture prevails more in the milk of camels and donkeys, cheesy moisture prevails more in sheep's milk, and fat in cow's milk.

And likewise, he explains in *De alimentorum* [*facultatibus* III.14.6], that the fatty part—that is, the butter—prevails in cows' milk. But in his *De victu attenuante* [12], he says the following, and these are his words: And that milk in which the cheesy part greatly prevails such as cows' milk. There is a point of doubt in that in the first statement he remarks that butter prevails more in cows' milk, while in the last statement he remarks that cheese dominates more in it. This ought to be contemplated.

(XXV.31) When he mentions the watery part of the milk in *De simplicium medicamentorum* [*temperamentis ac facultatibus*] X[.8], he says the following, and these are his words: The strength of the watery part of this milk which is free from butter and cheese is that it purifies and cleanses the viscera and expels the putrefying superfluities from them, if it is imbibed or taken as an enema. It achieves this with no biting effect; on the contrary, it is also very effective in alleviating biting pain. These are his words there. And in *De alimentorum* [*facultatibus*] III[.14.5], he says the following about the watery part of the milk, and these are his words: Do not be amazed that milk, once the watery part has been removed from it and water is again added to it, has a sympathetic quality. For the physicians do this not because they shy away from the watery part of the milk but because they shy away from its sharpness, which causes the bowels to be relieved. These are his words. The point of doubt is clear. In the first statement he says that it has no biting effect at all, but that on the contrary it alleviates biting pain, while in the last statement he says that he watery part of milk has a sharpness that causes diarrhea. This ought to be contemplated.

(XXV.32) In *De naturalibus facultatibus* I[.6], he makes the following statement, and these are his words: All the partly alterative faculties of the natural faculties produce the very substance of the two coats of the stomach, of the intestines, and of the uterus and make them what they are. In the same book [*De naturalibus facultatibus* I.13] he also makes the following statement, and these are his words: The urinary bladder is an extremely thick and solid body, hard and consisting of two strong coats. These are his words. And in [*De naturalibus facultatibus* III.11], he makes the following statement, and these are his words: For this reason, any organ—even if it has only one coat, such as the urinary bladder, the gallbladder, the uterus, and the non-pulsatile vessels—necessarily has both kinds of fibers together, that is, those that stretch in the length (longitudinal) and those that stretch in the width (transverse). The point of doubt is that whereas here he remarks that the uterus and the urinary bladder have one coat—and this is correct—in *De usu partium* [XIV.14], next to the earlier statement in *De* [*naturalibus*] *facultatibus* I, he says they have two coats. In my opinion there is no doubt that this is an error either the translators or an error made during the copying (by the copyists). If someone were to say that the urinary bladder really only has one coat, as mentioned by Galen, and that the upper coat is the membrane that covers every organ, this is problematical as well since every organ with two coats also has this membrane and he does not say that it has three coats. This ought to be contemplated.

(xxv.33) In [*De morborum differentiis* 5], he reviles those who sometimes call fever an illness and at other times—namely, when it is consequential upon a tumor—call it a symptom. He says that this is an error and that it is always an illness, and that sometimes illnesses come after other illnesses just as fever comes after a tumor. And in *Ad Glauconem* [*de medendi methodo*] I[.4], he makes the following statement, and these are his words: Fevers that flare up from the putrefaction of the humors are especially known by this name, that is, that of fevers. They are not symptoms of other illnesses, but are illnesses themselves. These are his words. One should contemplate how inconsistent he is in the terminology he uses.

(xxv.34) In *De alimentorum* [*facultatibus*] II[.37.2], he makes the following statement about *utrujj* (citron or lemon) peels, and these are his words: When used as a medicine, they are good for the digestion just as many other things that have a sharp, acrid quality. And in *De simplicium medicamentorum* [*temperamentis ac facultatibus*] VII[.18], he says the following, and these are his words: *Utrujj* peels have no cooling effect but a moderate or a little less than moderate effect. The point of doubt is that there he describes them as being among the sharp, acrid things, but here he describes them as being among the moderate things.

(xxv.35) When speaking about honey in *De alimentorum* [*facultatibus* III.38.7], he mentions the bile whose color is pale yellow and the bile whose color is yellow and remarks that there are other types of yellow bile besides these two. Then he says the following, and these are his words: We see with our own eyes how all these other types, except for the leek-green one, are evacuated from the body in the case of a severe and serious illness. Yellow bile, pale yellow bile and leek-green bile are often expelled through emesis and diarrhea while there is no illness. This is a clearly defined formulation as it can be found in ancient writings. The point of doubt is how he first stipulated in the case of leek-green bile that it is only emitted in a severe, serious illness and then remarks that the leek-green bile is often emitted without any illness. If we try to explain the contradiction by saying that the meaning of his words is that in the case of a severe, serious illness there is no leek-green bile and therefore it does not emerge and is not seen, this is even more problematic in trying to provide a reason for this. To sum up, it may be said that it is a point that should be contemplated.

(XXV.36) In *De usu partium* XVI[.2], he says the following, and these are his words: No special, separate nerve was made to reach the skin, but it is reached by certain subdivisions of the nerves from the parts that lie beneath it. These subdivisions go to these parts in order that they are bonds between the skin and the parts beneath it and serve as sensory organs for them. These are his words there. And in *De locis affectis* III[.14], he says the following, and these are his words: The physicians do not at all know that the nerves that are spread and distributed in the skin of the entire hand and provide it with sensation have special roots, and that the nerves for the movement of the muscles of the hand have other roots. These are his words as well. The point of doubt is very clear in that in *De usu partium*, he definitely states that the nerves of the skin are only subdivisions of the nerves that reach the muscles beneath the skin. And here in *De locis affectis* III, he says that the nerves that reach the skin of the hand are different from the nerves that reach the muscles that move the hand. I wish I knew whether this applies only to the hand among all the organs and if this is the case why he did not mention it.

(XXV.37) Says Moses: In my opinion, his statement in *De usu partium* is correct. The fact that the organ hidden beneath the skin can lose its sensation but not its motion is not caused by the nerves that are inserted into the muscle of that organ and that provide it with motion, but by the very nerves themselves (the part not inserted into the muscle), as he states in *De usu* [*partium*]. However, an affliction occurs in the ends of that fine nerve that is distributed in the skin, and therefore the sensation of the skin is abolished, but that affliction does not reach the root of that nerve—the root that is inserted in the muscle—and therefore motion is not abolished. This is in accordance with the principal rules that Galen taught us, namely, that the loss of function of a branch does not damage the root, but that the abolishment of the root necessarily causes loss of function of the branch.

(XXV.38) In [*De morborum differentiis* 2], he says the following, and these are his words: These humors are mixed with one another, and one only rarely finds one of them that is pure not mixed with another one. And in [*De causis morborum* 6], he says the following, and these are his words: Every singular one of these humors often streams to the organs while it is pure and unadulterated, not mixed with anything else. Sometimes, however, they stream into them, mixed with one another. These are his words there. The point of doubt is clear, namely, that in the first statement he considers the existence of one of the humors in a pure unadulterated form as a rare phenomenon, but then remarks in the second statement that more often one finds one of them streaming in an unadulterated form and that only occasionally one finds them mixed. What I observe constantly is in agreement with what he says in the first statement. This ought to be contemplated.

(XXV.39) In his *De atra bile* [3], he makes the following statement, and these are his words: Black chymes are often excreted with vomiting or diarrhea, and this can in some cases be a good sign. But when black bile is excreted with vomiting or diarrhea, it indicates death because its development in the body is a fatal sign. These are his words. He makes it absolutely clear in that statement that the appearance of this humor is a sign of death and that ignorant physicians think that the emission of this malicious humor is a good thing, but that this is not the case. In his *In Hippocratis Aphorismos commentarius* IV[.22], he states the following, and these are his words: Therefore, black bile—and every other humor with a similar bad condition—, if it appears at the end of the illness once signs of coction have become visible, it indicates that its evacuation has a wholesome effect. These are his words there. The point of doubt is clear, namely, that in this last statement he stipulates that the appearance of black bile after coction is a good sign, while in the first statement he states in a definite and absolute way that its excretion indicates death. It seems to me that the statement he makes in *De atra bile* is correct and that the statement that he makes in his *In Hippocratis Aphorismos commentarius* IV is only correct for the other black humors but not for black bile. One should contemplate this matter very well.

(XXV.40) In *De temperamentis* II[.3], he says the following, and these are his words: Of humors the most appropriate for the nature of human beings and the most beneficial is blood. Black bile is like a sediment and dregs of blood, and therefore it is colder and thicker than blood. Yellow bile is much hotter and drier than blood. Phlegm is colder and moister than all the humors in the body of a living being. The instrument to measure this as well is the sense of touch. These are his words. In [*De causis morborum* 6], he says the following, and these are his words: That which pours must inevitably and unavoidably be moist and fluid in its appearance, although it is not absolutely necessary that it is moist in its potency. Ancient physicians and philosophers speak about the potency of such humors. I too have commented upon the matter of this potency in the books in which I describe the subject of medicines and in other books. But what I need for my present subject in this book is what I am going to say now, namely, that the potency of yellow bile is hot and dry, that of black bile is cold and dry, that of blood is hot and moist, and that of phlegm is cold and moist. These as his words as well. The point of doubt is that in *De temperamentis* he explains that yellow bile is hot and dry as it is measured with the sense of touch, while here he says that it has these qualities potentially. The same is true for the other three humors: It is clear from his words in *De temperamentis* that these qualities are ascribed to them actually. But here he says that they are attributed to them potentially. This ought to be contemplated.

(XXV.41) In his *In Hippocratis De natura hominis commentarius* [I.34], he says the following, and these are his words: I explained in my book *De temperamentis* that spring is moderate, while Hippocrates says here that it is hot and moist. The matter is according to Hippocrates' statement. And in his *In Hippocratis De aere, aquis et locis commentarius* I, he says that spring is hot and moist with regard to its essence, but moderate in relation to the human body.

(XXV.42) Says Moses: This last statement is correct. He did not formulate all his previous statements as accurately as he did this last statement.

(XXV.43) When he describes in *De methodo medendi* VII[.4] the case of the man whose stomach was dried by the physicians to a degree that he suffered from marasmus, he says the following, and these are his words: Then, when they finally saw that his stomach could not digest any food at all, they prompted him to drink tanner's sumach juice and put all those medications on the outside of his stomach, which I mentioned before. By doing this they made him like someone whose body was wasted away and depleted of moisture until he was like dead. When I was charged with the treatment of this man, I started to moisten him in any possible way. These are his words.

When he started to mention the treatment of that man, he made the following statement, and these are his words: Just as I treated that man whom the physicians had dried out and who in terms of heat and cold was healthy since none of these prevailed over him, neither in his body in general, nor in his stomach, but suffered from extreme dryness, emaciation, and leanness of the body. These too are his words concerning this man. [*De methodo medendi* VII.6]. The point of doubt is very clear. How can a person whose body has become so utterly dry that he is like dead—as he says—have a moderate constitution between heat and cold? Rather, his body should be cold since the substance of the innate heat has dissipated.

In his discussion of this very same man in this treatise, he says the following, and these are his words: It is impossible that dryness remains on its own and by itself while heat and cold are counterbalanced without any blemish, for organs, if not nourished, become cold very rapidly. These too are his words there and this is correct. But when he remarked in his earlier statement about this man that he was healthy in terms of heat and cold in his body, he started to correct this with the following words: But in this case I only treated, as I said, from the beginning of the matter the dryness that prevailed on its own and by itself and that persisted for a long time without being followed by cold of a perceptible size. This is the end of his statement over there in his own words. [*De methodo medendi* VII.7].

I am even more doubtful now. I wish I knew the answer to the following: If in the case of someone whose body has become so dry that it is as if he is dead, there is no cold discernible in him, what is then the case of dryness that is necessarily followed by perceptible cold? Would you consider it to occur once he has died—being old and decayed? Even more amazing is his statement about him that he became utterly emaciated because of lack of food, while he says here that the organs, if they are not nourished, become cold very quickly. In general, this last statement is correct; there is no doubt about it.

(XXV.44) In *De puls*[*ibus libellus ad tirones* 12], he says the following, and these are his words: When the affliction is minor, it makes the pulse regularly unequal, and when the affliction is major, it makes that the pulse have an irregular inequality. These are his words there. In *De* [*praesagitione ex*] *puls*[*ibus* II.13], he makes the following statement, and these are his words: An irregularly unequal pulse indicates that the cause of the inequality shifts from organ to organ and is not stable. The illness may shift to an inferior organ and the patient is spared. But it may also shift to a noble organ and he dies. Therefore, one cannot use the irregularity of the unequal pulse as a genuine prognostic sign. This is his formulation, and the point of doubt is clear and evident. For in the first statement, he declares positively that irregularity of the unequal pulse indicates that the affliction is a major one, and in this last statement he says that it is neither a good nor a bad sign. The doubt can be solved by saying: Irregularity of an unequal pulse indicates that the current affliction is severe but that one cannot know what will really be in the end. This too ought to be contemplated.

(XXV.45) In his *De* [*totius*] *morb*[*i*] *temporibus* [4], he starts to explain that every illness from which one can be healed has four stages—beginning, increase, climax, and decline—and that in the case of some illnesses one thinks because of their short beginning that they do not have a beginning, while they do have a beginning without any doubt, but only a very short one. He then says the following, and these are his words: We find that in the case of an illness that is extremely detrimental—namely, apoplexy—its beginning and increase take place in a short time. The same holds true for epilepsy. These are his words and this statement is true without any doubt.

In *De crisibus* I[.4], when he began to explain that from the nature of an illness one can draw conclusions about its length or brevity, he makes the following statement, and these are his words: In the same way, in the case of the other illnesses, one can draw conclusions about their duration. Hectic fever, pleurisy, and pneumonia have a short beginning, but epilepsy, sciatica, arthritis, and nephritis have a long beginning. These are his words there.

The point of doubt is that in this last statement he makes the beginning of epilepsy long. What does he mean with this statement? If he means the beginning of an epileptic fit, it is impossible that the time is shorter than that, for then it would be imperceptible, as he explained in the beginning of his statement in that treatise. And if he means the beginning of the cause that produces epilepsy, the question arises as to what the observation of this matter has to do with the definition of the stages of an illness. The most probable solution in my opinion is that the epilepsy mentioned in *De crisibus* is originally a mistake by the copyist.

(XXV.46) In *De simplicium medicamentorum* [*temperamentis ac facultatibus*] IV[.19], he says the following, and these are his words: A similar effect as iron and a stone heated in the fire and the like is achieved by the drugs that kill through the corrosion they cause when they are brought to the same degree of heat as the body has. Examples are yellow vitriol, green vitriol, red vitriol, and mercury, for all such drugs that are coarse and have a hot potency burn the stomach and the adjoining parts of the abdomen. These are his words over there.

And in [*De simplicium medicamentorum temperamentis ac facultatibus*] IX, when speaking about mercury, he says: I do not know from testing or experience if it is fatal when it is ingested nor what effect it has if it is applied externally to the body. These, too, are his words concerning mercury. I wish I knew who is the authority he relies on for the judgment he passes on mercury in [*De simplicium medicamentorum temperamentis ac facultatibus*] IV, namely, that it kills by burning just like the different types of vitriol.

(XXV.47) He says the following in *De methodo* [*medendi*] XI[.15] and these are his words: It is most beneficial, as I have stated, to apply venesection not only in continuous fevers but in all fevers that arise from putrefaction of the humors.

(XXV.48) Says Moses: One may doubt Galen's approval of venesection in the case of all putrid fevers. In his *De* [*curandi ratione per*] *venae sectione*[*m* 10] and other places, he himself forbids venesection in pure phlegmatic fever because the humors are raw and crude. He also forbids bloodletting in pure quartan fever, unless there is a clear indication for excess of blood. To solve this doubt, it seems to me that when he speaks about all fevers that arise from putrefaction of the humors, he means that the putrefying substance consists of many humors and not one unadulterated humor. Thus, the meaning of his words is that in the case of every fever that arises from putrefaction of the blood, although that putrefying blood is mixed with an even larger quantity of phlegm or black bile, venesection is beneficial. But if only the phlegm or the black bile putrefies, one should not apply venesection. But he would still be inconsistent in his statements if he used the following words: However, all fevers arising from putrefaction of one single putrid humor, whatever humor it may be.

(XXV.49) In *De simplicium medicamentorum* [*temperamentis ac facultatibus*] VI[.13], while discussing the plant called Roman nettle when he mentions the benefits of its seed and leaves, Galen says the following, and these are his words: Moreover, they both have flatulent strength, and for this reason stimulate the sexual lust, especially when the seed of this plant is ingested with concentrated grape juice. These are his words. When he describes the effects of this plant more into detail, he makes the following statement, and these are his words: The flatulence that I said is produced develops only from the plant when it is digested in the stomach. The reason for this is that this plant is not flatulent actually but only potentially. These are his words.

(XXV.50) Says Moses: I can in no way understand what he said about this matter or what he is trying to say, and the way he expresses himself is confusing for the translator. The point of doubt is his statement that it is flatulent potentially but not actually; that is to say, that any substance is flatulent only potentially but not actually, neither this plant nor any other flatulent one. But how does he conceive that a drug can actually be flatulent? He himself explained for us in a previous chapter of this book that any property that is ascribed to a drug—as when we say that it is hot or cold—refers only to its potential effect, but not to the sensation of that drug as hot or cold. However, the heat of our body actualizes what is potentially in it. This ought to be contemplated.

(XXV.51) In his *In* [*Platonis*] *Timaeum commentarius* [II], Galen explains that only the liver transforms the food into blood and that the body of the vessels that contain the blood do not convert it into something blood-like. He says with the following words: We find that every bodily organ that feeds itself with blood transforms its nourishment and makes it similar to its substance so that, if it is completely without blood like bones, cartilage, nerves, ligaments, tendons, and membranes, it transforms the blood into its own nature. How is it then possible that the body of a vessel produces blood, since it is white and a type of membrane, so that it nourishes only itself by altering and transforming the food into its own nature? These words are sufficient to conclude that it is the liver that transforms the food into blood. So far, his words.

(XXV.52) In *De locis affectis* III[.13], when speaking about the pain of migraine, Galen states the following: If the pain is caused by wind, the patient feels a tension; if it originates from a surplus of superfluities, the patient also feels heaviness. In his *De* [*curandi ratione per*] *venae sectione*[*m* 7], he says the following, and these are his words: A special sign for the kind of overfilling that is commensurate to strength is weight, and a special sign for the kind of overfilling that is commensurate to the vessels is tension.

The point of doubt is that in the first statement he says that the sensation of heaviness that comes with the pain of migraine indicates a surplus of humors, while in the second statement he says that tension indicates overfilling that is commensurate to the vessels. And this overfilling originates without any doubt from a surplus of humors. It seems to me that the proof adduced in *De* [*curandi ratione per*] *venae sectione*[*m*] for two kinds of overfilling is valid only if the patient feels that heaviness or tension without pain, regardless of whether that sensation is only in one part or in the entire body. But if he feels a severe pain like migraine in a bodily part and next to the pain, he feels heaviness, it indicates a surplus of humors and not only malignancy of humors. For overfilling commensurate to strength is only caused by malignancy of humors, and this is harmful for the strength of the organ so that he has a sensation of heaviness, while it is not severe. Some people say that this applies to the head especially. This is confirmed by what Galen says in [*De compositione medicamentorum secundum locos* IV.1], and these are his words: A surplus of humors in the head produces heaviness but not a headache unless an obstruction results from it. These are his words. It is very difficult to provide a reason why only a surplus of humors, that is, overfilling commensurate to the vessels, causes heaviness in the head and tension in any other part of the body or in the entire body. This ought to be contemplated.

(XXV.53) In *De methodo medendi* V[.8], when he begins to describe how someone suffering from hemoptysis from the lungs should be treated, he says the following, and these are his words: Tell the patient not to take deep breaths and always to remain quiet, and immediately phlebotomize him from the vein at the inner side of the arm. These are his words there. And in his [*In Hippocratis*]

De humoribus commentarius I[.18], he makes the following statement, and these are his words: It is not proper for someone who emits blood from the larynx, lungs, chest, or windpipe to raise his voice or breathe deeply. But to move his arms is not bad for him, and it is even more appropriate in this regard to move his legs moderately so that his pulse does not become spasmodic. These are his words there. The point of doubt is that in the first statement he instructs the patient to adhere to a regimen of rest and repose, while in the second statement he allows moderate movement. This ought to be contemplated.

(XXV.54) When he mentions fleawort seed in *De simplicium medicamentorum* [*temperamentis ac facultatibus*] VIII[.23], he makes the following statement, and these are his words: The most beneficial part of this plant is its seed; it is cold in the second degree and is in the middle between moisture and dryness, balanced. These are his words there. In his *Ad Glauconem* [*de medendi methodo*] II[.3], when speaking about corrosive shingles he says the following, and these are his words: In this illness, be careful not to use cultivated lettuce, common knotgrass, fleawort seed, common duckweed, *nīlūfar* (blue Egyptian, European white, or yellow water lily), common purslane, *ḥayy al-ʿālam* (common houseleek or tree aeonium), or similar ingredients with cooling, moistening properties. These are his words in this place. The point of doubt is that in this last statement he explains that fleawort seed is cold and moist and counts it with cultivated lettuce, common purslane, common duckweed, and *nīlūfar* and says that all these have cooling and moistening properties, while in the first statement he says that fleawort seed is intermediate between dryness and moisture. This ought to be contemplated.

(XXV.55) In *De methodo* [*medendi*] XIII[.17], when speaking about the treatment of tumors of the liver and spleen and comparing their remedies, he says the following, and these are his words: That is that both these organs require remedies that, although of a similar kind, differ in strength and weakness. For the spleen needs stronger remedies because of the greater amount of thickness of its nourishment over the nourishment of the liver. These are his words there. And in *De usu* [*partium*] IV[.15], he makes the following statement, and these are his words: Note the following summary of my words to you concerning the nourishment of these three organs: the liver is nourished by thick, red blood; the spleen is nourished by thin, dark blood; and the lung is nourished by blood that is extremely well concocted, bright red, thin, and spirituous. These too are his words.

The point of doubt is that in *De methodo medendi*, he explains that the nourishment of the spleen is thicker than that of the liver, whereas in *De usu partium*, he explains that the nourishment of the spleen is thinner than that of the liver. His explanation in *De usu partium* is correct; there he compares the degree of thinness of the nourishment of the liver, spleen, and lung and says that the nourishment of the liver is thick according to its substance, the nourishment of the lung thin, and that of the spleen intermediate between these two, namely, thinner than the nourishment of the liver and thicker than that of the lung. Once he has compared the thinness of the blood, as we have just described, he compares the color of the blood of these three organs and says that the blood with which the lung nourishes itself is bright red, and that with which the spleen nourishes itself is dark, and that with which the liver nourishes itself is intermediate between these two, that is, less red than the blood of the lung and less dark than that of the spleen.

It seems to me that Galen did not forget all this, nor did he disregard it. But he expressed himself very carelessly in his statement in *De methodo* [*medendi*] and took the term nutrition in its most general sense, that is, something that has the property to turn into nutrition, just as one says of bread and beetroot that they are nutrition. There is no question that the substance that the spleen attracts before it transforms it and nourishes itself with it is thicker than that which is attracted by the body of the liver for nourishment. This is the matter he looked at in his statement in *De methodo* [*medendi*]. This ought to be contemplated.

(xxv.56) In *De* [*differentia*] *pulsu*[*um*] II.5], Galen makes the following statement, and these are his words: The language of the Greek is the most pleasant of all languages and the most universal for all people endowed with logic, the most eloquent and most human. For if you pay attention to the pronunciation of the words in the languages of other peoples, you will certainly discern that some of them are very much like the grunting of pigs, others resemble the croaking of frogs, and yet others resemble the sound produced by the green woodpecker. Then you will also find that these words originate in an ugly way in the movements of the tongue, lips, and entire mouth. For some people bring forth sounds mostly from deep within the throat as if they were snoring, others twist their mouth and whistle, others roar and scream at the top of their voice, others make no perceptible or discernible sound at all. Some of them open their mouth widely and stick out their tongue, and others do not stick out their tongue at all; it seems to be idle and difficult to move as it is heavy and tied.

(xxv.57) Says Moses: Al-Rāzī and others have cast doubt on these words of Galen. The thrust of their objection is that he makes the Greek language into a unique one among the languages spoken by men and regards all the other languages as ugly ones. It is well known that the languages are conventional and that every language is ugly, hard, and obscure for someone who does not know it and who has not been raised with it. This is the basic meaning of the words of every one who doubts this statement by Galen. It seems to me that what Galen said in this statement is correct—that is, that the difference in the pronunciation of the letters and the difference in the movement of the organs of speech during speaking are consequential upon the difference in climates, that is, the difference of the temperaments of their inhabitants and the difference of the shapes of their organs and their external and internal sizes.

(xxv.58) This was mentioned by Abū Naṣr al-Fārābī in the *Kitāb al-Ḥurūf* (*Book of Letters*). For as, in general, people living in the temperate climatic zones have more perfect intellects and better forms their shape and outline is more regular, their organs are better proportioned, and their temperament is more balanced than that of the inhabitants of the distant climatic zones in the extreme north and south, so the pronunciation of the letters by the inhabitants of the temperate climatic zones and the movement of their speech organs during speaking are more balanced and are closer to human articulated speech than the pronunciation of the letters and the movement of the speech organs of those people, I mean, the inhabitants of the distant climatic zones in the extreme north and south and their language, as Galen remarks. Galen does not mean the Greek language only, but it and similar ones, namely, the Greek language, Arabic, Hebrew, Syriac, and Persian since these are the languages of the inhabitants of these moderate climatic zones, and they are natural to them according to the difference of the places they live in, which are close to one another.

Regarding the Arabic and Hebrew language, everyone who knows these two languages agrees that they are undoubtedly a single language and Syriac is somewhat close to them and Greek is close to Syriac. The pronunciation of the letters in these four languages is the same, except for a few letters, perhaps three or four. Persian is more remote from these, and the pronunciation of its letters is very different. One should not be deluded by the fact that the current inhabitants of the climatic zone that is in the middle of the earth speak in a very bad language. For they are immigrants to that place from remote places, just as one finds a Hebrew- or Arabic-speaking person in the extreme north or south who there speaks in the language he was raised with in his homeland.

(xxv.59) Says Moses: It is a well-known saying of the philosophers that the soul can be healthy or ill, just as the body can be healthy or ill. These healthy and ill conditions of the soul they allude to belong to the field of opinions and ethical qualities of human beings and are characteristic of them, without any doubt. Therefore, I call untrue opinions and bad ethical qualities with their many varieties "human" diseases. Among all the human diseases there is one disease that is so common that almost no one can escape from it, except for a few individuals in long periods. This disease varies among human beings in the greater or lesser degree of its severity just like the other physical and mental diseases. This illness that I mean is that every person imagines himself to be more perfect than he is and that he desires and wishes that all his opinions that he acquired without any effort and exertion pass as perfect.

Because of this common illness, we find that individuals who possess cleverness and alertness and have learned one of the philosophical, theoretical, or speculative sciences, or one of the conventional sciences, and have become proficient in that science, that such a person expresses his opinion not only in that science that he has mastered but also in other sciences that he does not know at all or only knows deficiently and speaks about those sciences with the same authority as about the science in which he has specialized. This is especially the case if that person happens to achieve one of the alleged felicities of being regarded as someone with authority and preeminence and has become one of the great masters who only has to speak in order to make his words accepted. No one refutes his words or objects to them. And as that alleged felicity becomes more established and stronger, that disease becomes more severe and stronger as well, and that person begins, in due course, to talk nonsense and to speak whatever comes to his mind according to his phantasies or his dispositions, or according to the questions addressed to him. He answers whatever comes to his mind because he does not want to say that there is something he does not know. In some persons this illness becomes so inveterate that they are not content with all this, but begin to argue and explain that those sciences that they do not know are useless and needless and that there is no science worthy of a lifelong attention, except for that science that they know, be it a philosophical, or conventional science. Many have composed refutations of sciences that they have not mastered. To sum up, this disease is very widespread, and if you look at the words of a person with an impartial eye, the degree of severity of this disease will be clear to you and whether this person is close to health or ruin.

And this man Galen, the physician, was attacked by this disease in the same degree as others who were equal to him in science. That is, this man was very, very proficient in medicine, more than anybody we have heard about or whose words we have seen; he has achieved great things in the field of anatomy, and things became clear to him—and to others in his time as well—about the functions of the organs, their usefulness and structure, and about the different conditions of the pulse, which were not clear in Aristotle's time. He, I mean Galen, has undoubtedly trained himself in mathematics and has studied logic and the books of Aristotle on the natural and divine sciences, but he is defective in all that. His excellent intellect and acumen that he directed towards medicine, and his discoveries of some of the conditions of the pulse, anatomy, and the usefulness and functions of organs—which are undoubtedly more correct than what Aristotle mentions in his books, if one looks at them impartially—have induced him to speak about things in which he is very deficient and about which the experts have contradictory opinions.

So, he refutes, as you know, Aristotle in logic and speaks about the natural and divine sciences, as he does in *De propriis placitis*, and in *De placitis Hippocratis et Platonis*, and in the book *De semine*, which contain refutations of Aristotle. Likewise, he composed a book on motion, time, the possible, and the first mover, and about all these things he comes with opinions that are well known to the people of that branch. This led to the point where he composed his famous book *De demonstratione* and maintained that the physician is not perfect in medicine unless he knows this book and that it is very useful for the physician. He limited himself to those syllogisms that are necessary for demonstration, maintaining that those syllogisms are useful in medicine and in other branches, and omitted the other syllogisms. But the syllogisms that he mentioned are not at all the demonstrative syllogisms, and he omitted those syllogisms that are very useful in the medical art and claimed that they are not at all useful and that Aristotle's and other people's study of them is a waste of time.

All this was explained by Abū Naṣr al-Fārābī—that is, that Galen omitted the hypothetical and the mixed syllogisms and confined himself to the absolute syllogisms (the hyparctic) and did not pay attention to the fact that demonstrative syllogisms are necessary ones and not hyparctic ones and that that which is useful in medicine and in most arts is the hypothetical and mixed syllogisms. Hear the words of Abū Naṣr on this matter. He says in his great commentary on *Analytica* [*priora* I.1] when he begins to explain the preliminary exposition that Aristotle has made on the possible and the hypothetical syllogisms.

Abū Naṣr says: The question here is not as Galen the physician thinks, because in his book called *De demonstratione*, he mentions that the study of the possible and of the hypothetical syllogisms that are derived therefrom is superfluous. Galen the physician is one of the people for whom it would have been most proper to study the hypothetical syllogisms; even more so, he should have directed most of his attention in his book called *De demonstratione* to the hypothetical syllogisms; for he pretends that he composed his book *De demonstratione* in order that it might be useful in medicine. And the syllogisms that the physician uses for extracting the different parts of the medical art and the syllogisms that he employs for recognizing the internal diseases and their causes in every one of his patients whom he wants to cure, all these are hypothetical syllogisms, and there is no necessary syllogism among them, except for exceptional cases that are practically outside the medical art. Therefore, he should have spoken in his book called *De demonstratione* about the kinds of the hypothetical syllogisms only and not about those of the hyparctic syllogisms, and if he has confined himself in his book to the hyparctic kinds in order to restrict himself to those syllogisms that are useful for demonstrations, then one has to say that the kinds relating to existence are not destined for demonstrations, because demonstrations are not made from this matter but are made from the necessary kinds only. End of the quotation from Abū Naṣr.

(xxv.60) When Aristotle begins to explain the syllogisms which are mixed from hypothetical and absolute ones, Abū Naṣr says the following in his commentary to this statement, and these are his words: This chapter is extremely useful and more useful than the chapter on the plain hypothetical ones because all the practical arts make use of this chapter, especially in finding out whether the individual phenomena that are in the future will occur or not, in medicine, agriculture, navigation, politics, rhetorics, general premisses, and in all the activities in which one needs prognostics; all that which can be found in the book *Prognostic* of Hippocrates the physician and in similar books resolves itself into these syllogisms. End of the quotation from Abū Naṣr. This ought to be contemplated.

(xxv.61) One should be astonished by the words of this man Galen, of the fact that he exaggerates in his praise of logic in all his books and says that the affliction that has affected contemporary physicians, and the cause of their deficiency, is simply their lack of knowledge of logic, and that the cause of his skill lies in the fact that he was well trained in logic and that he always endeavors to show that the physician has need of logic. But when he composed this book, he not only did not mention one single kind of syllogism of the different kinds of hypothetical and mixed syllogisms that alone are useful in medicine, but rebuked him who studies them and said that there is no need for them at all. No one doubts that Galen studied Aristotle's books on logic and understood them better than others who are inferior to him. But because of that common illness we are speaking about, he imagined that the understanding of the art of logic and the other theoretical sciences is like the understanding of the medical art and that his skill in all those sciences is like his skill in medicine. Therefore, he exposed himself to all these errors.

He did not stop at this limit, but because of the excessive pleasure he took in what became evident to him about some of the uses of organs, he pretended to be a prophet and said that an angel came to him from God and taught him such and such and ordered him such and such. If only he had stopped at this point and had arranged himself among the majority of the prophets—peace be upon them—and had not burst out against them. However, he did not do so; on the contrary, a wrong evaluation of his own value led him to eventually compare himself with Moses—peace be upon him—and to attribute to himself perfection and to Moses—peace be upon him—ignorance. God is exalted above the sayings of the ignorant.

Therefore, it seems to me a good thing to let you know the text of his own words—he who quotes the words of an unbeliever is not an unbeliever himself—and to refute him; although it is not a refutation of someone who committed an enormity like this, for Moses—peace be upon him—is not to him what he is to us, the community of followers of Divine Laws. Rather, in this my refutation I will explain that the ignorance that he attributes to our prophet Moses—peace be upon him—does not pertain to him, but that Galen is, in reality, the ignorant one. I will make my own judgment of both of them as if I am judging between two learned men, one of whom is more perfect than the other, and not as if I were deciding between the words of a great prophet and those of a medical practitioner, because this is the correct procedure if the matter is looked into.

(XXV.62) I say that when Galen began to explain, in *De usu partium* XI[.14], the usefulness of the fact that the hair of the eyebrows does not grow long and hang down like the hair of the head, and the usefulness of the fact that the hair of the eyelids is rigid and does not grow long, he says the following, and these are his words: Do you say, then, that the Creator has commanded this hair to remain at all times at one and the same length and not to grow longer and that the hair has accepted that order, obeyed, and remained at the same length, without deviating from what it had been ordered either out of fear and apprehension to offend against the command of God or because of politeness and awe before God who gave this command, or that the hair itself knows that it is more appropriate and better to do so? This is the opinion of Moses about the natural things, and I think that this opinion is better and more appropriate to be adopted than that of Epicurus, even though the best thing is to refrain from both and to maintain that God—may He be exalted—is the principle of the creation of all created things as Moses—peace be upon him—has said, but to add to this the material principle from which they were created.

Our Creator has made the eyelashes and eyebrows feel the necessity of remaining at one and the same length since this was more appropriate and better. And since He knew that it was necessary to make them so, he placed under the eyelashes a hard body similar to cartilage that extends along the eyelid, and spread under the eyebrows a hard skin adherent to the cartilage (the superficial fascia) of the eyebrows. And this because it would not have been sufficient, in order to retain this hair in one and the same length, that the Creator would have wished it to be so. In the same way, if he would wish to turn a stone into a man all of sudden, without making the stone undergo the appropriate alteration, this would not be possible.

The difference between the belief of Moses—peace be upon him—and our belief and that of Plato and the other Greeks is the following: Moses claims that it is sufficient that God wishes to give shape and form to the matter in order to let it take shape and form instantly. This is because he thinks that all things are possible with God, and that if He wishes to create a horse or an ox from ashes instantly, He can do so. But we do not approve of this, but say that there are some things which are impossible in themselves and these God never wishes to occur, but he wishes only possible things to occur, and from the possible things he only chooses the best, most appropriate, and excellent. For this reason, as it is most appropriate and proper for the eyelashes and eyebrows to be always and forever of the same length and number, we do not say about this hair that God wished it to be so, and that straightaway it became as He wished it to be. For, if He had wished the hair to be so a million times, it would never have been so, once He had let it grow from soft skin; if he had not planted the roots of the hair in a hard body, they would—while greatly changing from their initial condition—not have remained erect and rigid.

And since this is the case, we say that God has accomplished two things: firstly, the choice of the best, most suitable and most appropriate condition for what he was going to do; and secondly, the selection of the appropriate material. Therefore, since it was most proper and good that the eyelashes be erect and rigid and that they remain always of the same length and number, he made the planting ground and center of the hair in a hard body. If he had planted them in a soft body, He would have been more ignorant than Moses and more ignorant than a foolish army commander who laid the foundations of the walls of his town or fortress in soft ground which is submerged by water. Similarly, the fact that the hair of the eyebrows remains always in the same condition, only comes from His choice of the right material. End of the quotation from Galen.

(xxv.63) Says Moses: If a man, a philosopher, who is familiar with the basic rules of the Divine Laws known in our times, looks into these words, the confusion of this man becomes evident to him. For his words on the whole are neither congruous with the opinion of the followers of Divine Laws nor with that of the philosophers, because the rules of both opinions are neither well established nor accurately defined with Galen. Rather, he speaks about things the premisses of which he does not understand, as I am going to explain to you now. For he ascribed to Moses—peace be upon him—in that statement by Moses that he refers to, four opinions; one opinion of the four is really the opinion of Moses—peace be upon him—but the remaining three opinions are not those of Moses. But Galen, through his lack of an established and accurate knowledge of all things about which he is talking, except medicine, thought that the four opinions that he mentioned are only one. I also want to say that that one opinion that is the opinion of Moses—peace be upon him—as mentioned by Galen is a necessary consequence of the principle and basic rule of his Divine Law and that of his ancestor Abraham—peace be upon them. Therefore, his words are neither confused nor contradictory, but follow the premisses and consequences of his Divine Law. But all the assertions which Galen has made for himself and claims to be his faith are not the consequence of his own fundamental belief, but what he says is the consequence of the belief of others. Therefore, his words are confused and his conclusions do not conform to his principles.

(xxv.64) I will now begin to explain those four opinions which he ascribes to Moses—peace be upon him—in that statement quoted above. The first one is his saying that God commanded the hair of the eyebrows not to grow long, and that it obeyed him; he says that this is the opinion of Moses regarding natural things. But in reality, this is not the opinion of Moses, for according to Moses, God only gives orders and prohibitions to intelligent beings. The second opinion is his saying that Moses believes that all things are possible with God; this, too, is not the opinion of Moses, but his opinion is that the power to do impossible things cannot be ascribed to God. Galen, because of his distortion of the facts, did not notice the point where opinions differ. For there are things of which Moses says that they are possible and of which others say that they are impossible. This difference of opinion concerning these things is a necessary consequence of the difference in the principles. But Galen did not pay attention to this and did not know it, since he only proceeds at random.

The third opinion is his saying that Moses believes that God, if He wished to instantly create a horse or ox from ashes, He could do so. It is true that this is the opinion of Moses and it is a necessary consequence of one of his principles, as we are going to explain.

The fourth opinion is his saying that Moses believes that God does not choose the proper material for that which He wishes to come into existence in a certain manner, as, for instance, what he said about His choice of a cartilaginous body beneath the eyelashes. But Moses—peace be upon him—does not have a different opinion in this. One of the things that Moses—peace be upon him—clearly stated is that God does nothing in vain and by chance, but that He creates very well with justice and equity all that He creates, as I explained in my exposition of the principles of religion.

From all this one knows, of necessity, that the grape-like tunic of the eye has been perforated for the purpose of vision, that the bones are hard and dry in order to provide solid support, and likewise all that exists in the bodies of living beings, or rather everything that exists, as the prophets who came after Moses—peace be upon him—have said that God has made all that He created with wisdom. [*Proverbs* 3:19]. Galen understood only this one of Moses' opinions, that is, that something can suddenly exist in a manner contrary to the course of nature, like the transformation of a rod into a snake [*Exodus* 4:2, 3; 7:10] and of dust into lice. [*Exodus* 8:13]. Therefore, it is possible according to him that ashes are instantaneously transformed into a horse or an ox, and this is true and it is the opinion of Moses—peace be upon him. All these are necessary consequences of the principles in which Moses—peace be upon him—believes, and that is that the world was created. For the meaning of the world being created is that God—may He be exalted—alone, without anything beside Him, is the primordial and eternal one, that He has created the world after complete nonexistence and has brought into existence this heaven and all that is in it, and the first matter which is below the heaven, that He has formed from it water, air, earth, and fire, that He has shaped the celestial globe with its different spheres according to His will, and that He has shaped these elements and all that is composed of them with these different natures that we perceive, for He is the giver of forms by which they get their nature. This is the principle of the doctrine of Moses—peace be upon him. Since the first matter, according to Him, was brought into existence after nonexistence and was then shaped into its forms, it is possible that God, who brought it into existence, will destroy it once He has made it. Likewise, it is possible that He will change its nature and the nature of everything that is composed of it and will give it instantly a nature different from the regular one, just as He brought it into existence instantly.

Thus, according to Moses—peace be upon him—the change of anything that belongs to the natural world of coming into being and passing away from its present condition falls under the category of being possible, and God possesses the power and will to effect this. If God—may He be exalted—wishes to maintain this world in its present state for all eternity and forever and ever, He can do so. And if He wishes to annihilate it all so that nothing remains besides Himself—may He be exalted—He can do so and has the power for it. If He wishes to retain it in its present nature in all its particulars he can do so, and if He wishes to change an existing particular of an existing thing from its natural course, He can do so. All the miracles are of this kind. Therefore, the perception of one miracle on the part of him who perceives it is a stringent proof for the creation of the world. I mean by miracle here those cases in which there appears the existence of a thing not in accordance with the normal and permanent nature of its existence. It is of two types, either that of a thing that has the property of being always formed by certain degrees and under certain conditions is formed contrary to these normal conditions and is transformed instantly, like the transformation of the rod into a snake, of dust into lice, of water into blood [*Exodus* 7:20], of air into fire [*Exodus* 9:23], and the noble holy hand of Moses turning white [*Exodus* 4:6], all of which occurred instantly; or that of a thing the production of which cannot occur at all according to the nature of this established world, like the manna which was so hard that it could be ground and made into bread [*Numbers* 11:8], but melted and became liquid when the sun warmed it, together with the other miracles of the manna related by the Torah. All these and similar miracles fall under the category of the possible, because the existence of the world in the way in which it was produced is a possible thing itself. But according to the opinion of someone who professes that the world is eternal, all these things that are possible with us are impossible for him. For someone who believes in the eternity of the world says that this world, in its entirety, was made by God, that is, that He is the cause of its existence, and that this world in its present state is a necessary consequence of the existence of the Creator, just as the thing caused is a necessary consequence of the cause that is only to be found together with it, like the day being the necessary consequence of the sunrise and the shadow being the necessary consequence of an erect object, and similar cases.

(xxv.65) Someone who holds this opinion says that movement can neither be generated nor perish; therefore, the heaven is, according to him, eternal and the first matter neither generated nor perishable, but has been and will be forever in the same condition as it is. And all that differs from this natural world of generation and decay is impossible according to him. Therefore, it is impossible, according to him, that something is generated instantly whose nature is not such that it can be generated instantly, and that a thing can be generated whose generation does not belong to the nature of this matter, and that any condition of the conditions of what exists in the upper or lower world can be changed from its condition.

It is apparent to anyone who understands the necessary consequences of the opinions that for someone who believes in the eternity of the world in this manner God has no novel will nor choice, and nothing can possibly exist on which He can exert His power and will, so that, for instance, He cannot bring us rain on one day and withhold it on another day, according to His will, because the rainfall in this established nature is consequential upon the formation of the vapors and the air that bring it about or withhold it. All this is consequential upon the formation of matter over which God can exert no influence. This means that He cannot simply bring about that which is impossible in matter, and He cannot create anything that is impossible in its forms of existence, since the matter has not been created but exists necessarily in this manner for all eternity and forever and ever. It should thus be clear to you what the consequences are of the opinions of those who believe in the eternity of the world as well as the consequences of the opinions of those who believe in its creation.

(xxv.66) But this Galen, a feebleminded and inexact man, who is ignorant in most of the things he speaks about except for the medical art, repeatedly says and explains that he is skeptical on this point, namely, the fundamental principle of the creation of the world, and does not know whether it is eternal or created. I wish I knew how he can be skeptical on this principle when he has built his whole discussion of the hair of the eyelashes and eyebrows on the principle of the eternity of the world. Therefore, he says that anything that is impossible in matter is impossible for God to bring about and one cannot attribute to Him the power over it, even if He wished so a million times. He further states that His will is not sufficient, unless the matter is appropriate.

(xxv.67) He says that God is the principle of the creation of all created things, as Moses has said, in addition to the principle that resides in the matter from which they have been created. These are Galen's very words, and therefore he believes in the eternity of the world and, likewise, in the eternity of God, and that both of them are principles for the creation of everything that is created. This is the belief in the eternity of the world of which Galen says is subject to skepticism. Therefore, he should also have been skeptical whether the sudden creation of a horse from dust is possible, as Moses—peace be upon him—says, or impossible, as say those who pass judgment in favor of the eternity of the world. That he is skeptical about the principle but passes judgment in favor of the possibility of a necessary consequence is proof of his ignorance about the fact that that consequence is intrinsically connected to that principle.

Similarly, his statement that there are things that are impossible for God in themselves is an acknowledgment of the eternity of matter. The most amazing thing is his saying that God knew that it was best for the eyebrows not to grow long, and his saying that God only wishes possible things to occur, and from the possible things he only chooses the best. As to that knowledge, will, and choice that are attributed to God, according to him, and as to the existence of things which are possible for God to bring about: I wish I knew on which of the two fundamental principles he has based his saying and decided his judgment, on the belief in the eternity or on that in the creation of the world.

(xxv.68) I have explained to you that, according to the belief in the eternity of the world, there does not remain with God either will or choice, and there is no possible thing in existence that He could choose or produce. But what Galen has said in these sayings is correct according to the opinion that both world and matter are created. Therefore, you should consider how he confuses in what he says things that are consequences of the doctrine of the creation of the world with other things that are consequences of the doctrine of the eternity of the world and thinks that all this is one belief and one opinion, whereas he is skeptical about the question whether the world is eternal or created. All that he said in his confused statement is clear and evident to him, but they are his particular belief and something he is convinced of. This is clear proof that he is ignorant about the principles and their necessary consequences he is speaking about and that he pays only little attention to his own words.

This was my aim in this chapter and nothing else. I did not endeavor in this chapter to refute those who believe in the eternity of the world, to make them doubt and to expose them, as I have composed a number of expositions of these subjects in my writings on the Divine Law.

(xxv.69) Says Moses: In a previous aphorism I spoke about human diseases. My aim in this aphorism is to give you some very useful advice concerning your opinions and beliefs. That is that if any man informs you about things that he has witnessed and observed with his own eyes, even if that person is according to you most trustworthy and honest and has excellent intellectual and moral qualities, you should consider carefully what he tells you. If he wants with his account of his observation to strengthen an opinion that he has or a doctrine he believes in, distrust him in what he says that he observed and let not your mind become confused by those stories. Rather, consider those opinions and doctrines according to the requirements of sound judgment without paying attention to what he says that he saw with own eyes, regardless whether this assertion is advanced by a single person or by a group of persons holding that opinion. For the ambition to have his opinions accepted induces a person to ugly things, especially in the case of controversy and disputation.

(XXV.70) I have only made this statement as an introduction to what I will remind you of concerning the matter of Galen, this learned and eminent man. You know that according to his opinion there are three major organs—the heart, the brain, and the liver—and that none of these three fundamental organs derive their particular power from another organ in whatever way. But, as you know, the opinion of Aristotle and his followers is that the only major organ is the heart, and that the heart sends a power to every singular organ and with this power those organs perform their particular function. Therefore, according to Aristotle, the heart sends a power to the brain and with this power the brain performs its function, namely, providing sensation and motion to the other parts of the body. Similarly, concerning the faculties of imagination, rational thought, and memory that exist in the brain, these faculties exist in the brain and perform their functions thanks to that principle that the brain derives from the heart. And this is correct when one looks into it, because the brain—and similarly every organ—only carries out its functions while it lives its particular perfect life, and the heart is the organ that provides the brain with the power for its particular life.

(XXV.71) Others than us have sufficiently discussed this matter. Galen thinks this faculty of sensation and motion, as well as rational thought, memory, and imagination, has its first principle in the brain and that the heart does not participate in this at all, meaning that no power of sensation or motion reaches the brain from the heart. You know his constant argumentation concerning this opinion in all his books. His endeavor to proof the correctness of his opinion led him to relate the following in his *De placitis Hippocratis et Platonis* II[.4]. Listen to what he says there.

He says: It is possible to expose the heart, press it, crush it, or remove it completely without piercing the two chest cavities. It was a custom for most sacrifices to be offered in this way. And animals could be observed—once their heart was removed and placed on the altar—to breathe and bellow vehemently and to flee until they suffered from a hemorrhage and died. These are his words.

(XXV.72) Be amazed, you who belong to the community of those who engage in speculation. How can we believe him in what he says in this statement and at the same time believe him in what he says in *De locis affectis* V[.2], and this last statement be correct? For there he remarks that it is in any case unavoidable that the heart suffers harm when death occurs. And death is consequential upon an excessive dyscrasia of the heart. But a severe dyscrasia of the heart that is specific for the homogeneous parts is not followed by quick death. But when it is specific for the composite organs, it is followed by sudden death. These are his words there.

Galen wants us to believe in both statements at the same time. One statement is that if the heart suffers from a severe dyscrasia, because it is a composite organ, that is when superfluous matter streams into it that changes its temperament or causes a swelling and the living being dies suddenly. And the second statement is that the heart can be pressed or crushed or removed and thrown into a different place, yet the animal lives, bellows, runs, and breathes until he is killed by an excessive loss of blood, as he states in this other statement. Perhaps we could also say to him that, since his death only results from the harm caused by the loss of blood, if we would grasp the edges of the pulsatile vessels from which the blood is flowing with our hands for a long time, the animal would remain alive while he has no heart. This is astonishing!

Consider to what consequences a person is necessarily lead when he wants to support his opinion. One of the things that should be pointed out is that if what he says is correct, it would not be a decisive argument for refuting Aristotle's opinion that the principle of sensation and motion comes from the heart. For the truth is that the root (the heart) that provides a certain power may be eliminated and yet that power remains for a certain time but then ceases because that which replenishes it has ceased to be active. This is comparable to a well that is suddenly filled up and the water that flowed from it remains in channels that water and moisten the surrounding area until that water comes to an end.

One can also see how in the case of some dead persons their body remains warm for an hour like the heat of the body of living persons even though their heart has stopped beating. This is because that heat is that which emanated from the heart before it stopped, but then this heat dwindles away and dissolves because it finds none to replenish it. Likewise, some animals after being decapitated still move their limbs through that strength that remains in their nerves until it is exhausted. So, too, we say to him that the principle that the heart sends to the brain remains there for a short time after the heart is gone until that strength ceases to be. The only thing that befalls us from these stories by Galen is that they are repulsive and difficult to accept, nothing else.

But how can one take out the heart without perforating one of the chest cavities? This can only be done by splitting the site of the throat at the back of the neck and by gently pulling out the heart from its membrane therethrough.

And then the membrane of the heart is left as it is, connected to the back and chest. Such an operation is very difficult if one tries to do it after the death of an animal. But when the animal is still alive as Galen mentions, it is something that is most unlikely. He only made this assumption to support his opinion, nothing else.

God is all-knowing.

BOOK 6

On Coitus

First published in:

Maimonides
On Coitus

A New Parallel Arabic-English Edition and Translation
by Gerrit Bos,
with Editions of Medieval Hebrew Translations
by Gerrit Bos
and Medieval Latin Translations
by Charles Burnett
and a Slavonic Translation
by W.F. Ryan and Moshe Taube.

Leiden (Brill) 2019
MWMM 11

∴

(1) The most honored Lord—may God perpetuate his glory—has ordered me to relate to him the regimen that is helpful in increasing sexual potency, since he told me that that is his eager desire although his servant (Maimonides) drew his attention to the leanness of his body and diminution of his flesh to a degree that it approaches emaciation, while his temperament tends somewhat toward heat. He also told me that he does not want to abandon any of his habits concerning coitus, but that he especially wants this regimen because of fear for the emaciation of his body and because of his desire to increase his sexual vigor for the sake of the large number of slave girls. He also wanted that I only mention in this regimen those things that can be done easily and with little effort.

I thought it proper to select medications and foods that are beneficial for this and that can be easily found and that are regularly taken in this country of Egypt and that are not exceedingly hot, because of what was mentioned concerning the condition of his temperament. I also thought it appropriate to present him first of all with a general statement, namely, the following: It is well known to the physicians that in this matter foods are much more beneficial than medi-

 | DOI:10.1163/9789004498884_008

cines, since the sperm is a residue of foods that remains from that which the organs require with the third digestion. For this reason, the body becomes meager if one indulges excessively in sexual intercourse, next to the other kinds of harm resulting from that.

(2) Know that everything that cools the body or the procreative organs, and similarly everything that dries the body or those organs, is extremely harmful for sexual vigor. And know that among foods and medications everything that moistens and heats moderately, and likewise the rest of the regimen, is very beneficial in this regard. Similarly, joy, fun, laughter, jesting, leisure, and sleep that is not excessive are beneficial in this regard. But the opposite of these is extremely detrimental for stimulating lust, that is, sadness, worry, anxiety, continuous silence, toil, exertion, and sleeplessness. All these things abolish erection and dry the sperm. Similarly, speaking frequently about things pertaining to sexual intercourse and talking and thinking about it are among the things that are helpful for it, whereas directing one's thoughts away from it is among the things that make the male member flaccid and weaken its activity. In the same way, having sexual intercourse moderately is among that which strengthens the male member and helps to increase the sexual vigor, whereas having sexual intercourse immoderately weakens the male member, makes it flaccid, and diminishes sexual vigor. This is especially the case if this is combined with lack of thought and lack of activity, for this is the first thing that is being practiced by monks and ascetics to find relief from the sorrows caused by their having to abandon sexual intercourse altogether.

(3) It is well known that this activity (sexual intercourse) is not merely a natural activity, that is, erection is not equivalent to the activity of nutrition or the activity of growth, in which activities the animal soul plays no part. Rather, it is also an animal activity that is peculiar for to the animal soul, and therefore affections of the soul are very harmful or very beneficial in this regard. I mean that worry, anxiety, sorrow, and the disgust of the woman one intends to have intercourse with severely weaken the lust for sexual intercourse, while the opposite affections incite thereto and strongly stimulate the sexual lust. The physicians have stated that among the things that especially weaken the lust for sexual intercourse are intercourse with a virgin, an old woman, or a minor who has not yet reached puberty, or a woman who was unable to have sexual intercourse during a period of several years, or a menstruating or ill woman. More weakening the sexual lust than all these is sexual intercourse with an abhorrent woman for a man has to compel himself to do so, and nature gets accustomed and used to indolence when it is moved in this respect. And then it turns into

a habit for a person that every time that his soul desires sexual intercourse, he finds languor. These general introductory words are sufficient for deriving therefrom that which one has either to strive for or to avoid regarding this matter.

(4) Now I will start to relate particular detailed matters that fall under the general matters I have referred to before. The first matter is that of foods. One should know that the foods that are beneficial in this regard are all those that produce good, wholesome blood and all those that heat and moisten and that contain flatulence necessary for the erection that is released from the food with the third digestion.

Among the foods that are good for an erection are mutton, young pigeons, and all brains, especially those of chickens, sparrows, and pigeons. Rooster testicles are very beneficial in producing and increasing sperm for people of all temperaments and ages. And similarly beneficial are bone marrow, yolk of chicken eggs, partridge eggs, pigeon eggs, sparrow eggs, and fresh milk.

Among the plants that are beneficial are turnip, wild carrot, onion, especially the white variety, fennel, peppermint, chickpeas, broad beans, black-eyed peas, sesame, and asparagus.

Among the tree fruits: dried almond kernels, hazelnuts and pistachio nuts, grapes, large pine nuts, and coconut, and similarly *ḥabb al-zalam* (earth almonds), which are known as *fulful al-sudān* (Sudanese pepper). All these are foods that are easily found and that are beneficial in this regard; they help erection and they contain something that increases sperm, whether they are taken separately or in compounded form, according to their composition. A drink of hydromel helps erection.

More beneficial than any food or remedy in this regard is wine. There is nothing that can replace it in this respect, because the blood that is produced therefrom is abundant, hot, and moist, and it rejoices the soul and strongly incites to sexual intercourse—because of a specific property it has in addition to its nature, it fills the vessels with beneficial vapor and therefore stimulates an erection—if it is ingested with moderation and after a meal and after leaving the bath. Its effect in this regard is greater than that of anything else.

(5) Know that hot and dry seeds dry the sperm and weaken sexual intercourse, especially those seeds that have the property of expelling the flatulence necessary for an erection, such as common rue, cumin, black cumin, caraway, black pepper, mustard, and the like. Therefore, one should avoid all seeds and condiments with which foods are seasoned except for those that I am going to mention to you, namely, one ounce each of long pepper, greater galangal, ginger, and

bitter ginger; two ounces each of Chinese cinnamon and anise; one quarter of an ounce each of clove, and nutmeg. These medications should be pulverized and should be ready to season any dish that is to be cooked; the spice mixture should be sprinkled over any dish, according to the detailed instructions that will be given.

As to those foods and medications that should be avoided, these are all those that cool, dry, or expel the flatulence. Among these are the following that are common among us: lentils, Indian pea and cooling vegetables such as garden orach, spinach, and especially cultivated lettuce, because it is very harmful in this regard. Similarly, the smaller variety of cucumbers and normal cucumbers, *biṭṭīkh* (common melon or watermelon), and acid ingredients: all these are harmful—most of all, vinegar. I have said that all spices should be avoided except for those which I mentioned to you explicitly. So it is with turnip seeds since they cause headache and dry the sperm. And of the things which are common among us, one should greatly avoid *nīlūfar* (blue Egyptian, European white, or yellow water lily) because it has the specific property of annulling the production of sperm. It has such a contrary effect that even its smell weakens the lust for sexual intercourse—such is its specific property.

(6) It is appropriate that I mention the compounded foods and compounded medicines that are beneficial in this regard. I will start with the foods. *Tubāla*: It is prepared from the meat of two-year-old sheep (mutton), chickpeas, wild carrots or turnips or both together, white onions, and the yolks of chicken eggs; and the spices that we have mentioned before should be apparent. *Maḍīra*: It is prepared from mutton or the meat of castrated cocks or young pigeons with milk of a cow and spiced with the aforementioned spices. *Harīsa*: It is prepared from mutton or rooster testicles and spiced with the spices that we have mentioned; one may also sprinkle Chinese cinnamon over it. If one drinks one *raṭl* of hot milk on which is sprinkled a quarter of a *mithqāl* of ground and sifted clove, it is very beneficial and helps to get an erection and increases the sperm. Similarly, fried onion is very beneficial because of its specific property, especially if one sprinkles some of the aforementioned spices on it. It is mentioned that the consumption of fried onion with boiled egg yolk has a strong effect in this regard. Similarly, the yolk of soft-boiled eggs: if one sprinkles on them some of the aforementioned spices and eats about ten eggs when one goes to bed, it stimulates the lust for sexual intercourse.

Ibn Sīnā mentions an omelet (egg fritter) for strengthening the lust for sexual intercourse, which he composed himself, and this is its composition: Take a sum of fifty brains of sparrows and pigeons, twenty yolks of sparrow eggs, ten yolks of the eggs of young hens, and one bowl of the stock squeezed from pounded and well-boiled mutton; and three ounces of juice expressed from onions, five ounces of wild carrot juice, and the necessary quantity of salt and spices, and fifty *dirhams* of clarified butter. Prepare an omelet from this and eat it. Once it has been digested, drink strong fragrant wine tending toward sweetness. [*Kitāb al-Qānūn fī al-ṭibb* (*The Canon of Medicine*)].

Derived from Ibn Sīnā's treatise, I have made an omelet myself, which is easy to prepare and tastes delicious. The one to whom I prescribed it told me that he found it very effective. This is its composition: Take four onions, roast them in an oven until they are done, remove their outer peel, and pound them well. Likewise, take half a *raṭl* of meat that was roasted and broiled in its own broth until it was well done. Pound the meat and mix it with the roasted onions together with the remaining broth. Break twenty chicken eggs and add their yolks to it. Mix all this and add to it such a quantity of the aforementioned spices that their flavor can be clearly noticed, as well as some salt, and if the salt is from the skink, it is best. Roast this in sesame oil or clarified butter. One can also make another omelet that is exactly the same except that it is made with roasted wild carrots instead of the onions. One can also make it with both wild carrots and onions as I have described.

Another omelet: Take three ounces of rooster testicles, three ounces of sparrow brains, and twenty yolks of chicken eggs—and if they are pigeon eggs it is even better—and the aforementioned spices. Roast this mixture in sesame oil or in clarified butter. One may also prepare a cake with lamb brains instead of the meat, for it has a good effect.

(7) Ibn Sīnā and other physicians have mentioned different kinds of confections that are beneficial. From these I am going to mention one that is easy to prepare, tastes delicious, and has been verified by experience. Its composition is as follows: Take two ounces each of pine nuts, pistachio nuts, and almond kernels; one ounce each of roasted sesame with its shells, of garden rocket, and of *biṭṭīkh* (common melon or watermelon) seeds; and four *raṭls* of sugar and skimmed honey. All the kernels should be roasted in sesame oil and congealed into a confection in the usual way, but the fire should not be too strong.

Another confection: Take chickpeas, soak them in wild garden rocket juice until they swell up, peel them, and take one part thereof and one part of the aforementioned kernels, and roast all this in sesame oil and let it congeal into a confection. Know that all these foods, which serve to strengthen the lust for sexual intercourse, should be taken after bathing. If one can drink a measure of three ounces of fragrant wine thereafter, it is most effective in this respect and also for fattening the body of my Lord.

(8) Among the compounded medicines there is also an electuary of wild carrots and an electuary of sekakul parsnip, which are both of them prepared in the same way because sekakul parsnip is the same as "wild carrot." It should be prepared as follows: Take the outer part of the wild carrots and throw away what is inside—and the same should be done with sekakul parsnip—boil it, and let the water cool off, and press it out with the hand. Take one *raṭl* of either of them, then take three ounces each of garden rocket seed, peeled sesame, fruit of the ash tree, and pine nuts, and three *raṭl*s of skimmed honey. This should be prepared just as all stomachics are prepared. Then take three *dirham*s each of red behen (possibly Mediterranean sea lavender) and white behen, and similarly four *dirhams* each of greater galangal, cinnamon, long pepper, Chinese cinnamon, and great false leopardbane. Pulverize all these ingredients, sift them, and mix them with the stomachic once you have taken it from the fire, and season it with one eighth of a *mithqāl* of musk, and take a spoonful thereof every day for it will have a good effect, nearly as good as that of the skink.

Another remedy for someone whose temperament is hot: Take one *raṭl* of fresh milk, dissolve forty *dirham*s of manna in it, and boil it until it thickens; take a third of a *raṭl* thereof every day. This is how the physicians mention it. But I added a quarter of a *dirham* of pulverized clove to it and it had a good effect.

Another remedy: Five *dirham*s each of asparagus seed, sekakul parsnip, and ginger; three *dirham*s each of white and red hedge mustard, white behen and red behen (possibly Mediterranean sea lavender), roasted sea squill, and the parts beneath the navel of the skink; two *dirham*s each of lucerne seed, garden rocket seed, fruit of the ash tree, Roman nettle seed, and radish seed; and fourty *dirhams* of sugar. This should be taken in a dose of four *dirham*s.

Among the beneficial medicines the physicians mention is the kernel electuary. Its composition is one part each of almonds, hazelnuts, pistachio nuts, peeled and scraped coconuts, pine nuts, wild senna seed—meaning that which the druggists sell instead of balsam seed—*ḥabb al-zalam* (earth almonds), that is, *fulful al-sudān* (Sudanese pepper), and fruit of the turpentine tree; and ten parts each of long pepper and ginger. Pulverize all these ingredients, knead them with *fānīdh*, and take a dose equal to an egg every day.

A potion of which the physicians say that it increases the lust for sexual intercourse and also increases the sperm: Take turnips, walnuts, and figs; cook them well in water, strain this and throw pitted raisins into the water. Cook this well, strain it and throw *fānīdh* into it, and leave it on the fire until it boils and turns into *nabīdh*; drink this.

The following remedy was mentioned by them as effective because of its specific property: Take the penis of an ox, dry it and pulverize it, and sprinkle some of it on a soft-boiled egg; slurp it.

The matter of the beneficial effect of the meat of the skink is well known, especially of the parts beneath the navel, and similarly of its salt which, if its inner parts are stuffed with it, and then the food is steeped and boiled in it, greatly strengthens the lust for sexual intercourse. The same holds good for the varan because its meat has a beneficial effect.

Ibn Zuhr has mentioned the following remedy and said: An electuary that is beneficial for lack of erection (impotence) and lack of sperm and lust: One part each of thick salep, ginger, long pepper, turnip seed and radish seed; half a part each of sekakul parsnip, pine nuts, and hazelnuts; half a part each of borage blossom, giant fennel, and garden rocket; and a third of a part of skink. Grind these separately, sieve what should be sieved, and knead these ingredients with apple juice. Administer a dose from three to four *dirhams*.

(9) He also said that since there are many people who wish the erection to continue even when they do not have an ejaculation of sperm anymore, it is appropriate that he list the following remedy, which is a wonderful secret that has not been revealed by anyone previously. Take one *raṭl* each of wild carrot oil and radish oil and a quarter of a *raṭl* of mustard oil; mix these ingredients and put half a *raṭl* of live yellow ants into it. Set the oil apart in the sun between four and seven days. Then use some of it and smear it on the penis about three or two hours before sexual intercourse, then wash the penis with hot water and it will remain erect after the ejaculation of sperm. No one has ever applied such a remedy for this matter.

Another aphrodisiac mentioned by other physicians: one *dirham* of pellitory, half a *dirham* of resin spurge, and a quarter of a *dirham* of musk. Pulverize all these ingredients and mix them in one ounce of *zanbaq* (white or Arabian jasmine) oil, and smear this every day on the pubes, anus, penis, and testicles.

(10) The regimen which one should adhere to, next to the frequent consumption of the foods and medicines that we have mentioned, should consist of entering the bathhouse every five days—and not staying there for a long time—and treating oneself with different kinds of hot aromatics, such as musk, ambergris, and *galia*. After the bath one should feed oneself and then drink, if possible, a cup of fragrant *nabīdh* or a honey drink. And, after washing them with warm water, one should massage one's feet every night until they become red before one goes to sleep. One should do so continuously, in summer and winter, because whenever the feet become cold or dry the erection subsides or decreases. Similarly, one should constantly aim at warming and oiling the lumbar region. This is the most important thing to do in this regard.

In our opinion the best treatment for this is to massage the entire lumbar region, when one wakes up from one's sleep, with a coarse cloth until it becomes warm. Then one should massage it strongly with the palm of the hand with ben oil scented with musk. One should also massage the anus and perineum because this is the most effective treatment for warming the genitals and attracting good blood to them, strengthening them, and strengthening the erection. Similarly, one should constantly try to drink iron water, as is prescribed to those suffering from intestinal abrasion. Let it become cold and drink it when one needs it. And if it is possible that the broth of every dish one eats consists of iron water, it is most beneficial for strengthening the erection and for strengthening all internal organs.

Know that the physicians only apply the name "exhilarating drink" to the drink prepared from borage. The ancient physicians have tried this; that is, if one puts some borage in *nabīdh* and leaves it there until its strength is extracted, one finds that it greatly increases pleasure and strengthens the lust for sexual intercourse. And if one takes the well-known iron water and boils in it four *dirhams* of borage, half an ounce of *utrujj* (citron or lemon) peel, and half a *dirham* of crushed clove, and mixes with this water two *raṭls* of wine or one *raṭl* of bees' honey for someone who cannot take wine, and drinks this little by little, it will be greatly beneficial.

This much is sufficient for what your Servant was ordered to do. And let my Lord choose from it that which is easy to carry out, and do sometimes this and sometimes that.

May God lengthen his life in happiness and enjoyment
and join this for him with eternal happiness,
in His grace.

BOOK 7

On the Regimen of Health

First published in:

Maimonides
On the Regimen of Health

A New Parallel Arabic-English Edition and Translation
by Gerrit Bos,
with Critical Editions of Medieval Hebrew Translations
by Gerrit Bos
and Latin Translations
by Michael R. McVaugh.

Leiden (Brill) 2019
MWMM 12

In the Name of God,
the Merciful, the Compassionate

(N) The command of the most eminent Master and Sovereign—may God exalt him and sustain him—has reached this minor Servant Mūsā ibn ʿUbayd Allāh the Israelite from Córdoba. Sent by a messenger, it requests of him to relate a regimen to be relied upon for curing the illnesses that happened to my Master—may God keep diseases away from his high abode and may health and peace always accompany him. The messenger who brought the high command related that my Lord complained that his stools are most of the time so dry and hard that it is almost impossible to excrete them except with effort. He also mentioned that sometimes my Lord is affected by depression, evil thoughts, loneliness, and foreboding of death, and that he often suffers from indigestion and has a feeble digestion most of the time. This is what he mentioned and this Servant thought that the right thing to do was to compose four chapters concerning this regimen.

The first chapter on the regimen of health in general, with respect to all people, in a few words.

 | DOI:10.1163/9789004498884_009

The second chapter on the regimen of sick people in general, when no physician can be found or when the available physician is deficient and his knowledge cannot be relied upon.
The third chapter on the regimen of my Master in particular, according to the symptoms he complains about.
The fourth chapter consists of sections in the form of hortatory rules that are useful in general and in particular for healthy and sick people in all places and all times.

Let not someone who looks into this treatise and in all that which I have composed criticize me for the fact that some sections of this treatise have already been mentioned in other treatises that I composed earlier because each treatise was written by me according to the request of an individual, not as a composition intended to teach the art of medicine to people in general. I ask God for success in what is right.

∴

Chapter One

On the regimen of health in general, with respect to all people, in a few words

(I.1) Our intention in this chapter is to give rules that are easy to remember, while their application is of great benefit in the regimen of health. These are general statements of the great physicians. One of these is the statement by Hippocrates: The preservation of health consists of being on one's guard against satiation and to give up laziness for exertion. [*Epidemics* VI.4]. Note how Hippocrates summarized the entire regimen of health in two rules, namely,

1. that a person should not eat until he is satisfied and
2. that he should not neglect exercise.

For satiation, that is eating until one loses one's appetite and one begins to detest it, requires filling the stomach to the utmost of its capacity and distending it. When any organ is distended, its continuity is dissolved and its vigor is necessarily weakened. The stomach will not digest that food properly at all; inertia, weakness of movement, and heaviness of food will occur, especially when one drinks much water after the satiating meal, which is necessarily required in satiety because nature requires water to float the meal in order to ease the burden on the stomach.

(I.2) Of necessity, one of two things will happen: either an indigestion, a severe one that is fatal or a mild one causing illness, or a bad digestion. The kinds of bad digestion vary greatly according to the various types of food, the various temperaments, and the various dispositions of the organs to diseases. When the food is badly digested in the stomach, its second digestion in the liver is necessarily also bad, and its third digestion in all the other organs will be worst of all. This is the cause for all kinds of diseases, in their great variety. Similarly, Galen has said and these are his very words: If someone wishes not to fall ill at all, he should endeavor not to suffer from indigestion and not to move after a meal. [*De bonis malisque sucis* III]. Because of this grave danger, all physicians have warned against satiation and ordered a person to stop eating while there is still appetite left, before it departs, and to guard against distending the stomach and overfilling.

(I.3) All physicians agree that the consumption of a small amount of foods of a bad quality is less harmful than the consumption of a large amount of good and healthy foods because if someone takes bad foods but does not eat from them until he is satisfied, these foods are well digested and the organs are nourished from them with whatever is beneficial. The expulsive faculty is strengthened and expels their bad superfluities, and no harm occurs at all or the harm that occurs is insignificant. But in satiation, even if it is from bread that has been well prepared and from good meat, the food is not digested well at all and we have already mentioned the cause of this. To guard against satiation, the physicians have forbidden to eat many dishes but to limit oneself to one dish with every meal so that one does not eat too much and the appetite subsides before satiation occurs. By doing so, one will also be free from a diversity of digestions because different dishes are digested in different digestions, every dish according to its nature.

(I.4) The view of this Servant regarding the determination of the quantity of food for someone who wishes to preserve his health, is that he should eat, when the weather is temperate, a quantity that does not distend his stomach, does not burden it, and does not fail to digest. And when it is clear to him that this is a good amount—and this is the case when he does not belch badly nor suffer from thirst, but experiences energy and lightness and his stools become moderate, cohesive, and slightly tending towards softness—then this is a good amount, which he should keep on taking. As the weather becomes warmer, he should reduce the amount of food because the digestions are weak in the summer because of the dissolution of the innate heat. And as the weather becomes colder, he should increase the amount of food because the digestions are strong in the winter because of the increase of the innate heat inside the body, due to the constriction of the pores, and satiation will not be attained.

(I.5) This Servant says: If someone would conduct himself in the same way as he manages the animal on which he rides, he would be safe from many diseases, that is, you do not find anyone who gives his animal fodder at random, rather, he measures it out for her according to what she can tolerate. He himself, however, eats at random, with no calculation. But he checks the activity of his animal and trains her so that she does not stand still forever and her health is ruined. But he does not do so for himself, nor does he consider physical exercise, which is the cornerstone of the preservation of health and the repulsion of most diseases.

(I.6) We have quoted Hippocrates' statement above, that the preservation of health consists of giving up laziness for exertion. There is nothing that can replace exercise in any way, because through exercise the innate heat flares up and all the superfluities are expelled, while through rest the flame of the innate heat is extinguished and superfluities develop in the body, even if the food is of the very best quality and of a moderate quantity. Exercise repels the harm done by most bad regimens that most people adhere to.

(I.7) Not every movement is exercise according to the physicians. What they call exercise is a strong or fast movement or a combination of both, that is a vigorous movement whereby breathing changes and a person begins to heave deep sighs. Whatever exceeds this is exertion, that is to say, that very strong exercise is called exertion. Not everyone can tolerate exertion nor does he need it. It is nevertheless better in the preservation of health than the neglect of exercise. One should not take exercise except on an empty stomach once the superfluities have been expelled, that is, the urine and the feces. One should not exercise in intense heat nor in intense cold, the best time for exercise is in the beginning of the day when one awakens from one's sleep after the expulsion of the superfluities, as we mentioned.

(I.8) Among Galen's general statements concerning the regimen of health is the following: Just as movement before the meal is completely good, so movement after the meal is completely bad. Know that any movement after the meal is very harmful, I mean no strenuous movement, no sexual intercourse, no bath, because the harm caused by these is great, especially for someone whose vessels are narrow and thin by nature. The affliction it brings with it is severe. But one should move a little after the meal one from one side of the room to the other to the extent that the food settles in the bottom of the stomach and stays there until it is digested. Sleep helps the digestion, especially for someone who is used to sleep during the day.

(I.9) One of the rules in the regimen of health is that one should not consume meal after meal, and that one should not eat except after true hunger when the stomach is empty and the saliva is being drawn to the mouth and the hunger is real. This is the time that nourishment is beneficial. One should not drink except when one is truly thirsty, that is, that when one is hungry or thirsty, one should wait a while because it may be a false hunger or a false thirst that arises because of a bad humor that irritates the cardia of the stomach. If this (the false hunger or thirst) subsides, one should not eat or drink anything, but when the hunger or thirst intensifies, then he should eat or drink. Drinking water after a meal is bad; it corrupts the digestion except for someone who is used to do so. One should not drink during the meal or afterwards as long as the food is still in the stomach, except pure, cold water that should not be mixed with anything.

(I.10) One of the rules in the regimen of health is that one should not retain a superfluity in any way, when there is need to expel it, one should do so quickly. One should not take a meal, go to the bathhouse, have sexual intercourse, sleep, or take exercise until one examines oneself and tries to expel the superfluities. Similarly, after these five things one should examine oneself again.

(I.11) One of the rules in the regimen of health is also that one should look into the quality of the food. This is a very broad subject that requires knowledge of the natures of all the foods, of each and every kind. The physicians have composed a number of lengthy books on this subject and they were right to do so since it is something that is absolutely necessary. We however—according to the intention of this treatise and according to the foods that are common with us and can be found in many places—will give some useful summarizing rules.

(I.12) One of these is that the excellent foods on which everyone who desires to stay healthy should rely upon are well prepared wheat bread, the meat of sheep (mutton) in their first or second year, the meat of the chicken, francolin, *ṭayhūj*, turtle dove, partridge, and the yolk from chicken eggs. With well-prepared bread I mean that it should be made from fully ripened wheat after the superfluous moistures have been dried out but which is not so old that it begins to spoil. The bread should be made of coarsely ground grain, I mean that it should not be peeled and that its bran should not be removed through sifting. It should be clearly raised and salted and well worked during kneading and baked in an oven. This is well-prepared bread according to the physicians; it is the best of foods.

(I.13) You should know that everything that is prepared from wheat other than this bread is not good food in any way. On the contrary, very bad foods are made from it, such as *faṭīr*, dough cooked like *iṭriya* and *lākisha*—and this is what the Persians call *ṭuṭmāj*—, boiled flour such as *ḥarīra*, *ʿaṣīda*, dough that is fried like *zalābiyya* and bread that is mixed with olive oil or with other oils. All these are very bad foods for all people. Similarly, bread made from white flour (*ḥuwwārā*) and bread made from the finest white flour (*samīdh*) and from *harīsa*, are not good foods. Although they are good once they are digested, they require a stomach with a strong digestion and then they provide abundant, good nourishment.

(I.14) Those meats that we have mentioned are not all of one nature and are not equally laudable. But the best meat of land animals is that of sheep that graze in the field, that are in their first or second year and moderately fat. The best part of this meat is the front part and that which is attached to the bone. All that which is in the abdomen is bad, and all fat is bad; it satiates, causes indigestion, spoils the appetite, and produces phlegmatic humor. Similarly, the heads of all animals have more superfluities than the rest of their bodily parts. The extremities of animals, that is, their shanks, are free of superfluities and their nourishment is not bad. Lamb has many superfluities, there is no good in it. But the suckling kid is good nourishment and digests quickly. The meat of birds in general is lighter than that of land animals and is digested quicker. The best meat of birds is that which we have mentioned.

(I.15) Fresh milk is a good nutrient for someone if it does not turn sour in his stomach, nor becomes vaporous or flatulent, nor produces flatulence in the hypochondrium. One should add a little honey and a grain of salt, as Galen has mentioned, so that it does not curdle in the stomach. The best milk is the thinnest, such as goat's milk, the milk of a she-camel is also good.

(I.16) All that is made from milk or mixed in it is very bad, that is *rāʾib*, *khilāṭ*, and *shīrāz*; similarly, what is boiled from milk or cooked in it, all that is bad nutrition. As for the different types of cheese, they are all very bad and thick nutrients, except for the cheese that is fresh, white in color, sweet of taste, and light of fat. Galen says that it is a good nutrient and praises it. But what is different from it is very reprehensible, especially old cheese with much fat. As for fresh butter and clarified butter, they are not bad foods; they are allowed to all people.

(I.17) Bees' honey is good nourishment for old people but bad for young people, and especially for those with a hot temperament, because it changes into yellow bile.

(I.18) Most fish are bad nourishment, especially for people with a moist temperament and for old people; especially bad among them are fish with a large body, and salted ones, and those that live in bad waters, and that are very fat and very viscous. But fish that have a small body, white flesh that falls apart easily, and that tastes sweet, or fish that live in the sea or in streaming waters such as those that are called *būrī* (black mullet) or *rāy*, are not bad nourishment, but one should limit their consumption.

(I.19) It is known among all the physicians that the best of all nutriments is that which is widely known as being prohibited in Islam (wine). It unites the good qualities of all foods—since it nourishes with good, abundant, and fine nourishment—, is quickly digested, and at the same time assists the digestion, expels the superfluities from the pores, and induces micturition and perspiration. It has other virtues besides these and many other benefits enumerated by the physicians. But speaking about something the consumption of which is illicit is futile, and therefore we have omitted mentioning its varieties and the manner of its usage with respect to the regimen of health.

(I.20) Those vegetables, which are bad for all people in general and in particular, are garlic, onion, leek, radish, cabbage, and eggplant. They are extremely bad for whoever wishes to preserve his health. Small cucumbers (*khiyār*) and cucumbers (*faqqūs*) are less harmful. As for the yellow common melon, if it is consumed alone at the beginning of the day on an empty stomach and there is no harmful humor in the stomach that has flowed into it, nor is there a bad temperament in it, then it will be well digested; cool the body a little, induce micturition, cleanse the vessels, and evacuate what is in them. Then its nourishment is not bad. I have mentioned it only because all people eat it frequently.

(I.21) As for fresh fruits, know that all that trees produce is discommended as foodstuff for people in general, although some are worse than others. Some of them are very bad nourishment, such as carob, *nabiq* (the fruit of Christ's thorn jujube), and common medlar, and some of them are only slightly harmful, close to being good, such as figs and grapes. Galen says that figs and grapes are like princes to the rest of the fruits and they are less harmful. Nevertheless, they are not free from the censure that adheres to feeding oneself with any fruit. Let not the observer err in my statement that all that the trees produce is discommended as foodstuff, since fruit conserves, their syrups and the electuaries made from them are beneficial in specific diseases because the consideration of nutrients, in their capacity of nutrients, is different from their consideration as medicines. This is clear to someone who knows the principles of the art of medicine.

(I.22) Galen has a saying in which he tells people in the form of an advice and swears by God that it is the ultimate advice in which he forbids people to eat fruit. He said that he used to suffer from fever every year, and that when his father told him not to eat any fruit at all, he was saved from the fever during that year. He continued not to eat fruit during the whole of his life, and he swore that he did not suffer from fever from then on until the time that he wrote down that statement, except for an ephemeral fever. [*De sanitate tuenda* V.1; *De bonis malisque sucis* I]. What he states is the truth because summer fruit is the substance of fevers. It is not an argument against us that many people eat fruit and do not suffer from fever, since customs and difference in dispositions have different laws. If a Hindu would eat well-prepared bread and mutton, he would necessarily fall ill. And if one of us would constantly eat rice with fish as the Hindus always do, he would necessarily fall ill. But the purpose of this treatise does not require to communicate the reasons for this; rather, the intent is to make it known that fruits in general are bad and that one should limit their consumption. One should not combine them with a meal at all. One should eat all those fruits that are softening, such as plums, grapes, and figs before the meal, and should not eat a meal after them until they have left the stomach. One should consume all those fruits that are astringent, such as quinces and pears, after the meal, and one should only take a little, that is, an amount that strengthens the cardia of the stomach. Just as the best of fruits are figs and grapes, so the worst of them are peaches and apricots. The digestion cannot master these two kinds in any way, and of necessity some of the watery superfluity will remain in the vessels mixed with the blood and will boil. This is a major cause for the generation of putrid fevers. But dry fruits, such as raisins, dry figs, dry almond kernels and pistachio nuts are not bad. It is good to take of them after the meal, especially raisins and pistachio nuts, because they are very beneficial for the liver, and our life lies in the health of the liver, as Galen has also said. Similarly, the consumption of a few sweets after the meal is good, so that the stomach retains the meal and digests it.

This is what I held for good to mention in this chapter. It is sufficient for our purpose.

∴

Chapter Two

On the regimen of sick people in general, when no physician can be found, or when the available physician is such that one cannot rely upon his knowledge

(II.1) Those engaged in speculation have taught that the art of medicine is very necessary for man, and especially for people of the cities, because of the abundance of foods, and that the physician is indispensable at any time or in any condition. This is because the art of medicine comprises three regimens, of which the first and most noble is the regimen of the healthy, that is, the regimen of the existing state of health, so that it is not lost. The second is the regimen of the sick, that is, the activities of the craft to restore lost health, and this is what is known as the art of cure. The third is the regimen that Galen calls "vivification," that is, the regimen of those who are neither perfectly healthy nor sick, such as the regimen of the convalescent and the old. [*De sanitate tuenda* V.4]. It is thus clear that a human being requires the guidance of a physician in any circumstance and at any time. But the need for a physician during illness is stronger, and the lack of a physician at that time is more dangerous. Therefore, people in general think that they do not need a physician except during illness, and not otherwise. But people often fall ill during a journey or in a town where there is no physician, or there is a physician but one cannot trust his knowledge. Therefore, this Servant thought it a good thing to give advice as to what should be done in such a case.

(II.2) And I say that Galen has explained to us that all the ancient Greeks, when a disease was obscure to them, would not treat it with anything, but left the patient to nature, because she is sufficient to cure diseases. Hippocrates has praised nature at great length in a number of places in his books, stating that she is skillful and sagacious; that she does what is proper, and that she does not need anything else beside her for the cure of diseases. [*Epidemics* VI.5.1]. The physician only has to support nature, nothing else, and to follow in her path.

(II.3) Al-Rāzī has said in one of his well-known aphorisms, that when the disease is stronger than the strength of the patient, there is no hope for saving the patient and the physician is of no use to him at all; and when the vigor of the patient is stronger than the disease, there is no need for a physician at all, for nature will cure him. But when they are equal, then the physician is needed to support the strength of the patient. This is so if the physician is accomplished and knows how to aid and support nature and how to remove that which hinders her. But most physicians err greatly in this matter and think that they help the strength of the patient, while in reality they destroy it or hinder it or confuse its way. Therefore, Aristotle says in his book *De sensu et sens*[*ibilibus*] that most of those who die, indeed die from the treatment because of the ignorance of the physicians about nature. When using the term "nature" in this connection, physicians mean the power that governs the body of a living creature; its existence and the soundness of its actions have been demonstrated in the scholarly books on sciences composed by the ancients. For these reasons, kings take a number of physicians and select from them those who have acumen and long experience, because by their combined discernments they will perhaps be saved from error.

(II.4) It is clear from all that I have mentioned above, that it is proper to leave the patient to nature when an accomplished physician cannot be found. The meaning of leaving it to nature is that one should not take a medicine other than that which healthy people use to take and that one does not give up taking food altogether, but drinks when one is thirsty and eats when one is hungry at the time that one is used to eat. At that time, one should eat the lightest meal that one is used to eat. One should know that even if one is attended by a well-known physician or by a number of physicians, one should not resign and undergo strong treatment except on the advice of a very accomplished physician whose knowledge has been verified and whose experience has been attested. Otherwise, one should be guided by a mild treatment, not a strong one.

(II.5) I will explain what a strong treatment is. It includes: bleeding with the extraction of much blood; evacuation by strong attracting purgatives, such as colocynth pulp and scammony; evacuation by emesis using strong remedies, such as the two hellebores (black and white false hellebore), and the poison nut (*nux vomica*); sharp enemas containing colocynth, sagapenum, castoreum, and the like; the deprivation of nourishment altogether and the instruction to the patient not to eat anything at all; the prohibition of drinking water and the endurance of thirst; the ingestion of the multi-beneficial great electuaries, such as the theriacs, the Mithridates, and Theodoretus, and the like. All these things are a very strong form of treatment, and one should not apply any of them except on the advice of a physician of superior knowledge, because these things, if they hit their mark, heal the patient immediately or within a short time, or save him from death. But if they miss their mark, they mostly kill immediately or impart a disease that ultimately leads its host to death; therefore, one should beware of them.

(II.6) As for the mild treatment, it consists of: the extraction of blood through scarification of the thighs or the upper parts of the body; softening the stool with two kinds of manna, plums, cherries, violets, refined rose syrup, and the like; emesis with barley gruel, or oxymel, or radish, or garden orach seeds, or *biṭṭīkh* (common melon or watermelon) roots, and the like; mild enemas, such as the injection with barley gruel, or a decoction of bran, or honey water, or with olive oil alone, and the like; softening the food by taking the usual drinks prepared from sugar, or bees' honey, or barley gruel, or barley groats, or the soaked soft part of bread, or by taking a little bread with one of the vegetarian dishes for the sick; medication with healthy remedies, that is things that are often taken by the healthy, such as the well-known syrups like the syrup of oxymel, roses, *utrujj* (citron or lemon), violets, and the robs that are similar, that is preserved roses, preserved violets, preserved chebulic myrobalan, and the like; taking decoctions compounded from mild and safe remedies, such as licorice, maidenhair fern, borage, *hindibā'* (endive or chicory) seed, *utrujj* peel, field eryngo, asparagus roots, the bark of *hindibā'* roots, fennel, celery, cucumber seed, common purslane seed, small cucumber seed, *biṭṭīkh* seed, the stem of the common marshmallow and its seed, and the like; infusions compounded from fruits, seeds, and flowers that are usually taken by the healthy; and an infusion of tamarind. All these are different sorts of mild treatment. If they hit their mark, they are beneficial and cure a mild illness and in time may cure a severe illness. And if they miss their mark, they do not kill and do not cause serious harm. Thus, one finds that most physicians rely on this form of treatment in seeking safety.

(II.7) As for the evacuation with *hiera*s, agarikon, St. Thomas lidpod, and the like, and similarly purging cassia, the situation is an intermediate one. They are not of the kind of remedies that cause a strong evacuation nor of those that are part of a mild treatment. Purging cassia: although it may cause distress and in some cases abrasion, it is nevertheless a very reliable remedy. Similarly, agarikon: although it is reliable as a purgative, it can nevertheless cause serious harm because of its refining properties and its severely drying effect when we need to moisten either the entire body or a single part. Similarly, the harm caused by *hiera*s and the different kinds of *iṭrīfal* to those suffering from fever is severe most of the time.

(II.8) The warning we gave against taking the theriac and Mithridates, except on the advice of an accomplished physician, is only for the sick. As for the healthy, it has been mentioned that it is part of the regimen of health to take the theriac every ten days. Thus, it was stated by the physicians; however, there is not one directive in the field of medicine that is an absolute one, but for every rule issued by them, there are necessary conditions, as where they stated to take the theriac every ten days with regard to the regimen of health. For it should not be taken by someone who has a hot temperament, nor should it be taken at the time of intense heat, nor should it be taken by someone who has any kind of bad humor in his stomach. As to their statement that emesis once or twice a month is very good in the regimen of health, it also has conditions attached to it, namely, that the person should not have a weak chest, nor be someone whose head becomes congested quickly or suffers from headache most of the time. Emesis is also not beneficial at a time of severe cold. Similarly, every rule issued by them has its conditions, as we exemplified.

(II.9) Our instruction to apply a mild treatment—some matters of which we have mentioned—when a skilled physician cannot be found and one follows the directions of the attending physician, whoever he is, only replaces what would have been necessary, because even such a treatment can be harmful when the physician is mistaken and applies it out of place. Galen has explained to us that sometimes a patient is ordered to drink water until he is satiated and his body becomes wet with sweat, his stools become soft, his fever departs, and he is completely healed, while at other times he is allowed to drink water at an inappropriate time and this causes the patient to perish or to get a chronic disease from which he never recovers. I have already explained all the conditions under which the drinking of water is allowed or prohibited. If this is the case with drinking water, how much more so with other things.

(II.10) When the symptoms are contradictory and it is difficult for us to determine whether the drinking of water should be allowed or prohibited, the patient should be allowed to drink water, but not to excess. Similarly, if it is difficult for us to determine whether one should feed the patient or whether this should be prohibited altogether, we feed him with some light food. In the same way it is proper that the regimen, when a skillful physician cannot be found, should always be according to what is customary in health. One should take a little bit of what one usually takes and always maintain one's strength by taking nourishment, either light nourishment, such as chicken soup, meat broth, the yolk of soft-boiled eggs, and wine for him who may take it, or nourishment that is heavier than these, such as meat of young chickens and bread.

(II.11) One should never neglect to strengthen the natural faculty with nourishment; and to strengthen the psychical faculty with fragrant odors: either hot, such as musk and ambergris and bush basil in cold diseases, or cold, such as rose, *nīlūfar* (blue Egyptian, European white, or yellow water lily), myrtle, and violet in hot diseases; and to strengthen the animal faculty with musical instruments by telling the patient joyful stories that dilate his soul and chest, by telling him tales that divert him and make him laugh, and by the presence of someone who dilates his soul by his company. All this is necessary in every disease when there is no physician who is capable to do what should be done.

(II.12) The physicians have instructed every physician not to treat a patient with medication, if he can be treated only by a dietetic regimen. If one cannot manage without treating him with medication, one should treat him with things that are customary, such as medicines with nutritional properties and nutrients with medicinal properties. But if one cannot manage without a purely medicinal treatment, one should start with the mildest remedies, and if this is sufficient, it is good. But if it is not sufficient for the disease, one should resort to stronger remedies and then to even stronger ones. Whenever it is possible to treat a disease with a simple drug, one should not treat it with a compound drug. But if one cannot manage without a compound one, one should treat the disease with the least compound one. One should not resort to very complex remedies except when absolutely necessary. If these rules hold good with respect to an eminent physician, how should it be when there is no physician? One should be very careful and never rush to use stronger remedies and one should not turn away from what is proper regarding the application of multiple drugs but be content with what is customary from the lighter kinds of treatment. This is the measure of what I considered proper to give counsel concerning this matter.

∴

Chapter Three
On the regimen of my Master in particular, according to the symptoms he complains about

(III.1) The physicians agree that the first thing to look after in the regimen of health is that the stools be soft. [*Kitāb al-Taysīr fī l-mudāwāt wa-l-tadbīr*]. When the stools become dry, let alone if they are retained, very bad vapors develop, ascend to the heart and the brain, corrupt the humors, make the pneumas turbid, produce depression, evil thoughts, stupefaction, and indolence, and prevent all the superfluities of the digestions from being expelled. Therefore, one should take utmost care to soften the stools.

(III.2) Abū Marwān ibn Zuhr—may God have mercy with him—has said that the best thing for softening the stools is an infusion of rhubarb with tamarind. [*Kitāb al-Taysīr fī l-mudāwāt wa-l-tadbīr*]. But what this minor Servant considers the best, according to what was mentioned to him about the temperament of our Master, is to soften the stools with a lemon dish (*laymūniyya*), prepared with a fat hen, with much safflower seed, sugar, lemon juice and beetroots that were boiled—and their juice should not be discarded. He should also make it his habit at mealtime to first eat vegetables spiced in barley gruel and fragrant olive oil before the meal. Then our Master can take whatever food he likes. After finishing his meal, he should suck on a quince, pear, apple, or a pomegranate with its seeds. The vegetables that he should take first are chard, garden orach, spinach, or purple amaranth, whatever is available, spiced with fragrant olive oil and barley gruel. When it is necessary to soften the stools with medication, take one *dirham* of good rhubarb and crush it, and one ounce of tamarind, cleaned of its peel and seeds, cut as thin as possible. Macerate these for a night in one and a half *raṭl* of hot water that has been boiled thoroughly. The next morning, filter this over three ounces of refined rose syrup. He should take this in the morning and he should not eat thereafter until six hours of the day have passed.

(III.3) If the stools become as hard as stone, there is no alternative but to take purging cassia. The manner of its preparation is as follows: Take four *dirham*s of borage, three *dirham*s each of licorice, peeled and crushed, maidenhair fern, and barberry seeds, five *dirham*s of common marshmallow seeds, seven flowers of fresh roses, when they are available, and seven kernels of fennel. Macerate all this in one and a half *raṭl* of hot water for a day and night. Boil, stir, and filter it over twenty *dirham*s of the scales of purging cassia, four *dirham*s of almond oil, and two ounces of sugar. Take this and wait until its action is completed and then take to finish it off boiled chicken. If it is not the time to find fresh roses, filter it over three ounces of refined rose syrup. I know that he who might look into this treatise will be confused and say: Why should he use barberry seeds, which are constipating, in a preparation with which he wants to relieve the bowels? He should know that barberry seeds have the specific property of preventing the distress caused by purging cassia and that they strengthen the intestines so that abrasion will not occur; this is what we have learned from the Elders of the Art.

(III.4) The physicians have mentioned the oxymel syrup of roses as a purgative; it should also be in the possession of our Master and he should take it for softening the stools during the time of intense heat. Its composition is: Take one *raṭl* of very strong vinegar, throw into it one hundred petals of fresh roses, and put it in the sun for one day. The next morning, press out the roses, throw them away and throw into that vinegar other roses, as above; do not stop to change the roses in this way for forty days. Then take this vinegar and thicken it into syrup, one *raṭl* of sugar to every three ounces of this vinegar.

(III.5) Ibn Zuhr has compounded the oxymel syrup of raisins and it is very good. Our Master should use it occasionally during the summer. Its composition is:

Clean the black raisins of their seeds and throw half a *raṭl* of the raisins in each *raṭl* of vinegar, and let them soak in it for two days. Then put it on a fire, boil it a few times, filter it, and thicken this vinegar into oxymel. This compound was indeed composed with good consideration, because the vinegar cuts the phlegm and opposes the putrefaction of the humors in an unequalled way. It is of a very fine substance and cools the temperament, and for this reason oxymel is very beneficial for all fevers. However, the vinegar is very harmful to the liver; it scrapes and emaciates it and whitens its blood. Galen has explained that the maintenance of health of a human being lies in the health of the liver, and vinegar weakens its strengths. Raisins are friends of the liver; they fatten and strengthen it, they color the blood and ripen the humors. However, they heat it, and if one takes too much of it, they burn the blood. But if the syrup is compounded from vinegar and raisins, just as that eminent physician (Ibn Zuhr) has compounded it, we obtain the beneficial effects of the vinegar and are saved from its damage to the liver. We also obtain the beneficial effects of the raisins and are saved from its heating effect. This is extraordinary syrup that one should keep in readiness.

(III.6) This Servant thought it proper to compound for his Master two syrups and an electuary in accordance with those symptoms that were mentioned. One of the syrups should be taken regularly, at all times. Its effects are that it clarifies the blood, removes its turbidity and cleanses it of its melancholic vapors, so that the soul is dilated and gladdened, the chest widened, and the sadness and anxieties referred to disappear. The description of its preparation is: Take one *raṭl* of fresh rose leaves, half a *raṭl* of borage, two ounces of French lavender, one ounce each of raw silk, chopped seeds of common fumitory, and *utrujj* (citron or lemon) peel. Steep all these in six *raṭl*s of hot water for a day and a night. Then boil all this a few times, macerate it and filter it through a sieve, throw over it six *raṭl*s of common sorrel syrup, put it on a low fire that it attains the consistency of a syrup, and season it with one quarter of a *mithqāl* of Iraqi musk. This is a syrup of which no equal can be found, to our Servant's opinion, in gladdening, strengthening, and invigorating the heart. It is moderate and it does not heat nor chill, and therefore it can be taken at any time. The amount to be taken is two to three ounces with cold water in the summer, or hot water in the winter.

(III.7) As for the second syrup, which our Servant thought proper to compound, it is a syrup that softens the stools very much and that may in some cases require two or three sittings, according to the preparation. It strengthens the expulsive faculty, which is in the stomach and the intestines, gently expels the phlegm and black and yellow bile, but does not harm the digestive organs. One should take three to four ounces of it with hot water in which anise has been boiled until its properties changed. One should not take this constantly, but only take it when one needs to expel the retained residues. If our Master makes it his habit to take it once a week, it strengthens the intestines and removes from them that disposition which causes dryness of the stools. The stools become soft and return to their normal nature. Its composition is: Take common polypody from which the upper skin has been peeled, two ounces of pounded and crushed pistachio nuts, one ounce each of senna of Mecca and borage, half an ounce each of pounded licorice and pounded common marshmallow stem, a handful of fresh fennel, and twenty flowers of fresh roses. Steep all this in four *raṭl*s of hot water for a day and a night; then boil it the next morning, stir and filter it over thirty *dirham*s of the scales of purging cassia, cleaned and mixed with half an ounce of almond oil. Filter this and set it aside. Then take ten *dirham*s each of cleansed chebulic myrobalan, Indian and emblic myrobalan; pound the myrobalans and steep them in one and a half *raṭl* of hot, intensely boiling water for a day and a night. The next morning stir the myrobalans well, filter them and add them to that decoction containing the purging cassia that had been put aside. Take the two combined liquids and pour this over four *raṭl*s of violet syrup; place this on a low fire and suspend in it a bag of fine linen containing two *dirham*s each of spikenard and mastic, three *dirham*s of pounded rhubarb. Do not stop squeezing the bag with a spoon until the powers of the medicaments, which are in it, have emerged. When the liquid has attained the consistency of syrup, take it from the fire, put it in a pitcher, and use it when necessary as I have mentioned.

(III.8) As for the electuary referred to by your Servant, it is the great *iṭrīfal*, which your Servant has compounded in the past for someone who needed it. It improves the three digestions, strengthens all the intestines in general, and the heart and stomach in particular. It delays aging, dissolves the phlegm, prevents the vapors from flowing into the brain, strengthens all the senses and removes their dullness, aids coitus, and dilates the soul. Its composition is: One ounce each of chebulic, Indian, and beleric myrobalan; two ounces of emblic myrobalan; one ounce each of *utrujj* (citron or lemon) peel, borage, French lavender flowers, common hedgenettle and *antula* (yellow monkshood); one ounce of leaves of red roses; half an ounce each of fruit of the ash tree, sekakul parsnip, asparagus seed, wild carrot seed, garden rocket seed, the two behens (white behen and red behen, possibly Mediterranean sea lavender), anise, mastic and Mecca myrrh peel; an eighth of an ounce each of cubeb, black cardamom, clove, cinnamon, greater galangal, long pepper, ginger, spikenard, great false leopardbane, and fragrant agarwood; and three ounces of pine nuts. The dry medications should be pulverized and sifted, the seeds and the pine nuts should be pounded until they become very fine, the myrobalans should be stirred time and again with half a *raṭl* of almond oil or pistachio oil, and the whole should be mixed and kneaded with three *raṭl*s of julep and two *raṭl*s of bees' honey from which the foam has been removed, and placed in a vessel manufactured in Āmid. The amount that should be taken is four *dirham*s to half an ounce, in the wintertime with hot water in which anise has been boiled. When the weather is moderate it should be taken as a linctus. It should not be used in a time of extreme heat; at other times it should not be used frequently, but once a week. These are the syrups and electuary of which this Servant thinks that they should always be found in the blessed royal treasury of al-Afḍal, may God preserve it together with a long life of its king.

(III.9) It is known to my Master—may God prolong his days—that the passions of the soul produce changes in the body that are great, clear, and evident to all people. As evidence thereof, you can see a person with a strong physical constitution, a loud voice, and a radiant face. If news reaches him all of a sudden, which grieves him very much, you see that his color becomes ash-grey at that moment, his face loses its radiance, his posture droops, and his voice becomes weak. Even if he wants to raise his voice and tries to do so, he cannot. His strength diminishes and sometimes he trembles from weakness. His pulse becomes small, his eyes become sunken, his eyelids become too heavy to move, the surface of his body cools and he loses his appetite. The cause of all these symptoms is the withdrawal of the innate heat and the blood into the interior of the body.

Contrary hereto, you may see someone with a weak body, a pallid color and a soft voice. If news reaches him that causes him great rejoicing, you see that his body becomes strong, his voice becomes loud, his face brightens, his movements become faster, his pulse becomes greater, the surface of his body becomes warmer, pleasure and joy overwhelm him so much that he cannot hide them. The cause of all these symptoms is the move of the innate heat and the blood to the exterior of the body. The state of someone who is afraid and anxious, and of someone who is confident and hopeful, is known. Likewise, the state of the defeated and victorious is clear. The defeated can hardly see anything because of the diminution and dispersal of the visual pneuma. As for the victorious, the light of his vision has so much increased, that it seems to him that the light of the day has increased and grown. This matter is so clear that it is not necessary to elaborate thereon.

(III.10) Because of this, the physicians instruct us to always look after and attend to the matter of the movements of the soul. One should see to their balance in the state of health as well as during any disease and not let any other regimen take precedence over this in any way. The physician should aspire that every sick and healthy person has a cheerful and dilated soul at all times, and that they should be relieved from passions of the soul that cause constriction of the soul. Because in this way the health of the healthy is preserved and it is the foremost principle in curing any patient, especially someone whose illness is psychic, as those who suffer from hypochondria and melancholic delusion, for looking after the movements of the soul in these is most pressing. And the same holds good for someone who is overcome by anxiety, constant worry, or fear of something that normally he would not be afraid of, or by a lack of joy of something that normally he would enjoy. In all of these, the skillful physician should not let anything precede the rectification of the state of their soul by the removal of these passions. But the physician, inasmuch as he is a physician, his art does not demand knowledge of the stratagem to remove these passions. Because this matter is only attained by practical philosophy and by the admonitions and disciplines of the Law.

(III.11) For just as the philosophers have composed many books in the various sciences, so they have composed many books dealing with the improvement of morals and the discipline of the soul so that it will acquire moral virtues until nothing will come from it but good actions. They warn against moral imperfections and teach the way to remove them from the soul of any person who finds any of these bad virtues in himself until that habitus, which prompts them to all evils, departs. Similarly, the disciplines of the Law and the admonitions and laws received from the Prophets—peace be with them—or from their followers, and the knowledge of their virtuous ways improve the moral qualities of the soul until it acquires a virtuous disposition, so that nothing comes from it but good actions. Therefore, one finds that these passions only make a very strong impression on people who have neither knowledge of ethical philosophy, nor of the disciplines and admonitions of the Law, such as children, women, and the ignorant. For these, because of the softness of their soul, are anxious and fearful. One finds that, when harm befalls them, or there comes to them a calamity of the calamities of the world, their anxiety is great, they cry out, weep, slap their cheeks, and beat their chests. Sometimes the affliction is so great upon them that one of them dies—either suddenly or after some time—from the anxiety and worry that overtook him. Similarly, if these individuals acquire a good from the goods of the world, their joy increases therein and one of them thinks—because of the lack of discipline of his soul—that he has acquired a very great good. His conceit and delight increase in his exaggeration of what he has acquired. He becomes severely affected by this, his laughter and exuberance increase to a degree that some of them die from an excess of exultation, because of the dissolution of the pneuma through the intensity of its sudden deflection to the outside, as Galen has mentioned. [*De locis affectis* v.1]. The cause of all this is the softness and ignorance of the soul.

(iii.12) As for people trained in ethical philosophy or in the disciplines and admonitions of the Law, their soul acquires courage and they are the truly courageous, so that their soul is influenced and affected as little as possible. The more a person is disciplined, the less he is affected in both these states, namely, the state of prosperity and the state of vengeance. This is the case so much so that if he acquires a great good from the goods of the world and these are those, which are called imaginary goods by the philosophers, he is neither affected by that nor are those goods magnified by him. Similarly, if he is afflicted by a great evil of the evils of the world, and these are called imaginary evils by the philosophers, he is neither anxious nor fearful, but bears it well.

(iii.13) Indeed, a human being will acquire this disposition of his soul through consideration of the truth of things and through knowledge of the nature of that which exists, because the greatest good in the world—even though it endures with someone all his life—is a very basic thing, as it is something that is perishable; and what is there in it for a human being, compared to the fact that he must die like the other species of animals? Similarly, the greatest evil in the world, if compared to death from which there is no escape, that evil is without any doubt less than death. Therefore, one should be less affected by such an evil, as it is less than the evil from which there is no escape.

(iii.14) In truth, the philosophers have called the good and evil things of the world imaginary good things and imaginary evil things, because how many of its good things are supposed to be good, while in truth they are evil, and how many of its bad things are supposed to be bad, while in truth they are good! And how often has someone acquired much wealth, and how often has someone acquired futile possessions, and this became the cause of the corruption of his body, the deformation of his soul through moral defects, the shortening of his life, his separation from God—Who is exalted—, and the intervention of a barrier between him and his Creator. And what is there in it for him, in comparison to eternal misery? And how much wealth someone was deprived of, or property taken from him, and this became the cause of the improvement of the condition of his body, and the adornment of his soul with moral virtues, and the prolongation of his life, bringing him close to his Creator through his devotion to His worship! And what is there in it for him, in comparison to eternal happiness?

(III.15) Indeed, what this Servant has said about that, through which one has a long life or a short life, is according to the opinion of the physicians and philosophers and some of the experts in the religious laws that preceded Islam. On the whole, most of the things that people in general consider to be fortunate, are in truth unfortunate and most of the things that they consider to be unfortunate, are in truth fortunate. But it is not the intention of this treatise to explain the truth of these things, to expound them, and to teach its ways, for much has been compiled about this subject at all times and in every wise nation that studied the sciences. This Servant has only referred to these things to stimulate training of the soul in freedom from emotion by studying those books on ethics, the disciplines of the Law, and the admonitions and laws spoken by the sages, so that the soul will be strengthened and see the true as true and the false as false, and the passions will diminish, evil thoughts will depart, fear will pass away, and the soul will dilate, whatever the condition someone is in.

(III.16) Here, reflection is very good. Evil thoughts, anxieties, and worries will be less through it and sometimes cease completely if a person holds the following consideration before his mind's eye, namely, that whenever someone thinks about something and he becomes sad because of it and anxiety, worry, and grief befall him, this is unavoidably the result of one of two things. Either because he thinks about something that has passed like someone who thinks about the loss of wealth he had, or the death of a person who was dear to him, or because he thinks about things that he anticipates and fears their coming to pass, like someone who thinks and reflects about what he dreads that might happen to him as a result of misfortune. It is known through rational contemplation that thinking about something that has passed and has gone by is of no benefit at all, and that grief and worry about things that have gone by are something that those do who have a deficient apprehension. It makes no difference whether someone is sad because of wealth that he lost, and the like, or that he is sad because he is a human being and not an angel or a star, and similar thoughts about impossibilities. As for acts of thinking that bring about constriction of the soul (anxiety) about what one dreads that might happen in the future, they should also be abandoned with the consideration that everything that someone anticipates belongs to the category of something possible that may happen or may not happen. And just as someone may be sad and distressed lest something he dreads might occur, in the same way one should dilate one's soul with lasting expectation and hope that perhaps the opposite of what he anticipates might occur; since both what he anticipates and its opposite are possible. This is the measure of what the Servant saw necessary in this chapter.

∴

Chapter Four

Consisting of sections in the form of hortatory rules that are useful in general and in particular for healthy and sick people in all places and all times

(IV.1) One should first pay attention to the improvement of the air, then to the improvement of the water, and then to the improvement of the foods we take. This is so because what the physicians call "pneumas" are fine vapors found in the bodies of living creatures. Their origin and most of their substance come from the air inhaled from outside. The vapor of the blood found in the liver and in the veins originating therefrom is called "natural pneuma," and the vapor of the blood found in the heart and the arteries is called "vital pneuma," and the vapor found in the ventricles of the brain and that which is transmitted from it into the cavities of the nerves is called "psychical pneuma." All these pneumas and their substance originate from the air inhaled from outside, and—if this air is putrid, evil-smelling, or turbid—all these pneumas are altered and their condition becomes the opposite of what it should be.

Galen said: Pay attention to the matter of the essence of the air that reaches the body through inhalation, so that it will be utterly balanced and free from all that what might pollute it. [*De methodo medendi* VIII.6].

Says the author: The finer the pneuma is, the more it changes with changes in the air. The natural pneuma is coarser than the vital pneuma, while the vital pneuma is coarser than the psychical pneuma, so that with the slightest change in the air the condition of the soul changes perceptibly. Therefore, one sees that many people notice a deterioration in their psychical functions with the corruption of the air, that is to say, that they suffer from dullness of understanding, lack of comprehension, and loss of memory, although their vital and natural functions are not perceptibly changed.

(IV.2) The relationship between the air in cities and the air in deserts and steppes is comparable to the relationship between water of a coarse, turbid substance and fine, pure water. In the city—because of its high buildings and narrow streets, the large amount of refuse and waste of its inhabitants, their dead and the carcasses of their animals, and the putrefaction of their food—the air becomes stagnant, turbid, thick, misty, and foggy. The pneumas gradually become like that as well, although a person might not realize what has befallen him. If we cannot escape from this, since we have grown up in cities and are used to them, one should at least choose a city with open horizons, especially towards north and east, high on the mountains or hills, sparse in trees and waters. If you have no choice in this either, that is, if you cannot choose to move to another city, you should at least try to live on the outskirts of the city, facing north and east. The dwelling place should be a tall building with a wide court, so that the north wind can traverse it and sunlight can enter it, because sunlight dissolves the putrefied air and makes it fine and clear. One should strive to put the toilet as far as possible from the place where one lives. And one should endeavor to improve the air and dry it with fragrant odors, vapors, and fumigation, as is proper according to the changes in the air. This is a fundamental rule with which every regimen of body or soul should start.

(IV.3) Even if you are careful and on your guard as much as you can be, there is no escape from minor ailments constantly occurring in the human body. For instance, sometimes the stools become a little bit soft and sometimes a little bit dry, or one finds a feebleness in his digestion one day, or suffers from a mild headache or a mild pain in some part of his body. There are many minor ailments like these. One should be extremely careful then, not to be hasty in treating this minor ailment by taking medicines to eliminate it. The most eminent physicians have warned against it, because one's nature alone is sufficient in things such as these and does not need the assistance of medicines; rather, one should adhere to a healthy, good regimen. For once you start to treat that minor ailment, you do one of two things: either your action is a mistake and contrary to the tendency of your nature, so that you confuse it and aggravate the ailment; or your action is correct and you restore the natural functions of your nature but at the same time you teach your nature passivity and you accustom it not to do what is required except with external assistance. You can compare this, as they say, to someone who accustoms his animal not to move except with a spur, for the animal stands still forever until it is spurred. It is also similar to the situation that you find when the stools have softened in an unusual way even though you did not change your regimen in any way; this may last for two or three days without pain or weakening of your stamina. And if you hasten to use astringents and thus stop this diarrhea, your nature returns to its normal condition by means of medication. But sometimes the cause of this is a natural movement of the expulsive power, which moves to expel that which should be expelled, so that the stools become soft. But when nature is restrained in such a case, it is harmed, its proper activity is suspended, and that which should have been expelled is retained, so that harm is being done. At other times that softness of the stools is caused by the weakness of the retentive power, and if it had been left alone it would have awakened and the organ would have returned innately to its natural action. But when this power is strengthened by means of drugs whenever it is weakened, this will become a custom and a habit; whenever this power is deterred from action, it will need an external stimulant. It will thus be clear that the proper thing to do is not to do anything. This should be done in every case where there is no danger to life.

(IV.4) Abū Naṣr al-Fārābī has mentioned in this connection that in the art of medicine, in seamanship, and in agriculture, the outcome does not necessarily depend upon the efforts invested. For the physician may do whatever is necessary in the best possible way, without any error committed neither by him nor by the patient, yet he does not attain the cure, which is the ultimate goal. The reason for this is clear, for the active factor in this case is not medicine alone, but medicine and nature. Sometimes nature does not react for a number of reasons, some of which have been mentioned in this treatise. Similarly, the farmer may do all that is necessary, but the seed does not prosper. Similarly, the seaman may navigate his ship in the best possible manner, build it with the best construction, and sail the sea at the usual time, yet the ship may perish. The reason for all these failures is that the goal is achieved only through the action of two agents, one of which does whatever is necessary, while the other falls short in its action.

(IV.5) If you consider the contents of the preceding chapter, you will realize that sometimes the disease is mild and that nature is stronger than it and has begun to remove it and to do all what should be done, yet the physician may err in his treatment or the patient may err, and the actions of nature come to nothing. This happens in the majority of cases in all places and at all times.

(IV.6) In one of his aphorisms, al-Rāzī makes a statement with the following meaning, saying: When the disease is more manifest than the strength of the patient, medicine is of no use at all, and when the strength of the patient has the upper hand over the disease, there is no need for a physician in any way. But when they are equal, then the physician is needed to support and promote the strength of the patient against the disease. [*Kitāb al-Murshid aw al-fuṣūl*].

(IV.7) Says the author: From the words of this man, who is perfect in his art, one can also learn that when one draws an analogy with all the diseases, one can do without a physician more often than one needs him, even when he is excellent and knows how to support nature and does not confuse it and divert it from its proper way.

(IV.8) Careless physicians often commit very grave errors against the people; yet the sick do not die, but recover. I have seen several times, how someone administered a strong purgative to a person who did not even need a weak purgative. As a result, this person lost much blood from below, which condition lasted for several days and he suffered from severe dysentery; yet he recovered afterwards. I have also seen how someone bled a person suffering from indigestion at a time when he did not know about his indigestion. As a result, the patient lost consciousness, his strength diminished, and his illness became protracted and worsened, yet he recovered in the end. However, one should not take an example from this and think that physicians' errors do little harm. Nor should one say: If they commit such grave errors and the patient does not die, why should he die if the physician errs in determining the correct amount of nutrition or of mild decoctions? The matter is not so, however; for the case of these preceding internal causes of illness is rather like that of the following external causes. You see with your own eyes, people whose arms are cut off below the elbow or whose legs are cut off below the knee, or whose eyes are extracted, or who are stricken in battle with severe blows in the cavity of the body and who do not die but live, as God wills. And on the other hand, you see a person pricked by a thin needle or thorn that hits one of his nerves and he has spasms and dies. The same applies to errors by physicians: A physician may commit a grave error and yet the patient is saved; or he may disregard something, which both he and the patient consider a minor thing, and yet it becomes the cause of the patient's death. This should be taken into consideration by every thinking person.

(IV.9) It is well known that all men suppose eating the usual food, drinking the usual water, bathing in cold water for one who is used to this, and bathing in the bathhouse, are all matters that are not very dangerous for the sick, even if done improperly. But this is not so. Galen has explained to us that among those suffering from fever there are some in whom the drinking of cold water—which they are allowed to drink—causes their humors to become crude and fires their fever, so that they perish. And there are others for whom the drinking of cold water is a cure: it softens their stools and extinguishes the fire of their fever and they recover; if water is withheld from them, they perish. Similarly, some patients with fever recover and are saved when one lets them enter cold water, while others perish by it. Similarly, bathing in the bathhouse cleanses the body of some of those with fever and enables their complete recovery, while in the case of others it increases their putrefaction, gives them a bad fever, and kills them. The same holds true for food: withholding it from a patient can be the cause of his recovery or the cause of his death; and giving it freely to the patient can be the cause of his recovery or the cause of his death.

The rules for all these matters and the conditions under which every single one of these actions should be allowed or prohibited have already been given and explained and proof has been given for the reasons behind them. Understanding all this from books is very easy for everyone who is in full possession of his faculties, but applying it in an individual case is very difficult for a conscientious scholar. But, for those who are ignorant of the principles of this art and for those who are reckless with this art, nothing seems difficult and they do not see that there are diseases that require consideration.

(IV.10) In one of his aphorisms, al-Rāzī has said: Medicine is a studied art and is subject to claim by the riff-raff; however, how difficult is its attainment for the skillful physician.

(IV.11) Says the author: Concerning the matter discussed by al-Rāzī in this aphorism, Galen has remarked many times in his books that the crafty find this art easy and insignificant, while Hippocrates finds it difficult and time-consuming. But do not think, dear reader, when you consider my words that this is unique to medicine. If you look into the natural sciences, or the conventional ones, or the ones on the religious law, you find the same. The more accomplished a person is in that science, the more precise his investigation becomes; doubts and difficult questions arise in him; he becomes deliberate in his investigation and hesitant in some of his answers. The less a person knows, the more he considers all that which is difficult to be easy and holds all that which is distant to be near. Such a person makes many nonsensical and pretentious remarks and gives prompt nonsensical answers to that which he does not understand. But let me return to my subject and reiterate what I said about the ease with which the medical art is understood by those who have a good intellect, and about the difficulty they have in practicing it, which has already been mentioned by Galen in a statement with the following words.

(IV.12) Galen said: Therefore, it is easy to say that it is correct to rub the elderly in the morning with oil and massage them, but to do this properly is a most difficult thing. [*De sanitate tuenda* V.4].

(IV.13) Says the author: Consider, O possessors of fair judgement, if the procedure of rubbing with oil and massage is, according to Galen, one of the most difficult things to put into practice—that is to say, its practical individual application—and likewise the drinking of water or abstention therefrom, as we explained, how much more so is this the case for bloodletting; for evacuation by means of pulp of colocynth, juice of the squirting cucumber, and the two hellebores (black and white false hellebore); for the enemas with castoreum and opopanax; for cautery, lancing and cutting! Are all these procedures really easy for a physician, or difficult?

(IV.14) Ibn Zuhr has said in one of his extant and well-known books: I have never administered a purgative without thinking about it for days before and after. [*Kitāb al-Tadhkira*].

(IV.15) The attitude of all men regarding coitus is known. That is that no one desires it in order to preserve his health or to have progeny, but merely for pleasure. For this reason, they try to satisfy their desire at all times and at every opportunity. There is clear evidence for those who know that sexual intercourse is harmful for all men except for a few individuals whose temperament demands it to a degree that a little bit of it does no harm. But men differ only in the degree of harm, some among them are greatly harmed by it, while others are only harmed a little. Its harm to young men who have a moist temperament is only little, while the harm it does to the old, the convalescent, and to anyone with a dry temperament is very great. We have seen among the convalescents those who copulated and died the very same day, while others suffered from syncope and recurrent fever, and died after a few days. In general, sexual intercourse is life-threatening for the sick and convalescent and very harmful for the elderly and for every one with a dry temperament. No one should have sexual intercourse before the food is digested in the stomach, nor when he is hungry or thirsty, nor in a state of drunkenness, nor after leaving the bath, nor after physical exercise or before it, nor for one day before bloodletting or for one day thereafter. Whoever wishes to remain healthy should turn his thoughts away from coitus as much as he can.

(IV.16) The benefits of wine are very many when taken properly, for then it is a major factor in the preservation of health, and in the cure of many diseases. However, it is well known how people in general consume wine. That is, they only intend to get drunk, yet drunkenness is harmful to all people. He is wrong who thinks that getting drunk once a month is beneficial, for drunkenness is an indigestion that pervades the whole body and especially the brain. The small amount that is beneficial should be taken once the food has left the stomach. Children should not drink it because it is very harmful to them, because it destroys their body and soul. Galen has said that the young should not consume any of it, except after three sabbaths, that is, twenty-one years. [*De sanitate tuenda* V.5; *Quod animi mores corporis temperamenta sequantur* 10]. The more one is advanced in years, the more beneficial wine becomes for him. Those who need it most are the old.

(IV.17) Going to the bathhouse is greatly needed in the regimen of health and in the healing of diseases. The physicians prescribe going to the bathhouse in the case of illness according to the different types of illnesses, according to the seasons, and according to the different ages. As for the regimen of health they said that it is proper to go to the bathhouse every ten days. [*Kitāb al-Taysīr fī l-mudāwāt wa-l-tadbīr*]. The physicians have mentioned that frequenting the bathhouse every day putrefies the humors. This statement is correct for someone who stays in the bathhouse for such a long time that he sweats profusely. But if someone enters the bathhouse and does not stay there for a long time, but washes and leaves, it is beneficial even if he does so every day, and especially for the elderly and for those with a dry temperament. No one should go to the bathhouse before the food has left his stomach. But if one enters when the stomach is empty and before feeling hungry, it is good for all people, but after feeling hungry it is not proper to enter except for someone who wishes to make his body lean. The description of its usage is that he should first sweat and wipe his sweat with a clean linen cloth. As the sweat flows, he should wipe it until the cloth, with which he wipes himself, becomes soaked. Then he should clean the skin and after this he should have a massage and wash with hot water that does not cause horripilation of the skin. Then he should diminish the heat little by little until he finally washes himself with lukewarm water that is almost cold, but not so cold that it causes horripilation of the skin. Then he should descend into the bathing basin, the water of which should be the same. But he, who wishes to make his body lean, should use hot water and descend into water that is as hot as he can bear.

(IV.18) As for the head, one should never wash it with cold water or with lukewarm water, but with water that is so hot that it nearly burns the skin of the head. For even though cold water strengthens the brain, it retains and cools its superfluities and cools the brain itself. Consequently, all the nerves are cooled, since the brain is their origin, and all movements become difficult. Sometimes, this may cause hemiplegia, or paralysis of the facial nerve, or sudden spasms; therefore, one should be very cautious about this. Similarly, tepid water adds coldness and softness to the brain, so that all the movements and senses are weakened. But very hot water strengthens the substance of the brain, expels its superfluities, and improves its temperament, so that all the movements and senses are strengthened.

(IV.19) One should go to sleep after leaving the bath. Galen said: For cocting what can be cocted and for dissolving what can be dissolved, I deem nothing better than sleep after leaving the bath. [*De sanitate tuenda* IV.4]. But sleep in the bathhouse is very bad. Sometimes it produces syncope because of the conflict resulting between the sleep and the heat of the bath. Because the heat of the bath attracts the innate heat to the external surface of the body, while sleep requires the heat to sink deep into the body.

(IV.20) One should be very careful not to drink cold water after leaving the bath. Galen has mentioned people who drank cold water after leaving the bath and whose kidneys were consequently chilled immediately and they suffered from dropsy. [*De locis affectis* V.7]. Therefore, a person should endure thirst until his body cools and the heat that the organs acquired from the bath dissipates. Then he can drink water. If he cannot bear to wait because of his severe thirst, he should mix the water with syrup of *utrujj* (citron or lemon) peel or mastic syrup or syrup of rose buds, and then drink it. Similarly, drinking a brew prepared with pomegranate seeds and sugar spiced with musk, agarwood, and clove after the bath is not harmful. And if he waits after the bath until the heat of the bath disappears from the body, and then takes it, it is beneficial, that is, that brew or the other drinks mentioned before.

(IV.21) People often neglect catarrhs because they do not know what may result from them. What results from them in most cases is either a rheum when it descends to the nose, or hoarseness and cough if it descends to the trachea. [*Airs, Waters, Places*; *De symptomatum causis* I.11]. My advice is to be careful and to be on one's guard for catarrhs in the winter and in the summer, and to wear one's clothes when sweating inside the bathhouse, and to always protect the head from the intense cold which causes catarrhs, and, similarly, from the intense heat, because the heat melts the coagulated superfluities in the brain, so that they descend; these are the hot catarrhs.

(IV.22) All catarrhs, hot and cold, often stream into the cavities of the lungs and fill them all at once, because of the abundance of the descending humor and the weakness of the receiving organ. The expulsive power is too weak to expel that humor through coughing, so that the patient suffocates and dies or suffers from the illness of orthopnea. Sometimes they descend to the cavity of the stomach and cause lientery; this is a disease that is hard to cure. At other times they descend to one of the joints and cause arthritis. They may also descend to the substance of the internal organs, to their cavities, and cause a swelling in those organs, pleurisy, pneumonia, swelling of the liver, swelling of the stomach, or of the other organs. Therefore, one should beware of catarrhs.

(IV.23) Guarding against catarrhs means to beware of heating or cooling the head excessively, as we have mentioned, to avoid eating that which fills the head, such as the different kinds of milk and inflating seeds such as broad beans and Indian pea, not to go to sleep immediately after a meal, especially at night, not to consume intoxicating drinks in a quantity that alters the mind even slightly, and to strengthen the substance of the brain by smelling aromatic plants and spices according to the temperament and season. Among the prescriptions with specific properties for strengthening the brain is the following: Pulverize clove as fine as dust and put it on the parting of the hair during the entire winter. Similarly, anointing the brain with spiced ben oil during the winter strengthens it. But at the time of intense heat, one should perfume the head with water of roses and dog roses, and sprinkle on the head some mace that has been thoroughly pulverized.

(IV.24) It is not proper for anyone in any place or at any time to consume food that has begun to spoil—even when it is minimal—, or water that is turbid, altered in odor, or lukewarm, or anything putrid like *kawāmikh*, *ṣīr*, *ṣaḥna*, *khilāṭ*, and the like. Because these are the substances that give rise to fevers and they are like poisons. The eminent physicians have warned against the consumption of food left overnight, or meat left overnight, because the putrefaction has already begun even though it is not apparent to the senses. [*Kitāb al-Taysīr fī l-mudāwāt wa-l-tadbīr*]

(IV.25) One should endeavor to take sweet foods, for the sweet is what nourishes, as Galen has mentioned. [*De simplicium medicamentorum temperamentis ac facultatibus* IV.15]. Similarly, one should drink water that is the sweetest, clearest, and coolest. If one dislikes sweet foods, one should temper their sweet taste with a little of the sour or with that which has a clear salty or astringent taste, such as a dish cooked in juice of unripe, sour grapes, vinegar, lemon, barley gruel, tanner's sumach, quinces, or pomegranate seeds. These foods, though they are not really sweet and only have little nutritious value, are nevertheless beneficial. First, they are not loathsome. Then, some of them dissolve the phlegm in the stomach and whet the appetite, such as a dish cooked with barley gruel. Some of them resist putrefaction and have a cleansing effect, such as dishes to which vinegar and lemon juice have been added. And some of them strengthen the stomach and its cardia, such as dishes cooked in tanner's sumach, pomegranate seeds, quinces, and the juice of unripe, sour grapes. One should rely on these foods as much as possible.

(IV.26) Habit is fundamental for the preservation of health and the cure of diseases. No one should give up his healthy habits all at once, neither in eating, drinking, sexual intercourse, going to the bathhouse, nor in exercise. In all these activities one should observe one's habits, even if the thing one is accustomed to is contrary to the medical rules. One should not abandon it for what is required by these rules, except gradually and over a long time, so that one does not notice the change. If someone changes his habit in any of these all at once he will perforce fall sick. As for sick people, they should not change their habit in any way, that is to say, that one should not even start at the time of illness to change one's habit, even for the better.

(IV.27) It is known that there are animals whose meat has a temperament that is very contrary to the nourishment of human beings, such as the meat of wolves and foxes, while there are other animals whose meat is very suitable, such as mutton. The same rule applies to the hair of animals used for for clothing. Because the most suitable for human beings are clothes [made] from lambskin, and the most harmful for them are clothes made from the fur of foxes. The skillful physicians have stated so and it is the truth. In this regard, this Servant has observed that the garment, which is called *qarṭāsī*, is objectionable. The fur of the squirrel has been praised by the physicians. They also stated that wearing furs from the skins of cats causes illness, just as smelling their breath. [*Kitāb al-Taysīr fī l-mudāwāt wa-l-tadbīr*]. Therefore, they recommend to keep away from them and the smell of their breath, just as they recommend to smell the breath of pigeons and to keep them in the house. Because this, they said, protects against all diseases of the nerves, that is, hemiplegia, paralysis of the facial nerve, spasms, tremor, and the like. Whoever keeps pigeons is safe from all these illnesses, on the condition that he bewares of their excrement and does not leave it to accumulate in any way, because it putrefies the air and corrupts it. Similarly, the consumption of young full-fledged pigeons cures diseases of the nerves.

(IV.28) The best of game meat is the gazelle; similarly, the hare. It has virtues that have been verified by experience, that is, eating its brain is beneficial for tremor, and in the same way its flesh in general is good for tremor and diseases of the nerves. The fur of hares heats greatly and is beneficial for diseases of the nerves, especially in old people. The wild ass has a great specific property in strengthening vision; this has been verified by experience. The consumption of its flesh and holding one's eyes over the vapor of its cooking meat strengthens vision and opens obstructions of the hollow nerves, and if one looks into the eyes of the wild ass for a long time, it strengthens vision and removes its defects. This has been verified by experience. [*Kitāb al-Taysīr fī l-mudāwāt wa-l-tadbīr*].

This is the measure of what the Servant has now presented, of what our Master—may God give that his rule lasts forever until all times—needs. May God—He is exalted—lengthen the days of my Master and give him everlasting health and may He—He is exalted—grant him the ultimate happiness in both worlds, as he, with his noble character and generosity, has benefitted servants and subjects through his benevolence and munificence.

Praise be to God, Lord of the two worlds.

BOOK 8

On the Elucidation of Some Symptoms and the Response to Them (Formerly Known as *On the Causes of Symptoms*)

First published in:

Maimonides
On the Elucidation of Some Symptoms and the Response to Them
(Formerly Known as *On the Causes of Symptoms*)

A New Parallel Arabic-English Edition and Translation
with Critical Editions of the Medieval Hebrew Translations
by Gerrit Bos.

Leiden (Brill) 2019
MWMM 13

∴

In the Name of God,
the Merciful the Compassionate

(0) A letter has come to this minor Servant, which contains a detailed statement of all those afflictions that have occurred to my Master—may God perpetuate his days—along with an explanation of the causes of all those afflictions and the times of their occurrence, information about every particular one, which the physician has to inquire about, and a description of his reflections at each time upon every affliction. He has also written down in it what the physicians advised that should be done, and wherein they agreed or disagreed.

This minor Servant knows for certain that this letter was dictated by our Master, without any doubt, and this Servant swears by God—Who is exalted—that eminent physicians in our time lack the knowledge necessary for systematizing such complaints, let alone explaining and organizing them in such a fashion. Therefore, this minor Servant deems it proper to answer him who holds him in bondage—may God perpetuate his shadow—in the words of one physician to another, not in the words of a physician to someone who does not belong

 | DOI:10.1163/9789004498884_010

to those who practice this art, since it is clear to this Servant that the knowledge of my Master about those afflictions and their causes is perfect. And as this Servant knows about those afflictions, which are now firmly established, the removal of what is to be desired, and as our Master has mentioned to his minor Servant what advice was given by every physician and has ordered him to commend upon the statement of each of them, he will follow his command and say the following.

(1) As to the statement by the physician who said that those afflictions now present would disappear if the blood would flow now from the openings of the vessels as it has already done at times: it is true, without any doubt. This is so because the blood flowing out is only the turbid part of the blood and its sediment, and nature expels it because of its badness in the form of a crisis. As to the physician who advised to open the openings of the vessels by means of water in which one sits, or cataplasms on which one sits, he is mistaken. This Servant does not agree with it in any way for a number of reasons that he will explain. First, because those things, which are applied below or in the water in which one sits, are hot and may heat the temperament and burn the humors. Second, when nature opens these vessels, she opens them in the required measure. But if we open them ourselves with medications, they may open more than they should and the flow of blood becomes excessive and is difficult to stop. This may also happen with someone whose blood flows by itself, namely, that it becomes so excessive that it cannot be stopped. Third, if these vessels open by themselves, what comes out of them is mostly what should come out, because nature has driven it to the farthermost parts and the expulsive faculty has moved to expel it. But if we open them ourselves, something may come out that should not come out. And if something comes out, it is mostly part of that which should not come out. In general, we do not resort to such an action unless those places are swollen and they have become very painful. Then we resort to opening them with medications so that the blood that was dispelled there and that caused those places to swell flows out. Our action at that time is similar to the action of someone who lances a tumor when nature cannot open that which overlies the tumor and expels what is in it. However, our Master should not do this at all. But if the blood comes out by itself, as it has flowed out several times, it should not be stopped at all, unless it is excessive, God forbid.

(2) Our Master then mentioned that some physicians advised him to take some wine with borage juice a few hours after the meal and when he goes to bed so that he may have a deep sleep, but that other physicians gave him the opposite advice saying that there is no reason to use it, since the unmixed wine heats

the temperament, while the mixed wine generates winds and flatulence. As this Servant sees it, the first view is the correct one; that is, if the food has begun to be digested, a little bit of wine, namely, a Syrian ounce or the like, helps the digestion and the discharge of superfluities through stimulating micturition and removes the smoky vapors from the blood, which produce all the afflictions that occur presently, especially if the wine is mixed with borage juice. If borage itself is steeped in it, in a measure of two *dirhams* per ounce, it is most effective and its dilation of the soul is greater. When the physicians speak of the beverage that exhilarates generally, they especially mean by that the syrup of borage. If borage is put in wine, it increases its dilating and exhilarating effect on the soul. Drinking wine moistens the body with a good moisture. Galen has mentioned this in his *De sanitate tuenda* [1.11]. But if someone believes that it heats, he is mistaken, for wine is a food not a medicine. It is a very good food and the good foods neither heat nor cool, but medicines heat and cool. Indeed, it produces wholesome blood, of the nature of natural blood, which is hot and moist.

As for mixing wine, there is no doubt that this generates winds. Sometimes it generates tremor. Nevertheless, Ibn Zuhr, who was unique in his generation and one of the greatest observers, mentioned that the mixture has this effect if it is mixed and drunk immediately. However, if one mixes it and leaves it for twelve hours or more and then drinks it, it is very good, because the wine part prevails over the watery part, transforms it and improves its temperament. This Servant recommends that what ought to be used of the borage are the barks of its roots, not its leaves as the people of Syria-Palestine and Egypt do. So too, we observed, was the practice of all the eminent Elders (senior physicians) in the land of al-Andalus. And all the Arab physicians prescribe the bark of its roots, not the leaves. Our Master should have this herb always with him because it has the specific property of dilating the soul, effacing the black bile and eradicating its traces. This Servant has tried and verified as true, without any doubt, that light wine, when mixed with a little rose water, about a tenth, dilates the soul, does not intoxicate, does not harm the brain, strengthens the stomach, and increases all the virtues ascribed to wine. Therefore, this Servant advises that one add ten *dirhams* of rose water and twenty *dirhams* of borage juice to one Syrian ounce of wine. It should be set aside for about ten hours and then it should be taken. As for taking it also at bedtime, this is an excellent idea from various viewpoints; it gives a deep sleep, eliminates evil thoughts, improves the digestion, and repels the superfluities.

(3) When the physicians agreed that the temperament of our Master tends towards heat and that he should take that which cools and moistens, they were

correct stating so, but their statement is too general and should be put forth in greater detail and should mention the specific regimen. As to one of the physicians who advised to drink *hindibā'* (endive or chicory) juice with sandalwood syrup, and the infusion of tamarind, plums, and common jujube, it seems to this Servant that this is a grave error, because as phlegm is dominant in your basic temperament, such absolute cooling ingredients are not at all appropriate, especially the plums and jujubes. Because such a regimen weakens the stomach, causes severe harm, and shortens the digestions, and when the stomach is moistened and weakened, the three digestions are corrupted. Such a regimen is only beneficial for someone who is dominated by yellow bile. But that physician has not mentioned anything that indicates a dominance of yellow bile at all. Rather, the implication of all the symptoms mentioned is the generation of black vapors caused by the black bile originating from the burning of phlegm that recurs periodically.

(4) As for the physician who advised to drink an infusion of rhubarb in *hindibā'* (endive or chicory) juice one day and its omission for two days, if he intended by that to soften the stools, then he is correct. This Servant has mentioned a prescription for softening the stools with rhubarb in the third chapter of his treatise that was presented in an audience granted by our Master.

(5) As for the physician who advised bathing every three days, exercising every day, and anointing with oil of violets, all this is correct. This Servant will speak about this in greater detail and with a proper evaluation.

(6) As for the physician who advised to place cloths with sandalwood upon the liver, and similarly he who advised to eat the smaller variety of cucumber, cultivated lettuce, regular cucumber, common purslane, spinach, and garden orach; all this is absolutely wrong, for this is a regimen that suits those who suffer from extremely inflaming ardent fevers, when these occur to those who have a hot temperament during the summer. And still worse than this is the error of the physician who advised drinking fresh milk, because he has perceived the matter of its moistening effect, but overlooked its quick transformation into any humor whatsoever, and did not consider the substance that caused the illness, namely, the inflamed phlegm.

(7) He who advised to use oxymel of quinces one hour after the meal is correct; it is a good regimen that improves the digestions. But adding juice of barberry to such a beverage after the meal is an uncommon regimen not in accord with the syllogistic reasoning, which is customary in medicine, that is, taking bar-

berry juice while the food is still in the stomach. Even when the stomach is empty, the juice should not be introduced in this disease.

(8) Whoever advised drinking the exhilarating drink of Ibn al-Tilmīdh [*Al-Aqrābādhīn al-kabīr*] or someone else, and similarly he who advised syrup of common sorrel, apples, borage juice, *rayḥān* (myrtle or basil) seed, and lemon balm seed, all this is correct. However, the addition of fleawort seed is not regarded by this Servant as correct, because I do not think that extreme cooling is a good thing in the case of this disease and temperament.

(9) The suggestion by one physician to take barley gruel, opium poppy and cucurbit seed is strange, as he mentioned that the sleep of my Master is balanced (healthy). To him, the moistening effect of the barley gruel is so insufficient that he supported it with seed of cucurbits. Even stranger than this is the suggestion of the one who advised taking plums after the barley gruel. I do not think that for these physicians there is any organ of the body lower than the stomach, and that they do not take into consideration whether the stomach is weakened or not, and whether there is moisture in it or not. Perhaps they do acknowledge the eminence of the stomach and its general usefulness, and that one should always look after it, for which reason the most eminent physicians have devoted treatises to it. Nevertheless, according to them, this regimen strengthens the stomach, improves its digestion, dries its moisture, cuts the viscosity of the phlegm, which evidently never stops to accumulate in it, and thins its thickness. With this regimen, I mean the aforementioned regimen prescribed by one of them, namely, barley gruel with cucurbit seed and opium poppy, and plums for dessert. This Servant denounced in this section what ought to be denounced so that my Master will be extremely careful, and will not feel any need whatsoever to follow any of their statements.

(10) The consumption of apples and quinces, and sucking pomegranate seeds after the meal are recommended for everyone as part of the regimen of health. There is nothing superfluous in it in relation to this disease, except what was mentioned regarding taking coriander after the meal. This is truly ridiculous, as it was proposed because coriander thickens the vapors and prevents them from ascending, which is right, but it should be taken as part of medicines such as powders and the like, or cooked with the food. As to taking coriander alone after the meal, if it does not cause vomiting, it undoubtedly causes nausea and corrupts the food. Occasionally taking common purslane seed with sugar apart from the meal is good. Even if it is taken with the meal, it would not harm its cooling and strengthening effect on the heart.

(11) Our Master has mentioned that the physicians advised to take apricots, pears, and quinces after the meal, and grapes, *biṭṭīkh* (common melons or watermelons), and pomegranates before it. This Servant does not understand the meaning of this advice. If there is need to induce appetite or a habit of taking fruits, and thus one should take before the meal what softens the stools and after the meal those fruits in which there is astringency, such as pear, quince, and apple, then the intent is correct. But if they advised that taking these fruits is beneficial for this disease, this is an error, for all the fresh fruits are bad for everyone—healthy or sick—if they are taken as foods, especially melons and apricots, because they are rapidly transformed into whatever bad humor there is in the body. Peaches are also very bad and are the substance of bad malignant fevers. Galen mentioned, that from the time he stopped eating all fresh fruits, he never had a fever to the end of his life. [*De sanitate tuenda* V; *De bonis malisque sucis* I]. He told his story into detail as an admonition to the people, as expressed in his treatise. Therefore, our Master should avoid fresh fruits all he can.

(12) The physician who advised against the use of game meat, cured (jerked) meat, eggplant, and everything that heats the body is right, because all these increase the afflictions of which our Master has complained. He who advised exercising every day gave most appropriate advice. Likewise, he who forbade travelling to hot countries gave good advice with his suggestion. He who assumed that hot countries dissolve the vapors, is only correct with regard to those vapors that ascend to the surface of the body if they are cold and moist. As for the vapors that arise from thick turbid blood, those countries increase the thickness of the blood and roast it and increase its vapors. When health is reestablished—God willing—our Master may travel wherever he wishes until God fulfills his expectations in both worlds.

(13) This Servant does not approve of evacuation with lapis lazuli nor with the Armenian stone; with lapis lazuli because of its vehemence, and with the Armenian stone because its color is unknown, and because the eminent physicians have doubts regarding it, most of them believing that it is not the stone that is designated with this name. This Servant also approves of the opinion of the physician who forbids to apply strong purgatives and to restrict oneself to rhubarb or whey or senna of Mecca and the like; all of this is correct. This Servant does not approve of the infusion of peaches or *biṭṭīkh* (common melon or watermelon) juice, because of their harm to the stomach. The afflictions he complained of do not involve burning heat or thirst. He also does not approve of the excessive use of *nīlūfar* (blue Egyptian, European white, or yellow water

lily) because it thickens the blood and loosens the stomach. This is only good for those who suffer from acute, burning fevers, as this Servant has mentioned. This Servant does also not approve of the use of a decoction of dodder because of its distressing and drying effect. If one steeps dodder in one hundred *dirham*s of whey and takes this twice or three times in the springtime and once or twice in autumn, it is good, but there should be fifteen days between one time and the other. The dodder should be pounded in almond oil, wrapped in a finely woven piece of cloth, and then steeped for one night in the whey.

(14) Our Master mentioned that once he had a vessel opened and there came out blood as thick as that of the spleen, and because of this the physicians advised additional bloodletting. As for the overfilling that manifests itself from time to time, it undoubtedly requires bloodletting, and the blood should be withdrawn proportionally. One should constantly strive for the clarification of the blood and the equilibration of the temperament of the liver so that it produces good blood. This Servant has explained in his previous treatise how this can be done through the syrups that he has compounded.

(15) He who suggested that the nourishment should consist of peach and tamarind with kid is correct for the summertime. But one should not neglect to add cinnamon, mastic, spikenard, and the like to these dishes so that they do not harm the stomach. The same applies to the consumption of cooling boiled vegetables, which they recommended in the summertime, for they are wholesome, provided that one does not take too much of them. They should not be taken deliberately, because the intention of this Servant is the equilibration of the temperament, not an increase in cooling, for the basic cause of his afflictions is the burning of the phlegm.

(16) He who recommended the exhilarating drink and the electuary in which there are jacinth (red zircon), emerald, gold, and silver; all this is correct and useful, because these are cardiac medicaments that are beneficial through their specific property, that is, their specific form which is the whole of their essence, and not through their sheer quality.

(17) Our Master has mentioned his frequent use of borage and *nīlūfar* (blue Egyptian, European white, or yellow water lily), without, however, eliminating the root (cause) of the disease. The reason for their little effect is that they have been used continuously. Similarly, the remedies that are extremely powerful, if one uses them continuously—nature gets used to them, and she is not at all affected by them, and they turn into nourishment or the like of nourishment.

Galen has mentioned this. [*De antidotis* 1.1]. This is all the more so if these are weak remedies that are close to being nutriments. For if these are taken continuously for a week, their medicinal actions are abolished and not a trace of them appears thereafter. Therefore, one should change from one remedy to another, omitting one remedy for a few days and then returning to it.

(18) Our Master has mentioned a reduction in coitus from what was customary; what a good action is this and what a great benefit comes from this reduction. Going to the bathhouse, on the other hand, should never be neglected, whether during an attack of fever or during abatements. It is wholly a blessing that sleep is regular, and a clear proof that these melancholic vapors have not hurt the brain or changed its temperament, although they are especially harmful for the heart. As to what our Master has mentioned regarding the presence of weakness after exercise, the cause of this is its omission and remission. If he resumes it gradually, little by little, he will find, following it, the strength and the vitality that should be found after all exercise that is carried out properly.

(19) As this minor Servant has responded to all the sections of that noble letter, as commanded, he will now compile a concise statement in one chapter in which he will explain what the regimen of our Master should be, according to the symptoms that can be found at the moment. This might well have been made obvious by what this Servant has mentioned in these sections and by what he mentioned in that treatise, but these were statements that were dispersed and not properly organized. But before I start with this section, I would like to say that there should be two electuaries in the treasury of our Master, in addition to those syrups and the great *iṭrīfal*, which this Servant mentioned in the third chapter of his previous treatise.

(20) One of these is the cool musk remedy which the elder (senior) experienced physicians have tested and found it to have such an extraordinary action that they do not permit to substitute it with anything else or to prescribe its individual ingredients separately. [*Kitāb al-Aghdhiya* (*Book on Foodstuffs*)]. Rather, some among them presented it as an electuary. It is the remedy composed by al-Rāzī in his book [*Manāfiʿ al-aghdhiya wa-dafʿ maḍārriha* (*The Benefits of Nutrients and the Repulsion of their Harmful Effects*)]. And this is its composition in his own words: Take one part each of pounded roses, tabasheer (a white substance obtained from the nodal joints of bamboo), dry coriander, and amber, half a part of small pearls, one sixth of a part of good and pure musk. Then take some crystalline sugar and dissolve it in sour, pressed, and sieved apple juice and cook this until it attains the consistency of honey. Then

throw *utrujj* (citron or lemon) leaves therein and knead the mentioned ingredients in it. Someone suffering from this affliction should take this remedy frequently because it is an excellent remedy for strengthening the heart without heating, and it is beneficial for palpitation and throbbing of the heart with heat.

(21) The second remedy is the jacinth electuary composed by Ibn Sīnā in his famous treatise *Fī aḥkām al-adwiya al-qalbīya* (*On Cardiac Remedies*); he mentioned three recipes for it, the first cold, the second hot, and the third temperate. The one that this Servant considers appropriate to use for our Master is the temperate one, and this is the description of the third in his own words. He said: There is another excellent compound that I have tried as an electuary and as pastilles and I added to it and deduced from it according to the individual temperament of the patient. It is very good for strengthening the heart. These are its basic ingredients: one and a half *dirham* each of pearl, amber, and coral; one *mithqāl* and a *dāniq* each of crushed silk, and burnt river crabs; five *dirhams* of borage; two *dāniqs* of gold filings; three *dirhams* each of seeds of *faranjamushk* (possibly wild basil), *bādharūj* (sweet basil), and lemon balm; one *mithqāl* each of red behen (possibly Mediterranean sea lavender), white behen, Indian agarwood, Armenian stone, washed lapis lazuli, mastic, Chinese cinnamon, cinnamon, saffron, common cardamom, large cardamom (black cardamom), and cubeb; two and a half *dirhams* of dodder; three *dirhams* of French lavender; one *mithqāl* of zedoary, and if it is not available, then instead of it two *mithqāls* of bitter ginger; two *mithqāls* of great false leopardbane; five *dirhams* of *hindibā'* (endive or chicory) seed; four *dirhams* of cucumber seed; ten *dirhams* of manna; four *dirhams* of red roses; two *mithqāls* of musk; one *mithqāl* of camphor, one *mithqāl* of ambergris; two *dirhams* each of spikenard, and Indian malabathrum. These are its essential and basic ingredients. They can be made into pastilles or combined with honey; both of them can be prepared to suit a patient with a moderate temperament, but one should not change anything of it. It can also be prepared for someone with a hot bad temperament (dyscrasia) or for someone with a cold bad temperament (dyscrasia). As for the moderate temperament, it should be left as it is. When one makes it into pastilles, each pastille should be of one *mithqāl*. The whole should be kneaded with three equal parts of honey. If one wants it to be fermented and then to be used, one should throw five *dirhams* of opium into it, and the same amount of pulverized castoreum. It should not be used except after at least six months, that is, if one adds the opium and castoreum to it.

(22) For someone who is dominated by a hot bad temperament (dyscrasia), one should restrict the saffron and musk, which one puts into it, to half a *mithqāl*, omit the dodder and put instead of it five *dirhams* of common fumitory and four *dirhams* of senna of Mecca into it. One should throw in it ten *dirhams* of roses, eight *dirhams* of common purslane seed, five *dirhams* of tabasheer, two *dirhams* of asphodel seed, and three *dirhams* of sandalwood. The other ingredients should stay as they are. It should be made into pastilles and kneaded with honey, thoroughly skimmed of its foam.

(23) For someone who is dominated by a cold bad temperament (dyscrasia), add to the remedies above one *dirham* each of nutmeg rind, *utrujj* (citron or lemon) peel, balsam wood, ginger, and black pepper; and two *mithqāls* of castoreum; the camphor should be restricted to half a *mithqāl*. Whoever has a hot temperament should proceed to take half a draught of this with one *mithqāl* of tabasheer in apple rob. If someone has a cold temperament, he should take a draught of it with two *ṭassūj* of castoreum.

(24) I have treated some of those who follow the same course as kings for severe melancholy, which tends towards mania, that is wild frenzy with this remedy, and added to the temperate recipe one *dirham* of thoroughly pulverized jacinth of exquisite pomegranate color, and they benefited greatly from it after despair.

(25) As to the compound specific for those who have a hot temperament and are attacked by palpitation and weakness of the heart because of their hot bad temperament (dyscrasia), there is a compound with the following composition: five *dirhams* each of cultivated lettuce seed, seeds of the *biṭṭīkh* (common melon or watermelon), *qarʿ* (field pumpkin or winter squash) seed, peeled cucumber seed; four *dirhams* of common purslane seed; one *mithqāl* each of pearl, amber, coral, burnt river crabs, and crushed silk; one *mithqāl* of the thickened juice of frankincense, and if that is not available, three *mithqāls* of the wood of frankincense; two *dirhams* each of Indian agarwood, great false leopardbane, bitter ginger, and white behen; three *dirhams* each of tabasheer and common cardamom; seven *dirhams* of red stalkless roses, dried in the shade; half a *mithqāl* of saffron; pulverized camphor with a tenth of its weight of thoroughly pulverized musk, and a sixth of ambergris, one and a half *mithqāl* of the whole; five *mithqāls* of borage. All of this should be made into pastilles, as we have explained, and kneaded with rob of apple, rob of quince, or rob of pomegranate in parts equal to the quantity in which it is kneaded.

(26) There is also a julep of the above; it should be prepared with borage juice or an equal quantity of *hindibā'* (endive or chicory) juice, a fourfold quantity of apple juice, twice the whole of rose water, and one sixth of the whole of crystalline sugar; it should be cooked gently until thickened. The julep that is prepared with leaves of *badharanjūya* and cooked in rose water until it takes on its power, or with juice of *badharanjūya* put into rose water, one third to two thirds, is beneficial to all those who have a weakness of the heart, especially if it contains borage, which, if dry, should be cooked with it in rose water, and if fresh, should be mixed with its juice. If the temperament is extremely hot, reduce the juice of *badharanjūya* and increase the borage juice; if not, both should be taken in equal quantities.

(27) I should also mention a number of foods that one should regularly consume. The first is bread. One should be concerned about the quality of the flour, and not make it from white flour (*ḥuwwārā*); by that I mean that it should not be immersed in water as the custom goes, and it should not be sifted so thoroughly that nothing of the bran remains. It should be kneaded extremely well and it should be clearly salted and clearly raised. The loaves should be free of crumbs, and it should be baked in the circular earthen oven, excavated in the ground (*tannūr*), or in a baking oven (*furn*); the earthen oven is the best.

(28) The meat: One should always intend that the meat that one eats is that of chickens or young chickens and one should always drink their broth, for this kind of bird has the specific property of improving the corrupt humors, whatever the corruption may be, and especially the melancholic humors, so much so that the physicians have mentioned that chicken broth is beneficial for elephantiasis. Of this species, one should neither take the too old, which has attained two years, nor the too young, in which mucus is predominant; neither the too lean, nor those that have been force-fed, but rather those that are fat by nature and not stall-fed. The manner of their management is the following: The chickens and young chickens that are ready to fly should be let loose in a spacious chicken coop in which there is no dunghill or dirt and which should be tended with cleanliness and constant sweeping. The food that they eat, should be given to them in the beginning of the day in vessels; it should be barley meal kneaded in fresh milk, and if dried figs are chopped and mixed with it, it is even better. Food should be given to them only in an amount that fills their crops. Water should be given to them. After some hours, one should scatter before them wheat that has been soaked in water for hours. At the end of the day, one should give them once again barley meal and chopped figs kneaded with milk. In chickens and young chickens thus managed, one finds the white and deli-

cious suet, which is cocted very quickly and greatly moistens the temperament and brings it into balance. These things have been verified and their usefulness is clear. If one is fed up with the constant consumption of one and the same variety, there is no harm in taking francolin or *ṭayhūj* on some days. As for the turtle dove, there is dryness in it, although it has the wonderful specific property of sharpening the mind. Similarly, I do not recommend partridge, because it causes constipation. If the spirit craves for meat of land animals, it should be that of a suckling kid. If sometimes mutton cannot be avoided, one should take lamb that is not yet one year old, but is close to it. One should especially take the front part of the meat; it should not be exceedingly fat, but from grazing animals. One should not take anything of these, unless one is fed up with chickens and young chickens.

(29) Wine: One should provide oneself with the white colored one, as far as possible. It should be fine in consistency and good in taste. If there is a little astringency in it, it is not harmful, providing it has a good aroma and is one year old or approximately so. One should beware of wine that is deep red, or of a thick consistency, or of altered aroma, or old and very bitter. One should not approach any of these kinds at all.

(30) Dishes: One should always intend that the dishes are sweet in taste and that they contain little sourness or nothing sour at all. I will mention a number of dishes so that our Master may select from them according to the different times of the year, since our Master knows the powers of most of these foods and a physician is always at hand to assist in this matter. The first of these is chickens or young chickens, boiled or stewed or steamed, or cooked with fresh coriander or with some fresh fennel cast into the water in which it is cooked. These dishes are appropriate for the wintertime. Those cooked in water to which lemon juice, or the acidic inner part of the *utrujj* (citron or lemon), or compounded lemon is added, are suitable in the summertime. Those prepared with almonds, sugar, lemon juice, and wine are suitable at any time of the year. Those prepared with raisins, almonds, and a little bit of vinegar are good at any time of the year. Those prepared with *isfīdabāj*, chard, or cultivated lettuce, or those prepared with cucurbit, or spinach, or purple amaranth, or plums, which the people of Syria-Palestine call *khawkh* (peach), are all good in the summer. But it is absolutely necessary to spice them with Chinese cinnamon bark, mastic and spikenard to prevent them from harming the stomach. Also good are those dishes prepared with tamarind and sugar, and those prepared with common purslane seed and sugar, but they should not be used except in the summer. Also good are those prepared with rose preserves, but they are better in the

winter. Also beneficial are those prepared with pistachio nut and sugar, but they should have a little bit of lemon juice added to it.

(31) A dish eaten in cold weather should not be free from the good wine described above. The meat should be roasted in it if it is a cooked dish, or it should be added to the boiled food, if it is a boiled dish. Likewise, when the weather is hot one should add to all the dishes during cooking twenty *dirhams* of wine and five *dirhams* of rose water. If the dishes are to be sour, one should add twenty *dirhams* of the wine, five *dirhams* of rose water, and five *dirhams* of lemon juice. If the meat one wants to roast is chicken, it should be roasted on a spit, as is customary, and continuously basted during the roasting with wine and lemon juice or wine alone.

(32) If the soul craves for roast meat of land animals, it should be the suckling kid, basted with wine and a little saffron during the roasting. If one wants to add a little bit of saffron to every meal that one prepares, one should do so, because it is an exhilarating cardiac remedy. But one should not take too much of it because it has the specific property of quieting the appetite for food. This is what this Servant now presents on the dishes of food, which suit our Master, may his days be prolonged.

(33) Galen, and those who preceded him among the physicians, mentioned a drink that they name in their language "hydromel" [*De sanitate tuenda* IV.6; *De alimentorum facultatibus* III.38]; they used to prepare it from bees' honey and thin white wine, as they used to prepare oxymel from vinegar and honey. But their successors, as they prepared oxymel from sugar and vinegar, prepared hydromel from sugar and wine. This is a most excellent drink, beneficial in strengthening the stomach and the heart, improving the digestion, and dilating the soul. It eases the egress of the two superfluities with good effect. I have tested it, and so have others, several times.

(34) The description of its preparation is: Take five Egyptian *raṭl*s of sugar, cook it as syrups are cooked, take the foam away from it, and continue cooking it until it assumes a good consistency. Then cast into it one Egyptian *raṭl* of the wine described before and thicken it into a syrup with the consistency of syrup of roses. This Servant has only mentioned this syrup along with the foods because it is similar to them. It should always be taken daily at the beginning of the day, in wintertime in hot water and in the summertime in cold water. One should take three or four ounces at a time, because this drink is not like the drink of oxymel and other similar drinks, because these drinks are medicines requiring

apportioning and discernment regarding the person for whom they are good. This drink is an excellent nutriment because the sugar by itself is already a nutriment even if it has some medicinal effect. Similarly, the wine is an excellent nutriment, without any doubt. The most wonderful thing about it is, they say, that it is not harmful for those with a hot temperament. The reason for this is that its basic ingredients are familiar good nutriments. This is the measure of what this Servant considered proper to present before mentioning the concrete arrangement of the regimen.

(35) On the arrangement of the regimen for our Master with respect to that he complains about, may God remove his pains and lengthen his days:

There is no doubt that this treatise will reach our Master at the approach of winter and therefore he thought it proper to start with the sort of regimen he should follow in cold weather. This Servant hopes that if our Master perseveres in this regimen, his health will return to normal very soon, God—Who is exalted—willing. This Servant does not know the habits of our Master when he is healthy, whether he eats once a day or whether he eats breakfast and supper. Therefore, he will mention a regimen appropriate for both conditions.

(36) I say that one should always try to awaken from sleep at sunrise or a little before that, and at that time one should take two or three ounces of the hydromel drink. He should then wait one hour and then go riding. He should ride leisurely without stopping and then gradually quicken the pace until the members of his body are warmed and his respiration changes. Then he should dismount and rest until none of the changes caused by the exercise remain on the skin of the body and in the respiration. After that, he should feed himself with one of the dishes mentioned above, and take a little of the astringent fruits, as has been said, or pistachio nuts and raisins, or a little of dry sweetmeats, or a little rose preserve, all this according to what he is now used to. Then he should recline to sleep and a singer should sing while playing on a stringed instrument, raise his voice, and sing at a high pitch for an hour, then lower his voice gradually and lower the sound of the stringed instrument and soften his melody until he falls into a deep sleep, whereupon he should stop. Physicians and philosophers have stated that sleep in this manner, when the melody of the stringed instrument induces sleep, endows the soul with a good moral habitude, dilates it greatly, and thereby improves its management of the body. When he wakes up, let him spend the rest of the day with reading whatever he wishes or by being in the company of someone whose company he prefers. This is the best, I mean the company of someone whose company he prefers because of his vir-

tues or because of the delight of seeing him or because of the lightness of his mind. All these dilate the soul and expel evil thoughts from it.

(37) But if he is used to take another meal for supper, he should take fifty *dirhams* of the wine described above, mixed with ten *dirhams* of rose water and twenty *dirhams* of borage; this should be taken little by little until the time for supper arrives. Then he should wait for half an hour until the wine has left the stomach and then eat supper as is his custom, from one of the dishes mentioned above. Then the singer should attend and entertain him with songs for two hours after the meal. Then he should recline and tell the singer to lower the sound of the stringed instrument and his melodies until he falls into a deep sleep. Then the singing should be stopped, as it was done in the daytime.

(38) If there is no supper and he does not take a second meal after that taken during the day, he should mix the wine according to the aforementioned ratio. He should continue taking it little by little, while listening to the sound of the stringed instrument, until it is time to go to sleep, either after two hours of the night or three or four, as long as it pleases him to stay up. There is no need for him to pay attention to the quantity of the aforementioned mixed wine, if he does not eat supper. Even if he takes two hundred or three hundred *dirhams* of it, or a little bit more than that on winter nights, it is good and has a moistening effect on the body. If it is his habit that he takes nothing after the wine for dessert but a few roasted pistachio nuts with lemon juice or salt, or some lemon peel preserved in sugar, or roasted myrtle seed, or roasted coriander, it is the best. If it is his habit to take some food with the wine, the best thing to take is young chickens roasted on the spit. These should be those young chickens that were fed with what we mentioned, namely, with barley meal, milk, figs, and grains of wheat. Let no one suppose that taking lemon peel preserved in sugar heats the temperament because lemon peel is intermediate between the hot and the cold; it is a cardiac remedy, and one should rely upon taking it for dessert. If this would be his very regimen from tomorrow upon awakening from sleep, he should not change anything from it during the cold season.

(39) He should examine his condition upon arising from sleep. If he is thirsty, drinking oxymel of roses is preferable to drinking hydromel. If there is a little bit of uncocted matter in the urine flask, drinking oxymel of raisins is preferable. If there is overfilling of the stomach, taking ten *dirhams* of rose preserves and four *dirhams* of that *iṭrīfal* is preferable. If his stools are retained or are hard as a stone, he should take less wine during the night, or give up supper if he has

a habit of eating supper. He should take a laxative when it has cooled down and on such a day no physical exercise should be done. We have explained in the third chapter of that treatise and in these chapters all those ingredients that should be used for softening the stools. The attending physician should at all times give advice regarding those remedies that are beneficial in that regard.

(40) On the day on which he intends to take a bath, he should first take the drink as mentioned above, and reduce the vigor of the exercise and shorten its duration. He should take a bath immediately after the exercise, then leave the bath and drink a brew prepared with pomegranate seeds, sugar, many spices, and hot choice spices such as clove and mace, or syrup of roses and common sorrel with borage juice, or the syrup that we have compounded and mentioned in the third chapter of that treatise. He should sleep immediately after the bath. Galen said: I have never seen anything more effective in cocting what needs to be cocted and in dissolving what can be dissolved than sleep after the bath. [*De sanitate tuenda* IV.4]. Upon awakening, he may take food and occupy himself the rest of the day and an hour of the night with what we mentioned. When the food begins to leave the stomach, he should begin to take that mixed wine, little by little. And the singer should sing until he falls into a deep sleep in the manner described. He should have no supper at all that night. But if he is used to have supper, he should postpone the meal until after arising from the sleep that follows the bath.

(41) Regarding the time he intends to have sexual intercourse, there are two periods, either after the digestion of the food once he has taken that small quantity of wine before supper or late at night. The crux of the matter is that this activity should neither take place when one is hungry and has an empty stomach, nor when the stomach is filled with food. The same applies to the drinking of wine. He should neither drink it as long as the food in the stomach has not been digested because the wine will keep it uncocted and will expel it before it has been cocted, nor when the stomach is empty and in need of food, for then it heats the temperament and causes headache and burns the humors. Rather, it should be taken when the food begins to be digested.

(42) On every Friday morning he should take one *mithqāl* of that temperate electuary, which is made with jacinth—and he should not exercise on that day—or with the *iṭrīfal* mentioned above, or with one of the recipes of the musk medicaments that are mentioned in the *Kitāb al-Qānūn fī al-ṭibb* (*The*

Canon of Medicine). He should not, under any circumstances, take an electuary in which there is any castoreum. Castoreum should be omitted from any musk remedy that our Master takes. This is the regimen for the time of the year in which the weather is cold.

(43) In the hot season one should not awake from sleep except after one hour of the day and take the syrup of oxymel of roses and raisins and the syrup that we mentioned in the third chapter of that treatise. He should exercise when the weather is cold and feed himself with dishes tending towards coldness. He should sleep for a long time after listening to the stringed instrument of which we spoke earlier. He should only take a little of that mixed drink. He should not stay awake at night and reduce sexual intercourse from what he is used to in winter. He should take the cool musk remedy we have mentioned instead of the temperate jacinth remedy. If he likes to drink some wine, let him do so at the end of the day, so that he will take the measure of it that we mentioned, and sleep at the beginning of the night or at the end of its second hour. It is good for him to take the cool jacinth remedy. The brew that he drinks after the bath should be of tamarind, sugar, musk, and some camphor. Softening of the stools, when needed, should be done by an infusion of rhubarb and tamarind as we mentioned in the third chapter of that treatise, as well as with the syrup that we have compounded.

(44) If the heat increases, it is unavoidable to take a compound with barley groats, which is prepared every day when one gets up one hour before the exercise instead of the aforementioned drinks. Or take it at bedtime and sleep on it, instead of the stomach being occupied with the digestion of foods or beverages. Its composition according to the needs of our Master is as follows: Take forty *dirhams* of peeled barley, six months after it is harvested; four *dirhams* each of crushed common fumitory seed, crushed *hindibāʾ* (endive or chicory) seed, and borage; two *dirhams* of crushed Iraqi opium poppy seed; one *dirham* of oily Indian sandalwood; a quarter of a *dirham* of spikenard; half a *dirham* of dill flowers; three *dirhams* of fragrant olive oil from the Maghreb or Syria-Palestine, yellow of color and free from bitter taste. Put all these all at one time into an earthen pot, pour one thousand *dirhams* of water into the pot, and place it on a charcoal fire until half of the water has evaporated. Then pour into it six *dirhams* of vinegar. Its cooking is completed when less than a quarter of it remains and its color appears red. Then filter it and add to the filtrate half a *dirham* of salt. It should be taken alone without a drink. An hour after it is taken, one should lick one spoonful of lemon syrup.

(45) Our Master should be very strict concerning this prescription; he should keep it in mind and turn its use into a regular habit, because it resists the dryness of the melancholic humor, brings the disordered humors into balance, removes their burning, thickens those vapors that arise to the heart and brain, prevents their ascent, cools the temperament through bringing it into balance, and improves the condition of all that of which our Master complains. Because Hippocrates states among all the virtues that he enumerates of barley groats, that it conveys what should be conveyed to where it should be conveyed. [*Regimen on Acute Diseases* 11.40]. Our Master should not neglect to take it regularly in the summer in any manner, unless he suffers from constipation or acidity in the stomach, or flatulence is produced in the hypochondrium. For then our Master should not take it.

(46) This Servant knows that because of the excellence of the intellect of our Master and the soundness of his perception, he is capable of adhering to a regimen as is proper according to that preceding treatise and these chapters, and all the more so if there is at hand someone who can guide him and help him by his knowledge and familiarity with the art.

(47) God—Who is exalted—is witness and He is a sufficient witness, that it was the highest hope of this minor servant to attend to the service of his Master with his body and speech, not with paper and pen. However, his fundamental bad temperament and weak natural constitution—even when he was young, how much more so in his old age—stood between him and many pleasures. With pleasures I mean nothing else but good deeds, the greatest and highest of which is to attend to the service of Our Master. But God be thanked for all what occurs generally in the universal existing things and in the particular existing things, namely, in every single individual, according to His will, which follows His wisdom, the depth of which man cannot fathom. Praise be to God, always, in any circumstance, whatever turn events may take.

(48) Our Master should not criticize his minor Servant for what he mentioned in this his treatise about the use of wine and song, both of which the religious Law abhors, because this Servant has not commanded that this should be done, but has mentioned what his art requires. The lawgivers know as well as the physicians, that wine can be beneficial for men. The physician, inasmuch as he is a physician, must give information about the form of the beneficial regimen, no matter whether it is forbidden or permitted, while the patient has the option to act accordingly or not. If the physician refrains from prescribing all that is beneficial, whether it is forbidden or permitted, he acts dishonestly, and

does not give true counsel. It is known that the religious Law commands what is beneficial and forbids whatever is harmful in the next world, while the physician gives information about what benefits the body and about what is harmful to it in this world. The difference between the commandments of the religious Law and the counsels of medicine is that the religious Law commands adherence to what is useful for one's lifespan and compels it, and forbids that which harms one's lifespan and punishes for it, while medicine merely recommends what is beneficial and warns against what is harmful, but does not enforce it nor punish for it. Rather, it leaves the matter to the patient in the form of an advice; he has the choice.

(49) The reason for this is clear. In medicine, the harm of what is harmful and the benefit of what is beneficial are immediate and tangible and there is no need for coercion and punishment. However, the harm and benefit of religious commandments and prohibitions cannot be clearly distinguished in this world. Rather, the ignorant sometimes imagines that all what is said to be harmful does not harm, and all what is said to be beneficial does not benefit, because he cannot see these things as he can see those that are tangible. Therefore, the religious Law compels one to do good and punishes for evil, as good and evil can only be ascertained in the next world. All this is out of beneficence towards us and favor upon us and compassion with us because of our ignorance and mercy with us because of the weakness of our understanding. This is the measure of what this Servant thought proper to present to him who holds him in bondage.

May God perpetuate his days;
the judgment of our Master is supreme and perfect.

BOOK 9

Commentary on Hippocrates' Aphorisms

First published in:

Maimonides
Commentary on Hippocrates' **Aphorisms**

A New Parallel Arabic-English Edition and Translation with Critical Editions of the Medieval Hebrew Translations by Gerrit Bos.

Leiden (Brill) 2020
MWMM 14

∵

In the name of God,
the Merciful, the Compassionate

(N) (1) Says the master, the erudite, the eminent, the leader, Mūsā ibn 'Ubayd Allāh, the Israelite from Córdoba, may God bless his soul: I do not think that any scholar who composes books would write a book in any kind of science with the intention that the contents of his book cannot be understood, unless they are explained. If any author would have such an intention, he would thwart the purpose of his composition, because an author does not write a book so that he alone will understand its contents. However, he writes a book so that others will understand it. And if a book he wrote can only be understood by another book, he has thwarted the purpose of its composition.

(2) In my view, there are four reasons why later authors were prompted to explain the books of earlier authors and to comment upon them:

The first reason is the perfection of the degree of knowledge of the author. Because of his excellent intellect, he speaks briefly about things that are obscure, hidden, and difficult to understand for others, but which are clear to him so that he does not need to use more words. If someone in a later generation wants to understand those matters that were written down in such a concise

 | DOI:10.1163/9789004498884_011

way, it is very difficult for him. A commentator must add an explanation to his words so that the meaning of the matters, which the first author had in mind, can be understood.

(3) The second reason is the omission of premisses in a book. For the author sometimes composes a book assuming that the reader will have preliminary knowledge of certain premisses. But if someone who does not know those premisses wants to understand that book, he is unable to do so. Then the commentator has to supply and explain those premisses or to refer the reader to books in which those premisses are explained and to direct him to them. For the same reason, the commentator has to explain the causes of things that were not mentioned by the author.

(4) The third reason is the correct interpretation of a statement. For most statements in any language can be interpreted in various ways. They can have meanings that are different and sometimes even opposite or contradictory. Consequently, disagreement arises between those who look at that statement. One person gives it a certain interpretation and says that the author only meant this, and another person gives it another interpretation. The commentator of that statement must declare one interpretation for correct and adduce proof for its correctness and declare the other interpretations for false.

(5) The fourth reason is the errors that befall the author, or words that are repetitive or even utterly useless. The commentator must draw the reader's attention to these words and prove that they are futile, useless, or repetitive. This should not really be called a commentary, but a refutation or annotation. However, when people study a book and most of its contents is correct, they usually consider the annotations to the few erroneous places to be part of the commentary, in which it is said: the error of the author is such and such and the truth is such and such, or: this should not have been mentioned, or: this is repetitious; all this is explained. However, if the contents of that book is mostly mistaken, then the later work, which exposes those mistakes, is called a refutation, not a commentary. When the work with the refutation cites a correct statement, it will say: such and such statement is correct.

(6) It seems to me that all the commentaries on the books of Aristotle were composed for the first and the third reason. All the commentaries on the books on the mathematical sciences were composed for the second reason, although it is also possible that some mathematical statements have been commented upon because of the fourth reason. For the book called *Almagest*, in spite of the

eminence of its author (Claudius Ptolemy), has errors that were pointed out by a group of Andalusian authors in the books they composed regarding that matter. And all the commentaries written on the books of Hippocrates are mostly composed for the first, third, and fourth reason, while some of its statements are commented upon for the second reason.

(7) However, Galen denies this and does not think in any way that the works of Hippocrates contain errors. [*De usu partium* 1.8]. But Galen offers explanations, which cannot be supported by the text and provides commentaries to certain statements that are not alluded to by those statements. We can see how he did so in his *In Hippocratis De humoribus commentarius*, even though he was doubtful whether this book was written by Hippocrates or by someone else. He was prompted to do so because of the confusion in matters discussed by him and because it resembles the works of the alchemists or is even worse than these. In my opinion, it would be more correct to call it "The Book of Mental Confusion." However, because of the fame of Hippocrates and the ascription of the book to him, Galen composed this strange commentary. Everything that Galen said in that commentary is correct from a medical viewpoint; however, the text that he commented upon does not indicate (relate to) anything of the commentary that he wrote. His commentary should not really be called a commentary, because a commentary brings to actuality that which can potentially be understood from a text, so that, if you look once again at that commented text—once you have understood the commentary—you will see that that text indicates (relates to) what you have understood from the commentary. This is what should be called a real commentary, but this is not the case if someone makes true statements and maintains that they are a commentary to the words of the author, as Galen did with regard to some of the statements by Hippocrates. The same holds good for those who draw conclusions from the words of a certain person and call it a commentary. In my opinion, it is not a commentary but another work, like most of the commentary by al-Nairīzī on Euclid. I do not call that whole work a commentary.

(8) Similarly, we find that Galen, in his commentaries on the works by Hippocrates, explains certain statements contrary to their meaning so that he turns that statement into a correct one. He does so in the book [*In Hippocratis*] *De septimanis* [*commentarius*], where Hippocrates says that the earth surrounds the water. Galen explains this statement by saying that it is possible that he meant with this statement that the water surrounds the earth. He says all this so that he would not have to say that Hippocrates made a mistake or committed an error in this statement. And when the matter baffled him because he found

a statement that was clearly mistaken and he did not find any other way out, he would say that this statement is falsely ascribed to Hippocrates and interpolated into his words, or that these are the words of a *certain* Hippocrates but not *the well-known* Hippocrates. He did so in his [*In Hippocratis*] *De natura hominis commentarius*. He did all this to defend Hippocrates; although Hippocrates is without any doubt one of the most eminent physicians, such a defense is not a virtue, even in the case of an eminent man.

(9) It is well known that not everything in a book that has been commented on, or that will be commented, on needs an explanation. There are inevitably statements in it that are clear and do not need an explanation. However, the goal of the commentators with their commentaries is comparable to the method of the authors in their compositions. Some authors strive for brevity, which does not affect the meaning so that if, for instance, to fulfill the purpose of the composition in one hundred words they would not use one hundred and one words. Other authors aim at long-windedness and verbosity at composing a voluminous work of many parts, even though the total work does not have much content. The same applies to commentators: Some of them explain something that needs to be explained as briefly as possible and omit the rest; others are long-winded and explain that which does not need to be explained or explain that which needs to be explained more verbosely than necessary.

(10) I thought that Galen is a very verbose commentator, as most of his commentaries are very lengthy until I noticed what he remarks in the beginning of his commentary on Plato's *Laws*, and these are his words:

I have noticed that a commentator explained the following statement of Hippocrates on more than one hundred folios without any reason to do so and without any actual content:

When the disease reaches its climax, then the regimen of the patient should be extremely thinning. [*Aphorisms* I.8].

(11) Says Moses: When I saw this statement of Galen, I excused him for his works and commentaries as I realized that he had been very brief therein in comparison with the works of his contemporaries. On the other hand, these works are so verbose that it can only be denied by someone who is biased. I am only speaking to those who are free of unfounded predilections and who seek the truth in everything. Galen remarks in *De methodo medendi* VI[.1] that his colleagues discussed these statements by Hippocrates lengthily.

(12) And since I consider Hippocrates' *Aphorisms* to be the most useful of the books he composed, I decided to explain them; for these are aphorisms that every physician should know by heart. I have even seen how non-physicians have schoolchildren memorize them, so that subsequently people who are not physicians know many of these aphorisms by heart from learning them as young children at school.

(13) Among these aphorisms of Hippocrates are some that are problematic and require explanation, some that are self-evident, some that are repeated, some that are useless for the medical art, and some that are completely mistaken. However, Galen denies this and explains such statements as he wishes. But I will explain them in a fair (honest) way, that is, I will only explain that which needs an explanation, and will comply therein with Galen's goals (opinions), except for a few aphorisms, where I will give my opinion, in my name. Every explanation that I will mention anonymously is that of Galen, according to its sense (figuratively), for I do not envisage (intend) to be meticulous in quoting his words as I did in the *Epitomes* [*from the Works of Galen*]. In this commentary, my only intention is to abbreviate so that it will be easy to memorize the meaning of those aphorisms that require explanation. To achieve that I try to use as few words as possible, except for the first aphorism on which I will dwell a little longer. I am not doing so in order to compose a true commentary on that aphorism, but in order to inform the reader about some things in it that occurred to me as useful, regardless whether Hippocrates intended them so or not.

Now it is time to start with the commentary.

∴

The First Part of the *Commentary on Hippocrates'* Aphorisms

(1.1) (14) Says Hippocrates: *Life is short, and the art is long, and time is limited, and experience is dangerous, and judgment is difficult. One* (*the physician*) *should not be content with the intention to do what is necessary without the patient and his attendants doing the same; and the external matters also.*

Says the commentator: It is well known that short and long are adjunctive attributes. If he wants, by saying "life is short," to refer to the art of medicine, then his statement "the art is long" is a repetition that is unnecessary, and there is no difference between this and saying "Zayd is shorter than ʿAmr" and "ʿAmr is longer than Zayd." But if he meant to say that the life of an individual is short in comparison to perfection in any science and that the art of medicine is long in comparison to the other arts, then this reiteration is useful, as if he says how far man is from being perfect in this art—all this to urge persistence in it.

(15) As for the fact that the medical art is longer than the other theoretical and practical arts, this is obvious, because it is an art that cannot be comprehended nor perfection attained in it, except through its many parts. But the life of a single person is not sufficient to comprehend all those parts in a perfect and complete way. Abū Naṣr al-Fārābī has mentioned that there are seven parts, the knowledge of which constitutes the art of medicine. The first part, pertaining to the physician, is the knowledge of the object of his art, namely, the human body, that is, the science of anatomy, and the knowledge of the temperament of each of the organs in general, and the knowledge of its function and usefulness and the condition of its substance in firmness, softness, density, and looseness, and the form of each of the organs, and the location of the organs (parts), both internal and external, and the connection of the organs to each other. Every physician should have this degree of knowledge about everything of it or in it, although it may take a long time to acquire this knowledge, as long as it does not concern things that are hidden. [*Risāla fī al-ṭibb*].

(16) The second part related to our subject is the condition of the body, that is the knowledge of the different kinds of health of the whole body, in general, and the different kinds of health of every singular organ.

The third part consists of the knowledge of the different kinds of disease and its causes, and the pertinent symptoms in the whole body, in general, and in every singular part of the body.

The fourth part consists of the knowledge of the rules of deduction, that is, how to select from those afflictions affecting the subject, the indications from which one can draw conclusions about each and every kind of health and about each and every kind of disease, whether in the entire body or in any of its parts and how to distinguish between one disease and another when most of the indications are similar.

The fifth part consists of the rules of the regimen of the health of the body in general and the health of each of its organs for every age and for every season of the year and according to every place, so that every body and every organ will maintain the health specific to it.

The sixth part consists of the knowledge of the general rules according to which the illness should be treated so that the missing health is restored to the entire body or to the ailing organ.

The seventh part consists of the knowledge of the instruments that the physician uses to preserve health when it is present or to restore it when it is lost, that is, the knowledge of the different kinds of the foods of man and his medicines, both simple and compound; binding, bandaging, and douching are also part of this. Likewise, the instruments with which the flesh is lanced and cut, the hooks that are used for suspension, and the other instruments that are used for wounds and for eye illnesses, all these belong to this category. Included in this part of the art of medicine is the knowledge of the form of every plant and mineral used in it, because if you know only their name you cannot gain their end. Likewise, you also need to know their various names in various places so that you know in each place with which name to ask for it.

(17) It is well known that by knowing all these seven parts and by memorizing them from the books composed for each part, the physician will not attain the goal of his action, nor will the physician who has this knowledge acquire perfection in the art, until he attends to individual persons, both when they are healthy and sick, and until he acquires the skill to recognize the symptoms from which he can draw whatever conclusions and knows readily the condition of the temperament of that person and the condition of the temperament of each of his organs in what kind of health or illness it is, and, similarly, the state of function of each organ of that person and the condition of the substance of his organs. Likewise, through prolonged observation of a person and through those forms impressed in his mind, he will readily know how to use those instruments, that is, foods, medicines, and the other instruments. This requires an extremely long time.

(18) It will be clear to you that the knowledge of these parts in general and the memorization of these rules, until nothing is lacking therefrom, needs a very long time. Likewise, attending to individual persons until one is trained in regimenting the health of one individual after another, in managing the cure of the diseases of one individual after another, in applying those instruments in individual cases, that is, one time using them alone and another time combining some of them with others, and in selecting a particular medicine or food over another of its kind, all this requires a very long time. It was rightly said that this art is longer than every other art for him, who aims at perfection therein. Galen has said in his [*In Platonis*] *Timaeum commentarius*: No one can master the art of medicine completely.

(19) Says the author: To be honest, you should know that every physician who is not perfect in the art does more harm than good because whether a person is healthy or sick, it is better not to be treated by a physician at all than to be treated according to the opinion of a physician who makes a mistake;

his mistakes will be in proportion to his inadequacy and if he happens to do something right, then it is by accident. For this reason, that eminent physician (Hippocrates) began his book with the exhortation to be perfect in this art by saying:

Life is short, and the art is long, and time is limited, and experience is dangerous, and judgment is difficult.

As to experience being dangerous, that is clear, but I will add an explanation.

(20) As to his statement "time is limited," it seems to me that he means with this that the time for treating the disease is far too limited to experiment. If you do not know all matters already verified by experience (*tajriba*), but begin now to experiment with certain matters on this patient, time is too short for that and there is danger in beginning to experiment on this patient. All these words are in exhortation to be perfect in the art, so that all that has been tried throughout the years is present in your memory.

(21) As to his statement "judgment is difficult," it seems to me that he means by this the judgment whether the disease tends towards the patient being saved or perishing or to another kind of change. In general, prognosis is very difficult in the art of medicine because the elements of the body are in a state of constant change and rarely remain in the same condition. You already know that most of the natural matters are not constant. How many times are the indications extremely bad, yet the patient is saved, and how many times one takes the favorable indications as a good omen, yet what they indicated does not come true. Therefore, lengthy training is needed in the observation of individual symptoms, because then you will be able to judge what will occur with a good intuition that approaches the truth. This saying also urges to apply oneself with persistence and perseverance to this art.

(22) The meaning of "danger in experience" is as I will describe now. Know that in every natural body there are two kinds of accidents: accidents that adhere to it with respect to its matter and accidents that adhere to it with respect to its form. Man is an example of this: Health and illness, sleep and wakefulness adhere to him with respect to his matter, that is, with respect to his being a living being, and it adheres to him that he thinks, reflects, wonders, and laughs with respect to his form. Those accidents that adhere to his body with respect to its form are those that are called "specific properties," because they are specific to this species alone. Likewise, every plant, every mineral, and every organ of a living being has these two kinds of accidents.

(23) To each of these accidents belongs a certain action in our body. The actions performed by a drug in our body with respect to its matter is that it heats, or cools, or moistens, or dries. These are the actions that the physicians call "the primary powers" and say that this drug heats or cools by its nature. They also say that it does so by its quality. Similarly, the actions that result from these primary powers, those which the physicians call "the secondary powers," such as when a drug hardens, or softens, or loosens, or thickens, and the other actions, which they enumerated—all of them are effected by the drug with respect to its matter.

(24) The actions that a drug performs in our body with regard to its specific form, are those, which the physicians call "specific properties." Galen expounds this kind of action by saying that it acts by the whole of its essence, that is to say, it performs its action with respect to its specific form through which that body is constituted as a substance. This present action does not result from its quality. They also call these "tertiary powers," and these are, for instance, the purgative effect of purgatives, the emetic effect of emetics, the lethal effect of poisons, or the life-saving effect of drugs for the ingestion of a poisonous substance or for the bite of a poisonous animal. All these actions result from the form of the remedy, not its matter.

(25) Nutrients are also of this kind, that is to say, the fact that certain species of plants serve as nourishment for certain species of animals is not only attributable to the first qualities and also not to the hardness, softness, thickness, or looseness that follow from them. Rather, it is an action of the entire substance, as Galen says. Consider how we are nourished by things that are close to the nature of wood and on which our stomach acts upon and changes, such as dried sweet chestnuts, dried acorns, and dried carobs. But our stomach does not at all change the peel and pits of grapes, nor the peel of apples, and their like. As these enter the body so they leave, for it is not in their essence to be influenced (affected) by the stomach in any way.

(26) In his famous book *De simplicium medicamentorum* [*temperamentis ac facultatibus* IV.26], Galen has explained how to deduce from its taste the nature and action of a drug resulting from its quality. As to the knowledge of what the drug does with respect to its specific form—and this is, what is said above, that it performs this action with its entire substance—we have no indication whatsoever, nor any other way by which to draw conclusions about this action, except by experience (*tajriba*). How many drugs are bitter and extremely foul-smelling, and yet are beneficial drugs. But one may also find a plant that tastes

and smells like the other nutrients, yet is a lethal poison or a plant of which one thinks that it is one of the different kinds of nutrients, except that it is wild and not cultivated, yet it is a lethal poison. The danger of applying a certain medication based on experience should be clear to you; there is nothing more dangerous than it. Yet there is a great need for it, for the nutritional power of all the nutrients was not learned except by experience. Likewise, the actions of most drugs were not learned except by experience. Therefore, you should not give precedence to experimentation, but first seek help by remembering all that others have tried.

(27) Know that there are drugs whose action in our bodies, which occurs as a result of their matter, is clear and manifest, while their action that results from their form is very much hidden so that it is not perceived, like most drugs to which no specific property is ascribed and to which no specific action is attributed. But there are also drugs whose action in our body, which occurs as a result of their form, is very clear, like purgatives, poisons, and antidotes. These affect our bodies with respect to heating and cooling only very little, either because of the small quantity taken of them—even though they are warming or cooling—or because they do not have a predominant manifest quality. In any case, it is absolutely necessary that these two actions are present, namely, that which results from the matter and that which results from the form. Because of the action that results from the form, there are drugs that are specific for the stomach, drugs that are specific for the liver, drugs that are specific for the spleen, drugs that are specific for the heart, and drugs that are specific for the brain. And because of the specific form, the actions of the drugs are diverse, even though their nature is the same. If you look well, you will find numerous drugs that have exactly the same degree of heat and dryness, for instance, and each of these drugs has actions other than those of the other drug. All this was indeed brought out by experience in the course of time.

(28) Because of his great moral virtues, Hippocrates ordered in this aphorism, with which he began, that the physician should not be content with doing what is necessary only and stop there, because that is not sufficient for the attainment of health for the patient. Because the goal will only be achieved and the patient healed, if the patient and all those around him will also do what is necessary and remove all external impediments that prevent the cure of the illness. It is as though he is commanding in this aphorism that the physician should apply his abilities to manage his patients and make their treatment easy with, for instance, the ingestion of bitter medicines, clysters, lancing, cautery, and the like. He should admonish and warn the patient and those around him

against making mistakes, and make those around him take care of the treatment of the patient, as is proper when the physician is absent. Similarly, he should remove the external impediments as well as he can, according to each individual case. For instance, if the patient is poor and he is in a place that increases his illness but he cannot afford another place, the physician should move him from that place to another one. Likewise, he should provide him with nourishment and medication if the patient does not have that. These and their like are the things that exceed a physician's duty with respect to his art, yet are necessary for the attainment of the goal that the physician wants to attain for this patient. Only to prescribe what is necessary to do with regard to the medical art and to leave it at that, the physician should not do so, because then the goal intended will not be attained.

(1.2) (29) Says Hippocrates: *If the material that is evacuated from the body during diarrhea or during vomiting, which happen spontaneously, is from the kind that should be purged from the body, it is beneficial and easy to bear. But if this is not the case, the contrary holds good. The same applies to the artificial emptying of the vessels. If they are emptied from the material they should be free from, it is beneficial and easy to bear. But if this is not the case, the contrary holds good. One should also consider the current time of the year, the place where one lives, the age and the diseases as to whether the intended evacuation should be carried out or not.*

Says the commentator: The statement "the same applies to the emptying of the vessels" means through micturition, or perspiration, or through flow of blood (nosebleed or menses), or the opening of the orifices of the blood vessels. All these are things that occur spontaneously. As for Galen, he says that with the "emptying of the vessels," he means the evacuation by means of a drug. In his opinion, the last part of Hippocrates' statement is repetitious, so that it needs an explanation. Then he states that if you intend an evacuation of a humor, which is of the kind that should be evacuated when the signs of its domination are clear to you, you should also take into consideration the current time of the year, the place where one lives, the age, and the nature of that disease and deal with the matter accordingly. Because the evacuation of yellow bile in winter, or in cold places, or in old age, or in diseases caused by cold is difficult and cannot be tolerated by the patient. Likewise, the evacuation of phlegm in summer, or in hot places, or in the case of young people, or of diseases caused by heat is difficult and cannot be tolerated by the patient. [*In Hippocratis Aphorismos commentarius* 1.2].

(1.3) (30) Says Hippocrates: *In those who do physical exercise, extreme stoutness of the body is dangerous if they have reached the very limit therein. For they cannot stay or remain in that condition, and since they cannot stay in that condition and cannot become healthier, their condition can only become worse. For this reason, one should reduce the stoutness of the body without delay so that it can start again to assimilate the food, but the reduction should not be extreme, because that is also dangerous. It should only be to the degree, which can be tolerated by the nature (constitution) of the body, which one wants to reduce. Similarly, any evacuation carried out to the extreme is dangerous and any feeding that is extreme is also dangerous.*

Says the commentator: With "those who carry out physical exercise," he means wrestlers and the like, among those who choose hard physical exercise for their profession. When their blood vessels are filled more than necessary one cannot be sure that they will not burst or that the innate heat will not be strangled in them, so that it becomes extinguished and they die. For the blood vessels need a vacuum to receive the food that reaches them.

(1.4) (31) Says Hippocrates: *A strict regimen is undoubtedly dangerous in all chronic diseases, and in acute diseases when it is not endured. A regimen that is extremely strict is undoubtedly difficult and reprehensible.*

Says the commentator: A regimen that is extremely strict is that in which one absolutely abstains from taking any food; a regimen that is very strict but not extreme is the imbibition of honey water and the like. A regimen that is strict but not very strict consists of barley gruel and the like.

(1.5) (32) Says Hippocrates: *In a strict regimen, patients sometimes make mistakes, which cause severe harm to them. For all that happens to them as a result of a strict regimen is more serious than what happens to them as a result of a regimen of food that is slightly thickening (nourishing). For this reason, a strict regimen is also dangerous for healthy people, but they endure the harm resulting from a mistake in a thickening (nourishing) regimen more easily. Therefore, a strict regimen is in most cases more dangerous than a regimen that is slightly more thickening (nourishing).*

Says the commentator: This is clear and evident.

(1.6) (33) Says Hippocrates: *In extreme diseases, the best regimen is that which is extreme.*

Says the commentator: Extreme diseases are those, which are extremely acute.

(1.7) (34) Says Hippocrates: *When the disease is very acute, extreme pains appear in the beginning and it is necessary to apply an extremely strict regimen. If this is not the case, and a more thickening (nourishing) regimen is possible, the relaxation of the extremely strict regimen should be according to the mildness of the disease and its deviation from the extreme.*

Says the commentator: Extreme pains are severe pains, such as those occurring during fever attacks and all other afflictions. They happen during the culmination of the disease, for the culmination is that phase of the disease that is most powerful in the disease's symptoms. His statement "in the beginning" should be understood as referring to the first four days or a little bit later.

(I.8) (35) Says Hippocrates: *When the disease has reached its culmination, one should apply a regimen that is extremely strict.*

Says the commentator: This is because of the severity of the symptoms at that time, and so that the illness can be concocted. For nature should not be diverted through the concoction of new food that is delivered to it from the concoction of the humors that produced the disease. Because at that time nature is wholeheartedly engaged in that with all its powers and it only needs to do a little more until it has subdued the humors completely.

(I.9) (36) Says Hippocrates: *One should also examine the strength of the patient and find out whether it can remain firm until the culmination of the disease, and investigate whether the strength of the patient will dwindle before the disease becomes extremely severe, and his strength will not last on that diet, or whether the disease will decline first and lose its severity.*

Says the commentator: This is evident.

(I.10) (37) Says Hippocrates: *The regimen of those whose illness reaches its climax right in the beginning should be strict straightaway. The regimen of those whose illness culminates later on should be more thickening (nutritious) in the beginning and then, when the culmination of the illness approaches, the regimen should be restricted slowly in a way that the strength of the patient lasts. One should stop the administration of food during the culmination of the illness, for an increase in food is harmful.*

Says the commentator: This is evident.

(I.11) (38) Says Hippocrates: *If the fever has cycles, one should stop the administration of food during its attacks, for an increase in it is harmful.*

Says the commentator: This is evident.

(I.12) (39) Says Hippocrates: *The paroxysms and course of a disease are indicated by the diseases themselves, the seasons of the year, the increase in the cycles—*

whether they come every day or every two days or at a longer interval. They are also indicated by the symptoms that appear later; for instance, in patients with pleurisy, if expectoration appears straightaway in the beginning of the disease, the disease will be a short one, but if it appears later, the disease will be prolonged. When urine, feces, and sweat appear later, they may indicate whether the crisis of the disease will be benign or bad, and whether the disease will be short or prolonged.

Says the commentator: From the nature of the illness itself one can know whether the illness ends quickly or slowly. Pleurisy, pneumonia, and phrenitis are acute diseases; angina, cholera, and spasms are very acute diseases; dropsy, delirium, internal suppuration, and phthisis—which is an infection of the lungs—are chronic diseases. Fever attacks mostly occur on alternate days in the case of pleurisy and phrenitis. They are mostly quotidian, especially during the night, in the case of those who have a purulent abscess in the stomach or liver or who suffer from phthisis. Fever attacks occur every three days in the case of those who suffer from an illness of the spleen or an illness resulting from black bile. The same holds good for the seasons of the year. Quartan fever is mostly short in the summer and long in autumn, especially when it is nearly winter.

An increase in attacks (cycles) indicates an increase in the severity of the disease and imminence of its culmination. The increase in the second attack can be distinguished from the first attack by three things: the first is the time of the attack of the fever, the second is the length of the attack, and the third is its strength, that is, its severity.

(I.13) (40) Says Hippocrates: *Old people bear fasting most easily; then adults. Young people bear fasting less well and least of all children, and especially those children who have a very strong appetite.*

Says the commentator: The reason for what he said in this aphorism is mentioned by him in the next aphorism, namely, the stronger one's innate heat, the more food one needs, since the dissolution in the bodies of young people is stronger because of their moisture. And regarding his statement that old people endure fasting most easily, Galen said that this refers to old people who have not reached the stage of senility. [*In Hippocratis Aphorismos commentarius* I.13]. Extremely old people cannot endure fasting, but have to feed themselves with small quantities time and again, since their innate heat is close to extinction, and they consequently have a constant need for that which reinforces it little by little.

(I.14) (41) Says Hippocrates: *Bodies that are growing have the greatest amount of innate heat. For fuel they need more food than the other bodies. If they do not take the amount of food they need, their body wastes away and becomes emaciated. Old people have little innate heat and for this reason they only require little fuel, because their innate heat would be extinguished by too much fuel. For this reason, too, the fever of old people is less acute than that of young people, for their bodies are cold.*

Says the commentator: Galen says that the substance that contains the innate heat in the case of children is very large in quantity and this is what he means in all those cases in which he says about them that their innate heat is greater in quantity, as he explains in *De temperamentis* [II.2].

(I.15) (42) Says Hippocrates: *During winter and spring, the interior parts of the body are naturally the hottest and sleep is the longest. For this reason, one should take more food during these seasons, for during that time the body has much innate heat and thus needs more nourishment. This is proven by those who are young men and wrestlers.*

Says the commentator: This is proven by young men and wrestlers. Galen says: For young men have more innate heat and therefore need more nourishment. Wrestlers can also take more nourishment, since their innate heat increases because of their intensive training. [*In Hippocratis Aphorismos commentarius* I.15].

(I.16) (43) Says Hippocrates: *Moist foods are appropriate for all those who suffer from fever, especially in the case of children and others, namely, those who are used to be nourished with moist foods.*

Says the commentator: This is clear; it is an example of a case from which the general rule is deducted that every disease should be treated by opposite means (*contraria contrariis curantur*).

(I.17) (44) Says Hippocrates: *To some patients, food should be given once, to others twice, in greater or smaller portions, while to yet others it should be given little by little. One should also consider the current time of the year (season), habit, and age.*

Says the commentator: After first giving the rules regarding the appropriate quantity of the food, and then regarding the quality, he here begins with giving the rules regarding the proper way of its administration. The basic rule is that one should consider the strength of the patient and the power of the disease. One should also consider the age and habits of the patient, and the climate. When the vigor of the patient is strong, his food intake should be all at one time, and when it is weak it should be little by little. When his body is lean and emaciated, one should give him much food, and when he is corpulent one should give him little food. It therefore follows that if his vigor is weak and his body lean, he should be nourished with small amounts of food at many times. But if his vigor is weak and his body is not lean, he should be nourished with little food only a few times. The same applies if his vigor is strong and his humors are plentiful. However, if the vigor of the patient is strong but his body is lean and its humors corrupt, he should be fed much food at many times because the condition of his body requires much food, and because his vigor is strong, he is able to digest the food. But if fever attacks prevent him from eating frequently, one should feed him only a few times.

This is the reasoning regarding the vigor of the patient and the disease. As for the current time of the year, the age and habits of the patient and similar factors, the reasoning is as follows: In summer one should eat more often but the amounts taken at each time should be smaller; in winter one should eat more food but less frequently. But after the middle of spring, when summer approaches, one should take little food at long intervals, because at this time the body tends to be full. This is because the humors that were congealed during winter, melt and dissolve. But if someone suffers from fever during autumn, he needs an ample portion of healthy additional food because of the corruption of the humors at that time. The matter of the age and habits of the patient is clear.

(1.18) (45) Says Hippocrates: *In summer and autumn, bodies can only tolerate food with great difficulty, while in winter and next in spring, it is very easy for them.*

Says the commentator: Galen remarks that Hippocrates' statement in this aphorism refers to sick people, while his earlier statement refers to healthy people. [*In Hippocratis Aphorismos commentarius* 1.18].

(1.19) (46) Says Hippocrates: *When fever attacks recur in cycles, one should not give the patient any food during the attacks nor force him to take anything; rather one should decrease the food portions before the times of separation (crises).*

Says the commentator: Galen says: With his statement "before the times of separation," he means "before the times of the attacks." Since during this time one should decrease the superfluous matters so that the fever does not get worse, far be it from you to increase them in any way through nourishment.

(1.20) (47) Says Hippocrates: *When a body suffers from a disease that is attained by a crisis or when the crisis has become full-blown, one should not disturb it, nor try any experiments, neither by purgatives nor other stimulants; rather, it should be left alone.*

Says the commentator: His words "that is attained" mean that the causes of the crisis are ready to bring the crisis about, and that its symptoms are apparent and that it is immanent. His words "nor other stimulants" refer, for instance, to inducing vomiting, perspiration, and micturition or menstruation, and to massaging. He stipulated that the crisis should be complete (full-blown). As to an incomplete crisis, one should complete what is missing and expel the remaining illness-producing humor in the easiest possible way. Galen says that a complete crisis is a combination of six things. The first is that it is preceded by concoction. The second is that this occurs on one of the days of the crisis. The third is that the crisis occurs with plain matter that is evacuated from the body, but not with an abscess. The fourth is that the evacuated matter only consists of the harmful matter that causes the illness. The fifth is that the evacuation is done correctly, from the side of the illness. The sixth is that it is accompanied by relaxation and lightness of the body.

Says Galen: If one or more of these conditions are missing, the crisis is neither perfect nor complete. [*In Hippocratis Aphorismos commentarius* I.20].

Says the commentator: At this point one should ask and say: How can the very illness-producing humor be evacuated, after its concoction on the day of the crisis, correctly, without being followed by lightness and relaxation of the body? Since Galen stipulates a sixth condition, namely, that it is accompanied by lightness and relaxation, it is proof that sometimes the five conditions can be fulfilled without occurring relaxation there. The answer is that this is possible if the evacuation is excessive. Although it is a kind of evacuation that comes with the other conditions being fulfilled, yet, if it is excessive, it is not followed by lightness or relaxation, but by weakness and limpness of the body, and sometimes by a severe feebleness. You should know this.

(I.21) (48) Says Hippocrates: *The matters that should be evacuated, should be evacuated from the sites to which they tend mostly and through those organs that are appropriate for their evacuation.*

Says the commentator: Galen says that the matters that should be evacuated are the humors that produce those illnesses that have an incomplete crisis, and that the sites that are suitable for their evacuation are the intestines, stomach, urinary bladder, uterus, and skin. And the palate and the nostrils as well, if we want to cleanse the brain. The physician should seek for an evacuation that is based on his knowledge of the tendency of nature. If he finds that it tends in a direction that is appropriate to evacuate that which he wants to evacuate, he should provide it with that which she needs and help it. But if he sees that the opposite is the case and sees that nature's movement is harmful, he should prevent it and divert it and draw it in the direction that is opposite to the one nature tends to. I will give you an example of this: If there are humors in the liver that have produced an illness, it is good if they tend to either one of two sides (directions); one is that of the stomach. If they tend to that side, their evacuation through purgation is better than that through emesis. The other side is that of the kidneys and urinary bladder. But it is not good if they tend to the side of the chest, lungs, or heart.

(I.22) (49) Says Hippocrates: *One should only administer drugs and move (disturb) the body once the humors that cause the illness are concocted. As long as they are crude and in the beginning of the illness one should not administer drugs, unless the illness is stirred up; but in most cases, it is not stirred up.*

Says the commentator: With the word "drugs," he means purgatives, and "the illness that is stirred up" is an illness in which the humors disturb the patient and harm him with their heat that is severe and their flow from organ to organ in the beginning of the illness. Consequently, they oppress the patient and disturb him and do not let him rest, as they move and stream from organ to organ. But this happens most rarely. In most cases, the humors are motionless and stay in one organ, and in that organ their concoction takes place during the whole duration of the illness until they decrease.

(I.23) (50) Says Hippocrates: *One should not conclude to the measure of that which should be evacuated from the body from its large quantity. But one should take the opportunity to evacuate, as long as only that is actually evacuated that needs to be evacuated, and as long as the patient endures it easily and comfortably. When necessary, one should carry out the evacuation until the patient faints, but only if he can tolerate it.*

Says the commentator: Galen says that if the prevailing superfluous matter is that which is being evacuated, then the body of the patient feels lighter than before. But if, together with the unnatural matter, natural matter is evacuated, then the patient will necessarily lose strength, his vigor will weaken, and he will feel heaviness and anxiety. The evacuation should be carried out to the point of fainting in the case of extremely large inflammations, and extremely ardent fevers, and extremely severe pains. But one should only resort to this amount of evacuation if the vigor of the patient is strong. I have tried this innumerable times and found it to be highly beneficial. I do not know any remedy that is stronger and more effective in the case of extremely severe pains than evacuation up to the point of fainting. But one may only do so once one has investigated and determined whether one should apply phlebotomy or purgation up to the point of fainting. [*In Hippocratis Aphorismos commentarius* I.23].

(I.24) (51) Says Hippocrates: *In the beginning of acute diseases, one should only rarely use purgatives and one should only do so after a proper examination of the patient.*

Says the commentator: He explained to us that we are not allowed to apply purgation in the beginning of diseases, except for some acute diseases and these are those that are stirred up, as he mentioned before. Moreover, one should only do so very carefully and cautiously and after preparing the body as much as possible and after ascertaining the thinness (consistency) of the humors.

Galen says that the danger (risk) of an improper use of purgatives in the case of acute diseases is very great for the patient, because all purgatives are warming and drying and because fever in its capacity as fever does not need anything that heats and dries; rather it needs that which is the opposite, that is, something that cools and moistens. Purgatives are only used because of the presence of a humor that activates the fever. The benefit to be derived from the evacuation of the humor that produces the illness should be greater than the harm done to the body in that case as a result of the application of purgatives. And the benefit will only be greater if the harmful humor is evacuated completely without causing harm to the body. But one should first consider whether the body of the patient is prepared and ready for such a purgation. Those whose illness starts from frequent indigestions or from viscous thick foods and those who suffer from stretching or swelling in the hypochondrium, or from an extremely severe heat of the urine, or from an inflamed tumor in one of the viscera; the body of none of these persons is ready to be purged. None of these afflictions should be present and the humors in the body of the patient should be as fluid as possible, that is to say, they should be thin and not at all thick. And the passages through which the evacuated matter has to pass should be widely open; there should not be any obstruction in it. We have to do these things and we have first to prepare the body by bringing it into this condition when we want to purge it. [*In Hippocratis Aphorismos commentarius* I.24].

(I.25) (52) Says Hippocrates: *If the body is purged from the kind of matter, it should be purged from, it is beneficial and easily borne* [*by the patient*]*; but if the opposite is the case, it is borne with difficulty.*

Says the commentator: In my opinion, this aphorism is not a repetition of the contents of the second aphorism, because that aphorism deals with that which is evacuated spontaneously, whereas this aphorism deals with that which we evacuate by means of drugs. Since Galen thought that the second aphorism deals with both matters, he sought to give a reason for the repetition of this aphorism. [*In Hippocratis Aphorismos commentarius* I.25].

This is the end of the first part.
Praise be to God alone.

In the name of God,
the Merciful, the Compassionate

The Second Part of the *Commentary on Hippocrates'* Aphorisms

(II.1) (53) Says Hippocrates: *If sleep causes pain in a certain disease, it is a fatal sign. But if sleep is beneficial, it is not a fatal sign.*

Says the commentator: With the term "pain," he means harm, because there are illnesses and cases in which sleep is harmful. Therefore, the patient should be ordered to stay awake during them, for if he sleeps, he will suffer harm. On the other hand, there are also cases in which sleep is beneficial, but if the patient sleeps and suffers harm, it is a fatal sign; we hoped that sleep would be beneficial, but it was harmful. This happens especially when the humors of the body are very bad and suppress the innate heat. However, illnesses in which sleep is always harmful are when one sleeps in the beginning of internal tumors and when superfluous matters stream into the stomach, or in the beginning of a fever attack, especially when it is accompanied by cold and shivering. The times during which sleep is beneficial are at the end of the beginning of an attack or tumor, especially during the climax. Sleep is most beneficial during the decline of a disease. If it is harmful at that time, it is a fatal sign. If it is beneficial, according to what is known of its benefit during this time, it does not tell us anything more than that.

(II.2) (54) Says Hippocrates: *When sleep puts an end to mental confusion (delirium), it is a good sign.*

Says the commentator: This indicates that the innate heat has prevailed over the humors and has subdued them.

(II.3) (55) Says Hippocrates: *If both sleep and sleeplessness exceed the measure of moderateness (become immoderate), it is a bad sign.*

Says the commentator: This is clear.

(II.4) (56) Says Hippocrates: *Neither satiation nor hunger nor anything else is good when it exceeds the measure of nature.*

Says the commentator: This is clear.

(II.5) (57) Says Hippocrates: *Spontaneous fatigue indicates illness.*

Says the commentator: This indicates that the humors move along channels that are not natural to them and therefore cause pain to the organs, either because of their bad quality or because of their large quantity. For this reason, they indicate illness.

(II.6) (58) Says Hippocrates: *If someone has a painful spot in his body, but does not feel the pain in most cases, he suffers from mental confusion.*

Says the commentator: With "pain," here he means the cause of the pain. For instance, when the patient is affected by a hot tumor, erysipelas, wound, bruise, crushing of a limb, and the like, and does not feel it, then he suffers from mental confusion.

(II.7) (59) Says Hippocrates: *Bodies that become emaciated over a long period should be slowly restored with nutrition to their normal corpulence, while bodies that become emaciated over a short period should be restored quickly.*

Says the commentator: For bodies that become emaciated in a short time are affected by that emaciation and leanness because of the evacuation of humors, and not because of a dissolution of the solid organs. But bodies that become emaciated and lean over a long period, their flesh is dissolved and the other organs in which digestion, distribution of the food in the body, and production of blood take place become thin and emaciated, so that they cannot concoct the amount of food that the body needs. For that reason, their corpulence should be restored over a long time.

(II.8) (60) Says Hippocrates: *If a convalescent takes food but does not become stronger, it is a sign that he burdened his body* (ate) *more than it can tolerate. But if this happens while he takes none, it is a sign that evacuation is required.*

Says the commentator: He explains the reason in the aphorism in which he informs us that the more one feeds a body that is not clean, the more harm one does.

(II.9) (61) Says Hippocrates: *If one wants to purge a body, one should take care that that, which one wants to be purged, should flow through it easily.*

Says the commentator: This is done by opening all its passages widely and by diluting, thinning, and dissolving its humors, if they have any sort of thickness and viscosity.

(II.10) (62) Says Hippocrates: *A body that is not clean, the more you nourish it the more you harm it.*

Says the commentator: The reason for that is clear: This happens mostly if the stomach is full with bad humors; for then that happens what Hippocrates has mentioned regarding a convalescent who cannot take any food.

(II.11) (63) Says Hippocrates: *It is easier for a body to be full with drink than with food.*

Says the commentator: With drink, he means liquids and beverages that are nutritious for our bodies. For liquid food, especially if it is hot by its nature, is the easiest and fastest food for the body.

(II.12) (64) Says Hippocrates: *Remnants of diseases left behind in the body after a crisis usually cause a relapse.*

Says the commentator: Those remnants mostly putrefy in the course of time and thereby produce fever because every remaining humor that is strange to the nature of the surrounding body cannot feed it and therefore eventually putrefies in most cases. And if, next to this, the site in the body—in which the humor collects—is hot, its putrefaction occurs most rapidly and powerfully.

(II.13) (65) Says Hippocrates: *If a crisis reaches someone, the night before the paroxysm of the fever is difficult for him, but the following night is mostly easier.*

Says the commentator: When nature separates bad matter from good matter and prepares it for expulsion and evacuation, the body is in a state of disturbance. When this disturbance happens, the patient is necessarily restless (anxious) and the illness is difficult for him. People usually sleep at night. If that disturbance prevents a patient from sleeping, it is extremely clear that this happens because of his restlessness (anxiety) and because of the severity of his disease. Sometimes, this occurs during the day, when the crisis is about to occur in the following night. He says that in the night following the paroxysm, the crisis is mostly easier because that crisis mostly results in health (recovery).

(II.14) (66) Says Hippocrates: *In the case of looseness of the bowels, a change in the various kinds of the stools may be beneficial, unless they change into bad ones.*

Says the commentator: This is so, because many different kinds of stools indicate the evacuation of many different kinds of humors. The bad kinds of stools are those, in which there is some indication of the dissolution of the body, namely, fatty stools, or some indication of putrefaction, namely, a bad smell.

(II.15) (67) Says Hippocrates: *If a person suffers from pain in the throat, or if pustules or abscesses appear on the body, he should examine and look at that which is excreted from the body. If bile prevails therein, then the rest of the body is affected in addition to that spot. But if that which is excreted from the body resembles that which is excreted by the body of a healthy person, one should feel safe to resort to feeding the body.*

Says the commentator: Galen says that the throat also receives the humors that descend from the brain and that pustules and abscesses indeed occur when the blood is heated through the yellow bile. Then, one should examine and look whether nature has expelled all the superfluities to the diseased parts. You will know that this is the case if that which is excreted from the diseased body resembles that which is excreted from the body when it is healthy. In that case, there is no danger in feeding the patient. But if one has not completely cleansed the body of the humor, one will find bile prevailing in the excretion of the body. In that case, one should cleanse and purge the body of the patient before feeding him, because the more one feeds a body that is not clean, the more one harms it. [*In Hippocratis Aphorismos commentarius* II.15].

(II.16) (68) Says Hippocrates: *When a person is hungry, he should not tire himself out.*

Says the commentator: With a small intake of food, one should avoid physical exercise. The reason for this is clear.

(II.17) (69) Says Hippocrates: *If the body receives an amount of food that is much larger than is natural for that body, it produces disease, as the recovery shows.*

Says the commentator: It seems to me that his intention in this aphorism is to tell us that if the intake of food is much larger than is natural—whether in quantity or in quality—it produces disease. The severity of the illness is according to the degree of deviation of the intake of food from what is natural. If the deviation is large, it produces a severe illness. But if the deviation that produces the illness is small, then the illness will be light. He also said that the degree of deviation is indicated by observing the body's recovery: If the deviation is small, the recovery is quick.

(II.18) (70) Says Hippocrates: *Foods that nourish quickly and all at once are also quickly excreted.*

Says the commentator: That which nourishes most quickly and suddenly is wine. The meaning of the term "quickly" is a short time after ingestion. The term "suddenly" means that once one starts to feed the body, it uses up (assimilates) all the food all at once and does not attract it little by little.

(II.19) (71) Says Hippocrates: *To predict either death or recovery in the case of acute diseases is not quite safe.*

Says the commentator: Galen says that fever, in the case of an acute illness, is most often continuous, for only a small number of acute illnesses, such as apoplexy, occur without fever. [*In Hippocratis Aphorismos commentarius* II.19].

(II.20) (72) Says Hippocrates: *He who has loose bowels when he is young will have constipated ones when he grows old, and he who has constipated bowels when he is young will have loose bowels when he grows old.*

Says the commentator: When I tried to verify this statement, I found that it is not universal and therefore it is a false assertion without any doubt. In my opinion, the truth is that Hippocrates saw one or two persons in whom this happened and turned that into an indefinite verdict, as was his habit in the major part of his book *Epidemics*, because on the basis of the investigation of the condition of one or two persons his assertion turns into a judgment regarding the whole category (species). These are, in my opinion, the true facts. If you do not want to acknowledge this, but prefer to give this incorrect statement a semblance of truth by attaching certain conditions and prerequisites to it, then you should look into what Galen said in his commentary to this aphorism. [*In Hippocratis Aphorismos commentarius* II.20].

(II.21) (73) Says Hippocrates: *Drinking* sharāb *alleviates* (*cures*) *hunger.*

Says the commentator: With *sharāb*, he means "wine" and with "hunger," here he means "canine appetite," for the drinking of wine, which has a strong warming effect, relieves this hunger. Canine appetite originates either from a cold temperament of the stomach alone or from an acid humor that has been absorbed by its substance. Wine, as mentioned, cures both conditions together.

(II.22) (74) Says Hippocrates: *Illnesses that arise from repletion are cured by depletion and those that arise from depletion are cured by repletion. All diseases are cured by opposites.*

Says the commentator: This is clear.

(II.23) (75) Says Hippocrates: *Acute diseases come to a crisis in fourteen days.*

Says the commentator: Galen says that none of the acute diseases that have a uniform movement and continuous pace (progress) goes beyond this limit. In many acute diseases, the crisis may come on the eleventh, ninth, seventh, or fifth day. In some of them it may occur on the sixth day, but this is not a good crisis. Hippocrates is used to generally call those illnesses that have a complete crisis on the fourteenth day or earlier "acute diseases." As for diseases in which there is an incomplete crisis on one of the first days of the crisis, and in which there remains a part of the crisis, and which complete their crisis on one of the subsequent days, up to the fourteenth day, he calls them "acute diseases whose crisis occurs on the fourteenth day." [*In Hippocratis Aphorismos commentarius* II.23].

(II.24) (76) Says Hippocrates: *The fourth day is indicative of the seventh; the eighth day is the beginning of the second week; the eleventh day is indicative of the fourteenth because it is the fourth day of the second week. The seventeenth day is also a day of prognostic indication since it is the fourth day from the fourteenth and the seventh day from the eleventh.*

Says the commentator: Galen says that the seventeenth day is indicative of the twentieth because the twentieth day is a day of crisis and it is the end of the third week. [*In Hippocratis Aphorismos commentarius* II.24].

(II.25) (77) Says Hippocrates: *The summer quartan fevers are mostly short and the autumn ones long, especially those contracted when winter is near.*

Says the commentator: Not only quartan fever is short in summer, but all other diseases, because the humors liquefy and are dispersed throughout the whole body and dissolve. As a result, all summer diseases are of a short duration. However, Hippocrates only speaks about the longest disease as an example. And in winter, the opposite is the case, that is to say, that the humors remain in the depth of the body as if they were petrified and their strength retains its vehemence. The diseases do not end since the humors that produce them are still there. The patients do not die since their strength remains and does not dissolve.

(II.26) (78) Says Hippocrates: *It is better that the fever occurs after the spasm than the spasm after the fever.*

Says the commentator: A spasm occurs either because of overfilling or of evacuation. If the spasm occurs because of overfilling, the nerves are filled with cold, viscous humor, with which they are nourished, and if fever occurs after the spasm, the fever often heats, dilutes, liquefies, and dissolves the humor. But if a person is affected by ardent fever, it dries his whole body and his nerves, and then the spasm occurs because of the dryness and the affliction is severe.

(II.27) (79) Says Hippocrates: *One should not be deceived by alleviation of a disease occurring to a patient, when it is illogical (irregular), nor should one fear a deterioration when it is illogical (irregular), because most such occurrences are uncertain and are hardly ever permanent and protracted.*

Says the commentator: When a serious disease occurs and then there is an alleviation all of a sudden without previous concoction or evacuation of the humors that produce the illness, one should not rely thereon, because the humors have become slow and subsided and their movements have diminished; that's all. Likewise, if a clear concoction precedes and then there occurs bad (difficult) breathing and mental confusion (delirium) and the like, one should not be afraid, because it is not permanent and often indicates a beneficial crisis.

(II.28) (80) Says Hippocrates: *If someone suffers from a fever that is not very light and his body remains as it is and it does not lose any weight and does not waste more than necessary, it is a bad sign, because the former indicates a long disease and the latter indicates that the strength of the body is weak.*

Says the commentator: Emaciation of the body is always a bad sign and indicates weakness of the strength of the body, regardless whether the fever is not very light (mild) or is very strong.

(II.29) (81) Says Hippocrates: *If you think that you can move something, do so, as long as the disease is in the beginning. But if the disease reaches its culmination, the patient should rest and repose.*

Says the commentator: The reason for this is given by him in the next aphorism. With the statement: "If you think that you can move something, do so," he especially means bleeding and sometimes one may also apply purgation. But none of these should be applied in the time in which the disease reaches its culmination, because the concoction of the disease takes place at that time and the psychical faculty is mostly exhausted at the time of the climax. To apply evacuation in the beginning of the disease is the best help for a concoction as quickly as possible, so that the superfluous matter causing the disease is diminished. The vital faculty and the natural faculty retain their strength at the time of the climax.

Says the commentator: He has already stated before that one should not purge in the beginning of a disease except for diseases that flare up. For this reason, here he remarks that if you think that you can move something you should do so.

(II.30) (82) Says Hippocrates: *All things are weaker at the beginning and end of the disease, but stronger at its culmination.*

Says the commentator: With "things," he means symptoms, because these, that is to say, the fever attacks, sleeplessness, pain, distress, and thirst, are milder at the beginning and end of the disease. The condition, from which these symptoms originate—namely, the disease—is necessarily at its best at the time of the culmination when the patient is one of those who are saved.

(II.31) (83) Says Hippocrates: *If the convalescent has a good appetite, but his body does not put on any weight, it is a bad sign.*

Says the commentator: This is clear and the matter has already been mentioned before.

(II.32) (84) Says Hippocrates: *In most cases, if someone with a bad constitution has a good appetite at the beginning of a disease, but does not put on any weight, he will lose his appetite in the end. However, if someone has a strong aversion of taking food in the beginning, but has a good appetite in the end, he will be better off.*

Says the commentator: He is speaking here about a convalescent. It is clear that—because of a bad temperament or because of a remnant of superfluous humors—his organs are not nourished, although he has a strong appetite in the beginning. And when he eats, his humors increase and his bad temperament becomes worse, so that he loses his appetite. But if he does not have an appetite in the beginning, because nature is busy with the concoction of the food, one should know that from the time when he starts to have an appetite, his humors have been concocted and his condition will mostly continue to improve.

(II.33) (85) Says Hippocrates: *A healthy state of mind is a good sign in every illness, and likewise a good appetite. The opposite is a bad sign.*

Says the commentator: This is clear. I have explained the reason for this in the aphorisms that I composed.

(II.34) (86) Says Hippocrates: *When the illness corresponds to the nature, age, and complexion of the patient and to the current time of the year, the danger is less than when the illness does not correspond to one of these factors.*

Says the commentator: This is clear, because if it does not correspond, it indicates that the temperament of the patient is very unbalanced.

(II.35) (87) Says Hippocrates: *In all diseases it is best that the parts around the navel and the lower abdomen keep their fullness. If they are very thin and emaciated, it is a bad sign. Moreover, if the latter is the case, purgation is dangerous.*

Says the commentator: The lower abdomen is the area between the genitals and the navel. The abdomen has three parts: the hypochondrium and the parts around the navel and the lower abdomen. If these regions are fuller, it is better, but if they are leaner, it is worse. The latter is a bad sign and a bad cause for the illness. It is a bad sign, because it indicates the weakness of those parts that are emaciated and dissolved. It is a bad cause, because the digestion of the food in the stomach and the production of the blood in the liver are not as they should be in this condition. These two organs benefit from the thick and fat layer that covers them because it warms them.

(II.36) (88) Says Hippocrates: *If someone with a healthy body is treated with a purgative or emetic, he will quickly faint. The same occurs to someone who feeds himself with bad food.*

Says the commentator: "The same occurs to someone who feeds himself with bad food." This means that if he is treated with an emetic or purgative, he will quickly faint because his body contains a surplus of bad superfluities. If the remedy only irritates it a little bit, then the bad condition of his body becomes clear and apparent. This is Galen's argumentation. But in my opinion, it is caused by the fact that, if someone constantly takes bad foods, his blood becomes extremely bad and its quality is corrupted. And if the medicine that he takes attracts the bad blood through its attractive power, it moves all the blood in his body and attempts to cleanse it of all its corrupt parts. These are extremely numerous and amalgamated; moreover, they are the vessel of the life of this person with this corrupt regimen. Fainting necessarily occurs because of the power of the attraction and because of the large quantity of amalgamated, mixed bad blood that the medicine attempts to attract.

(II.37) (89) Says Hippocrates: *If someone is in a good bodily condition, it is hard to purge him.*

Says the commentator: If a healthy person takes an emetic or purgative, he will suffer from dizziness, colic, and a difficult evacuation. He will also faint easily because the medication attempts to attract the appropriate humor. If it does not find so, it attracts the blood and the flesh and forces from them the extraction of that which is appropriate to it.

(II.38) (90) Says Hippocrates: *With regard to food and drink one should prefer something that is slightly inferior but tastes better above something that is better but tastes worse.*

Says the commentator: This is clear, because something that is more pleasant is better digested.

(II.39) (91) Says Hippocrates: *In most cases, old people fall ill less often than the young, but when they contract chronic ailments, they mostly die while still suffering from them.*

Says the commentator: Old people are stricter in their regimen than young people. However, their bodily strength is weak and unable to quickly concoct the diseases. All chronic ailments are cold and therefore lead necessarily to their death.

(II.40) (92) Says Hippocrates: *Hoarseness and catarrhs are not concocted* (*do not ripen*) *in the very old.*

Says the commentator: This holds good not only for these ailments but with all other ailments caused by cold humors.

(II.41) (93) Says Hippocrates: *If someone suffers from frequent and severe fainting without obvious cause, he will die suddenly.*

Says the commentator: If someone suffers from fainting under the following three conditions: there is no apparent cause, it is severe, and it occurs often, it will happen to him because of a weakness of the vital faculty.

(II.42) (94) Says Hippocrates: *If a stroke is severe, it is impossible for the patient to recover, and he will not recover easily if it is a mild one.*

Says the commentator: A stroke only occurs when the psychical pneuma is unable to stream into that part of the body that is below the head. This happens either because of a type of swelling occurring in the brain or because the ventricles of the brain are filled with phlegmatic moisture. If a stroke patient is unable to move his chest (cannot breathe), it is a stroke that is most severe and most dangerous. If he breathes with extreme coercion (difficulty), the stroke is also severe but not as severe as the previous one. If he breathes without exertion and coercion (difficulty), but the breathing is unequal and irregular, the stroke is also severe, but less severe than the previous one. If the stroke patient breathes regularly, the stroke he suffers from is light. If you proceed cautiously in the matter in all that is necessary to do, you may cure him.

(II.43) (95) Says Hippocrates: *Those who are strangled by hanging and lose consciousness but are not dead yet will not recover if they have foam at the mouth.*

Says the commentator: Galen mentions that some of those who were strangled by hanging or who strangled themselves (committed suicide) and foam appeared in their mouth, yet recovered. But that this is exceptional. [*In Hippocratis Aphorismos commentarius* II.43].

(II.44) (96) Says Hippocrates: *If someone is naturally very fat, he is apt to die earlier than someone who is lean.*

Says the commentator: The reason for this is clear, namely, the narrowness of the vessels and their width as Galen explained in *De temperamentis* [II.4].

Galen further states: If the body is well-fleshed and balanced so that it is neither fat nor lean it is best, for then a person will possibly live long and reach extreme old age. [*In Hippocratis Aphorismos commentarius* II.44].

(II.45) (97) Says Hippocrates: *If someone suffering from epilepsy is young, he is above all cured from it by a change in age, place, and regimen.*

Says the commentator: Epilepsy and apoplexy are both produced by a cold, thick humor. If someone's age, place, and regimen change into one that is hot and dry, and if there is also a change in the bad diet that produced this humor to the opposite thereof, he may recover.

(II.46) (98) Says Hippocrates: *If someone suffers from two pains at the same time, but not in the same place, the stronger one obscures the other.*

Says the commentator: When nature turns towards the organ in which there is the pain that is more severe, the sensation of pain in the other place becomes less, so that the patient may not feel that pain anymore.

(II.47) (99) Says Hippocrates: *Pain and fever occur when pus is forming rather than when it has been formed.*

Says the commentator: This happens because then the site of the swelling stretches more and more and the pain gets worse. The heat tends towards the pus in order to concoct it and spreads more and more and the fever intensifies.

(II.48) (100) Says Hippocrates: *In every movement of the body, rest at the beginning of pain will prevent further pain.*

Says the commentator: This is clear.

(II.49) (101) Says Hippocrates: *If a person is used to a certain labor, even if he has a weak body or is old, he is better able to bear it than someone who is not used to it, even if the latter is strong and young.*

Says the commentator: This is clear.

(II.50) (102) Says Hippocrates: *If someone has been used to something for a long time, even if it is more harmful than something to which he has not been used to, it will be less harmful to him. But sometimes it may be necessary to change to things one is not used to.*

Says the commentator: He has laid down a correct premise and has drawn conclusions from it. This premise also implies that regarding the preservation of health in all circumstances one should accustom oneself to change from habit to habit, but only gradually so.

Galen says that it is best for everyone to attempt trying everything to which he is not accustomed, so that when he encounters something unusual—which inevitably happens—it will not cause him severe harm. He should do so by not always adhering to the same habits but by sometimes attempting to do the opposite.

(II.51) (103) Says Hippocrates: *It is dangerous to suddenly fill the body excessively, or to empty it, or to heat it, or to cool it, or to move it with any type of movement. Everything that is excessive is hostile to nature. But that which is done gradually is safe, especially if you want to change from one thing to another or if you want something else.*

Says the commentator: This is clear.

(II.52) (104) Says Hippocrates: *If you do everything that should be done according to the medical rules, but do not get the result that you should have according to the medical rules, do not change to another treatment as long as your original diagnosis remains.*

Says the commentator: This aphorism comprises a major rule regarding medical treatment. In his commentary on this rule, Galen does not go far enough (does not cover everything necessary).

The meaning of this aphorism is as follows: If the symptoms tell you, for instance, that one should apply heating medications, and you did so for a long time but the patient did not recover, you should not change to another regimen, but continue to apply heating medications as long as the symptoms suggesting these medications remain. This is the meaning of his statement: "as long as your original diagnosis remains." And this is the meaning of his statement: "do not change to another treatment," that one should not change from one type of treatment to another type of treatment. However, it is certainly appropriate to change from one heating medication to another heating medication and to alternate between all simple and compound medications that have a heating effect, because when a body becomes used to one and the same medicine that has been taken constantly, its effect on the body becomes less. Moreover, to alternate between different types of medications that have the same quality is extremely appropriate for every temperament of every singular person, and of every singular organ, and for the afflictions coming with every singular disease. This is a major principle of the secrets of treatment. Exactly the same method should be applied with regard to nutrition, the different kinds of evacuation of the humor that causes the illness, and with regard to medications that dissolve, refine, concoct, or thicken matter, or medications that are astringent. Always adhere to the type of therapy that is indicated by symptoms that remain the same and alternate between the different medications and nutrients that are of the same kind. Understand this.

(II.53) (105) Says Hippocrates: *If someone has loose bowels, as long as he is young his condition will be better than that of someone who has hard bowels. But when he gets old his condition will be worse, because his bowels will be hard as is mostly the case in old people.*

Says the commentator: He has already spoken before about looseness and hardness of the stool during youth and during old age. Galen attempts to give the reasons for this repetition. [*In Hippocratis Aphorismos commentarius* II.53]. I have already given my opinion about this statement by Hippocrates. Moreover, loose bowels are always, in all ages, one of the reasons for lasting health and hard bowels are bad both for healthy and for ill people.

(II.54) (106) Says Hippocrates: *A large body is not unpleasing when one is young, on the contrary, it is desirable; however, when one is old, it is a burden and hard to use (inconvenient). It is worse than a body that is less in size.*

Says the commentator: Galen holds the opinion that with the term "largeness of the body," Hippocrates means its length so that this proposition is not merely a presumption (supposition).

This is the end of the second part of the commentary on the Aphorisms.

In the name of God,
the Merciful, the Compassionate

The Third Part of the *Commentary on Hippocrates'* Aphorisms

(III.1) (107) Says Hippocrates: *Especially the changes of the seasons of the year produce diseases and in every singular season, the great changes in cold or in heat, and similarly all other changes in the weather follow the same rule.*

Says the commentator: With a change in the nature of the seasons, he means that, for instance, the winter season is hot or the summer season cold, and the like. Similarly, a change in every singular season means that a big change in its normal temperament produces diseases, even though the other seasons do not change.

(III.2) (108) Says Hippocrates: *There are some people whose natures are in a better condition in summer and in a worse condition in winter, and there are others whose natures are in a better condition in winter and in a worse condition in summer.*

Says the commentator: With the term "natures," he means the temperaments of people and this is clear because in winter, the condition of people with a hot temperament is better and in summer, the condition of people with a cold temperament is better. In this way one should draw an analogy.

(III.3) (109) Says Hippocrates: *The condition of every singular disease is better or worse in relation to another. Similarly, someone's age is better or worse in relation to the seasons of the year, the places where one lives, and the kinds of regimen one adheres to.*

Says the commentator: If you properly arrange the words of this aphorism, it will be very clear. Similarly, if you arrange every singular illness, its condition in relation to every particular age, or place, or season of the year, or regimen will be better or worse. For instance, the condition of someone suffering from a cold disease will be better when he is young, when it is summer, when he lives in a hot place, and follows a hot regimen. But in the opposite conditions, it will be worse. In general, something is better for something else, when they are opposites. And something similar and unbalanced is very bad for something else that is similar to it and unbalanced in the same aspect. But for someone whose temperament is balanced because of his age, a moderate regimen, temperate season and place are most appropriate. Only the condition of someone with such a temperament is improved by similar things. For those whose temperament is unbalanced, opposite places, seasons, and kinds of regimen are most appropriate.

(III.4) (110) Says Hippocrates: *If during any season of the year now heat and now cold occurs on the same day, you must expect the occurrence of autumnal diseases.*

Says the commentator: This is clear.

(III.5) (111) Says Hippocrates: *The south wind causes hardness of hearing, dimness of vision, heaviness of the head, indolence and relaxation* (*weakness*). *When this wind becomes strong and prevails, these symptoms occur to those who suffer from diseases. The north wind causes cough, a sore throat, dryness of the abdomen* (*constipation*), *dysuria, shivering, pain in the ribs* (*sides*) *and chest. When this wind becomes strong and prevails, one should expect these symptoms to occur in illnesses.*

Says the commentator: The south wind is hot and moist and therefore it produces dimness of the senses and moistens the origin of the nerves. As a result, indolence and difficulty of moving occur. The north wind is cold and dry and thus causes rawness of the throat (hoarseness) and chest (cough), dryness of the abdomen (constipation), thickness (obstruction) of the passages, and consequently all the symptoms mentioned above occur.

(III.6) (112) Says Hippocrates: *When the summer is similar to the spring, expect much sweating during fevers.*

Says the commentator: When the summer is severely dry, perspiration necessarily evaporates and moisture dissolves. When the summer resembles spring, the moisture is necessarily drawn towards the area of the skin, because of its heat, but summer cannot dissolve the moisture in the way of vapor because of its fluidity. Since the moisture is evacuated suddenly during the crisis of the illness, much sweating occurs from it.

(III.7) (113) Says Hippocrates: *During droughts, acute fevers occur and if the year is extremely dry and a dry condition of the air is produced, these diseases and their like should be expected most of all.*

Says the commentator: It is clear that during droughts, the humors become dry and sharp and that consequently fevers are less frequent but qualitatively more acute.

(III.8) (114) Says Hippocrates: *If the seasons of the year are regular and come with the things that are proper to them, the illnesses that occur in them are regular and have an easy crisis. But if the seasons of the year are irregular, the illnesses occurring in them are irregular and their crises are bad.*

Says the commentator: This is clear.

(III.9) (115) Says Hippocrates: *In autumn, illnesses are most acute and, in general, most fatal. Spring is the healthiest season and least fatal.*

Says the commentator: Spring is moderate and in autumn the weather is extremely dissimilar (variable).

(III.10) (116) Says Hippocrates: *Autumn is bad for those who suffer from phthisis.*

Says the commentator: Because autumn is cold and dry and variable in temperament, it is very harmful for those who suffer from phthisis.

(III.11) (117) Says Hippocrates: *As for the seasons of the year, if the winter comes with little rain and the wind is northerly and the spring is wet and the wind south-*

erly, acute fevers, ophthalmia, and dysentery necessarily occur in the summer. Dysentery mostly affects women and those with moist natures (constitutions).

Says the commentator: This is clear once you know the principles of the medical art.

(III.12) (118) Says Hippocrates: *If winter comes with south winds; if it is rainy and mild and spring comes with little rain and north winds: women whose term of delivery happens to be around spring will have a miscarriage from the slightest cause, while those who do deliver, give birth to children that are weak and sickly, so these children either die immediately, or—if they survive—are emaciated and sickly all their lives. The rest of the population is affected by dysentery and dry ophthalmia, while old people suffer from catarrhs that quickly are fatal.*

(III.13) (119) Says Hippocrates: *If summer comes with little rain and with north winds and autumn is wet with south winds: severe headache, cough, hoarseness, and rheums occur in winter. Some people suffer from phthisis.*

(III.14) (120) Says Hippocrates: *But if autumn comes with north winds and is dry, it is beneficial to those whose nature (constitution) is moist and to women. Others suffer from dry ophthalmia, acute fevers, chronic rheums, and some of them suffer from melancholic delusion caused by black bile.*

(III.15) (121) Says Hippocrates: *Of the conditions of the weather during the year, less rain is—in general—healthier and less deadly than more rain.*

(III.16) (122) *Says Hippocrates: The illnesses that mostly occur during a lot of rain, are chronic fevers, diarrhea, putrefaction, epilepsy, apoplexy, and angina. The illnesses that occur during a lack of rain are phthisis, ophthalmia, arthritis, strangury, and dysentery.*

Says the commentator: All what Hippocrates mentions in these five aphorisms concerning certain diseases that occur to certain people under certain weather conditions, is not the rule by any means. For this reason, it is not necessary to give the causes for these diseases as is well known to someone who studies philosophy (logic). However, Galen attempts to give the cause for all these diseases and to inform us that—in general—with the knowledge regarding the natures of the seasons and the individual persons and regarding the causes of the diseases, which is fundamental in the art of medicine, and with the knowledge that moisture is the substance of putrefaction and that heat activates it, it is easy to give the causes of all the diseases that Hippocrates mentions, when they occur. [*In Hippocratis Aphorismos commentarius* III.12–16].

(III.17) (123) Says Hippocrates: *As for the daily conditions of the weather: A north wind braces the body, makes it vigorous and strong, improves its movement and complexion, clarifies one's hearing, dries up the bowels, and causes stinging of the eyes. If there is a pre-existing pain in the region of the chest, it is stimulated and aggravated by it. However, a south wind makes the body loose and relaxed, moistens it, causes heaviness of the head, hardness of hearing and vertigo, and difficulty of movement of the eyes and of the whole body, and looseness of the bowels.*

Says the commentator: It has already been noted that the north wind is cold and dry and that the south wind is hot and moist. All this is clear.

(III.18) (124) Says Hippocrates: *As to the seasons of the year, in spring and the beginning of summer, children and those next to them in age enjoy the greatest well-being and the most perfect health. During the rest of summer and the first part of autumn, old people enjoy the greatest well-being. During the rest of autumn and winter, those of intermediate age enjoy the greatest well-being.*

Says the commentator: I have already given the reason for this in the aphorism in which I altered the order of his words.

(III.19) (125) Says Hippocrates: *All diseases occur during all seasons of the year, but some of them are more likely to occur and to flare up in certain seasons.*

Says the commentator: This is clear.

(III.20) (126) Says Hippocrates: *In spring, the following diseases may occur: melancholic delusion, madness, epilepsy, hemorrhages, angina, rheum, hoarseness, cough, peeling of the skin, eczema, alphos, many ulcerative eruptions, tumors, and arthritis.*

Says the commentator: This aphorism explains in detail what has been said in the previous aphorism, namely, that every kind of disease can occur in every season of the year, but that some diseases are more likely to occur during certain seasons and those are the ones that mostly occur during that season. He concluded this matter by stating that in spring, which is the most moderate season, the following diseases may occur: diseases caused by black bile, such as melancholic delusion and madness; diseases caused by phlegm, such as epilepsy, rheum, hoarseness, and cough; diseases caused by yellow bile, such as ulcerative eruptions and tumors; and diseases related to blood, such as hemorrhages and angina. However, the diseases that are specific to spring, are those that occur as a result of the dissolution of humors and their excretion and the movement of nature to expel them forcefully. Likewise, the next aphorism is based on our explanation that illnesses sometimes occur contrary to the nature of the season of the year.

(III.21) (127) Says Hippocrates: *During summer, there occur some of the diseases just mentioned as well as continuous fevers, ardent fevers, and many tertian fevers, vomiting, diarrhea, ophthalmia, earache, ulcers in the mouth, putrefaction in the genitals, and heat-spots.*

(III.22) (128) Says Hippocrates: *In autumn occur most summer diseases as well as quartan and mixed (irregular) fevers, affections of the spleen, dropsy, phthisis, strangury, dysentery, lientery, pain in the hip (sciatica), angina, asthma, the severe colic that the Greeks call "ileus," epilepsy, madness, and melancholic delusion.*

Says the commentator: All this is clear from what we said before.

(III.23) (129) Says Hippocrates: *In winter occur pleurisy, pneumonia, rheum, hoarseness, cough, pains in the sides and loins, headache, dizziness, and apoplexy.*

Says the commentator: This too is based on what has been stated before, because during winter, diseases occur that are mostly specific to it, such as rheum, hoarseness, and apoplexy, but also diseases that are not specific to its nature, such as pleurisy.

(III.24) (130) Says Hippocrates: *In the different ages, the following diseases occur: Small children and new-born infants suffer from aphthae, vomiting, cough, sleeplessness, fright (nightmares), inflammation of the navel, and discharge from the ears.*

Says the commentator: They suffer from aphthae because of the softness of their bodily parts and the sharpness of the milk; vomiting occurs to them because of excessive nursing, the weakness of the retentive faculty since they have too much moisture. They suffer from cough because of the moisture of the lungs and the large quantity of moisture streaming to the lungs from the brain. This is also the cause of the discharge from the ears, because superfluities of the brain stream towards them. They suffer from inflammation of the navel because of the shortness of time since it was cut. Fright occurs mostly during sleep because the digestion of the food in the stomach is corrupted so that vapors arise to the brain and cause frightening imaginations (illusions). As for sleeplessness, Galen did not know its cause, but said that what is specific to children is that they sleep much. [*In Hippocratis Aphorismos commentarius* III.24]. This is correct. However, they often suffer from sleeplessness and cry all night long. The reason for this is their excessive sensitivity due to the softness of their bodies. Moreover, their powers are weak and not firm and the slightest pain will wake them up. It only happens rarely that they do not suffer from a poor digestion and restlessness caused by a bad digestion of the food in their stomach because they suckle too much. The pain resulting from this wakes them up and keeps them awake. If the pain becomes a little bit stronger, they cry. This is what we always see happening in little children and new-born infants.

(III.25) (131) Says Hippocrates: *When a child gets near to the time that he gets teeth, he suffers from irritation in the gums, fevers, cramps, and diarrhea, especially when the canine teeth begin to erupt. This also happens in the case of fat children and those who have constipated bowels.*

Says the commentator: All this occurs because the teeth break through and perforate the flesh of the gums and widen the opening. The resulting pain is followed by fever and cramps. Diarrhea occurs because the food is not well digested due to the pain and sleeplessness. Cramps occur mostly to fat children and those who have constipated bowels because of the excess of superfluities in their bodies.

(III.26) (132) Says Hippocrates: *When a child gets older, he is affected by inflammations of the throat, inward thrust (curvature) of the vertebrae of the neck, asthma, stones, roundworms, other intestinal worms (flatworms), warts, scrofula, and other tumors.*

Says the commentator: After dentition until nearly thirteen years of age, children take much food and drink a lot; they take food after food and do much exercise after a meal. This whole regimen corrupts the digestions and increases the humors, while their bodies are still moist and their organs soft and all the afflictions we mentioned necessarily occur to these children. When the muscles of the throat swell, they pull the vertebrae of the neck because of the softness of their ligaments.

(III.27) (133) Says Hippocrates: *As for those who are older than thirteen and approach the growing of pubic hair (puberty), many of these illnesses occur to them and also fevers that last longer and nosebleeds.*

Says the commentator: At this age, the blood increases and flows in these children and therefore nosebleeds occur to them when they are ill.

(III.28) (134) Says Hippocrates: *In most cases diseases occurring to children reach the crisis in some in forty days, in some in seven months, in some in seven years, and in some at the approach of puberty. However, those diseases that persist and do not dissolve at the time of puberty in boys or at the time of the menstruation in girls, have the property (tend) to become chronic.*

Says the commentator: With the term diseases, he means chronic diseases.

(III.29) (135) Says Hippocrates: *Young people suffer from hemoptysis, phthisis, acute fevers, epilepsy, and other diseases, but mostly they suffer from the diseases we have mentioned.*

Says the commentator: Galen has explained that epilepsy is in no way specific to young people, but is also one of the diseases occurring to children. [*In Hippocratis Aphorismos commentarius* III.29].

(III.30) (136) Says Hippocrates: *Those who are beyond that age suffer from asthma, pleurisy, pneumonia, fever associated with sleeplessness, fever associated with mental confusion (phrenitis), ardent fever, cholera, chronic diarrhea, abrasion of the intestines, lientery, and hemorrhoids.*

Says the commentator: It is known that in this age, namely, that of people past their prime, black bile is mostly very evident and therefore mental confusion (delirium), sleeplessness, and hemorrhoids are peculiar to them during fevers. As to the other illnesses enumerated by him, these are not peculiar to people of this age.

Galen maintains that he has given specific reasons for the illnesses of this age, but that is not so. [*In Hippocratis Aphorismos commentarius* III.30].

(III.31) (137) Says Hippocrates: *Old people suffer from difficulty of breathing and catarrhs associated with cough, strangury, dysuria, arthritis, nephritis, dizziness, apoplexy, bad tumors, pruritus of the body, sleeplessness, loose bowels, watery discharge from the eyes and nostrils, dim-sightedness, cataract, and hardness of hearing.*

Says the commentator: The reasons for these diseases are all of them clear from what is known from the condition of the temperament of old people.

This is the end of the third part of the
commentary on the Aphorisms.
Praise be to God alone.

In the name of God,
the Merciful, the Compassionate

The Fourth Part of the *Commentary on Hippocrates'* Aphorisms

(IV.1) (138) Says Hippocrates: *It is proper to administer purgative drugs to pregnant women when the humors in their body flare up, from when the fetus is four months old until it becomes seven months old. But in the latter case, one should proceed to administer a smaller dose. When a fetus is younger than four months or older than seven months, one should be very careful in the administration of these drugs.*

Says the commentator: This is clear because at the beginning, the fetus is weak and can be easily aborted, and at the end of the pregnancy, it is heavy and large and thus contributes to a miscarriage because of its heaviness.

(IV.2) (139) Says Hippocrates: *Drugs should be administered to evacuate from the body such substances, which—if spontaneously excreted—would be beneficial. But substances of an opposite character should be stopped.*

Says the commentator: This is clear.

(IV.3) (140) Says Hippocrates: *If the body is purged from such substances as should be evacuated, it is beneficial and easily borne. But if the opposite is the case, it is borne with difficulty.*

Says the commentator: He tells us this here so that it can serve as a diagnostic sign through which we know whether our conjecture was correct or whether we erred, that is to say, whether the patient bore the evacuation with ease or with difficulty.

(IV.4) (141) Says Hippocrates: *Evacuation by drugs should be effected more from above in summer and more from below in winter.*

Says the commentator: The yellow bile and the heat that dominate in summer cause the humors to move upwards continuously. Therefore, evacuation through emesis is to be preferred. During winter, the opposite is the case.

(IV.5) (142) Says Hippocrates: *After the time of the rising of the Dog Star (Sirius), during the time of its ascent, and before it, evacuation through drugs is difficult.*

Says the commentator: That is the hottest time of summer; the powers of the body are extremely weak and the heat of the air opposes the attracting force of the remedy, so that nothing results from it except weakness and disturbance.

(IV.6) (143) Says Hippocrates: *Those who have a lean body and thus easily vomit should be evacuated with emetic remedies from above, but beware of doing so in winter.*

Says the commentator: The condition of lean persons is always similar to that of most people in summer. The prohibition against the application of emesis in winter has already been stated before.

(IV.7) (144) Says Hippocrates: *If vomiting is difficult for a person and he is moderately corpulent, one should evacuate him with purgative remedies from below, but beware of doing so in summer.*

Says the commentator: This is clear.

(IV.8) (145) Says Hippocrates: *If you evacuate those who suffer from phthisis with purgative remedies, beware of evacuating them from above.*

Says the commentator: He means those who are predisposed to get phthisis, namely, those who have a narrow chest. Since they also have narrow passages in their lungs, you should not convey to them superfluous matters.

(IV.9) (146) Says Hippocrates: *Those whose temperament is dominated by black bile should also be evacuated from below with a remedy that is more solid (stronger), if one applies the same reasoning to these two opposite cases.*

Says the commentator: With a more solid remedy, he means a stronger remedy. The yellow bile streams upwards and the black bile sinks downwards. The same reasoning is to be applied by choosing one of the two opposites for each of these two humors, since we evacuate each humor from the spot where it is most likely to exit the body.

(IV.10) (147) Says Hippocrates: *In the case of very acute illnesses, one should apply evacuating (purging) remedies from the first day when the humors flare up, because it is bad to delay their application in such cases.*

Says the commentator: This is clear. One should be cautious not to leave behind these humors, which stream from site to site and do not rest. One should beware of letting them settle in a noble organ, but hasten to evacuate them before they weaken the strength of the patient or settle in the site of a noble organ.

(IV.11) (148) Says Hippocrates: *Those who suffer from colic, pains around the navel, and pain in the loins that are lasting and are not alleviated neither with purgatives nor with something else, will eventually develop dry dropsy.*

Says the commentator: If those pains are not alleviated through medical treatment, it indicates that a bad temperament prevails in those organs and has settled in them. This results in tympanites and this is the hydrops that he calls "dry," contrary to ascites in which there is water. Ascites originates from excessive cold.

(IV.12) (149) Says Hippocrates: *If someone suffers from lientery in winter, it is bad to evacuate him with medications from above.*

Says the commentator: This means that even if the lientery is caused by a sharp, thin humor that floats and requires evacuation by emesis, since it is winter, one should not apply emesis, as was mentioned before.

(IV.13) (150) Says Hippocrates: *If someone needs to be administered a hellebore potion and evacuation from above does not come to him easily, his body should be moistened with increased food and rest before he is administered the potion.*

Says the commentator: This is clear.

(IV.14) (151) Says Hippocrates: *If you administer a hellebore potion to someone, your intention should be to make that person move his body more and sleep and rest less. Travelling by boat too indicates that movement stirs up the body.*

Says the commentator: It is known that hellebore is a strong emetic. Movement of the body by local transport is also something that helps emesis, as can be concluded from the case of someone travelling by boat.

(IV.15) (152) Says Hippocrates: *When you wish that hellebore has a stronger evacuating effect, move the body; and when you wish it to stop, make the patient sleep and do not move him.*

Says the commentator: This is clear and repetitious.

(IV.16) (153) Says Hippocrates: *The ingestion of hellebore is dangerous to those who have healthy flesh, since it induces spasms.*

Says the commentator: This is clear.

(IV.17) (154) Says Hippocrates: *If someone has no fever, want of appetite, cardialgia (palpitation or heartburn), dizziness, and a bitter taste in the mouth, it indicates that he should be evacuated by a medication from above.*

Says the commentator: *Fu'ād* means the "cardia of the stomach," and *nakhs* means "stinging, biting," and *sadar* (dizziness) means that it seems to the patient as if everything he sees is turning around him and he suddenly loses the sense of sight so that he thinks that everything he saw is covered with darkness. These afflictions occur when there are bad humors in the cardia of the stomach that have a biting effect on it. Therefore, these humors should be evacuated through emesis, when these afflictions appear.

(IV.18) (155) Says Hippocrates: *Pains above the diaphragm indicate a need for evacuating (purging) through medication from above; pains below the diaphragm indicate a need for evacuating (purging) through medication from below.*

Says the commentator: To whatever side the humors tend to stream and settle, from that side one should evacuate with an emetic from above or purgative from below. During the time that the humors are actually flowing, one should attract them to the opposite side.

(IV.19) (156) Says Hippocrates: *If someone ingests a purging medicine and is being purged but is not thirsty, one should not stop the evacuation (purgation) until he becomes thirsty.*

Says the commentator: If thirst after the ingestion of a purgative medication does not result from the heat or dryness of the stomach or from the sharpness of the medication or from the fact that the evacuated humor was hot, this indicates that the organs have been cleansed and emptied from that humor, which one wanted to evacuate.

(IV.20) (157) Says Hippocrates: *If a person free from fever is affected by a colic, and heaviness in the knees, and pain in the loins, this indicates that he needs evacuation through a medication (purgation) from below.*

Says the commentator: This is clear.

(IV.21) (158) Says Hippocrates: *A black stool that resembles blood and comes spontaneously, either with or without fever, is one of the worst signs, and the more evil the colors of the stool, the worse the sign. If such stools occur after the ingestion of a purgative medication, it is a better sign and the more numerous the colors, the less evil it is.*

Says the commentator: This is clear.

(IV.22) (159) Says Hippocrates: *If, at the beginning of any illness, black bile is evacuated either from below or from above, it is a fatal symptom.*

Says the commentator: As long as the disease is in the beginning stages, nothing from what is excreted from the body of the patient is excreted through the movement of nature (in a natural way), rather, the excretion is an accident that is closely associated with the unnatural conditions of the body. The black bile mentioned by Hippocrates is the coarse humor, which—when it is burned—is similar to the lees of wine and has ceased to be the natural black bile. The excretion of these bad humors before they are concocted indicates that they bite (irritate) the organs because of the strength of their badness, and the organs are not capable to hold them until they are concocted.

(IV.23) (160) Says Hippocrates: *If someone has become weakened because of an acute or chronic disease, or miscarriage, or any other cause, and then passes black bile or something resembling black blood, he will die the next day.*

Says the commentator: The nature of someone with such a condition is so weakened that it cannot concoct nor select nor evacuate the humors, bad as they are. And because of the severity and gravity of the illness, they flow and pour forth since nothing can withhold them. His statement "something resembling black blood" means "black stools." The difference between black bile and black stools is that black bile is soluble, that it has a polishing and biting effect, similar to the biting of vinegar, and that it strips (scrapes) off the ground when it falls on it. None of these characteristics applies to black stools.

(IV.24) (161) Says Hippocrates: *If dysentery begins with the passage of black bile, it is a fatal sign.*

Says the commentator: If the discharge of yellow bile has come first and abraded and inflamed the intestines, and blood comes later, it is possible to cure this abrasion. However, if the black bile has abraded the intestines and then inflamed them until the dysentery began, the abrasion cannot be cured, because the intestines will be affected by something similar to cancer that occurs on the surface of the body.

(IV.25) (162) Says Hippocrates: *The evacuation of blood from above, whatever it is, is a bad sign; but its evacuation from below is a good sign if black humors are evacuated with it.*

Says the commentator: "From above" means through emesis. The evacuation from below is only good if nature expels it in the manner of cleansing superfluities as in the case of hemorrhoids, but on the condition that there is only a little.

(IV.26) (163) Says Hippocrates: *If someone has dysentery and he discharges something similar to pieces of flesh, it is a fatal sign.*

Says the commentator: This is so because it indicates that the tumor settled in (penetrated) the intestines to the point that it pierces its substance, and it is impossible for that flesh to be regenerated.

(IV.27) (164) Says Hippocrates: *If someone loses much blood from any site during fevers, he will suffer from loose bowels more than is normal if he is nourished during convalescence.*

Says the commentator: Because of the weakness of the innate heat in his body through the loss of blood, the attraction of the food to the intestines and their digestion in them weakens as well and, consequently, he suffers from loose bowels. [*In Hippocratis Aphorismos commentarius* IV.27].

(IV.28) (165) Says Hippocrates: *If someone who suffers from bilious diarrhea develops deafness, the diarrhea ceases; and if someone who is deaf is affected by bilious diarrhea, the deafness ceases.*

Says the commentator: The reason for this is clear, namely, the streaming of the superfluous matter in the opposite direction. It is also clear that it is a matter of deafness that occurs all of a sudden during illness, especially when the crisis is near.

(IV.29) (166) Says Hippocrates: *If rigor occurs to someone suffering from fever on the sixth day of his illness, the crisis will be hard.*

Says the commentator: If a rigor occurs during fevers, especially ardent fevers, it is usually followed by a crisis. The matter of the harmfulness of the crisis on the sixth day is well known and this is what he means with the term "hard."

(IV.30) (167) Says Hippocrates: *If someone has a fever illness with paroxysms, and if the fever returns on the next day at the very same hour that it left him on the previous day, his crisis will be difficult.*

Says the commentator: It is clear that if all the paroxysms of the fever are always the same in their beginning and end, it is an indication that the illness will be prolonged. And this is the meaning of his statement that the crisis will be difficult. It is as if he says that it will be difficult for this kind of fever to end with a crisis, because a crisis occurs, rather, in acute illnesses, whereas chronic illnesses dissolve over a long time.

(IV.31) (168) Says Hippocrates: *If someone with fever suffers from fatigue, abscesses will appear especially in his joints and near to the jaws.*

Says the commentator: Because of the heat of the fever and the heat of the organs in a patient with fatigue, the superfluity is expelled to the joints and to the upper part of the body where it is absorbed by the soft flesh in the joints of the jaws.

(IV.32) (169) Says Hippocrates: *If someone is recovering from an illness and a part of his body suffers pain, he will develop an abscess in that part.*

Says the commentator: He states that if a convalescent suffers from fatigue in one of his organs (parts) and develops pain in it, an abscess will form there. The reason for this is clear. Galen remarks that the occurrence of pain is also called "fatigue." [*In Hippocratis Aphorismos commentarius* IV.32].

(IV.33) (170) Says Hippocrates: *But if someone already suffered from pain in any organ (part) before he became ill, the illness will settle (establish itself) in that part.*

Says the commentator: This is clear. He refers here to the fatigue (pain) that precedes the illness, until it becomes the cause of the illness. In the previous aphorism, he speaks of the fatigue (pain) that occurs after leaving the disease behind (recovering from it). In the third aphorism before our aphorism, he mentions the fatigue (pain) that occurs during the disease itself. However, one should expect all the abscesses mentioned by him to occur in the case of crises that are not accompanied by a clear evacuation.

(IV.34) (171) Says Hippocrates: *If someone who is suffering from fever but has no swelling in the throat is suddenly seized by suffocation, it is a deadly symptom.*

Says the commentator: A sudden suffocation especially occurs as a result of the closure of the larynx, and the fever patient needs to inhale much cold air. If the air is prevented from passing, he will die without any doubt. He stipulated that there should be no swelling, because fever sometimes happens following a swelling in the throat. In such a case the suffocation develops slowly in relation to the growth of the swelling, and when the swelling reaches its acme, it may decrease slowly and the patient is saved.

(IV.35) (172) Says Hippocrates: *If someone is affected by fever and his neck is twisted around so that he can only swallow with difficulty, but no swelling is visible, it is a fatal sign.*

Says the commentator: The twisting of the neck and the difficulty to swallow result from straining a dorsal vertebra. The straining sometimes happens because of a swelling and sometimes because of the domination of dryness. The type of straining he means here is the one arising from the domination of dryness, for this indicates that the bad temperament has settled in the organs and that dryness is dominant.

(IV.36) (173) Says Hippocrates: *Perspiration is beneficial in a fever patient if it begins either on the third day, the fifth, the seventh, the ninth, the eleventh, the fourteenth, the seventeenth, the twentieth, the twenty-fourth, the twenty-seventh, the thirty-first, or thirty-fourth day, because perspiration on these days brings the disease to a crisis. However, perspiration not occurring on these days indicates evil and a lengthy disease.*

Says the commentator: This rule applies not only to perspiration but to all discharges during which there is a crisis. The nature of these critical days became known through experience. Every crisis occurs with perspiration or with another discharge. It has been established through experience that it mostly occurs on these days.

(IV.37) (174) Says Hippocrates: *If cold sweat occurs with high fever, it indicates death, but if it occurs with mild fever, it indicates that the disease will be prolonged.*

Says the commentator: The severity of the fever extinguishes the innate heat, so that the very cold humors, which are at the outside of the body and from which the cold sweat emerges, cannot be concocted. An indication of the crudeness of these humors and the severity of their cold can be derived from the fact that the high fever cannot heat those humors that emerge from the body.

(IV.38) (175) Says Hippocrates: *On whatever part of the body there is sweat, it indicates that the illness is in that part.*

Says the commentator: For this reason, the sweat only comes from that part where the humor is retained.

(IV.39) (176) Says Hippocrates: *Whatever part of the body is hot or cold, the disease is in that part.*

Says the commentator: This is clear.

(IV.40) (177) Says Hippocrates: *When changes occur in the whole body, if the body is sometimes cold and sometimes hot, or now has this color and then another color, it indicates a prolonged disease.*

Says the commentator: When the illness consists of many different kinds, it always lasts longer than the illness that is of one kind.

(IV.41) (178) Says Hippocrates: *Copious sweat occurring after sleep without any obvious cause indicates that someone has burdened his body with more food than it can tolerate. But if it occurs to someone and he is not taking any food, know that his body needs evacuation.*

Says the commentator: This is clear.

(IV.42) (179) Says Hippocrates: *Copious sweat, whether hot or cold, that flows constantly, indicates, when it is cold, that the illness is more serious, and when it is hot, that the illness is less serious.*

Says the commentator: He means that when the sweat that occurs during the days of the illness—other than as part of a crisis—is cold, the illness is more severe because it indicates coldness of the superfluous matter.

(IV.43) (180) Says Hippocrates: *If the fever is unremitting and grows worse every other day (turns into a tertian fever), it is exceedingly dangerous. But if it is intermittent in whatever way, this indicates that it is not dangerous.*

Says the commentator: The fever that is continuous is the one that grows worse every other day, and that is dangerous is the one called "semi-tertian."

(IV.44) (181) Says Hippocrates: *If someone is attacked by protracted fever, he will develop tumors or pain in the joints.*

Says the commentator: The duration of the fever depends upon the quantity of the superfluous matter, or the coldness of the matter, or the thickness of the humors. When this is the condition of the superfluous matter, it is mostly repelled to an organ where it causes a tumor or to a joint cavity where it causes pain in the joints.

(IV.45) (182) Says Hippocrates: *If someone is afflicted by a tumor or pain in the joints after the fever, he takes more food than he can tolerate.*

Says the commentator: "After the fever" means after the complete abatement of the fever, while the patient is still recovering.

(IV.46) (183) Says Hippocrates: *If a rigor occurs to someone who suffers from unremitting fever and has been weakened, it is a fatal sign.*

Says the commentator: Galen says that Hippocrates' words "when a rigor occurs to someone" indicate that it occurs continuously time and again and that its repeated occurrence—while the fever remains uninterrupted—indicates that nature tries to eject and expel the illness-producing humor, but cannot do so because it is firmly established in the organs and remains in them. The strength of the body is damaged and dwindles away more and more because it cannot tolerate the tremor of the rigor and its shaking effect on the body. [*In Hippocratis Aphorismos commentarius* IV.46].

(IV.47) (184) Says Hippocrates: *In unremitting fevers, livid expectorations that are similar to blood, or are fetid or bilious, are all bad. But if they are properly expelled, they are favorable. The same holds good for feces and urine. If something is excreted from one of these sites (the bowels and the bladder)* [*Aphorisms* VII.70] *from which excretion is not beneficial, it is bad.*

Says the commentator: This statement means that, in general, bad things that are evacuated indicate bad conditions in the bodies from which they are evacuated. But sometimes their evacuation is like the evacuation of serum from putrid ulcers, the evacuation of which is not beneficial in that disease. And sometimes their evacuation is like the evacuation of pus from an abscess that has broken and results in a beneficial cleansing for the diseased organ. The signs that indicate that the evacuation of a superfluous matter is beneficial are, above all, its concoction, that the body easily tolerates its excretion and that it finds relief through it, and also that it is according to the nature of the illness, and hereafter that it is according to the current time of the year, the place of living, and the nature of the patient.

(IV.48) (185) Says Hippocrates: *In an unremitting fever, if the external parts of the body are cold but the internal parts burning hot and it is accompanied by thirst, it is a fatal sign.*

Says the commentator: Galen says that this occurs only in some unremitting fevers and that it is caused by an inflammation in an internal part of the body, whereby the blood and the pneuma are attracted from the whole body to the diseased part. As a result, the internal parts of the body are burning hot but the skin is cold, as happens in the beginning of fever attacks. This is Galen's argumentation. [*In Hippocratis Aphorismos commentarius* IV.48]. But this is not true, because if this would follow necessarily, this affliction would inevitably be associated with every inflammation that occurs in the internal parts of the body. However, we always see that the skin of those who suffer from pleurisy, pneumonia, and liver complaint, is extremely hot, like the inside of their bodies. It seems to me that the reason for this is that the substances, which are in the external parts of the body, are very thick and very cold. The heat of the putrid humor that produces the fever that putrefies within the body cannot overcome them. The more this putrid substance becomes heated and its heat rises to the external parts of the body as it is looking for openings through which to breath, the more it finds itself up against a cold barrier which prevents the heat from emerging to the surface of the body. As a result, the heat is reversed and returns with the strongest possible force so that the inside of the body is burned even more and the thirst gets worse. And then something occurs to the heat, which is similar to what happens when blacksmiths sprinkle water on the fire in a smelting furnace until the internal heat of the fire becomes so strong that it melts the iron. This is without any doubt the real natural cause.

(IV.49) (186) Says Hippocrates: *If in an unremitting fever the patient's lip, eye, nose, or eyebrow is distorted; if the patient, being already weak, does neither see nor hear, whatever of these things occur, death is near.*

Says the commentator: This is clear, because when these symptoms occur in combination with a weakness of the strength of the patient and when fever preceded, one can learn from this that dryness prevails over the origins of the nerves and that this causes the distortion and the other afflictions mentioned by him.

(IV.50) (187) Says Hippocrates: *When difficulty of respiration and mental confusion (delirium) occur during unremitting fever, it is a fatal sign.*

Says the commentator: This is clear because the heat has taken possession of the organs to the point that also the nerves that move the chest and the diaphragm have weakened, so that respiration is difficult.

(IV.51) (188) Says Hippocrates: *An abscess, which occurs during a fever and is not dissolved at the time of the first crisis, indicates a long illness.*

Says the commentator: This is clear.

(IV.52) (189) Says Hippocrates: *If tears, which flow during a fever or during other illnesses, are shed by a patient of his own will, it is not extraordinary. But if the tears are shed involuntarily, it is worse.*

Says the commentator: This is clear because of the weakness of the retentive faculty. The word "worse" indicates that the first case is also bad, that is to say, that although he cries of his own will it is an indication that his heart is weak. For this reason, he is quickly affected by emotions that make him cry.

(IV.53) (190) Says Hippocrates: *If the teeth of someone suffering from fever are covered with viscous matters, his fever is high.*

Says the commentator: These viscous matters especially develop from strong heat, which acts upon phlegmatic moistures until they become dried out.

(IV.54) (191) Says Hippocrates: *If someone with ardent fever suffers from a frequent dry cough that only irritates him slightly, he will hardly suffer from thirst.*

Says the commentator: Galen says that it is impossible during coughing, even if there is no expectoration, that the trachea should not become moistened through the moisture that is attracted to it during coughing, and therefore the patient is not thirsty. [*In Hippocratis Aphorismos commentarius* IV.54].

(IV.55) (192) Says Hippocrates: *Any fever that comes with a swelling in the soft flesh of the groins (bubo) and the like is bad, unless the fever is ephemeral.*

Says the commentator: If the fever is caused by a swelling in the soft flesh of the groins and the like, it is ephemeral fever. However, if the fever is due to another cause and is associated with a swelling in the groins and the like, it is bad because in that case, the swelling in the groins is associated with a swelling in one of the intestines. And this internal swelling is the cause of the fever mentioned before, and therefore it is dangerous.

(IV.56) (193) Says Hippocrates: *If someone with a fever perspires but the fever does not abate, it is a bad sign because it announces that the disease will be prolonged and it is a sign of excessive moisture.*

Says the commentator: This is clear.

(IV.57) (194) Says Hippocrates: *If someone suffers from spasms or tetanus and then gets a fever, his illness will dissolve.*

Says the commentator: There are three types of spasms: backwards spasm (opisthotonos), forwards spasm (emprosthotonos), and tetanus, in which no cramps are visible in the parts of the body because they are stretched backwards and forwards equally. [*De tremore, palpitatione, convulsione et rigore*; *De locis affectis* III.7]. All types of spasm occur either because of overfilling or depletion of the neural parts. A spasm following ardent fever is necessarily caused by dryness. [*De tremore, palpitatione, convulsione et rigore*]. A spasm that occurs first and suddenly necessarily results from overfilling. If this spasm is followed by fever, it dissolves part of the superfluous moisture and concocts part of its coldness.

(IV.58) (195) Says Hippocrates: *If someone with ardent fever is affected by rigor, the fever will abate.*

Says the commentator: When the bilious humor moves to be evacuated, it causes rigor and this is followed by vomiting of yellow bile and diarrhea to evacuate the superfluity that produces the fever. When the vessels of the patient are clean, his fever abates.

(IV.59) (196) Says Hippocrates: *A tertian fever comes to a crisis, at the latest, in seven cycles.*

Says the commentator: Galen says: We have observed and investigated the crisis in quartan and tertian fevers and found that it occurs according to the number of cycles and not according to the number of days. Thus, the seventh cycle in tertian fever falls on the thirteenth day from its beginning. In most cases, the crisis and end of the illness occur on that day and one does not have to wait for the fourteenth day. Hippocrates is speaking here about simple tertian fever. [*In Hippocratis Aphorismos commentarius* IV.59].

(IV.60) (197) Says Hippocrates: *If someone with acute fever is afflicted by deafness and blood flows from his nose or he suffers from diarrhea, the illness will subside as a result of that.*

Says the commentator: The reasons for that have already been mentioned above.

(IV.61) (198) Says Hippocrates: *If the fever does not leave the patient on one of the odd days, it usually relapses.*

Says the commentator: Galen says that this is an error of the copyist and that Hippocrates is speaking about one of the days of the crisis regardless whether it is an even or an odd day. [*In Hippocratis Aphorismos commentarius* IV.61].

(IV.62) (199) Says Hippocrates: *If jaundice occurs during a fever before the seventh day, it is a bad sign.*

Says the commentator: Sometimes jaundice occurs in the way of a crisis, but a crisis with jaundice does not occur before the seventh day. The only exception is when it is caused by an affliction of the liver and for this reason it is a bad sign.

(IV.63) (200) Says Hippocrates: *If someone with fever suffers from rigor every day, the fever abates every day.*

Says the commentator: With the words "abates every day," he means that it leaves him and departs from him every day with the evacuation of the humor that caused the rigor and its movement to be excreted. The same holds good for tertian and quartan fevers.

(IV.64) (201) Says Hippocrates: *If jaundice occurs during a fever on the seventh, ninth, or fourteenth day, it is beneficial, unless the right side of the hypochondrium becomes hard. If that is the case, it is not beneficial.*

Says the commentator: The reason for this is clear from the preceding.

(IV.65) (202) Says Hippocrates: *If someone with fever has a sensation of severe heat in the belly and of cardialgia (palpitation or heartburn), it is a bad sign.*

Says the commentator: If with the term *fuʾād*, he means the cardia of the stomach, then *khafaqān* refers to a burning sensation in the cardia of the stomach because it is being soaked by bilious humors. If with the term *fuʾād*, he means the heart, the latter is afflicted by palpitations because the heat has taken possession of it. Both afflictions are extremely bad. [*In Hippocratis Aphorismos commentarius* IV.65].

(IV.66) (203) Says Hippocrates: *In acute fevers, cramps and pains in the intestines are a bad sign.*

Says the commentator: An extremely high fever dries the nerves like fire; it stretches and distends them and—in this manner—fatal cramps occur. Sometimes, also pain in the intestines occurs from precisely this condition, that is to say, from the extreme heat and dryness.

(IV.67) (204) Says Hippocrates: *Fear or cramps occurring to someone with fever on waking from sleep, are bad signs.*

Says the commentator: If the body is full with humors, the head becomes filled therewith during sleep and the brain becomes heavy. If the dominant humor tends towards black bile, fear ensues from it. But if this is not the case, pain and cramps happen from it. Galen says that he has often observed that fear, pain, and cramps occur as a result of sleep in the case of fatal illnesses and that it seems that this happens during sleep when the harmful humor reaches the brain. [*In Hippocratis Aphorismos commentarius* IV.67].

(IV.68) (205) Says Hippocrates: *If the air (respiration) changes during its passage through the body, it is a bad sign because it indicates spasms.*

Says the commentator: With "air," he means the air of respiration. If it meets an obstruction during its passage so that it is cut off in its entrance or its exit or both together it is a bad sign.

(IV.69) (206) Says Hippocrates: *If someone's urine is thick, similar to blood clots, and of small quantity, and his body is not free from fever, he will benefit if he urinates a large amount of thin urine. This type of urination happens mostly to someone in whose urine a sediment settles from the beginning of his illness or shortly thereafter.*

Says the commentator: Most patients with fever have thin urine in the beginning of the illness. The closer they get to the end, the thicker its consistency. Hippocrates informs us about something rare, namely, that sometimes the urine resembles mud and that its quantity is small in the beginning of the disease. The reason for its small quantity is that it only passes through the kidneys with difficulty. When the major part of the bad humor has been evacuated and the remainder thereof concocted, the patient urinates thinner urine and in a larger quantity.

(IV.70) (207) Says Hippocrates: *If someone with fever urinates turbid urine, similar to that of a beast of burden, he suffers from a headache at that moment or will so later on.*

Says the commentator: The urine is only like that when the heat acts on a large amount of thick superfluous matter. Especially when matters with this property are acted upon by extraordinary heat, vapors originate from them so that the urine becomes turbid like wax, pitch, and pine tree resin. The thick vapors and the heat quickly ascend to the head. Sometimes one can discern that the headache occurs at the same time as the turbid urine; sometimes earlier and sometimes later.

(IV.71) (208) Says Hippocrates: *If someone has a crisis on the seventh day, a red cloud will appear in his urine on the fourth day. Other symptoms are analogous.*

Says the commentator: The fourth day is the day that foretells what will happen on the seventh. Every important sign that clearly indicates concoction on this day indicates a crisis occurring on the seventh day. However, a white cloud is a more appropriate sign for this, and an even more appropriate sign is a white cloud suspended in the middle of the urine. If the disease moves quickly, only a change in color and in consistency is a sufficient indication for the crisis to occur on the seventh day. Galen says that Hippocrates mentions the red cloud, which is the weakest sign, so that one can learn from it about the matter of the other signs that are stronger. Because they indicate that the crisis is imminent. The signs that appear during the prognostic days in the stool or sputum can be interpreted according to the same analogy. [*In Hippocratis Aphorismos commentarius* IV.71].

(IV.72) (209) Says Hippocrates: *If the urine is transparent and white, it is bad, especially in patients with fever associated with an inflammation of the brain.*

Says the commentator: This urine is extremely far from being concocted and it indicates that the illness will be prolonged. It also indicates that all the yellow bile moves upwards, in the direction of the head.

(IV.73) (210) Says Hippocrates: *If the hypochondrium in a patient is swollen and if there are rumblings in it, and if he is then affected by pain in the lower back, his bowels will be loose unless many winds escape from him or unless he passes much urine. This occurs in fevers.*

Says the commentator: If the wind descends and moves downwards together with the moisture that causes the intestinal rumblings, the swelling descends to the region of the lower spine and the parts, which are there, are stretched so that pain occurs. Sometimes the moisture reaches the vessels and exits with the urine. In that case, the winds exit alone. Sometimes, the wind and the moisture exit together from the intestines and the bowels become loose. Sometimes, the moisture and wind go into the vessels and then pass easily through to the urinary bladder. Especially in the case of someone with a fever, one can rely on these symptoms and be aware that nature is determined to expel the harmful matter through the urine or stool.

(IV.74) (211) Says Hippocrates: *If an abscess is expected to develop in someone's joints, he may be saved from that abscess by an abundant flow of thick, white urine, like that which sometimes begins on the fourth day in some people who suffer from fever associated with fatigue. And if he has a nosebleed, his illness ends very quickly.*

Says the commentator: This is clear.

(IV.75) (212) Says Hippocrates: *If someone urinates blood or pus, it indicates that there is an ulceration in the kidneys or urinary bladder.*

Says the commentator: This is clear.

(IV.76) (213) Says Hippocrates: *If someone with thick urine passes small pieces of flesh or hair-like substances, they are a discharge from the kidneys.*

Says the commentator: The small pieces of flesh derive from the very substance of the kidneys. But the hair-like substance can neither be from the substance of the kidneys nor from the substance of the bladder. Galen says that he has seen that it happened to people that they urinated this hair-like substance, some of which was about half a cubit long, because they took foods that produce a thick humor. When the heat acts upon this thick humor until it burns and dries it in the kidneys, this hair-like substance originates from it. The cure of this illness confirms the correct deduction of the cause, for those who were affected by this illness were indeed healed by the application of refining, diluting medications. [*In Hippocratis Aphorismos commentarius* IV.76]. Hippocrates' statement that "they are a discharge from the kidneys" informs us about the site where this hair-like substance develops.

(IV.77) (214) Says Hippocrates: *If someone with thick urine passes bran-like particles, his urinary bladder is affected by scabs.*

Says the commentator: This is clear.

(IV.78) (215) Says Hippocrates: *If someone urinates blood without anything preceding it, it indicates that a vessel in the kidneys has burst.*

Says the commentator: This is clear.

(IV.79) (216) Says Hippocrates: *When someone's urine contains a sandy sediment, a stone will develop in the urinary bladder.*

Says the commentator: This is clear.

(IV.80) (217) Says Hippocrates: *If someone urinates blood with clots and has strangury and if a pain seizes him in the lower part of the abdomen and pubes, the parts about the urinary bladder are affected.*

(IV.81) (218) Says Hippocrates: *If someone urinates blood, pus, and scales, and his urine is foul-smelling, it indicates ulceration of the bladder.*

(IV.82) (219) Says Hippocrates: *If someone gets a tumor in the urethra, when it suppurates and bursts, the illness comes to an end.*

(IV.83) (220) Says Hippocrates: *If someone passes a lot of urine during the night, it indicates that the stool will be small.*

Says the commentator: All these aphorisms are also clear.

This is the end of the fourth part of the commentary on the Aphorisms.

In the name of God, the Merciful, the Compassionate

The Fifth Part of the *Commentary on Hippocrates'* Aphorisms

(V.1) (221) Says Hippocrates: *Spasms occurring from hellebore are a sign of death.*

Says the commentator: Spasms occur as a result of the ingestion of white false hellebore. And this is the one intended here, either because of its excessive evacuation or because of the strong movement of the emesis or because of the biting effect on the stomach. To heal this is difficult.

(V.2) (222) Says Hippocrates: *Spasms occurring as a result of a wound are a sign of death.*

Says the commentator: This happens because of the inflammation of the nerves and the pain ascends to the brain. Every time Hippocrates refers to something as a sign of death, he means that it is very dangerous and that the patient dies in most cases.

(V.3) (223) Says Hippocrates: *If much blood flows from the body and hiccups or spasms occur, it is a bad sign.*

Says the commentator: This is clear.

(V.4) (224) Says Hippocrates: *If spasms or hiccups occur after excessive evacuation, it is a bad sign.*

Says the commentator: This is clear.

(V.5) (225) Says Hippocrates: *If a drunken man suddenly becomes speechless, he will suffer from spasms and die, unless he gets a fever or recovers his speech when the effects of his intoxication disappear.*

Says the commentator: The spasms occur because of the filling of the nerves. Wine has the property to fill the nerves quickly because it enters in them quickly as a result of its thinness and heat. Therefore, if one drinks too much wine, it brings a spasm upon the nerves because of its large quantity. But through its quality, wine can also heal and restore that which was corrupted in the nerves since it can heat and dry them. If it cannot do so, the spasm resulting from too much wine will necessarily be followed by death. With the aforementioned property of wine to heal a spasm, it can also be healed by fever. Intoxication is the damage done to the head by the consumption of too much wine.

(V.6) (226) Says Hippocrates: *If someone is attacked by tetanus, he will die in four days, unless he survives these, for then he will recover.*

Says the commentator: Tetanus is a very acute illness because the nature of the patient cannot bear the strain of the stretching of the muscles caused by it, because it consists of backwards spasm (opisthotonos) and forwards spasm (emprosthotonos). It ends in the first of the cycles of the critical days.

(V.7) (227) Says Hippocrates: *If someone is attacked by epilepsy before the growth of pubic hair (puberty), he may experience a change of the disease (cure). But if it happens to someone after the age of twenty-five, he will die while still having this disease.*

Says the commentator: Galen says: With "change," he means the end of the illness. This occurs as a result of an improvement of the cold, viscous humor, which produces the epilepsy, that is the moist, phlegmatic humor, and this happens through a change of his temperament into dryness because of his age, through physical exercise, and through a drying regimen in combination with appropriate medications. In this aphorism, Hippocrates only refers to the change (cure) that occurs because of advancing age. The time of the growth of pubic hair (puberty) occurs between the end of the fourteenth year and the twenty-fifth year of age.

(V.8) (228) Says Hippocrates: *If someone is afflicted by pleurisy and is not cleansed thereof in fourteen days, his condition will lead to empyema.*

Says the commentator: Hippocrates calls "cleansing" the evacuation of the humor that produces pleurisy by expectoration.

(V.9) (229) Says Hippocrates: *Phthisis occurs mostly between the ages of eighteen and thirty-five.*

Says the commentator: He has already said before that phthisis is an illness of young people. He mentions it again since he discusses illnesses of the chest and lung.

(V.10) (230) Says Hippocrates: *If someone is afflicted by angina and is saved from it, but the superfluity that produced the illness turns to the lungs, he will die within seven days. If he survives these, he will develop empyema.*

Says the commentator: It is likely that Hippocrates had much experience with these and similar illnesses regarding this kind of change. There is no doubt that this change and similar ones are the rule.

(V.11) (231) Says Hippocrates: *If a person suffers from phthisis and expectorates sputum that is foul-smelling when it is poured on hot coals, and if the hair on his head is falling out, it is a fatal sign.*

Says the commentator: The foul smell is evidence of the corruption of the humors and their severe putrefaction. The loss of hair confirms what is already indicated by the corruption of the humors and also indicates that the organs lack nutrition.

(V.12) (232) Says Hippocrates: *If a patient with phthisis loses his hair and then suffers from diarrhea, he will die.*

Says the commentator: Diarrhea in these patients indicates that their strength is weak and this indicates that death is near.

(V.13) (233) Says Hippocrates: *If someone spits up frothy blood, the discharge comes from the lungs.*

Says the commentator: It is clear that when blood emerges that is frothy, it hails from the substance and essence of the lungs.

(V.14) (234) Says Hippocrates: *If someone with phthisis gets diarrhea, it is a sign of death.*

Says the commentator: Diarrhea in patients with phthisis is an indication of death. If this occurs with foul-smelling sputum and loss of hair, it indicates that death is near, as previously mentioned.

(V.15) (235) Says Hippocrates: *If the condition of someone with pleurisy results in empyema, the illness will end if he is cleansed from the pus within forty days from its outbreak. But if he is not cleansed within this period, he will develop phthisis.*

Says the commentator: If the matter (pus) that broke forth and occurred in the cavity of the chest is not excreted, it will putrefy and solidify and cause ulceration of the lungs.

(v.16) (236) Says Hippocrates: *Heat has the following harmful effects on those who use it frequently: It softens the flesh, weakens the nerves, benumbs the mind, it causes hemorrhages and fainting, and patients with these afflictions are overtaken by death.*

Says the commentator: He says that if someone uses heat excessively, it softens his flesh and weakens the nerves, that is to say, it makes them soft through the dissolution of its substance by the heat. Galen says that with the statement "it benumbs the mind," he means that it weakens the mind and takes away its strength by the dissolution of the substance of the nerves. And that it is clear that a hemorrhage is followed by fainting and fainting by death. [*In Hippocratis Aphorismos commentarius* v.16].

(v.17) (237) Says Hippocrates: *Cold produces spasms, tetanus, blackening of flesh from mortification, and rigors, which are accompanied by fever.*

Says the commentator: This is clear.

(v.18) (238) Says Hippocrates: *Cold is harmful for the bones, teeth, nerves, brain, and the spinal marrow. Heat, however, is good and beneficial for them.*

Says the commentator: This is clear.

(v.19) (239) Says Hippocrates: *Any part that is chilled should be heated, unless a hemorrhage has to be feared.*

Says the commentator: This is clear.

(v.20) (240) Says Hippocrates: *Cold has a biting effect on ulcers, hardens the skin, causes pain without suppuration, blackens the flesh from mortification, causes feverish rigors, spasms, and tetanus.*

Says the commentator: This is clear.

(v.21) (241) Says Hippocrates: *Sometimes, if one pours a large quantity of cold water—in the middle of summer—over a fleshy youth, who is suffering from tetanus without a previous ulcer, one brings a recovery of much heat, and he is saved by that heat.*

Says the commentator: This is clear.

(V.22) (242) Says Hippocrates: *Heat causes suppuration, but not in the case of every wound. When it does, it is one of the best indications that one can be confident and reassured to recover. It softens the skin, makes it thin, alleviates pain, annihilates the evil (harm) caused by rigors, spasms, and tetanus, and relieves heaviness occurring in the head. It is most beneficial for broken bones, especially when they are exposed, and above all for bones in the head. Also, for everything that is affected by mortification or ulcers because of the cold, for corroding herpes, for ailments of the anus, genitals, uterus, and urinary bladder—for those who suffer from these ailments, heat has a beneficial and healing effect, while cold is harmful and fatal for them.*

Says the commentator: The formation of pus is a good sign on which one can rely in the case of wounds, because it is a type of concoction, as you know. Not every wound forms pus. All bad wounds and corrosive wounds, which are difficult to heal, do not form pus. The rest of what he mentions is clear because every part of the body with nerves and every bone is harmed by cold.

(V.23) (243) Says Hippocrates: *Cold should be applied to the following parts of the body: to the parts where there is a hemorrhage or where it is imminent. One should not apply it to the actual spot from where bleeding occurs, but around whatever spot it comes from. It should also be applied to inflamed tumors and other inflammations that tend to red and to the color of fresh blood (when they are recent), because cold blackens inflammations when it is applied to them when the blood is old. It should also be applied in the case of the swelling called "erysipelas" when there is no ulceration, because it is harmful when ulcers have formed.*

Says the commentator: This is clear.

(V.24) (244) Says Hippocrates: *Cold things such as snow and ice are harmful to the chest, provoke cough, cause hemorrhage and catarrhs.*

Says the commentator: This is clear.

(V.25) (245) Says Hippocrates: *Swellings in the joints and pains in the joints without ulceration, and pains of those who suffer from gout or from bruises, which occur in places where there are nerves, and most similar cases, are relieved and reduced if one pours a lot of cold water over them. The pain is relieved because it causes numbness, for also a small amount of numbness relieves the pain.*

Says the commentator: The pain is relieved in such places because the cold puts an end to the pain itself, or because it benumbs one's sensation of pain.

(V.26) (246) Says Hippocrates: *Water that quickly gets hot and quickly gets cold is the lightest.*

Says the commentator: It is clear that with "heaviness" and "lightness," he means the rapidity with which it leaves the stomach or its delay there.

(v.27) (247) Says Hippocrates: *If someone desires to drink at night because of intense thirst and if he sleeps after that, it is a good sign.*

Says the commentator: If he sleeps after drinking the water, the humor that caused the thirst will be concocted during the sleep. But drinking water during the night should only be allowed in the case of severe thirst.

(v.28) (248) Says Hippocrates: *Fomenting with aromatic herbs brings about menstruation. It would also be beneficial in many other cases, if it did not cause heaviness in the head.*

Says the commentator: He says that fomenting with aromatic herbs induces the flow of menstrual blood or the blood of parturition if these are withheld, because it thins the blood if it is thick, or it opens an obstruction if it is there, or it widens the openings of the vessels if they are closed. It would also be beneficial for warming cold places or drying moisture (humors) if it did not fill the head, because everything that is hot ascends and causes headache.

(v.29) (249) Says Hippocrates: *It is proper to administer purgative drugs to pregnant women when the humors in their body flare up from when the fetus is four months old until it becomes seven months old. But in the latter case, one should proceed to administer a smaller dose. When a fetus is younger than four months or older than seven months, one should be careful with the administration of these drugs.*

Says the commentator: This aphorism is either repeated inadvertently by him, or he has done so on purpose to lead the discussion to that of women's diseases.

(v.30) (250) Says Hippocrates: *If a pregnant woman is bled, she will have a miscarriage, especially if the fetus is large.*

Says the commentator: This is clear.

(v.31) (251) Says Hippocrates: *If a woman is pregnant and attacked by one of the acute diseases, it is a fatal sign.*

Says the commentator: If it is one of the acute diseases that is accompanied by fever, it is fatal because of its bad temperament, which makes it necessary to inhale much air while the organs are compressed and because of the lack of nutrition. If, for instance, the disease is hemiplegia or spasms, she cannot bear the strong pain or the stretching of the muscles because of the heavy burden that she carries.

(V.32) (252) Says Hippocrates: *If a woman vomits blood and then begins to menstruate, the vomiting of blood will stop.*

Says the commentator: This is clear.

(V.33) (253) Says Hippocrates: *When menstruation stops, a nosebleed is good.*

Says the commentator: This is also clear.

(V.34) (254) Says Hippocrates: *If a pregnant woman suffers from constant diarrhea, one cannot be free from fear that she will have a miscarriage.*

Says the commentator: If the expulsive faculty becomes strongly active in those parts that are close to the uterus, it has to be feared that the expulsive faculty, which is in the uterus, will also become active.

(V.35) (255) Says Hippocrates: *If a woman who suffers from an affliction of the uterus or difficult labor has an attack of sneezing, it is a good sign.*

Says the commentator: With "an affliction of the uterus," he means hysterical suffocation and the sneezing indicates that nature is aroused to carry out its activities. It is also that which causes the organs to get rid of the harmful humors that stick and adhere to them. In a similar manner sneezing cures hiccups.

(V.36) (256) Says Hippocrates: *If the menstrual blood of a woman changes its color and does not always arrive at the normal time (is irregular), it indicates that her body requires cleansing.*

Says the commentator: This is clear.

(V.37) (257) Says Hippocrates: *If the breasts of a pregnant woman suddenly become thin, she will have a miscarriage.*

Says the commentator: The interrelationship between the breasts and the uterus is well known. When the breasts become thin, it indicates that only a small amount of food reaches them. If the nutrition that reaches the uterus also decreases, the fetus is aborted.

(V.38) (258) Says Hippocrates: *If a woman is pregnant with twins and one of her breasts becomes thin all at once, she will lose one of the twins. If the right breast becomes thin, she will lose the male child; if the left breast becomes thin, she will lose the female child.*

Says the commentator: In most cases, the male child is on the right side.

(V.39) (259) Says Hippocrates: *If a woman, who is not pregnant and has not given birth, produces milk, her menstruation has stopped.*

Says the commentator: Only rarely during amenorrhea do the vessels connected to the breasts become overfilled resulting in the production of milk due to the excess of blood reaching the breasts. It seems to me that this only happens when the body of the woman is extremely clean (free from superfluous humors) and her nourishment extremely good.

(V.40) (260) Says Hippocrates: *When blood congeals in the breasts of a woman, it indicates that her condition is one of madness.*

Says the commentator: It seems to me as most probable that he observed this only once or twice and yet made a definite statement about it as he usually does in his book *Epidemics*. Galen remarks that he has never seen this, and this is true, that is to say, that blood congealed in the breasts is never a cause of madness. [*In Hippocratis Aphorismos commentarius* V.40]. It must have happened accidentally once or twice and Hippocrates observed it and thought that it was the cause of madness.

(V.41) (261) *Says Hippocrates: If you want to know whether a woman is pregnant or not, give her honey water to drink when she wants to go to sleep. If she is attacked by a colic in the stomach, she is pregnant, but if she is not attacked, she is not pregnant.*

Says the commentator: He means with his formulation "when she goes to sleep" the time when she is rested and satiated with food. It is the honey water that gives rise to winds and receives help thereby from the filling of the stomach. If the winds do not find an outlet, because the uterus constricts their passage, a colic occurs.

(V.42) (262) Says Hippocrates: *If a woman is pregnant with a boy, her complexion is good, but if she is pregnant with a girl, her complexion is pallid.*

Says the commentator: All this is clear and applies in most cases.

(V.43) (263) Says Hippocrates: *If a pregnant woman suffers from the swelling called "erysipelas" in her womb, it is a sign of death.*

Says the commentator: From the writings of Galen, it is manifest that he means the death of the fetus. [*In Hippocratis Aphorismos commentarius* V.43]. The same applies to other hot swellings (inflammations).

(V.44) (264) Says Hippocrates: *If a woman, who is unnaturally thin, becomes pregnant, she will have a miscarriage before she will put on weight.*

Says the commentator: He says that if she becomes pregnant while she is extremely thin, the food that reaches the organs will be completely seized by those organs and there is nothing left with which the fetus can be nourished when it grows. Therefore, she miscarries before she reaches the point where she can put on weight, which would not happen during the time that she actually returns to the natural fatness of her body.

(v.45) (265) Says Hippocrates: *If a woman with a normal body has a miscarriage in the second or third month without any obvious cause, the fundus of the uterus is full of mucus and cannot retain the fetus because of its weight and the fetus breaks off from the uterus.*

Says the commentator: This is clear.

(v.46) (266) Says Hippocrates: *If a woman is unnaturally fat and cannot become pregnant, the inner membrane of the abdominal membranes, which is called* al-tharb (*fat; omentum*), *presses the mouth of the uterus and she will not become pregnant unless she becomes thinner.*

Says the commentator: The uterus has a long neck (cervix). The end of the neck, which is close to the vagina, and into which the penis enters, is called "the mouth (orifice) of the neck of the uterus;" it is also simply called "the mouth (orifice) of the uterus." But what is really called "the mouth of the uterus" is the beginning of the neck near the uterus, and this is what is pressed by the fat in an extremely obese woman.

(v.47) (267) Says Hippocrates: *When the uterus suppurates in the region where it lies close to the hip joint, it is necessary to perform an action.*

Says the commentator: With *ʿamal* (activity), he means "the activity of the hand" (surgery); namely, the insertion of lints. And when suppuration of an external site of the uterus occurs, then one also should apply lints.

(v.48) (268) Says Hippocrates: *In the case of a male fetus, it is better when it grows on the right side, and for a female fetus on the left side.*

Says the commentator: This is clear because the right side is warmer. Galen has mentioned that the semen that comes from the woman from the right side, from one of her ovaries, is thick and warm, while that which comes from the left side is thin and watery and colder than the other. [*In Hippocratis Aphorismos commentarius* v.48]. I wish I knew whether he received this knowledge by divine revelation or by analogical reasoning. If he has defined and formulated this argument through analogical reasoning, it is an astonishing and strange logical conclusion.

(v.49) (269) Says Hippocrates: *If you want to expel the placenta, put a sternutatory medicine into the nose and keep the nostrils and mouth closed.*

Says the commentator: This is in order to produce a stretching and tension in the abdomen, which helps to expel the placenta.

(V.50) (270) Says Hippocrates: *If you want to stop the menstrual bleeding of a woman, apply the largest available cupping glass to each of her breasts.*

Says the commentator: This is clear because it attracts the blood to the opposite side.

(V.51) (271) Says Hippocrates: *The mouth of the womb of a pregnant woman is closed.*

Says the commentator: This is clear.

(V.52) (272) Says Hippocrates: *If milk flows from the breasts of a pregnant woman, it indicates that the fetus is weak, but if the breasts are firm, it indicates that the fetus is healthier.*

Says the commentator: The milk of a pregnant woman rather flows because the vessels between the uterus and the breasts are filled to overflowing, and the blood is especially abundant there when the fetus is undernourished and is only provided with a very small amount of food from those vessels.

(V.53) (273) Says Hippocrates: *If the condition of the woman is such that it leads to a miscarriage, her breasts become thin. If the opposite is the case—that is, that her breasts become firm again—she will suffer from pain in her breasts, or in the hips, or in the eyes, or in the knees, but she will not miscarry.*

Says the commentator: Thinness of the breasts is an indication of lack of blood, as stated before; firmness of the breasts is an indication of a balanced amount of blood; hardness of the breasts is an indication of abundant, thick blood. For this reason, nature can push this excessive superfluity to another organ that is close to the uterus or to the breasts, and thus pain occurs to that organ. In general, all these indications are neither correct nor do they occur most frequently. In my opinion, all these aphorisms and their like follow from his observation of what happened only once or twice, for Hippocrates was merely a beginner in the medical art.

(V.54) (274) Says Hippocrates: *If the mouth of the womb is hard, it is necessarily closed.*

Says the commentator: This is clear.

(V.55) (275) Says Hippocrates: *If a pregnant woman catches a fever and the fever becomes extremely high without any obvious cause, her delivery will be difficult and dangerous, or she will have a dangerous miscarriage.*

Says the commentator: For an easy delivery it is necessary that both are strong, the body of the mother and the body of the child.

(v.56) (276) Says Hippocrates: *If a spasm and fainting occur after menstruation, it is bad.*

Says the commentator: This is clear.

(v.57) (277) Says Hippocrates: *When the menstruation is more copious than necessary, illnesses develop; when menstrual blood does not flow, illnesses occur from the side of the womb.*

Says the commentator: This is clear.

(v.58) (278) Says Hippocrates: *If an inflammation occurs in the rectum or in the uterus, it is followed by strangury. Similarly, if the kidneys suppurate, strangury results, and if an inflammation occurs to the liver, hiccups follow.*

Says the commentator: Strangury occurs because of a weakness of the retentive force of the urinary bladder or because of the sharpness of the urine. The weakness of the strength of the bladder results from a bad temperament or from the inflammation that occurs there. The sharpness of the urine occurs because of the admixture of biting humor therein. If there is an inflammation in one of these organs (the rectum or uterus) it is harmful for the bladder because of its proximity and it weakens its strength. If there is an illness in the kidneys, there is a biting sensation during urination. An inflammation of the liver is only followed by hiccups when it is severe.

(v.59) (279) Says Hippocrates: *If a woman does not become pregnant and you want to know whether she can become pregnant or not, cover her with clothes and then fumigate beneath her. If you see that the smell of the fumigation passes through her body until it reaches her nostrils and mouth, you should know that there is no reason why pregnancy is impossible for her.*

Says the commentator: The fumigation should be done with fragrant things that have sharpness such as frankincense, myrrh, and solid styrax.

(v.60) (280) Says Hippocrates: *If a pregnant woman has a regular menstruation, it is impossible that the fetus is healthy.*

Says the commentator: Galen says that it looks like the menstrual blood—in the case of a pregnant woman—streams from the vessels in the neck of the uterus because the placenta is attached to the mouths of all the vessels that are within the cavity of the uterus and it is impossible that any blood is expelled from there to the cavity of the uterus. [*In Hippocratis Aphorismos commentarius* v.60].

(v.61) (281) Says Hippocrates: *If a woman does not have a regular menstruation and she does not suffer from shivering or fever, but suffers from distress, nausea, and despondency, know that she is pregnant.*

Says the commentator: This is clear.

(v.62) (282) Says Hippocrates: *If the uterus of a woman is cold and dense, she will not become pregnant. If it is very moist, she will also not become pregnant because the moisture will drown, extinguish, and quench (destroy) the semen. Furthermore, when it is drier than it should be or when it is burning hot, she will not become pregnant, because the sperm is spoiled through lack of food. When the temperament of the uterus is balanced in the middle between these two conditions, the woman can get many children.*

Says the commentator: This is clear.

(v.63) (283) —

(v.64) (284) Says Hippocrates: *Milk is bad for those suffering from headache; it is also bad for fever patients, and for those whose hypochondrium is swollen and full of intestinal rumblings, and for those who are thirsty, and for those in whom the yellow bile prevails in their stool, namely, those who suffer from acute fever, and for those who have bloody diarrhea. Milk is beneficial for those who suffer from phthisis if they do not have a very high fever, and for those with a chronic, low fever, if it is not accompanied by any of the above-mentioned symptoms and their body is wasted more than the illness made necessary.*

Says the commentator: Milk is one of the substances that is changed quickly. If it is in a stomach that is cooler, it turns sour, and if it is in a stomach that is hotter, it becomes gaseous. If it is properly digested, it produces abundant good nutrition. But it may happen that during the process of digestion, flatulence is produced in the hypochondrium and pain in the head. This is its effect in healthy people; in sick people it effects all that has been mentioned above.

(v.65) (285) Says Hippocrates: *If someone suffers from a wound and then develops a swelling because of it, he will hardly ever be attacked by spasms or madness. If the swelling disappears suddenly and the wound is in the posterior part of the body, spasms or tetanus will occur to him. If the wound is on the front, he will suffer from madness or severe pain in the side, or suppuration or dysentery if that swelling is red.*

Says the commentator: I do not need to repeat that most of these assertions of Hippocrates are either mostly so or evenly so or not so; and upon verification, some of the statements are true only in a minority of cases. For if you look into them carefully, you will see that only some of his assertions are valid for very few cases. Perhaps he saw a case of illness once and then ascribed it to a cause by which it was not really caused.

The interpretation of this aphorism according to Galen is that with the term "swelling," he means the inflammation and any other unnatural thickening. The posterior part of the body contains nerves, but the front part is dominated by pulsating vessels. If the humor that produces the inflammation ascends to the brain, spasms occur, and if it ascends through the vessels to the brain, madness occurs. If that humor goes to the chest, it produces pain in the side. Patients with pain in the side often suffer from suppuration.

(v.66) (286) Says Hippocrates: *When severe, bad wounds occur but no swelling appears there, it is a bad affliction.*

Says the commentator: With bad wounds he means those that occur in the beginning or end of muscles or in muscles in which nerves dominate. If no swelling develops in wounds in which that is usually the case, one cannot be sure that the humors that stream to the wounds are not carried to a location that is more important than that of the wounds.

(v.67) (287) Says Hippocrates: *Soft swellings are good, crude swellings are bad.*

Says the commentator: Galen says that with the term "crude," he means "hard" and "resisting" cooking; it is the opposite of soft, because the humor of anything that is hard is not cooked. [*In Hippocratis Aphorismos commentarius* v.67].

(v.68) (288) Says Hippocrates: *If someone suffers from pain in the back of his head, he will benefit from an incision in the upright vein in the forehead.*

Says the commentator: The attraction of residues to the opposite site in the neck is from the back to the front and from the front to the back.

(v.69) (289) Says Hippocrates: *Rigors in women mostly begin in the loins and then ascend through the back to the head. In men too, they begin more often in the back of the body than in the front as, for instance, those that begin in the forearms and thighs. This is because the skin too—in the front part of the body—is porous, as is shown by the hairs.*

Says the commentator: The back is quickly affected by cold because its coldness is due to numerous bones there and to the paucity of flesh. Women are colder than men; he brings proof for the looseness of the skin of the front part of the body from the fact that the hair grows there.

(V.70) (290) Says Hippocrates: *If someone is afflicted by quartan fever, he is hardly attacked by spasms. If he is attacked by spasms before the quartan fever and then gets a quartan fever, the spasms will abate.*

Says the commentator: The interpretation of Galen is that this type of spasm is the one that arises from overfilling. It can be cured by the expulsion or concoction of the humor. In quartan fever it is expelled by the force of the spasm and concocted by the heat of the fever. [*In Hippocratis Aphorismos commentarius* V.70].

(V.71) (291) Says Hippocrates: *If someone's skin is stretched, dry, and hard, he dies without sweat. If someone's skin is soft and porous, he dies with sweat.*

Says the commentator: He means those people who are close to death and whose skin is as described.

(V.72) (292) Says Hippocrates: *If someone suffers from jaundice, he will hardly develop winds (flatulence).*

Says the commentator: One of the causes that give rise to winds is the phlegm, which is in the site of their origin. This does not happen in the case of jaundice because of the dominance of bile.

This is the end of the fifth part of the commentary on the Aphorisms.

In the name of God,
the Merciful, the Compassionate

The Sixth Part of the *Commentary on Hippocrates'* Aphorisms

(VI.1) (293) Says Hippocrates: *If acid eructations occur during the illness called "lientery" when it has become chronic and when these eructations did not happen before, they are a good sign.*

Says the commentator: If the cause of the lientery is the weakness of the retentive faculty and the food is excreted before it is properly digested and acid eructations occur thereupon, it is an indication that the food is staying sufficiently long in the stomach for a partial digestion to begin to a degree that the food turns sour. It is also an indication that nature is beginning to return to its normal activities.

(VI.2) (294) Says Hippocrates: *If a person's nostrils are excessively moist by nature and his semen is very thin (watery), his health leans toward sickness. But if the reverse is true in a person, he has a healthier body.*

Says the commentator: These are things that indicate moisture of the brain and dryness of the other organs and therefore his semen is thin.

(VI.3) (295) Says Hippocrates: *The abstention from food (loss of appetite) in chronic dysentery is a bad sign; if it is accompanied by fever, it is worse.*

Says the commentator: If dysentery is caused by protracted abrasion of the intestines, it increases the emaciation deep in the intestines and results in a putrid wound. The stomach will also hurt because of the sympathetic affection between the stomach and the intestines, and the digestion of food in it will be harmed. If the illness ascends to the cardia of the stomach, the appetite will be less. This is a sign that the illness has settled (established itself) and that its harm is spreading.

(VI.4) (296) Says Hippocrates: *If the area around ulcers peels or falls off, it is bad.*

Says the commentator: The fact that the hair around the ulcer falls out and that the skin peels off is an indication for the sharpness of the humor that streams into it; for this reason, the surrounding area is corroded eventually.

(VI.5) (297) Says Hippocrates: *One should observe about pains that occur in the ribs, in the front part of the chest, and in the other parts, whether they show great differences.*

Says the commentator: He means that one should not be content with observing the spot where the pain is without looking into the severity and mildness of the disease. One can conclude to that from the severity of the pain and the accompanying sensation of pricking, stinging, convulsive tension, and the like, that is, from the different symptoms and their severity that come with the pain in that organ.

(VI.6) (298) Says Hippocrates: *The illnesses that occur in the bladder and kidneys are difficult to cure in old people.*

Says the commentator: This is clear.

(VI.7) (299) Says Hippocrates: *Of the pains that occur in the belly, those that are located higher are milder and those that are not so are more severe.*

Says the commentator: Galen says that with "higher located," he means the pain that is close to the surface of the abdomen above the abdominal membrane (peritoneum). With his statement "those that are not so," he means the pain that is in the intestines and belly.

(VI.8) (300) Says Hippocrates: *Ulcers occurring on the body of those suffering from dropsy are not easy to heal.*

Says the commentator: Ulcers do not scar over (heal) until they have completely dried, and this is something that is not easy in those whose temperament is affected by dropsy.

(VI.9) (301) Says Hippocrates: *Broad pustules are hardly ever accompanied by itch.*

Says the commentator: When pustules and wounds stretch widely but do not swell, it is a sign that their substance is very cold. For that reason, itch does not occur because of the coldness of the substance.

(VI.10) (302) Says Hippocrates: *If someone suffers from headache and a severe pain in the head and pus or water flows from his nostrils or ears, his illness will be cured by that.*

Says the commentator: This is clear.

(VI.11) (303) Says Hippocrates: *When hemorrhoids develop in those who suffer from melancholic delusion or phrenitis, it is a good sign.*

Says the commentator: Melancholic delusion is the mental confusion (delirium) that occurs as a result of black bile. Its Greek name is *mālankhūliyā* (μελαγχολία). Phrenitis is an inflammation of the membranes in the brain. It is clear that the situation improves if the matter that causes the illness goes away to the opposite side and comes with an opening of the orifices of the vessels (arteries).

(VI.12) (304) Says Hippocrates: *If someone is treated for chronic hemorrhoids until he is cured and not a single one is left, one cannot be sure that he will not suffer from dropsy or phthisis.*

Says the commentator: The reason is that if not one hemorrhoid is left from which the turbid blood can be evacuated, that blood will return and become burdensome for the liver and extinguish its heat because of its large quantity and dropsy will occur. Alternatively, the blood may be sent through other vessels and a vessel in the lungs may burst and phthisis will occur. That is to say, that both illnesses may occur at the same time or that either of them may happen.

(VI.13) (305) Says Hippocrates: *If a person afflicted with hiccups develops sneezing, the hiccups will subside.*

Says the commentator: Hiccups mostly occur because of overfilling. This is cured by sneezing because those excessive fluids become less as the sneezing moves and expels them.

(VI.14) (306) Says Hippocrates: *If a person suffers from dropsy and water flows through his blood vessels to the abdomen, the illness will come to an end.*

Says the commentator: This is clear because nature does with these fluids what it does with the illness-producing matter in the crises of acute diseases.

(VI.15) (307) Says Hippocrates: *If a person suffers from prolonged diarrhea, spontaneous vomiting stops the diarrhea.*

Says the commentator: This is clear because nature attracts the matter that causes the illness to the opposite side.

(VI.16) (308) Says Hippocrates: *If a person is afflicted by pleurisy or pneumonia and then gets diarrhea, it is a bad sign.*

Says the commentator: Diarrhea is especially a bad sign in these two illnesses when the illness is so severe that the bowels become loose because of the weakness of the strength of the body.

(VI.17) (309) Says Hippocrates: *If a person suffers from ophthalmia and then gets diarrhea, it is a good sign.*

Says the commentator: This is clear.

(VI.18) (310) Says Hippocrates: *If a tear occurs in the bladder or the brain or the heart or the kidneys or one of the smaller intestines or the stomach or the liver, it is fatal.*

Says the commentator: Galen says: Hippocrates uses the term "fatal" for that, which kills necessarily always or kills in most cases. [*In Hippocratis Aphorismos commentarius* VI.18]. I have seen myself a man who was afflicted by a large, deep wound in his brain and yet he recovered. However, this only happens rarely.

(VI.19) (311) Says Hippocrates: *When a bone, cartilage, nerve, the delicate part of the jaw, or the foreskin is severed, it neither grows back nor unites.*

Says the commentator: "It does not grow back," this means that restoration similar to that in the case of a deep wound does not happen. If there was a split (crack), it (bone, cartilage, etc.) will not grow together again because these are dry organs. Also, when they are torn or cut, these parts separate widely.

(VI.20) (312) Says Hippocrates: *If blood streams into a cavity in an unnatural way, it must suppurate.*

Says the commentator: With "suppurate," he means that the blood changes and that its blood-like form is spoiled.

(VI.21) (313) Says Hippocrates: *If someone is attacked by madness and then has a widening of the veins, which are known as varicose veins or hemorrhoids, his madness disappears.*

Says the commentator: This is clear because of the turning of the matter that produced the illness to the opposite side, but on the condition that the humors that caused the madness flow to the loins. You should also know that Hippocrates' verdicts are not the general rule.

(VI.22) (314) Says Hippocrates: *Pains that descend from the back to the elbows are relieved by venesection.*

Says the commentator: If the causes of those pains are humors, which flowed to the elbow, and these humors are evacuated from the place they flowed to, it is beneficial without any doubt.

(VI.23) (315) Says Hippocrates: *If someone suffers from prolonged fear and despondency, it is caused by black bile.*

Says the commentator: If someone is affected by fear and despondency for no apparent reason, the cause is a sort of melancholy, even if those symptoms are not continuous. But when the beginning of these symptoms is for an obvious reason, such as anger, fury, or grief, and then the symptoms become lengthy and continuous, their continuity indicates a real melancholy.

(VI.24) (316) Says Hippocrates: *When one of the smaller intestines is severed, it does not unite.*

(VI.25) (317) Says Hippocrates: *When the inflammation known as erysipelas moves from the outside to the inside of the body, it is not a good sign; but when it moves from the inside to the outside, it is a good sign.*

Says the commentator: He mentions the inflammation of erysipelas only as an example. The same applies to any inflammation and any purulent matter that emerges from the inside to the outside, for it is a good sign. But if the opposite is the case, it is a bad sign because it indicates that nature is weak.

(VI.26) (318) Says Hippocrates: *If someone suffers from tremors during ardent fever, mental confusion (delirium) will relieve him from them.*

Says the commentator: Galen has already explained the confusion of what he says in this aphorism, namely, that when the matter that causes the ardent fever and that is in the vessels moves to the nerves, tremors occur. And when the matter settles in the brain, a mental confusion (delirium) develops and this is more dangerous than ardent fever. And in such a case, one should not say (it is not helpful to say) that the fever disappears because that which happens instead of it the supervening delirium is more dangerous and worse.

(VI.27) (319) Says Hippocrates: *If someone who suffers from an empyema or dropsy is cauterized or incised and then a large quantity of pus or water flows from him all of a sudden, he will die without any doubt.*

Says the commentator: Suffering from an empyema refers to everyone who has pus in the cavity between the chest and lung. Someone with this disease needs cauterization to dry that moisture, when he is unable to expel it through expectoration. Similarly, dropsy patients should be incised. He remarks that this sudden evacuation is fatal. He has the same opinion in the case of the other organs: When a large swelling occurs in one of them and then pus develops, the sudden evacuation of the pus from it is dangerous, because the patient will faint immediately and his strength will collapse. And afterwards he will remain in this weak condition that will be difficult to reverse.

(VI.28) (320) Says Hippocrates: *Eunuchs do not suffer from gout, nor do they become bald.*

Says the commentator: This is because they are like women. Just as women do not become bald because of their moist temperament, so too baldness does not occur to them. The rare occurrence of gout is as will be explained.

(VI.29) (321) Says Hippocrates: *Women do not suffer from gout, unless their menstruation has stopped.*

Says the commentator: He has implicitly given the reason for the rare occurrence of gout in women, namely, the evacuation of their superfluities through the menstrual blood.

(VI.30) (322) Says Hippocrates: *A young man does not get gout before sexual intercourse with a woman.*

Says the commentator: Galen says that having sexual intercourse has a very strong effect in producing gout, but does not say why. In my opinion, the most probable reason is that feet have very little flesh but many nerves and tendons and are exposed to the air. If sexual intercourse is harmful for the nerves in general, because of the evacuation of pneuma from them and because of their cooling, it is most harmful for the nerves in the feet. We always observe that when the feet are cold, the erection is less. This is an indication for their affinity of coitus and gout with regard to the nerves.

(VI.31) (323) Says Hippocrates: *Pains in the eyes are alleviated by drinking pure wine, or by bathing, or by fomenting, or by venesection, or by taking a purgative drug.*

Says the commentator: Galen has explained the kind of confusion of this aphorism and that it does not come in the way of teaching what is useful in the art of medicine. He said that if the superfluous matters are sharp and the body is clean, then bathing is useful, because then the pain is alleviated. And when the superfluous matters stop streaming while the body is clean, fomenting with hot water is useful. When the vessels of the eye are full, thick blood got stuck in them while the rest of the body is not full, and the eye is dry, drinking pure wine dissolves that thick blood, evacuates it, and removes it from the vessels in which it got stuck.

Galen said that these three kinds of treatment are very dangerous if they are not applied in the right situation. As for venesection, for overfilling with blood, or the evacuation of the prevailing humor through purgation, these are clear and correct methods that are always applied. [*In Hippocratis Aphorismos commentarius* VI.31].

(VI.32) (324) Says Hippocrates: *People who lisp are especially attacked by prolonged diarrhea.*

Says the commentator: Lisp is mostly caused by a large quantity of moisture and softness. For this reason, young people lisp because of their moisture and softness. People with this kind of temperament have mostly loose bowels.

(VI.33) (325) Says Hippocrates: *Those who suffer from acid eructations are hardly ever attacked by pleurisy.*

Says the commentator: Pleurisy mostly originates from a thin, sharp humor that flows to the membrane, which covers the ribs internally and gets stuck there. But this kind of humor only rarely originates in people who suffer from sour eructations.

(VI.34) (326) Says Hippocrates: *Bald people do not often have veins that become wide that are known as varicose veins, but if they get varicose veins their hair grows again.*

Says the commentator: Galen says that here, Hippocrates means the specific baldness caused by sores on the head. If the malignant matter that caused these sores moves downward, varicose veins develop and the hair grows back. [*In Hippocratis Aphorismos commentarius* VI.34].

(VI.35) (327) Says Hippocrates: *If someone who has dropsy develops a cough, it is a bad sign.*

Says the commentator: He means to say that it is a bad sign if dropsy is the cause of the cough. For this happens if the watery humors increase until they reach the windpipe and the patient is on the verge of being suffocated by that moisture.

(VI.36) (328) Says Hippocrates: *Venesection cures dysuria, and the incision should be in one of the inner veins.*

Says the commentator: Galen has corrected this aphorism by saying that sometimes venesection cures dysuria, namely, when it is caused by an inflamed tumor with an excess of blood. For the rest of the aphorism, he adds to the words of Hippocrates: In that case, the venesection should be from the back (hollow) of the knee (popliteal fossa). [*In Hippocratis Aphorismos commentarius* VI.36].

(VI.37) (329) Says Hippocrates: *If a swelling appears on the outside of the throat in the case of someone suffering from angina, it is a good sign.*

Says the commentator: It is clear that it is better when illnesses move from the internal organs to the external ones.

(VI.38) (330) Says Hippocrates: *If someone develops a hidden cancer, it is better not to treat him, because if he is treated, he will die. If he is not treated, he will survive for a long time.*

Says the commentator: With "hidden," he means the illness that is deep inside the body and that is not visible, or it is visible but not accompanied by ulceration. With "omitting treatment," he means the kind of treatment that involves surgery or cauterization but not the kind of treatment that consists of alleviating remedies.

(VI.39) (331) Says Hippocrates: *Spasms occur either because of overfilling or because of emptying, likewise hiccups.*

Says the commentator: The reason for all this is clear.

(VI.40) (332) Says Hippocrates: *If someone suffers from pain in the hypochondrium without inflammation and then gets a fever, it will relieve the pain.*

Says the commentator: If that pain is caused by wind or an obstruction, it is relieved by the fever. It is as if he had said: the fever may relieve the pain. The assertions of this man constantly follow this pattern. His verdicts are mostly missing the conditions under which they are valid or they are extraordinary; some of them are imaginary because they are based on chance (coincidence). He thought that because two things are connected by chance one of them is the cause of the other. This is what someone who is not biased would say. But someone who is biased can say anything he wants.

(VI.41) (333) Says Hippocrates: *If suppuration occurs in a certain place in the body but the suppuration does not show itself, this is due to the thickness of the pus or the thickness of the spot (part).*

Says the commentator: It is clear that it is difficult to recognize the suppurating substance because of its thickness or because of the thickness of the spot (part).

(VI.42) (334) Says Hippocrates: *If the liver is hard in someone suffering from jaundice, it is a bad sign.*

Says the commentator: This is clear.

(VI.43) (335) Says Hippocrates: *If someone suffering from an illness of the spleen is attacked by dysentery and this becomes chronic, dropsy or lientery supervenes and he dies.*

Says the commentator: A splenetic patient is someone whose spleen has been hard for a long time. If he develops dysentery, whereby those thick melancholic humors that got stuck in the body of the spleen are removed, he will benefit therefrom, as Hippocrates will explain later on. But if the dysentery becomes chronic and excessive, it undermines the powers of the intestines by transporting those bad humors through them and thus produces lientery. And the innate heat is extinguished. Because of the sympathetic affection between the intestines and the liver, the liver is weakened and dropsy occurs.

(VI.44) (336) Says Hippocrates: *If someone suffers, as a result of strangury, from a colic known as "ileus," which means "that from which ones seeks protection," he will die within seven days unless he develops fever and there is an abundant flow of urine.*

Says the commentator: Galen was in doubt about this aphorism and compelled himself to give farfetched interpretations in order to authenticate a statement that is clearly deficient and the product of those who pursue things that are vain (useless). [*In Hippocratis Aphorismos commentarius* VI.44].

(VI.45) (337) Says Hippocrates: *If ulcers last for a year or longer, the bone must necessarily exfoliate and—once the ulcer has healed—the scar must be depressed.*

Says the commentator: Ulcers mostly last a long time because of an affliction that reached the bone. When the corrupted bone has been expelled, the ulcer heals but the site remains hollow.

(VI.46) (338) Says Hippocrates: *If someone becomes humpback from asthma or cough before reaching puberty, he will die.*

Says the commentator: If a humpback develops without any initial cause, it comes from a hard tumor. Because of the curved spine, tightness of the lungs necessarily follows. During the growth of the body, the lungs enlarge but the chest cavity cannot expand and grow in its totality because of the humpback and its cause, and therefore the patient suffocates and dies.

(VI.47) (339) Says Hippocrates: *If someone needs to be bled or to be administered a purgative drug, he should be administered a purgative drug or bled in spring.*

Says the commentator: This is clear in the case of someone who needs that as a precautionary (prophylactic) measure, as healthy people always do.

(VI.48) (340) *Says Hippocrates: If someone suffering from an illness of the spleen develops dysentery, it is a good sign.*

Says the commentator: This has been explained before.

(VI.49) (341) Says Hippocrates: *When gout-like illnesses are accompanied by an inflammation, the inflammation subsides within forty days.*

Says the commentator: I have already described how he arrives at these incorrect definitions (conclusions).

(VI.50) (342) Says Hippocrates: *If someone suffers from a gash in the brain, he will unavoidably develop fever and bilious vomiting.*

Says the commentator: When the brain becomes swollen because of the gash, it is necessarily followed by fever and bilious vomiting because of the sympathetic affection between the brain and the stomach.

(VI.51) (343) Says Hippocrates: *If someone who is healthy suddenly gets a headache and immediately loses his voice and starts to breath stertorously, he will die within seven days, unless he develops fever.*

Says the commentator: The stertorous sound is an indication for the strength of the apoplexy, and you know that it is fatal unless fever develops, for sometimes the fever dissolves those thick humors or thick winds.

(VI.52) (344) Says Hippocrates: *One should observe the hidden part of the eye during sleep, for if part of the white of the eye is visible, while the eyelid is closed, and this does not occur after diarrhea or the ingestion of a purgative medication, it is a bad and exceedingly fatal sign.*

Says the commentator: The white of the eye becomes only visible when the eyelid is not closed. The eyelid does not close because of dryness and the dryness quickly affects the eyelids because of their natural dryness or because of the weakness of the strength of the body as occurs in patients who are too weak to close their mouths.

(VI.53) (345) Says Hippocrates: *When mental confusion (delirium) occurs with laughter, it is safer; but when it is accompanied by anxiety and sorrow, it is more dangerous.*

Says the commentator: There is not any type of mental confusion (delirium) that is safe. The worst kind is that, which comes with a desire to attack (fight) and aggressive behavior, and this is called "madness." The least detrimental is the type that comes with laughter and unusual pleasure, as in the case of someone who drinks wine. Intermediate is the type that comes with worry and fear and thought. All these occur because of a primary illness in the brain or because of the sympathetic affection with another organ. The type of mental confusion (delirium) that occurs because of heat (fever) only without the involvement of any humor is similar to the mental confusion (delirium) that occurs because of the drinking of wine. The type of mental confusion (delirium) that develops from yellow bile is accompanied by worry and fear. When the yellow bile becomes increasingly burnt and tends to black bile, the mental confusion (delirium) turns into madness.

(VI.54) (346) Says Hippocrates: *Respiration—that is broken as if by sobbing—in acute diseases accompanied by fever is a bad sign.*

Says the commentator: He means that the respiration of the patient stops and then returns like the respiration of someone suffocating from crying. This happens either because the patient is too weak to breathe fully or because the respiratory organs are so dry and hard that the patient has not the strength to expand them or because his condition is close to that of someone suffering from spasms. All these are bad during acute diseases.

(VI.55) (347) Says Hippocrates: *Gouty affections are active mostly in spring and autumn.*

Says the commentator: This happens in spring because the humors flow increasingly as they dissolve from their winter congelation, and in autumn because of the earlier consumption of summer fruit.

(VI.56) (348) Says Hippocrates: *In melancholic illnesses, one has to fear that they lead to apoplexy or hemiplegia or spasms or madness or blindness.*

Says the commentator: Galen says that apoplexy, hemiplegia, spasms, and blindness sometimes originate from phlegmatic humor and sometimes from melancholic humor. However, madness only occurs from the burning of yellow bile to a degree that it turns black. [*In Hippocratis Aphorismos commentarius* VI.56].

(VI.57) (349) Says Hippocrates: *Apoplexy and hemiplegia occur especially in the case of someone who is between forty and sixty years old.*

Says the commentator: Galen interprets this aphorism in a way that it is correct by saying: With apoplexy and hemiplegia, Hippocrates means apoplexy and hemiplegia that originate from black bile, because black bile dominates in people of that age. [*In Hippocratis Aphorismos commentarius* VI.57]. However, the truth of the matter is that the occurrence of these two illnesses as a result of black bile is extremely rare and that they occur mostly as a result of phlegm and from the age of sixty until the end of life.

(VI.58) (350) Says Hippocrates: *If the omentum protrudes, it will necessarily putrefy.*

Says the commentator: This is clear.

(VI.59) (351) Says Hippocrates: *If someone suffers from pain in the sciatic nerve and the hip joint dislocates and then returns again, mucous moisture is formed.*

Says the commentator: Because of the mucous moisture, the ligaments become moist and the head of the thigh bone dislocates from its socket in the hip bone.

(VI.60) (352) Says Hippocrates: *If someone suffers from chronic pain in the hip and the joint becomes dislocated, the leg wastes away completely and the patient becomes lame unless the part is cauterized.*

Says the commentator: That mucous moisture can be dried through cauterization, but if it is not dried through cauterization the patient becomes lame, and the leg is not nourished as it is normally so that it wastes away.

This is the end of the sixth part of the commentary on the Aphorisms.

In the name of God,
the Merciful, the Compassionate

The Seventh Part of the *Commentary on Hippocrates'* Aphorisms

(VII.1) (353) Says Hippocrates: *Coldness of the extremities in acute diseases is a bad sign.*

Says the commentator: This is, in my opinion, an indication for the weakness of the innate heat and that it does not spread to the extremities, while the illness with which it comes is acute, that is to say, "hot." Because Hippocrates sometimes calls those acute diseases "hot" that are associated with fever, which is continuous. The extremities are the tip of the nose, the ears, hands, and feet.

(VII.2) (354) Says Hippocrates: *If a bone is diseased and the color of the flesh is livid, it is a bad sign.*

Says the commentator: This color results from the extinction of the innate heat.

(VII.3) (355) Says Hippocrates: *The occurrence of hiccups and redness of the eyes after vomiting is a bad sign.*

Says the commentator: If spasms (hiccups) do not go away after vomiting, it is an indication that it is caused either by an inflammation in the beginning of the nerves, that is, the brain, or by an inflammation in the stomach. Redness of the eyes results from these two inflammations.

(VII.4) (356) Says Hippocrates: *If sweating is followed by shivering, it is not a good sign.*

Says the commentator: Hippocrates has already said that if the symptoms of a crisis do not result in a crisis, these symptoms indicate death or a difficult crisis because nature is weakened. [*Epidemics* II.1.76].

(VII.5) (357) Says Hippocrates: *If madness is followed by dysentery, dropsy, or confusion, it is a good sign.*

Says the commentator: The dropsy and dysentery cure the madness by removing the matter that produces the illness. Confusion cures madness because when the symptoms of confusion increase and become stronger, they constrain and move nature to expel all that is harmful in the way of a crisis. This is Galen's explanation of the aphorism. [*In Hippocratis Aphorismos commentarius* VII.5].

(VII.6) (358) Says Hippocrates: *In a chronic illness, loss of appetite and unmixed stools are a bad sign.*

Says the commentator: With unmixed stools he means those that are not mixed with any watery moisture, for only in this way the illness that is in the body can be expelled, whether it is a type of yellow bile or black bile. This is an indication that all the natural moisture that was in the body has been burnt by the heat of the fever.

(VII.7) (359) Says Hippocrates: *If rigor and mental confusion (delirium) occur from excessive drinking, it is a bad sign.*

Says the commentator: The combination of rigor and mental confusion (delirium) occurs only rarely, except in the case of some people who are often intoxicated. Then the innate heat is extinguished, rigor occurs, their brain is filled with hot blood or hot vapors so that mental confusion (delirium) develops.

(VII.8) (360) Says Hippocrates: *If an abscess breaks internally, it results in a collapse of strength and in vomiting and fainting.*

Says the commentator: This is clear; with *khurāj* he means *dubayla* (abscess). With "internally," he means "into the stomach."

(VII.9) (361) Says Hippocrates: *If mental confusion (delirium) or spasms occur as a result of a flow of blood, it is a bad sign.*

Says the commentator: After an evacuation of blood, a mental confusion (delirium) develops, because the brain is disturbed in its movements and is then constantly weak. Hippocrates calls a mild delirium "raving." [*In Hippocratis Epidemiarum commentarius* III.1].

(VII.10) (362) Says Hippocrates: *If vomiting, hiccups, mental confusion (delirium), or spasms occur as a result of a colic, may God protect us from it, it is a bad sign.*

Says the commentator: This is clear.

(VII.11) (363) Says Hippocrates: *If pneumonia occurs as a result of pleurisy, it is a bad sign.*

Says the commentator: If the humor that produces the pleurisy has not enough space, some of it flows to the lungs and causes pneumonia. But it is almost impossible that pneumonia leads to (causes) pleurisy.

(VII.12) (364) Says Hippocrates: *And it is a bad sign if phrenitis develops from pneumonia.*

(VII.13) (365) Says Hippocrates: *And it is a bad sign if spasms or tetanus develop from severe burns.*

(VII.14) (366) Says Hippocrates: *And it is a bad sign if a stupor or mental confusion (delirium) develops from a blow on the head.*

(VII.15) (367) Says Hippocrates: *And it is a bad sign if spitting of pus develops from hemoptysis.*

(VII.16) (368) Says Hippocrates: *And it is a bad sign if phthisis and flux develop from the spitting of pus. When the spitting stops, the patient dies.*

(VII.17) (369) Says Hippocrates: *And it is a bad sign if hiccups develop from an inflammation of the liver.*

(VII.18) (370) Says Hippocrates: *And it is a bad sign if spasms and mental confusion (delirium) develop from sleeplessness.*

Says the commentator: All these statements are clear. Their meaning is that if these illnesses become more severe and grave there may develop such and such conditions as mentioned. For instance, if the inflammation of the liver becomes more severe and harms the cardia of the stomach, hiccups develop. It is well known that spasms and mental confusion (delirium) may develop from dryness, and that dryness comes after excessive evacuation or the movements of the soul (emotions) and sleeplessness.

(VII.19) (371) Says Hippocrates: *And it is a bad sign if the swelling called "erysipelas" develops from the laying bare of a bone.*

Says the commentator: Galen has explained that this inflammation only rarely results from the laying bare of a bone. Therefore, Hippocrates mentions everything that can possibly happen as a result of the laying bare of a bone, even when it is most rare. [*In Hippocratis Aphorismos commentarius* VII.19].

(VII.20) (372) Says Hippocrates: *And it is a bad sign if putrefaction or suppuration develops from the inflammation called "erysipelas."*

Says the commentator: This is clear according to what I said on different occasions before, that it means that this may be the case.

(VII.21) (373) Says Hippocrates: *And it is a bad sign if a hemorrhage develops from violent throbbing in wounds.*

Says the commentator: This is clear because the severe pain causes the vessels to move (pulsate) strongly to expel the harmful matter.

(VII.22) (374) Says Hippocrates: *And it is a bad sign if suppuration develops from chronic pain in the parts about the belly.*

Says the commentator: An inflammation develops from chronic pain and that inflammation suppurates.

(VII.23) (375) Says Hippocrates: *And it is a bad sign if dysentery develops from unmixed stools.*

Says the commentator: He means that if the stools only consist of a certain humor, corrosion and wounds may occur in the intestines.

(VII.24) (376) Says Hippocrates: *And it is a bad sign if mental confusion (delirium) develops from the severing of a bone, if it reaches the cavity.*

Says the commentator: Galen says that if the bone of the head (skull) is severed to a degree that it reaches the cavity that surrounds the brain, mental confusion (delirium) develops.

(VII.25) (377) Says Hippocrates: *If spasms develop from the ingestion of a purgative drug it is fatal.*

Says the commentator: This is clear.

(VII.26) (378) Says Hippocrates: *If coldness of the extremities develops from severe pain in the parts about the belly, it is a bad sign.*

Says the commentator: This is clear.

(VII.27) (379) Says Hippocrates: *If a pregnant woman suffers from tenesmus, it causes a miscarriage*

Says the commentator: This is clear.

(VII.28) (380) Says Hippocrates: *If part of a bone or cartilage is cut through, it does not grow together again.*

Says the commentator: Galen has already affirmed that this aphorism is a repetition.

(VII.29) (381) Says Hippocrates: *If someone dominated by white phlegm is attacked by violent diarrhea, his illness will dissolve.*

Says the commentator: The white phlegm is the dropsy of the flesh (anasarca). Says the author (Maimonides): I have seen twice, that a patient suffering from dropsy of the flesh was cured through violent diarrhea.

(VII.30) (382) Says Hippocrates: *If someone suffers from diarrhea and the diarrhea is frothy, the cause of the diarrhea is moisture descending from the head.*

Says the commentator: The reason for the diarrhea to be frothy is that it is strongly mixed with air. Sometimes the airy moisture causing the diarrhea to be frothy descends from the head, sometimes it comes from the other organs, and sometimes it originates in the stomach and intestines.

(VII.31) (383) Says Hippocrates: *If someone with fever has sediments in his urine that resemble coarse meal, it is an indication that his illness will be protracted.*

Says the commentator: The humors of someone whose illness appears to be such are far from being concocted. For this reason, Hippocrates says that these patients mostly die and that he, who escapes, has a protracted illness, as he mentioned here. [*Prognostic* 12; *In Hippocratis Aphorismos commentarius* VII.31].

(VII.32) (384) Says Hippocrates: *If the sediment in the urine is dominated by bile and the upper part is thin (watery), it indicates that the illness is acute.*

Says the commentator: This is clear. With "thin," he means that the upper part of the sediment is thin and that its shape is like that of pine nuts.

(VII.33) (385) Says Hippocrates: *If someone's urine is heterogeneous, it indicates that there is a violent disturbance in his body.*

Says the commentator: It means urine consisting of different parts, and this is an indication for the variant activity of nature with regard to the humors.

(VII.34) (386) Says Hippocrates: *If there are bubbles on the surface of someone's urine, it is an indication that the illness is in the kidneys; it also tells us that it will be lengthy.*

Says the commentator: This is so because bubbles indicate thick wind (flatulence) within viscous humors, and this tells us that the illness will be lengthy.

(VII.35) (387) Says Hippocrates: *If someone observes that the surface of his urine is totally covered with a greasy substance, it indicates that there is an acute illness in his kidneys.*

Says the commentator: If the greasy substance turns up all at once, it is an indication that it comes from the melting of the fat of the kidneys. This is the meaning of the word "totally." But what turns up from the dissolution of the other organs comes little by little.

(VII.36) (388) Says Hippocrates: *When someone is affected by an illness in his kidneys and suffers from the aforementioned symptoms, and also suffers from pain in the muscles in the back, expect an external abscess, provided that the pain is in the external parts. But if the pain is in the internal parts, expect rather that the abscess will be internal.*

Says the commentator: This is clear.

(VII.37) (389) Says Hippocrates: *If someone vomits blood without fever, it is safe (not dangerous) and he should be treated with astringent ingredients. But if someone vomits blood while he has fever, it is a bad sign.*

Says the commentator: He means to say that if there is no inflammation in the stomach that would necessarily be followed by fever, and if the vomiting of blood is caused by a burst blood vessel or by a wound that has now developed, it is possible that the patient is cured quickly by means of astringent ingredients.

(VII.38) (390) Says Hippocrates: *Catarrhs that descend into the upper cavity suppurate within twenty days.*

Says the commentator: The upper cavity is the chest cavity in which the lungs are found. The twentieth day is the day of the crisis because it is the last day of the third week. Hippocrates says that this is the ultimate day in which a catarrh can concoct.

(VII.39) (391) Says Hippocrates: *If someone urinates blood with clots and he suffers from strangury and pain in the region of the anus and pubes, it indicates that there is a pain in the region of the bladder.*

Says the commentator: This aphorism is a repetition.

(VII.40) (392) Says Hippocrates: *When the tongue suddenly loses its strength or a limb of one's body becomes paralyzed, the illness is caused by black bile.*

Says the commentator: Galen has already affirmed that this condition does not necessarily and unavoidably result from black bile. [*In Hippocratis Aphorismos commentarius* VII.40].

(VII.41) (393) Says Hippocrates: *If an elderly person suffers from hiccups because of the emptying of the body through purging or emesis, it is not a good sign.*

Says the commentator: Hiccups after evacuations are bad because they follow dryness. In old people it is worse because of the dryness of their temperament due to their age.

(VII.42) (394) Says Hippocrates: *If a person is attacked by fever that is not caused by bile and one pours much hot water over his head, his fever will be dissolved.*

Says the commentator: Galen wants to explain this aphorism by saying that with the phrase "fever that is not caused by bile," Hippocrates does not refer to putrid fever but to some kind of ephemeral fever. There is no doubt that bathing is beneficial for it and that the fever is dissolved by it. [*In Hippocratis Aphorismos commentarius* VII.42].

(VII.43) (395) Says Hippocrates: *A woman does not become ambidextrous.*

Says the commentator: Galen says that the reason for that is the weakness of her nerves and muscles, for every ambidextrous person has strong nerves. [*In Hippocratis Aphorismos commentarius* VII.43].

(VII.44) (396) Says Hippocrates: *If patients with empyema are treated either by cautery or by incision and pure white pus flows out, they will be saved (recover). But if turbid and foul-smelling matter flows out, they will die.*

Says the commentator: Patients with empyema are those in whom much pus has accumulated between their chest and lungs. The ancient physicians used to cauterize them in order to eliminate that matter.

(VII.45) (397) Says Hippocrates: *If a patient has pus in the liver and is cauterized and clear white pus flows out, he will recover because that pus is situated in the membrane of the liver. But if it flows similar to lees of oil, he will die.*

Says the commentator: If the pus is in the membrane and the substance of the liver is healthy, recovery is possible.

(VII.46) (398) Says Hippocrates: *If someone suffers from pain in the eyes, administer him pure wine, then let him enter the bathhouse, pour much hot water over his head, and bleed him.*

Says the commentator: Galen says that this aphorism was ascribed to Hippocrates without proper authority (falsely ascribed to him). [*In Hippocratis Aphorismos commentarius* VII.46]. In short, it is totally incorrect, whoever said it for the first time.

(VII.47) (399) Says Hippocrates: *If a dropsical patient suffers from cough, there is no hope for him.*

Says the commentator: This aphorism is a repetition.

(VII.48) (400) Says Hippocrates: *Strangury and dysuria are alleviated by drinking wine and by venesection; one should open the internal veins.*

Says the commentator: This aphorism is evidently corrupt. But Galen took it upon himself to give a correct meaning (interpretation) to the first part by saying that if it is caused by cold or an obstruction due to thick blood while there is no overfilling in the body, then the drinking of much wine is beneficial. [*In Hippocratis Aphorismos commentarius* VII.48].

As for the latter part of this aphorism and likewise an earlier aphorism, where he states that one should open the internal veins, Galen has made it clear that this is not correct and that it is not the opinion of Hippocrates. [*In Hippocratis Aphorismos commentarius* VI.36].

(VII.49) (401) Says Hippocrates: *If a swelling and redness appear on the front of the chest in the case of someone suffering from angina, it is a good sign because the illness will have been diverted outwards.*

Says the commentator: This is clear.

(VII.50) (402) Says Hippocrates: *If someone is attacked in the brain by the illness called "sphacelus" (mortification), he will die within three days. But if he outlives these, he will recover.*

Says the commentator: This illness consists of a corruption of the substance of the brain for which there is no cure once it has become firmly settled. But here he wants to say that if this illness has begun and lasts longer than three days and the patient has not died, it is a sign that the illness is not firmly settled and that nature is powerful and will overcome the illness.

(VII.51) (403) Says Hippocrates: *Sneezing arises from the head when the brain becomes hot and the cavity in the head becomes moist; then the air that is inside descends and produces a noise because it passes through a narrow passage.*

Says the commentator: Sometimes sneezing occurs when the brain gets hot and the empty space in it becomes moist and that moisture dissolves in vapor. Sometimes, wind rises from below during coughing and when it arrives in the nasal passages it causes sneezing. The nasal passages lead to two places (organs): the mouth and the brain. The opening that leads to the mouth is cleansed by the wind that arises from below, while the passages that lead to the brain are cleansed by the wind that descends from it. With the term "the empty space," he means the ventricles of the brain.

(VII.52) (404) Says Hippocrates: *If someone suffers from a severe pain in the liver and then develops a fever it will relieve the pain.*

Says the commentator: A severe pain in the liver without fever is caused by thick wind (flatulence). For this reason, if fever supervenes, the wind (flatulence) is dissolved.

(VII.53) (405) Says Hippocrates: *If a patient needs venesection, one should bleed him in spring.*

Says the commentator: This is one of the aphorisms that are repetitious.

(VII.54) (406) Says Hippocrates: *If a person has phlegm confined in the area between the stomach and diaphragm and he suffers from pain because it has no outlet into either of the two cavities, the illness will resolve if the phlegm flows through the vessels into the urinary bladder.*

Says the commentator: It has been said that this aphorism is not by Hippocrates. Galen has said that it is not impossible that this humor can penetrate into the vessels through transudation, because nature is crafty in thinning superfluous matters and expelling them through any possible passage, even if it is extremely narrow, as it does to expel the pus accumulated in the area between the lung and chest. In general, what he says only happens rarely; it is therefore of very little benefit.

(VII.55) (407) Says Hippocrates: *Is someone's liver is filled with water and this water bursts into the omentum, the belly fills with water and he dies.*

Says the commentator: These watery vesicles often occur in the liver. His statement that "someone whose belly fills with water dies" means that this is mostly the case.

(VII.56) (408) Says Hippocrates: *Anxiety, yawning, and shivering are cured by wine when it is mixed with an equal part of water.*

Says the commentator: Anxiety mostly hails from harmful moisture in the cardia of the stomach. Drinking slightly diluted wine cures, as stated, all this because it washes (cleanses) the vessels and improves the humors.

(VII.57) (409) Says Hippocrates: *If someone gets a tumor in the urethra, when it suppurates and bursts, the pain comes to an end.*

Says the commentator: This aphorism is a repetition.

(VII.58) (410) Says Hippocrates: *If someone has a concussion of the brain, he will immediately become paralyzed.*

Says the commentator: A concussion of the brain or spinal cord is caused by a fall and the like.

(VII.59) (411) —

(VII.60) (412) Says Hippocrates: *If the flesh of someone's body is moist, he should starve because hunger dries the body.*

Says the commentator: This is clear.

(VII.61) (413) Says Hippocrates: *If changes occur in the whole body and it becomes very cold and then hot or it changes its color, it indicates a protracted disease.*

Says the commentator: This aphorism is a repetition.

(VII.62) (414) Says Hippocrates: *Much sweat that flows constantly—whether hot or cold—indicates that moisture should be evacuated from the body; in a strong person from above (through emesis) and in a weak person from below (through purgation).*

Says the commentator: His statement that the moisture of strong people should be evacuated through emesis and that of weak people through purgation should not always be carried out in this way. You already know Hippocrates' approach. Galen doubts whether this aphorism is by Hippocrates or by somebody else. [*In Hippocratis Aphorismos commentarius* VII.62].

This is the end of the seventh part of the commentary on the Aphorisms.
Praise be to God alone.

Glossary of Technical Terms

From: Faith Wallis (ed.), *Medieval Medicine: A Reader*, Toronto 2010 (*Readings in Medieval Civilizations and Cultures*, Vol. 15), 543–552

apoplexy cerebral hemorrhage or stroke.

bile, black → melancholy.

bile, red/yellow one of the four humors of the body; its temperament is hot and dry.

bole, Armenian earth containing iron oxide (from the Latin *bolus*, "clod of earth"). It was frequently employed in ancient and medieval pharmacy.

castoreum reddish glands found in the groin of the Eurasian beaver (*Castor fiber* Linnaeus, 1758) and widely used in medieval medicine, notable as an emetic.

cataract clouding of the crystalline lens of the eye resulting in loss of sight. The name derives from the theory that the eye was filling up with excess humor from the brain.

catarrh dripping from the nose; by extension, a head cold.

cautery the application of a heated metal instrument to the body to sear the tissue (e.g., in order to close off a ruptured blood vessel). In ancient and medieval medicine, cautery was also used to divert the flow of humors through the body.

cerate a thick, wax-based topical application.

chyle the initial product of the "first digestion" of food in the stomach: coarsely mashed and mixed food. The next phase is chyme.

chyme the pulpy, more liquefied stage of chyle as it is further digested.

clyster enema used to administer a purgative.

coction/concoction the action of the innate heat of the body in "cooking" food or morbific matter, permitting its digestion.

collyria medicated drops or ointment for the eyes.

complexion the blending of qualities or humors which is natural to an individual person, an organ of the human body, or a humoral type; temperament. The term survives today to denote the quality of the skin of the face, because pre-modern physicians made an initial determination of the patient's complexion from examining the face.

continuity → dissolution of continuity.

continuous fever → fever.

corrupt/corruption the state of a substance (e.g., air, food) or a humor that has been transformed into a morbid state through qualitative excess (e.g., too much heat), or through infection. The core metaphor is one of putrefaction: an internal disease is visualized as a collection of rotting organic matter that needs to be diverted away from important organs and then evacuated, or as an internal wound that is suppurating with diseased matter.

crisis a sudden change in the course of an illness which either restores the patient to health or leads to death.

critical day a day on which a crisis is likely to occur.

cupping the operation of evacuating blood through the skin by applying a heated glass cup to the surface of the skin (which may be scarified in advance).

decoction the fluid resulting from boiling an herb or other substance.

degree Galen assumes that each foodstuff or each basic ingredient of a compound medicine not only exhibits the primal qualities of heat, cold, moisture, and dryness, but does so to a greater or lesser extent. Arabic Galenists systematized this by positing four degrees for each quality, from barely perceptible (the first degree) to extremely intense (the fourth degree). Ingredients were held to possess two qualities, one from the hot-cold and one from the moist-dry binary.

determine in the jargon of the medieval university, to make an authoritative declaration on a topic, notably by resolving a disputed question or constructing a logical argument.

digest/digestion a term with both a primary and an extended meaning, digestion can refer to the physiological process of refining and transforming food, or even air, into a form the body could absorb. It is understood to proceed in stages: the first digestion in the stomach produces chyle, the second digestion in the liver produces blood, and the third digestion is when the blood is taken up into the members. All three produce waste products, which must be expelled by the body. Digestion also had an extended meaning when applied to pathology. A wound or internal disease required that the corrupt or peccant disease matter be "digested" and the body's normal continuity or temperament restored. Drug therapy and wound dressing in particular aimed to promote this digestion.

dissolution of continuity a rupture or dissolution of the continuity of bone or flesh, i.e., physical trauma in the form of breakage, tearing, or wounding.

dropsy accumulation of fluid in the abdomen.

dyscrasia disruption of an individual's complexional or humoral balance.

dyspnea difficulty in breathing.

electuary a drug administered in the form of a paste that was licked from a spoon.

emetic a drug that provokes vomiting.

ephemeral fever → fever.

erysipelas a streptococcal skin infection characterized by sudden high fever, malaise, and a painful, swollen rash with blistering and discoloration.

evacuate/evacuation any procedure designed to expel disease matter (e.g., corrupt or peccant humor) from the body. The body will do this naturally through vomiting, bowel movements, etc., but the physician may assist the weakened body at the suitable moment by administering a purge, or by opening a vein (bloodletting or phlebotomy).

experiment when applied to medicine, the word denotes a tried-and-true remedy, one that has been proven effective by experience (*experimentum*), but whose action cannot necessarily be explained by pharmacological theory.

fever unnatural heat of the body. Fevers were classified by the periodicity of their paroxysms: "continuous" fevers never broke, "quotidian" fevers peaked every day, "biduan" every other day, "tertian" fevers peaked every third day (counting inclusively), "quartan" fevers every fourth day, and so forth. Fevers were also classified according to the matter affected: "ephemeral" fevers attacked the spirits, "putrid" fevers the humors, and "hectic" fevers the solid parts of the body.

fistula an ulcer that takes the form of a channel or a pipe.

foment/fomentation a warm topical application, usually of a cloth steeped in water or a medical decoction.

form → specific form.

fumigation burning a medicinal substance to produce smoke, which is channeled into a body orifice. Fumigation was typically used to introduce medicine into the female reproductive organs. The patient would crouch on a stool over a small brazier.

hectic fever → fever.

hiera lit., "something holy". *Hiera* was a generic and honorific title for certain noteworthy compound medicines. The most widely known was *hiera picra* ("holy bitters"), a cathartic of which the principal ingredient was tincture of aloes.

homoeomerous having or consisting of similar parts.

humor depending on context, either (a) a moisture or fluid of some kind, or (b) one of the four bodily fluids deemed to constitute the physiological basis of human life. The classic humors are blood, red bile (also called yellow bile), phlegm and black bile (or melancholy).

hydromel a drink of honey mixed with water.

lientery diarrhea in which particles of undigested food can be observed.

melancholy black bile. One of the four humors of the human body, its qualities are cold and dry. It also refers to a disease state caused by excess of this humor, or by adust blood or black bile, and characterized by mental gloom, obsession, and other psychic disturbances.

mortify/mortification depending on context, "mortify" can mean either (a) to subdue or bring under control (a disease or a poison) or (b) to rot or corrupt (e.g., in cases of gangrene the flesh is "mortified").

natron hydrous sodium carbonate, a mineral salt found in dried lake beds, e.g., in Egypt.

ophthalmia an inflammation of the eye.

oxymel a medicinal drink made of wine and honey

phlebotomy bloodletting.

phlegm one of the four humors of the human body; it is cold and wet.

phlegmon an inflamed, red swelling, boil or tumor. The old-fashioned English equivalent was carbuncle, a word that also means "ruby."

phthisis synonym for consumption (from the Greek word meaning "wasting away").

potion internally administered medicine in liquid form; often generalized to cover any internally administered medicine.

powers (Latin *virtutes*) in Galenic medicine, the natural principles within the body that organize and execute the three major functions of life: nutrition, growth, and reproduction (natural power); respiration, heat, and emotion (spiritual or vital power); sensation, voluntary motion, and cognition (animal power). The powers are the manifestations of the spirits.

purge/purgative to "clean" or evacuate the body of disease matter or peccant humor by provoking vomiting (using an emetic or cathartic) or a bowel movement (using an enema). A purgative is a medicine administered to effect purging, or which has the property of purging.

putrid fever → fever.

quartan fever → fever.

quotidian fever → fever.

rheum a morbid discharge of phlegm in the head (e.g., a runny nose), eyes, joints, etc.

ripe/ripen the process whereby an aposteme reaches a mature state in which the morbific matter can be digested

scarify/scarification to make shallow cuts in the skin, or to raise a blister by the application of a hot iron, acid, or boiling pitch. The formation of liquid in the blisters was seen as a sign that the body was acting to drain away dangerous humors.

simple a drug composed of a single, usually herbal, substance; an herb used for medicinal purposes.

specific form a power that inheres in a substance by its very nature, and that is not reducible to the sum of the qualities of which it is composed. Also called "total species," this concept was used to explain, among other things, the specific action of drugs like theriac.

strangury difficulty in urinating.

syncope fainting.

synochous fever a kind of continuous fever, ascribed to putrefaction of the blood.

syrup in the medical sense, a drug administered in sugar syrup. The sugar syrup medium acted as a preservative agent, and thus the syrup itself was held to have medicinal, preservative effect.

temperament the proper or balanced mixture of the four elements, qualities (hot, cold, wet, dry), or humors. In pharmacy, the qualities of one ingredient will be tempered (mitigated, balanced out) by the addition of an ingredient of contrary qualities. With reference to human physiology and psychology, temperament can refer to generic type ("the melancholy temperament") or individual complexion.

tenesmus strong sensation of discomfort in the lower bowel and desire to defecate; straining results in the passage of mucus and often blood.

terra sigillata red clay, originally from the Aegean island of Lemnos, formed into tablets and impressed with a seal: a popular remedy in ancient Rome, and used in medieval medicine as an antidote and astringent.

tertian fever → fever.

theriac an elaborate compound drug, used as a panacea or universal antidote to poison.

vapors internal fumes produced by digestion. These could be benign or morbid, depending on the state of digestion or the predominance of certain humors.

ventricle a small cavity or hollow space within an organ. Medieval physicians recognized not only the ventricles of the heart, but also ventricles in the brain. To the three main ventricles, they assigned different cognitive functions (imagination, reason, memory).

Glossary of Weights and Measures

bean, Egyptian	2.34 g
dāniq	0.52–0.74 g
dirham	3.125 g
ḥabba	0.05 g
hazelnut	3.31–4.25 g
mithqāl	4.68 g
mudd	1.053 l
ounce	37.5 g
ounce, Syrian	Aleppo: 190 g
	Damascus: 154.166 g
	Ḥamā: 225 g
	Jerusalem: 208.33 g
qīrāṭ	0.176–0.186 g
raṭl	450 g
ṭassūj	0.18 g

Sigla

Ast	*On Asthma*
Coi	*On Coitus*
Com	*Commentary on Hippocrates'* Aphorisms
Elu	*On the Elucidation of Some Symptoms and the Response to Them*
Hem	*On Hemorrhoids*
Med	*Medical Aphorisms*
Poi	*On Poisons and the Protection against Lethal Drugs*
Reg	*On the Regimen of Health*
Rul	*On Rules Regarding the Practical Part of the Medical Art*

Index of Quoted Physicians, Philosophers, and Their Works

Pseudepigrapha are marked with *

Alexander of Aphrodisias **Ast** XIII.50
Maqāla fī al-qawl fī mabādiʾ al-kull ʿalā raʾy Arisṭaṭālīs al-faylasūf **Ast** XIII.50
al-Andalūsī, Abū al-Ḥasan Sufyān **Ast** XIII.38
Aristides **Med** XXIV.58
Aristotle **Ast** XIII.20–22; **Med** IX.127; XXV.25, 29, 59–61, 70, 72; **Reg** II.3; **Com** N (6)
Analytica priora **Med** XXV.59
De generatione animalium (= *De animalibus XV–XIX*) **Med** XXV.29
De sensu et sensibilibus **Ast** XIII.20; **Reg** II.3
Historia animalium (= *De animalibus I–X*) **Med** IX.127
Asklepios **Med** XV.63, 64; XXI.33
Avenzoar → Ibn Zuhr, Abū Marwān ʿAbd al-Malik
Avicenna → Ibn Sīnā

al-Biṭrīq **Med** XXIV.44, 59, 60

Epicurus **Med** XXV.62
Euclid **Com** N (7)

al-Fārābī, Abū Naṣr **Ast** XIII.6; **Med** N; XXV.58–60; **Reg** IV.4; **Com** I.1 (15)
K. al-Ḥurūf (*Book of Letters*) **Med** XXV.58
Risāla fī al-ṭibb **Com** I.1 (15)

Galen **Ast** N.4; I.1, 2, 4; II.2, 3; III.1–3; V.3–7; VI.2, 3; IX.2, 5–12; X.1, 3, 5, 6, 8; XI.2, 4; XII.3–5, 8; XIII.2, 11, 13–16, 18, 19, 22, 25, 29, 30, 32–34, 37–39, 44; **Poi** 20, 34, 39, 43, 53, 56, 70, 72; **Hem** I.3; **Med** N; I.20, 34, 38, 50; II.8; III.101; V.20; VI.8, 16; VII.8, 9, 12, 14, 15; VIII.49; IX.88, 127; X.33; XIII.6; XIV.10; XVI.19; XVII.2, 41; XIX.25, 26; XX.40; XXI.67; XXII.56; XXIII.1, 3, 20, 21, 22, 25, 31, 40, 50, 58a, 60; XXIV.1, 3, 4, 13–15, 17, 23, 26a, 39, 40, 44, 52, 53, 55, 57, 59; XXV.0, 1, 5, 11, 14, 15, 17, 20–23, 25, 29, 32, 37, 48, 49, 51, 52, 55–59, 61–64, 66–68, 70–72; **Reg** I.2, 8, 15, 16, 21, 22; II.1, 2, 9; III.5, 11; IV.1, 9, 11–13, 16, 19, 20, 25; **Elu** 2, 11, 17, 33, 40; **Com** N (7, 8, 10, 11, 13); I.1 (18, 24–26), 2 (29), 13–15 (40–42), 18–21 (45–48), 23–25 (50–52); II.15 (67), 19 (71), 20 (72), 23 (75), 24 (76), 36 (88), 43 (95), 44 (96), 50 (102), 52–54 (104–106); III.16 (122), 24 (130), 29 (135), 30 (136); IV.32 (169), 46 (183), 48 (185), 54 (191), 59 (196), 61 (198), 67 (204), 71 (208), 76 (213); V.7 (227), 16 (236), 40 (260), 43 (263), 48 (268), 60 (280), 65 (285), 67 (287), 70 (290); VI.7 (299), 18 (310), 26 (318), 30 (322), 31 (323), 34 (326), 36 (328), 44 (336), 56 (348), 57 (349); VII.5 (357), 19 (371), 24 (376), 28 (380), 40 (392), 42 (394), 43 (395), 46 (398), 48 (400), 54 (406), 62 (414)
Ad Glauconem de medendi methodo **Med** III.61; VII.3, 24; VIII.8, 34, 35, 58, 59, 65, 72, 73; IX.14, 62, 63, 105–107; X.8, 9, 25, 33–35, 41; XII.5, 41; XIII.38; XIV.4; XV.8–13, 45, 50–53; XVI.11, 22; XVIII.16; XIX.4, 23, 32, 33; XXI.95; XXII.17; XXIII.7, 37, 41, 47; XXV.33, 54
De alimentorum facultatibus **Ast** II.2; III.1–3; V.4; **Med** I.16, 17; II.11, 16, 17; XIV.7; XVII.15, 16, 25; XX.2–6, 13–17, 22, 23, 43–45, 54, 56, 62–65; XXI.9, 10, 14, 37; XXIII.104–106; XXIV.31–33; XXV.9, 22, 30, 31, 34, 35; **Elu** 33
De anatomia vivorum **Med** I.49
De anatomicis administrationibus **Med** XII.27; XXIV.5
De antidotis **Poi** 43, 53; **Med** XXI.32, 50; XXIII.97; **Elu** 17

De arte parva **Med** III.20; VIII.57, 64; IX.104; XV.49; XVII.8
De atra bile **Med** II.3, 14; III.50; VI.25, 26, 72; XV.59; XVI.31; XXV.39
De bonis malisque sucis **Ast** V.5; **Med** XVII.1, 3, 22; XVIII.1; XX.1, 19, 40, 41, 47, 48, 51, 58–61; XXI.2, 34; XXIII.102; XXV.10, 14, 30; **Reg** I.2, 22; **Elu** 11
De causis morborum (= *De morborum causis et symptomatibus II*) **Med** II.12, 22; VII.25, 67; XIX.6; XXV.5, 38, 40
De causis pulsuum (= *De pulsu magna III*) **Med** I.6; II.19; III.4; IV.5, 8–11, 21, 30–32, 37, 39, 41, 45–48; XXIII.27, 78; XXV.4
De circuitibus febrium **Med** X.24
De clysteribus et colica* **Med VII.65; VIII.27, 75; IX.91; X.52; XIII.34, 35; XXV.13
De compositione medicamentorum per genera **Med** III.114; XV.1, 2, 26, 32; XXIII.44, 98
De compositione medicamentorum secundum locos **Ast** XII.3; **Med** II.20; III.84–87, 109, 111; VI.59, 93; VII.33, 34; VIII.38, 39, 43, 66; IX.21, 22, 25–29, 37, 38, 50–53, 70–74, 87, 97, 121, 122; XII.30, 45; XIII.43; XV.27, 29; XIX.14, 15, 17; XX.31, 37, 55, 57; XXI.41–45, 47, 61; XXII.33, 34; XXIII.14, 24, 53, 54, 71–75, 79, 86–89; XXV.8, 52
De consuetudinibus **Med** VIII.22; XVII.23, 37; XXIII.9
De crisibus **Med** II.18; III.100–103; IV.29; V.1, 4–8, 10, 13–15, 17, 18; VI.28–30, 38, 73–77, 84–86; VIII.9; X.27–31, 39, 55; XI.1, 3, 6–16, 25; XXIII.30; XXV.45
De curandi ratione per venae sectionem **Med** III.8, 11, 46, 56; IV.4; VI.5; VIII.46; IX.2; XII.1–4, 6, 13–19, 22, 25, 26, 29, 31, 32, 35, 36, 38, 44; XIII.22; XVI.2, 13; XXIII.1; XXIV.7; XXV.11, 48, 52
De demonstratione **Med** XXV.25, 59
De diebus decretoriis **Med** X.21; XI.17–24
De differentia pulsuum (= *De pulsu magna I*) **Med** IV.2, 3, 33; XXIII.28, 29; XXIV.52; XXV.56
De differentiis febrium **Med** II.6; III.59, 68; IV.19, 35; V.2; X.6, 7, 10, 19, 20, 22, 23, 26, 38, 53, 54
De dignoscendis pulsibus **Med** IV.12–14, 36, 44
De examinatione medici **Med** IX.102
De extenuatione corporum pinguium* **Med IX.101
De febribus **Med** VII.44; X.58
De febrium differentiis **Med** VI.50; XXIII.26, 31, 39; XXV.5, 14, 23
De inaequali intemperie **Med** III.27, 64; X.36; XXV.21
De instrumento odoratus **Med** I.41; IX.12; XV.58
De libris propriis **Ast** XIII.30
De locis affectis **Med** I.32, 45–47; II.15; III.42, 43, 97, 104; V.11; VI.33–37, 42, 43, 51–58, 60–62, 78–83, 91, 92; VII.27–29, 35, 37, 47, 50, 52–54, 57; VIII.68; IX.15, 16, 43, 44, 65, 66, 79, 95, 109, 110, 113; X.42; XII.40; XV.14; XVI.5–7, 17–19, 24–27; XXIII.32, 50, 65, 66, 67, 77, 91, 93, 94; XXIV.8, 9, 30, 36–40; XXV.3, 19, 21, 28, 36, 52, 72; **Reg** III.11; IV.20; **Com** IV.57 (194)
De marcore **Med** III.3, 32; IX.100; X.57; XVII.36; XIX.2, 3, 31; XXIII.19, 20
De methodo medendi **Ast** XII.4; XIII.2, 32–34, 36; **Med** I.7, 60; III.13–15, 24, 30, 51, 67, 82, 83, 89–93, 105–108, 110, 113; VII.6, 9–15; VIII.10–12, 36, 37, 40–42, 47, 48, 61–63, 74; IX.17–20, 39, 46–49, 56, 57, 68–70, 75–78, 80, 86, 92, 114–120, 124–126; X.1–4, 15–18, 32, 47, 51, 60–71; XII.8–11, 20, 21, 24, 33, 34, 37, 46, 47; XIII.9, 13, 41, 42; XIV.6, 11; XV.15–25, 28, 33, 34, 36–43, 46–48, 54–57, 65; XVI.12; XIX.11–13, 16, 34–37; XX.8, 9, 30, 58; XXI.5, 6, 12, 16, 19, 27, 28, 39, 40, 92–94; XXIII.33, 42, 43, 52, 68, 97; XXV.7, 43, 47, 53, 55; **Reg** IV.1; **Com** N (11)
De morborum differentiis (= *De morborum causis et symptomatibus I*) **Med** II.12; VIII.44; XXIII.13; XXV.33, 38
De morborum temporibus **Med** VI.27
De motibus manifestis et obscuris **Med** VII.71; IX.11; XXIV.20
De motu musculorum **Med** I.9, 13–15, 24, 26–31, 33, 39, 40, 70, 71; VI.31; XXIV.21–23

De naturalibus facultatibus **Med** I.20, 50, 51, 57, 58, 66, 72–74; II.7–10, 23, 30; III.33, 60; XVI.21, 29; XX.18; XXV.3, 32
De nominibus medicis **Med** XXIV.3
De optico medico cognoscendo **Med** XXIV.24
De optima corporis nostri constitutione **Med** III.6
De optimo medico cognoscendo **Med** VIII.21; XIII.18, 30; XXIV.4
De parvae pilae exercitio **Med** XVIII.2, 3
De placitis Hippocratis et Platonis **Med** I.10–12; XXIV.55–57; XXV.59, 71
De plenitudine **Med** III.9; VI.6, 7, 9; VII.20, 22; XXIII.1–3
De praesagitione ex pulsibus (= *De pulsu magna IV*) **Med** I.65, 69; II.5; III.29, 70, 88, 98; IV.1, 6, 7, 18, 22–28, 38, 40, 42; VI.49; VII.1, 2, 30; IX.85; XXIV.41; XXV.44
De probis malisque alimentorum sucis **Med** II.24, 25
De propriis placitis **Med** XXV.59
De propriorum animi cuiuslibet affectuum dignotione et curatione **Med** XX.7; XXIII.95
De providentia creatoris **Med** I.21
De pulsibus libellus ad tirones **Med** III.69, 95; IV.15–17, 20, 34, 35; XVI.28; XXIII.22, 60, 85; XXV.44
De purgantium medicamentorum facultate **Med** XXIV.10
De remediis parabilibus **Poi** 34
De sanitate tuenda **Ast** I.1; IX.5; X.3, 5, 6, 8; XII.8; XIII.14; **Med** III.11, 12, 71–74, 81; VIII.60; IX.45, 55, 67, 112; XII.7, 23; XIII.10, 12, 31, 40; XIV.2, 5; XVII.5, 6, 10, 12–14, 17–20, 26–33, 35, 38–40; XVIII.6, 10–15; XIX.7, 8, 10, 18–22, 38, 39; XX.29, 38; XXI.4, 38; XXV.4, 6, 9; **Reg** I.22; II.1; IV.12, 16, 19; **Elu** 11, 33, 40
De semine **Med** III.19; VII.61, 73; XVI.10; XXIV.29, 30; XXV.25, 29, 59
De signis mortis* **Med III.76; VI.24, 48, 70, 71; X.14
De simplicium medicamentorum temperamentis ac facultatibus **Ast** XIII.30, 39; **Poi** 56, 72; **Med** III.94; IX.111; XIII.14–17, 39; XX.66; XXI.11, 18, 48, 49, 56–58, 62–66, 90, 91; XXII.18–22, 24–32, 56; XXIII.11, 99–101; XXIV.42, 43, 59; XXV.13, 31, 34, 46, 49, 54; **Reg** IV.25; **Com** I.1 (26)
De somno et vigilia* **Med III.58; VII.51; VIII.33, 56; XVII.4; XVIII.9
De symptomatum causis (= *De morborum causis et symptomatibus IV–VI*) **Ast** V.6; **Med** I.59; II.21, 26; III.41, 54, 55, 78; VI.88; VII.26, 32, 38, 46, 62, 63, 69, 70; IX.23, 54, 64, 94, 96; XVI.23; XXIII.22, 23, 70, 81–83, 92; XXIV.35; XXV.16, 17, 21, 27
De symptomatum differentiis (= *De morborum causis et symptomatibus III*) **Med** VII.55, 68; VIII.45; XXIII.12, 64, 80
De temperamentis **Med** XXV.6, 40, 41; **Com** I.14 (41); II.44 96
De theriaca ad Pamphilianum* **Med XXI.52
De theriaca ad Pisonem **Med** VII.31; IX.103; X.56; XVII.41; XXI.29, 30, 51, 53–55; XXII.1–16; XXIV.25–28
De totius morbi temporibus **Med** V.16; VIII.4–6; XI.2, 4, 5; XXV.45
De tremore, palpitatione, convulsione et rigore **Med** I.49; VI.8; VII.23, 36, 39, 40, 42–45; XXIII.21; **Com** IV.57 (194)
De tumoribus praeter naturam **Med** III.48; IX.98; XXIII.36, 38, 39a, 45, 46, 48, 51, 55–57; XXIV.11
De usu partium **Ast** IX.10, 11; **Med** I.1–5, 8, 18, 19, 22, 23, 42–44, 48, 52–56, 61–64, 66–68; II.8, 29; III.21–23, 34–40, 47, 52, 53, 62, 77; IX.90; XIV.1; XXIII.25, 69; XXIV.34; XXV.2, 32, 36, 37, 55; **Com** N (7)
De usu pulsuum **Med** I.20
De victu attenuante **Med** VIII.19; XVII.24; XX.28, 42, 49, 50, 52; XXI.8, 13, 17, 25, 31, 59; XXIII.103; XXV.30
De victus ratione in morbis acutis secundum Hippocratem **Med** XXI.24
De voce et hanelitu **Med** XXIII.76
In Hippocratis Aphorismos commentarius **Med** II.27; III.2, 31, 115; V.3; VI.1–3, 32, 63, 64, 89, 90; VIII.7, 12, 13, 50; IX.1, 40, 89; X.11; XI.28, 30; XII.12; XIII.7, 8, 11; XIV.3, 12; XV.4, 35; XVI.19; XVIII.4, 7;

XIX.1, 24; XX.24; XXIII.35, 50, 58a, 59, 61, 63, 96; XXIV.54; XXV.11, 39; **Com** I.2 (29), 13 (40), 15 (42), 18 (45), 20 (47), 23–25 (50–52); II.15 (67), 19 (71), 20 (72), 23 (75), 24 (76), 43 (95), 44 (96), 53 (105); III.16 (122), 24 (130), 29 (135), 30 (136); IV.27 (164), 32 (169), 46 (183), 48 (185), 54 (191), 59 (196), 61 (198), 65 (202), 67 (204), 71 (208), 76 (213); V.16 (236), 40 (260), 43 (263), 48 (268), 60 (280), 67 (287), 70 (290); VI.18 (310), 31 (323), 34 (326), 36 (328), 44 (336), 56 (348), 57 (349); VII.19 (371), 40 (392), 42 (394), 43 (395), 46 (398), 48 (400), 62 (414)

In Hippocratis De acutorum morborum victu commentarius **Ast** V.3; **Med** VI.44; VIII.1, 24–26, 52, 67; IX.81–83; X.5, 49; XIII.1, 2, 4, 5, 25–27, 33; XVII.11; XIX.25, 27–30; XX.25; XXI.3, 7, 15, 20–22; XXIII.33

In Hippocratis De aere, aquis et locis commentarius **Hem** I.3; **Med** II.28; III.16–18, 25; VII.16; IX.31; XV.3, 5; XX.10, 33–35; XXIII.15, 16, 34; XXV.18, 41

* *In Hippocratis De alimento commentarius* **Ast** II.2; **Med** III.7, 75; VII.20; XV.62; XVI.32; XVII.21, 34; XX.11, 12, 21, 40; XXI.1

* *In Hippocratis De humoribus commentarius* **Ast** IX.5, 6, 8; **Med** VI.22, 47; VII.4, 19; VIII.3, 16–18, 29, 31, 55, 71; IX.6–10, 34, 35, 59–61, 84; XII.43; XIII.20, 29, 37; XIV.3; XXIII.5, 8, 49; XXIV.19; XXV.53; **Com** N (7)

* *In Hippocratis De mulierum affectibus commentarius* **Med** II.26; XIV.9; XVI.1, 3, 9, 14–16, 20, 30, 35

In Hippocratis De natura hominis commentarius **Med** III.1; VIII.49; XIV.10, 13; XVIII.8; XX.32; XXV.41; **Com** N (8)

In Hippocratis De officina medici commentarius **Med** XV.30, 60, 61, 66–70

* *In Hippocratis De septimanis commentarius* **Com** N (8)

In Hippocratis Epidemiarum commentarius **Ast** I.4; XIII.19; **Med** II.1, 2, 5; III.28, 49, 65, 66, 80; V.12; VI.10–15, 17–21, 39–41, 45, 46, 65–68; VII.5, 17, 18, 41, 48, 49, 56, 58, 59, 64, 66; VIII.2, 14, 15, 20, 28, 30, 53, 54, 70; IX.3–5, 32, 33, 41, 42, 93, 99; X.13, 37, 40, 43–46, 48, 50, 59; XI.26, 27; XII.28, 39, 42; XIII.19, 21, 23, 24, 28, 32, 36; XV.6, 7, 44; XVI.8, 33, 34, 36, 38; XVII.2, 7, 9; XVIII.5; XIX.9; XX.20, 26, 27, 36, 39, 46; XXI.35; XXIII.4, 17, 18, 40, 58, 58a, 62, 90; XXIV.13, 16–18; XXV.12, 15, 18; **Com** VII.9 (361)

In Hippocratis Prognostica commentarius **Med** II.4; III.44, 63, 79, 96, 99; V.9; VI.4, 69; X.12; XI.29

In Platonis Timaeum commentarius **Med** VI.95; XXIII.6, 61, 109; XXIV.58; XXV.51; **Com** I.1 (18)

Introductio sive medicus **Med** IX.58

Mayāmir → *De compositione medicamentorum secundum locos*

Puero epileptico consilium **Med** IX.13; XXI.23; XXV.22

Qaṭājānas → *De compositione medicamentorum per genera*

Quod animi mores corporis temperamenta sequantur **Ast** I.2; **Med** VI.16; **Reg** IV.16

Hippocrates **Ast** I.4, 5; X.8; XI.4; XIII.13, 16–19, 22, 23, 29, 30, 44; **Med** N; VI.94; XIII.6; XV.63, 64; XVII.2, 28; XIX.25, 26; XXI.33; XXIII.40, 50; XXIV.1, 27; XXV.11, 29, 41, 60; **Reg** I.1, 6; II.2; IV.11; **Elu** 45; **Com** N (6–8, 10–13); I.1–25 (14, 19, 28, 29–52); II.1–54 (53–106); III.1–31 (107–137); IV.1–83 (138–220); V.1–62 (221–282), 64–72 (284–292); VI.1–60 (293–352); VII.1–58 (353–410), 60–62 (412–414)

Aphorisms **Ast** XI.4; XIII.29; **Med** N; **Com** N (10, 12); I.1–25 (14, 19, 29–52); II.1–54 (53–106); III.1–31 (107–137); IV.1–83 (138–220); V.1–62 (221–282), 64–72 (284–292); VI.1–60 (293–352); VII.1–58 (353–410), 60–62 (412–414)

Epidemics **Ast** I.4; V.5; XIII.17, 23; **Med** XVII.2; **Reg** I.1; II.2; **Com** II.20 (72); V.40 (260); VII.4 (356)

Diseases of Women **Med** XXIV.1; XXV.29

On Fractures **Med** XV.63, 64; XXI.33

Prognostic **Med** XXV.60; **Com** VII.31 (383)
Regimen on Acute Diseases **Med** XIX.25; **Elu** 45
Homer **Med** XXIV.57
Ḥunayn ibn Isḥāq (*lat.* Johannitius) **Poi** 45; **Med** XXIV.1, 44
K. al-Tiryāq **Poi** 45

Ibn Ayyūb, Solomon ben Joseph **Ast** XIII.38
Ibn Māsawayh, Yūḥannā (*lat.* Mesue)
Nawādir al-ṭibbiyya **Med** N
Ibn Māssa, Īsā **Med** XX.86
Ibn al-Mu'allim, Abū Ayyūb → Ibn Ayyūb, Solomon ben Joseph
Ibn Qamniel, Abū al-Ḥasan **Ast** XIII.38
Ibn Riḍwān, ʿAlī **Med** XXIV.14; XXV.1
Ibn Sīnā (*lat.* Avicenna) **Poi** 18, 38; **Hem** VI.8, 9; **Med** XXI.67, 80; **Coi** 6, 7; **Elu** 21
Fī aḥkām al-adwiya al-qalbīya (*On Cardiac Remedies*) **Elu** 21
K. al-Qānūn fī al-ṭibb (*The Canon of Medicine*) **Poi** 18, 38; **Hem** VI. 8, 9; **Med** XXI.67; **Coi** 6; **Elu** 42
Ibn al-Tilmīdh **Med** XXIII.107; **Elu** 8
Al-Aqrābādhīn al-kabīr **Elu** 8
Ikhtiyārāt al-Ḥāwī **Med** XXIII.107, 108
Ibn Wāfid **Hem** VI.6; **Med** XXI.67; XXV.13
K. al-Adwiya al-mufrada **Med** XXI.67
K. al-Wisād **Hem** VI.6
Ibn Zuhr, Abū al-ʿAlā' **Ast** XIII.16, 38; **Med** XIII.44; XX.67; XXII.35, 56; XXV.1; **Reg** IV.14
K. al-Tadhkira **Ast** XIII.16; **Med** XX.67; XXII.35, 54–56; **Reg** IV.14
Ibn Zuhr, Abū Marwān ʿAbd al-Malik (*lat.* Avenzoar) **Ast** IX.1; XII.6; **Poi** 19, 36, 78; **Med** VII.8; VIII.76, 77; XIII.44; XX.67, 81; XXI.26; XXII.35, 56; **Coi** 8; **Reg** III.2, 5; **Elu** 2
K. al-Aghdhiya (*Book on Foodstuffs*) **Med** XX.67; XXII.35, 46, 48–52; **Elu** 20
K. al-Taysīr fī l-mudāwāt wa-l-tadbīr (*Book on the Facilitation of Treatment and Diet*) **Ast** XII.6; **Poi** 19, 36; **Med** XXII.35–47, 53; **Reg** III.1, 2; IV.17, 24, 27, 28

Johannitius → Ḥunayn ibn Isḥāq

Mesue → Ibn Māsawayh, Yūḥannā

al-Nairīzī, Abū'l-ʿAbbās al-Faḍl ibn Ḥātim **Com** N (7)

Philo of Alexandria **Med** VIII.39
Plato **Med** XXIII.61; XXV.62; **Com** N (10)
Laws **Com** N (10)
Timaeus **Poi** 71; **Med** XXIII.61
Porphyry of Tyre **Med** XXIV.1
Ptolemy, Claudius **Com** N (6)
Almagest **Com** N (6)

al-Rāzī (*lat.* Rhazes) **Ast** XII.1, 2; XIII.8, 12, 13, 48; **Poi** 13, 33, 35, 56; **Hem** IV.5, 7; VI.7; **Med** N; XXV.1, 57; **Reg** II.3; IV.6, 10, 11; **Elu** 20
Fī man la yaḥduruhu ṭabīb **Hem** IV.5
K. al-Ḥāwī fī al-ṭibb **Ast** XII.1; **Poi** 35
K. al-Manṣūrī **Poi** 56
K. al-Murshid aw al-fuṣūl **Ast** XIII.8; **Med** N; **Reg** IV.6
Manāfiʿ al-aghdhiya wa-dafʿ maḍārriha (*The Benefits of Nutrients and the Repulsion of their Harmful Effects*) **Elu** 20
Rhazes → Al-Rāzī

Stratonicus **Med** XV.59
al-Sūsī, ʿAbd Allāh ibn Muḥammad al-Taqafī **Med** N

al-Tamīmī **Med** IX.30, 123; XIII.52, 54; XX.82, 86; XXI.96; XXII.57
K. al-Murshid fī jawāhir al-aghdhiya waquwā l-mufradāt mina l-adwiya **Med** IX.30, 123; XIII.52, 54; XX.82; XXI.96

Index of Diseases and Afflictions

abdomen → affection(s); ulcer(s); worms; wound(s)
- spitting of blood from the region of the ~ **Med** IX.37
- dryness of the ~ **Med** III.81; **Com** III.5 (111)
  - → constipation
- illness(es) in the ~ **Med** V.1; IX.50
- pain in the ~ **Poi** 77; **Med** VI.52; VII.2; XXII.26
- pain in the lower part of the ~ and pubes **Com** IV.80 (217)
- pain close to the surface of the ~ above the abdominal membrane (peritoneum) **Com** VI.7 (299)

abdomen, lower
- dissolution/emaciation/leanness/thinness/weakness of the parts around the navel and the ~ **Com** II.35 (87)

'abīṭ (congelation of copious blood) **Med** XXIII.36

abolishment → pulse(s); skin; speech

abrasion → intestines; liver

abscess **Rul** 83; **Med** III.24, 61, 102; V.18; X.41; XI.15, 20, 23, 28, 30; XV.20, 48; XXIII.39a; XXIV.11, 26, 38; **Com** I.20 (47); II.15 (67); IV.32 (169), 33 (170), 47 (184), 51 (188); VII.8 (360)
- → chest; ear(s); intestines; jaw; joint(s); *khurāj*; kidney(s); liver; lung(s); organs, respiratory; spleen; stomach
- bursting ~ **Med** VI.81
- cystic ~ → *dubayla*
- ~ deep inside the body **Med** IX.86, 87
- external ~ **Com** 36 (388)
- fatlike ~ **Med** XV.20
- honey-like ~ **Med** XV.20
- internal ~ **Med** IX.88; **Com** VII.8 (360), 36 (388)
- purulent ~ **Com** I.12 (39)

absconsio → *makhba*

accumulation → blood; breast(s); fluid; pus

ache → backache; earache(s); headache

acidity → stomach

activity
- lack of ~ **Med** IX.23; XXIII.27; **Coi** 2

activity, mental
- disturbance/loss of the ~ **Med** VI.94

affection(s) → bladder (, urinary); liver; soul; spleen
- abdominal ~ **Med** XXIII.93
- gouty ~ **Com** VI.55 (347)

affliction → bone(s); brain; diaphragm; eye(s); heart; hypochondrium; earhole; intestines; kidney(s); liver; nerve(s); skin; soul; uterus
- grave/severe ~ **Poi** 73; **Med** XII.21; XV.50; XVI.1; XXIII.20; XXV.44; **Reg** I.8; **Com** II.26 (78)
- major ~ **Med** XXV.44
- minor ~ **Med** IV.16; XXV.44
- respiratory ~ **Med** VI.45

aggressiveness **Med** VI.37
- → behavior

ailment → anus; bladder (, urinary); genitals; humors; kidney(s); liver; stomach; uterus
- chronic ~ **Com** II.39 (91)
- minor ~ **Ast** XIII.5; **Reg** IV.3

ākila (canker; ulcer in the flesh) **Med** XXIII.35, 48

alopecia **Med** XXII.2; XXIII.53
- → hair: loss of

alphos **Com** III.20 (126)

alteration → pulse(s)

amalgamation → blood

amenorrhea **Com** V.39 (259)

amentia **Med** VI.94; XXIII.64
- → reason(ing): loss of

anasarca (dropsy of the flesh) **Med** III.27; IV.41; IX.59; XXII.59; XXIII.3, 50; **Com** VII.29 (381)

aneurysm **Med** XII.38

anger **Ast** VIII.3; **Rul** 11, 31; **Med** VI.22; VII.3, 12; VIII.31; XVII.26; XXIV.56; **Com** VI.23 (315)

angina **Poi** 90; **Med** III.66; IX.32, 33; XII.22, 33; XXII.20; XXIII.77; XXV.11; **Com** I.12 (39); III.16 (122), 20 (126), 22 (128); V.10 (230); VI.37 (329); VII.49 (401)

annulling → sperm

ant(s) → pulse(s); sensation

anus → fissure; prolapse
ailment of the ~ **Com** V.22 (242)
discharge of blood through the ~ **Med** VI.81
diseases of the ~ **Med** IX.97
excrescences on the ~ **Med** XV.21
→ hemorrhoids
fistula surrounding the ~ **Med** XXII.63
pain in the region of the ~ and pubes **Com** VII.39 (391)
stretching/widening of the vessels of the ~ **Hem** II.1
tumors in the ~ and surrounding area **Med** III.105
ulcers in the ~ **Rul** 65; **Med** XIII.39
anxiety **Rul** 29–31; **Med** VII.2–4, 12, 37; VIII.8, 31; X.68; XXIII.86; **Coi** 2, 3; **Reg** III.6, 9–12, 16; **Com** I.23 (50); II.13 (65); VI.53 (345); VII.56 (408)
aphthae **Med** XXIII.75; **Com** III.24 (130)
apoplexy **Med** VI.1; XI.2; XII.14; XVIII.7; XXII.43; XXIII.61; XXIV.45, 58; XXV.45; **Com** II.19 (71), 45 (97); III.16 (122), 23 (129), 31 (137); VI.51 (343), 56 (348), 57 (349)
appearance
ashy/dust-colored ~ **Med** XXIV.48
appetite(s)
canine ~ **Med** XXIII.81; **Com** II.21 (73)
excessive ~ **Ast** V.6
diminishment of ~ **Med** III.28; VI.90; XX.65
disappearance of ~ **Med** XXIII.86
(total) lack of ~ **Med** VI.55, 57, 90; XI.17; XVI.23, 24; XXIII.87
loss of ~ **Ast** V.6; VIII.2; **Med** VI.67, 94; IX.47; XVI.5; XXIV.25; **Reg** I.1; III.9; **Com** II.32 (84); VI.3 (295); VII.6 (358)
ravenous ~ **Med** XVI.24
weak ~ **Ast** VII.4
arm(s)
~ cut off below the elbow **Ast** XIII.10; **Reg** IV.8
illness in the ~ **Med** IX.118
puncturing of the ~ **Rul** 83
trembling of the ~ **Med** VII.36
arm, upper
broken ~ **Med** XV.62
armpit(s)
inflammations in the soft flesh in the groin and ~ **Med** XXIII.56
swelling of the glands in the groin or ~ **Med** XIX.32
artery/arteries
blockage/heavy pressure in the ~ **Med** IV.31
injury of a ~ **Rul** 48
obstruction in/of the ~ **Med** III.59; IV.47
pain in the ~ **Med** I.6
softness of the organ (~) **Med** IV.39
weakness of the ~ **Med** VIII.44
arthritis **Ast** I.1; **Med** II.25; XI.25; XII.22; XXIII.14; XXV.45; **Reg** IV.22; **Com** III.16 (122), 20 (126), 31 (137)
ascites **Med** IV.41; XV.36; XXIII.50; **Com** IV.11 (148)
→ *jamʿ al-māʾ*
asthma **Ast** N.1, 2(, 3); I.1; IX.10(; **Rul** 0); **Med** II.25; VIII.19; XX.83; XXII.30; XXIII.78, 79, **Com** III.22 (128), 26 (132), 30 (136); VI.46 (338)
→ orthopnea
acute ~ **Med** XXIII.78
~ attack **Ast** N.2, 3; I.1; X.1–3, 7, 10; XI.4, 5; XII.1, 5, 6, 8
atheroma **Rul** 49
attack(s) → asthma; brain; fever(s)
stuporific ~ **Med** XXIII.68
→ stupor
aversion
~ of (taking) food **Med** IX.79; **Com** II.32 (84)

back
pain in the ~ **Med** III.66; XII.23; XXII.26
→ backache; ribs
pain in the lower ~ **Com** IV.73 (210)
pain descending from the ~ to the elbows **Com** VI.22 (314)
pain in the muscles in the ~ **Com** VII.36 (388)
rigor in the ~ **Com** V.69 (289)
tension in the ~ **Med** XII.23
backache **Med** XX.85
→ back: pain in the
baldness **Com** VI.28 (320), 34 (326)

bayḍa (headache affecting the entire head) **Med** XXIII.66
bed-wetting **Med** XXII.59
bee, honey → sting
behavior
aggressive ~ **Com** VI.53 (345)
insolent ~ **Med** VI.37
belly
drying of the ~ **Med** VIII.33
pain in the ~ **Com** VI.7 (299)
pain in the parts about the ~ **Com** VII.22 (374), 26 (378)
wound to the lower part of the ~ **Rul** 79
benumbing → mind; numbness; sensation; senses
beverages → craving
bile
emesis of ~ **Med** X.28
expectoration of a moisture resembling thin ~ **Med** XXIV.37
spitting up of ~ **Med** IX.84
vomiting of ~ **Med** VI.55, 57; **Com** VI.50 (342)
bile, black
diseases caused by ~ **Med** II.16; **Com** III.20 (126)
→ delusion: melancholic
illness caused by/resulting from ~ **Com** I.12 (39); VII.40 (392)
"~ illness" **Med** XXIII.63
→ melancholia/melancholy
irritation of ~ **Med** XX.88
palpitation caused by ~ **Med** XXII.66
putrefaction of ~ **Med** X.23; XXV.48
bile, yellow
discharge of ~ **Com** IV.24 (161)
diseases caused by ~ **Com** III.20 (126)
inflammation of ~ **Med** X.40
putrefaction of ~ **Med** X.23; XXV.12
putrefaction of ~ (in the (cardia of the) stomach) **Med** X.48; XXV.12
putrefaction of ~ (in the vessels) **Med** XXV.12
vomiting of ~ **Com** IV.58 (195)
bite (of a non-poisonous animal) **Poi** 59, 61, 62
~ of a crocodile **Med** XXI.54; XXII.16
~ of a domestic dog **Poi** 54, 59, 63; **Med** XXII.29
~ of a human being **Poi** 59
pain of a ~ **Poi** 54, 59
~ of a weasel **Med** XXI.54; XXII.16
bite (of a poisonous animal) **Poi** 4, 8–13, 15, 16, 18, 21, 30, 31, 36, 38, 39, 64, 65, 78; **Rul** 58; **Med** VII.14; IX.119; **Com** I.1 (24)
→ pain
~ of a mad dog **Poi** 54, 56–58, 63, 66; **Rul** 58; **Med** XXI.51
pain of a ~ **Poi** 10, 11, 13, 54, 64; **Med** XXI.54; XXII.16
~ of a *rutaylā'* (tarantula) **Poi** 47–49
~ of a scorpion **Poi** 16, 21, 41–44, 48, 64; **Med** IX.109
~ of a snake **Poi** 52
~ of vermin **Poi** 8, 52; **Med** XXI.50; XXII.64, XXIV.51
~ of a viper **Poi** 16, 52, 53; **Med** III.65; XXI.54; XXII.16, 64; XXIV.26a
blackening → blood; flesh; inflammation(s); limb(s); mortification
blackness → blood; *ḥumra*; sputum; stool(s); tongue; urine
bladder (, urinary)
affection of the ~ **Com** IV.80 (217)
ailment of the ~ **Com** V.22 (242)
diseases of the ~ **Med** XXII.51
illnesses in/of the ~ **Med** XXIII.94; **Com** VI.6 (298)
inflammation(s) in the ~ **Med** I.65; **Com** V.58 (278)
pain in the ~ **Med** I.69; **Com** VII.39 (391)
scabs in the ~ **Com** IV.77 (214)
sickness of the ~ **Med** VIII.15
~ stone(s) **Med** VI.92; XXII.10, 69; **Com** IV.79 (216)
→ urine
tear[2] in the ~ **Com** VI.18 (310)
tumor in the ~ **Med** III.105; XII.29
ulceration of the ~ **Poi** 89; **Com** IV.75 (212), 81 (218)
weakness of the ~ **Med** VIII.15; **Com** V.58 (278)
bleeding **Rul** 75–77, 84
blindness **Com** VI.56 (348)
blister **Med** XXIII.38
blockage → artery/arteries

blood → diarrhea; fever(s); nosebleed; tumor(s); vessel(s) (, blood)
accumulation of ~ **Med** XVI.38; XXIV.16
amalgamation of ~ **Com** II.36 (88)
bad ~ **Com** II.36 (88)
black ~ **Med** VII.24; XXIII.39; **Com** IV.23 (160)
blackening of ~ **Hem** II.3
clotted ~ **Med** VI.90
→ blood clots
coagulation of ~ **Rul** 72; **Med** VI.91; VII.24
congelation of ~ **Med** VI.91
congelation of ~ (in the breasts of a woman) **Com** V.40 (260)
congelation of copious ~ → *'abīṭ*
congestion of ~ **Med** XXIII.41; XXIV.16
corruption of the ~ **Med** VII.4; XVI.34
corruption of the ~ of the liver **Med** VI.58
coughing up ~ **Med** VIII.38
discharge of ~ (through the anus) **Med** VI.81
discharge/spitting of ~ (from the chest/larynx/ windpipe) **Med** IX.34, 37
discharge/spitting of ~ (from the lungs) **Rul** 72; **Med** IX.34, 37, 114
diseases related to ~ **Com** III.20 (126)
→ angina; hemorrhage(s)
expectoration of ~ **Med** XXIV.37
lividness of the color of the ~ **Med** XXIV.17
(frequent) loss of ~ **Med** VII.42; IX.65; XXV.72; **Reg** IV.8; **Com** IV.27 (164)
micturition of ~ **Poi** 89
old ~ **Com** V.23 (243)
spitting of/up ~ **Med** IX.37, 38
→ abdomen; chest; esophagus; intestines; larynx; lung(s); stomach; windpipe
spitting up frothy ~ **Com** V.13 (233)
thickening of the ~ **Elu** 13
thickness of the ~ **Elu** 12, 14
transudation of ~ **Med** IX.64
turbid ~ **Hem** II.1; **Med** II.15; **Elu** 12; **Com** VI.12 (304)
urination of ~ **Com** IV.75 (212), 78 (215), 81 (218)
urination of ~ with clots **Com** IV.80 (217); VII.39 (391)
→ blood clots
urination of the watery part of the ~ **Med** IX.64
vomiting of ~ **Poi** 91; **Med** VI.81; IX.114; **Com** V.32 (252); VII.37 (389)
blood, menstrual → amenorrhea; menses/ menstruation
congestion of ~ **Med** XXIV.16
drying of the ~ **Hem** II.3
excessiveness of evacuation/flow of ~ **Med** XVI.6, 15
putrefaction of ~ (in the veins) **Ast** VII.4; **Poi** 64; **Med** III.63; X.23; XII.14; XV.1; XXV.48
retention of ~ **Med** XVI. 3, 4
vomiting of ~ **Med** XXIV.1
blood clots **Com** IV.69 (206)
body → abscess; corpulence; disturbance; dryness; emaciation; fat(ness); feebleness; heaviness; lameness; leanness; limpness; looseness; meagerness; movement(s)/moving; obesity; pain; poison; pores; porousness; pruritus; putrefaction(s); side(s); skin; stoutness; strength; thinness; ulcer(s); wasting away; weakening; weakness
cold ~ **Med** XXIV.36
compression of the nervous parts of the ~ **Med** XXIII.23
corruption of the ~ **Reg** III.14
dissolution in the ~ **Com** I.13 (40); II.14 (66)
dissolution affecting a thin ~ **Rul** 40
inflammation in an internal part of the ~ **Com** IV.48 (185)
mortification of the solid parts of the ~ **Med** XXIII.51
→ gangrene; sphacelus
redness of the ~ **Poi** 88
boil **Med** XXIII.39
bone(s)
affliction that reached the ~ **Com** VI.45 (337)
broken ~ **Rul** 84, **Med** XV.63–65, **Com** V.22 (242)

caries in the ~ **Med** VII.25
corruption of the ~ **Coi** XXIV.5; **Com** VI.45 (337)
crushing of the ~ **Med** X.29
cutting through a part of a ~ **Com** VII.28 (380)
diseased ~ **Com** VII.2 (354)
exfoliation of the ~ **Com** VI.45 (337)
fissure of the ~ **Rul** (84)
fracture of the ~ **Med** IX.124
laying bare of a ~ **Com** VII.19 (371)
pain in the membranes surrounding the ~ **Med** VI.61; VII.27
perishing of the ~ **Med** XXIII.51
→ sphacelus
severed ~ **Com** VI.19 (311); VII.24 (376)
severed ~ of the head (skull) **Com** VII.24 (376)

bone, nasal
broken ~ **Med** XV.62

bowels
drying up of the ~ **Com** III.17 (123)
hard ~ **Com** II.53 (105)
looseness of the ~ **Com** II.14 (66), 20 (72), 53 (105); III.17 (123), 31 (137); IV.27 (164), 73 (210); VI.16 (308), 32 (324)

brain → brain, ventricles of the
affliction of the ~ **Med** VI.36, 94
attack in the ~ **Com** VII.50 (402)
coldness/cooling of the ~ **Ast** XII.5, 6; **Med** I.17; VI.2; **Reg** IV.18
concussion of the ~ **Com** VII.58 (410)
corruption of the substance of the ~ **Med** IX.15; **Com** VII.50 (402)
~ disease **Ast** IX.10; **Med** XXI.19
disturbance of the ~ **Com** VII.9 (361)
gash in the ~ **Com** VI.50 (342)
heaviness of the ~ **Ast** II.3; **Com** IV.67
illness ascending to the ~ **Med** XXV.28
illness (originating) in the ~ **Med** XXV.28; **Com** VI.53 (345)
inflammation of the ~ **Med** XXIII.67; **Com** IV.72 (209)
inflammation of the membranes of the ~ **Med** XXIII.67; **Com** VI.11 (303)
→ phrenitis
inflammation in the beginning of the nerves (~) **Com** VII.3 (355)
injury of the ~ **Med** XX.80
pain ascending to the ~ **Com** V.2 (222)
severing of the membranes surrounding the ~ **Med** I.49
softening of the ~ **Ast** X.4
softness of the ~ **Reg** IV.18
swelling in/of the ~ **Med** XXIII.61; **Com** II.42 (94); VI.50 (342)
swelling in the membranes of the ~ **Med** XXIII.60
tear[2] in the ~ **Com** VI.18 (310)
tumor(s) in the ~ **Rul** 63; **Med** III.82, 83; IX.17, 18; XXI.19
weakening of the ~ **Ast** XI.2
weakness of the ~ **Ast** II.3; **Com** VII.9 (361)
wound in the ~ **Med** XXIV.54; **Com** VI.18 (310)

brain, ventricles of the
obstruction of the ~ **Med** III.29
perforation in one of the two anterior ~ **Med** XXIV.6

breaking → arm, upper; bone(s); bone, nasal; collarbone; forearm(s); jaw; leg; ribs; thigh(s); tooth/teeth

breast(s)
accumulation of blood in the ~ **Med** XVI.38
cancer/tumor in the ~ (of women) **Med** XVI.22
emaciation of the ~ **Med** XVI.26
flow of milk from the ~ **Med** XVI.5; **Com** V.52 (272)
hardness of/pain in the ~ **Com** V.53 (273)
thinning of the ~ (of a pregnant woman) **Com** V.37 (257), 38 (258), 53 (273)

breastbone
wound in the ~ **Med** XXIV.5

breath
shortness of ~ **Ast** XII.3

breathing
bad (difficult) ~ **Com** II.27 (79)
~ with extreme coercion (difficulty) **Com** II.42 (94)
difficulty (of) ~ **Ast** XI.5; **Rul** 72; **Med** VI.1; VII.55; **Com** III.31 (137)
irregular ~ **Med** VI.1; **Com** II.42 (94)
stertorous ~ **Com** VI.51 (343)

unequal ~ **Com** II.42 (94)
weakness of ~ **Com** VI.54 (346)
bruise **Com** II.6 (58); V.25 (245)
bubbles → urine
bubo (swelling in the soft flesh of the groins) **Com** IV.55 (192)
bulimia **Med** IX.53; XXIII.85, 87
burn(ing) → head; hypochondrium; intestines; pain; stomach; uterus
~ sensation in the cardia of the stomach → *khafaqān*
severe ~ **Com** VII.13 (365)
→ sensation
bursting → abscess; kidney(s); lung(s); omentum; urethra; vessel(s) (, blood)

calcification → spleen
cancer **Rul** 52; **Med** II.16, 25; IX.98, 108, 120; XIII.20; XV.13, 18, 19; XXIII.46; **Com** IV.24 (161)
→ breast(s)
hidden ~ **Com** VI.38 (330)
large ~ **Med** IX.120
ulcerous ~ **Med** XXIII.46
→ ulcer(s)
canker **Med** XXIII.49
→ *ākila*; cankering
cankering **Rul** 56
→ canker
carbuncle(s) **Med** XV.2, 9; XXIII.38
→ *jamr*
putrefaction of ~ **Rul** 51
cardialgia **Com** IV.17 (154), 65 (202)
→ heartburn; palpitation(s)
caries → bone(s)
cartilage
cutting through a ~ **Com** VII.28 (380)
severed ~ **Com** VI.19 (311)
catalepsy **Med** XXIII.59, 64, 68
→ imagination(s): loss of
cataract **Med** VII.69, 70; XV.30, 31; XXII.4, 5, 37, 48; XXIII.69; XXV.17; **Com** III. 31 (137)
→ extension
catarrh **Rul** 31, 69–71; **Med** VI.41; XV.58; XVI.30; XIX.35; XXII.40; **Reg** IV.21–23; **Com** II.40 (92); V.24 (244); VII.38 (390)
cold ~ **Reg** IV.22
fatal ~ **Com** III.12 (118)
hot ~ **Reg** IV.21, 22
severe ~ **Med** VIII.38
~ associated with cough **Com** III.31 (137)
~ filling the cavities of the lungs **Reg** IV.22
cessation → pulse(s); respiration
chalazion (hailstone in the eyelid) **Med** XV.25
change → respiration
cheeks
leanness of the ~ **Ast** X.8
chemosis **Med** XXIII.70
chest
abscess in the ~ **Med** XXIV.9
coldness of the ~ **Med** I.17
discharge/spitting of blood from the ~ **Med** IX.34, 37
diseases of the ~ **Med** VI.4; XI.14; XXII.51
illnesses of the ~ and lung **Com** V.9 (229)
narrowness in the ~ **Med** XXIII.79
pain in the ~ **Med** XII.23; XXI.17; **Com** III.5 (111), 17 (123); VI.5 (297)
perforation of the ~ **Med** XXIV.5
perspiration on the ~ area **Med** VI.21
pus (in the area/cavity) between the ~ and the lung(s) **Med** XV.4; **Com** VI.27 (319); VII.44 (396), 54 (406)
putrefaction in the cavity of the ~ **Com** V.15 (235)
rattling sound in the ~ **Rul** 72
rawness of the ~ (cough) **Com** III.5 (111)
→ cough(ing)
redness/swelling on the front of the ~ **Com** VII.49 (401)
tension in the ~ **Med** XII.23
tumor in the ~ **Med** III.90; XII.33, 46
ulcer in the ~ **Rul** 72
weak ~ **Reg** II.8
weakening of the nerves that move the ~ and the diaphragm **Com** IV.50 (187)
wounds to the ~ cavity **Rul** 77
childbirth
difficult ~ **Med** XVI.33
→ delivery; labor
chilling → kidney(s)
choking **Med** IX.103; XXI.21; XXII.28
sensation of ~ **Med** XXIII.77

cholera **Med** III.60; VII.42; XXIII.83; **Com** I.12 (39); III.30 (136)
clay → craving
closure → larynx
cloud, black/red/white → urine
coercion → breathing
cold(ness) (of the body) → body; brain; chest; extremities; fingers; heart; liver; lung(s); organ(s); perspiration; stomach; stomach, cardia of the; sweat(ing); uterus
diseases caused by ~ **Com** I.2 (29)
extreme ~ **Poi** 65
sensation of ~ **Med** VII.46; X.29, 30, 36, 50
severe ~ **Poi** 16; **Med** I.38; III.83; VI.2; VI.84; VII.42; XII.5
colic **Poi** 77; **Med** IX.91; XII.7; XIII.34, 35, 52; XX.69; XXII.22, 31; **Com** II.37 (89); IV.11 (148), 20 (157); V.41 (261); VII.10 (362)
→ pain; stomach
pain of a ~ **Med** XXII.22
severe ~ **Poi** 89, 90, **Med** VIII.38; **Com** III.22 (128)
→ ileus
collapse → strength
collarbone
broken ~ **Med** XV.62
illness in the parts above/below the ~ **Med** XII.27
pain in the (right) ~ **Med** VII.54
collection → *kumna*; poison
colon
distension of the part of the intestines called "~" **Med** VII.65
pain in the ~ **Ast** V.6
stones in the intestines called "~" **Med** VI.92
complaint → liver
complexion
bad ~ **Med** II.25; XVI.6
dark ~ **Med** VI.47; X.18
faded ~ **Med** VI.47
green ~ **Med** VI.47
greenish yellow ~ **Ast** VII.4
lead-colored ~ **Med** X.18
pale ~ **Med** VI.47
pallid ~ **Com** V.42 (262)
red ~ **Ast** VII.4; **Med** VI.35
white ~ **Med** VII.56; X.18; XII.2
yellow ~ **Ast** X.8
yellowish white **Med** X.30
comprehension
lack of ~ **Ast** XIII.3; **Reg** IV.1
compression → body; organ(s); pulse(s); stomach, cardia of the
concussion → brain; spinal chord
consciousness
loss of ~ **Ast** X.9; XIII.10; **Med** XXIV.48; **Reg** IV.8; **Com** II.43 (95)
confusion (, mental) **Med** I.39; VI.3; XXIII.62, 64, 67; **Com** N (7); II. 6 (58); VII.5 (357)
~ (delirium) **Com** II.2 (54), 27 (79); III.30 (136); IV.50 (187); VI.11 (303), 26 (318), 53 (345); VII.7 (359), 9 (361), 10 (362), 14 (366), 18 (370), 24 (376)
→ delirium
~ (phrenitis) **Com** III.30 (136)
→ fever; phrenitis
congelation → blood
congestion → blood; blood, menstrual; head
conjunctivitis **Med** VI.13; XXIII.70
constipation **Med** VI.55; VIII.27; IX.47, 55; XIII.31, 40; XVII.19, 38; XIX.27; XX.68; XXI.29; **Elu** 28, 45; **Com** II.20 (72); III.5 (111), 25 (131)
→ abdomen: dryness of the
constriction → soul
consumption → poison
contraction → hypochondrium; uterus
contusion **Rul** 83; **Med** III.109
convulsion **Med** XXIII.22; XXIV.23
cooling → brain
cornea
collection/formation/originating of pus behind the ~/horn-like tunic/in the eye → *kumna*
corpulence **Med** X.4; **Com** I.17 (44); II.7 (59); IV.7 (144)
corrosion **Med** III.109; VII.60; IX.105; XV.7; XXIII.48, 75; XXV.46
→ flesh; hemorrhage(s); intestines; organ(s); skin; tooth/teeth; tunic, horn-like
corruption → body; blood; bone(s); brain; digestion; flesh; humors; liver; mind; sperm, female; ulcer(s); uterus

cough(ing) **Ast** IV.3; XII.2; **Rul** 63, 68, 69, 71; **Med** VI.43, 48, 54, 57; VII.50; IX.38; XXI.7, 27; XXIII.32, 82, 92; XXIV.19, 37; **Reg** IV.21, 22; **Com** III.5 (111), 13 (119), 20 (126), 23 (129), 24 (130), 31 (137); IV.54 (191); V.24 (244); VI.35 (327), 46 (338); VII.47 (399), 51 (403)
→ blood
benign/malignant ~ **Med** VI.41
catarrh associated with ~ **Com** III.31 (137)
chronic ~ **Med** VII.48
frequent dry ~ **Com** IV.54 (191)
mild ~ **Med** VI.55; IX.36
severe ~ **Med** VIII.38
cradle cap **Med** XXIII.54, 55
→ *saʿfa*
cramps **Com** III.25 (131); IV.57 (194), 66 (203), 67 (204)
→ stomach
craving
~ for bad and detestable beverages **Med** IX.54
~ for bad foods/things **Ast** IX.12; **Med** XVI.23, 24
~ for clay **Med** XX.84
crocodile → bite
crushing → bone(s); limb(s)
curvature → neck, vertebrae of the; spine
cutting off → arm(s); elbow(s); testicles
cutting through → bone(s); cartilage
cyst → *dubayla*

damʿa (rhyas) **Med** XXIII.71
damage → head; liver; muscle(s); nerve(s); organ(s); senses; strength
darkening → vision
darkness → urine
deafness **Med** XXII.47; XXIII.73; **Com** IV.28 (165), 60 (197)
death
condition similar to ~ **Med** XXIV.50, 51
state close to ~ **Med** IV.24
debility, mental **Ast** X.8
decay → lung(s); tooth/teeth
decrepitude **Med** III.14
defluxion **Ast** N.2; VIII.1; XI.2, 5; XII.1, 4, 5; **Rul** 70; **Med** III.66; IX.7; XIII.13; XXII.57
→ head
degeneration → flesh; ligament; nerve(s); organ(s); sinew
delirium **Rul** 77; **Med** III.77; VI.33, 37, 45, 46; VII.26, 35; IX.18; XV.15, 46; XXIII.58, 58a, 64; XXIV.22; **Com** I.12 (39); II.2 (54), 27 (79); III.30 (136); IV.50 (187); VI.11 (303), 26 (318), 53 (345); VII.7 (359), 9 (361), 10 (362), 14 (366), 18 (370), 24 (376)
mild ~ → raving
delivery
dangerous/difficult ~ **Com** V.55 (275)
→ childbirth; labor
delusion **Med** II.16; VI.33, 45; XX.74
melancholic ~ (caused by black bile) **Med** VI.11, 52; VII.26, 29; IX.16, 44, 79, 110; XII.40; XXIII.63; **Reg** III.10; **Com** III.14 (120), 20 (126), 22 (128); VI.11 (303)
→ bile, black
dementia **Med** VII.26
denseness → pulse(s); uterus
depression **Ast** X.8; **Med** IX.44; **Reg** N; III.1
derangement **Ast** V.6
→ mind
despondency **Med** VI.52; **Com** V.61 (281); VI.23 (315)
diabetes **Med** V.13; VII.57; VIII.68; XXIII.94; XXIV.39
→ thirst
diaphragm
affliction of the ~ **Med** X.60
inflammation of the ~ **Med** VI.53; XXIII.67
inflammation of the nervous part of the ~ **Med** IX.85
pain above/below the ~ **Com** IV.18 (155)
pain where the liver is connected to the ~ **Med** XXIV.7
stretching of the ~ **Med** XVI.15
tumor in the ~ **Med** XII.29
weakening of the nerves that move the chest and the ~ **Com** IV.50 (187)
wounds to the ~ **Rul** 77
diarrhea **Ast** V.3; IX.5; XIII.5; **Poi** 77; **Rul** 18, 23, 31; **Med** II.14; V.12; VI.12, 25; VII.14, 64; IX.62; X.8, 28, 67; XI.14; XII.5, 10; XIII.28, 47; XVII.37, 41; XIX.27; XXI.11, XXII.36; XXIII.83, 90, 95; XXV.31, 35,

39; **Reg** IV.3; **Com** I.2 (29); III.16 (122), 21 (127), 25 (131); IV.28 (165), 58 (195), 60 (197); V.12 (232), 14 (234); VI.15–17 (307–309), 52 (344); VII.30 (382)
→ lientery
bilious ~ **Med** VI.82; **Com** IV.28 (165)
bloody ~ **Med** VI.81, 82, 90; XXIV.10; **Com** V.64 (284)
chronic ~ **Com** III.30 (136)
constant ~ **Com** V.34 (254)
frothy ~ **Com** VII.30 (382)
prolonged ~ **Com** VI.15 (307), 32 (324)
severe ~ **Rul** 23, **Med** VII.12, 42; IX.47; XIII.47; XXII.61
violent ~ **Com** VII.29 (381)
~ of liquefied material **Med** X.59
~ of raw material **Med** X.45
~ of bilious matter **Med** XXII.58
~ caused by poisons **Med** XXII.36

difficulty → breathing; exhalation; eye(s); inhalation; movement(s)/moving; respiration; sensation; swallowing; tongue

digestion → organs, digestive
bad ~ **Ast** V.5, 6; **Hem** I.1; **Med** VI.76; VII.4, 15; XVII.1; XX.5; XXIII.80; **Reg** I.2
→ dyspepsia
corruption of the ~ **Hem** I.1; **Reg** I.9; **Elu** 3; **Com** III.24 (130), 26 (132)
diminished ~ **Med** III.28; XXI.5
feeble ~ **Ast** XIII.5; **Reg** N; IV.3
poor ~ **Med** XVI.6; XVII.6; **Com** III.24 (130)
slow ~ **Med** IX.67
weak(ness of) ~ **Ast** V.1; X.8; XIII.38; **Reg** I.4
weakening of the ~ **Com** IV.27 (164)

dim-sightedness **Com** III. 31 (137)

diminishment/diminution → appetite(s); digestion; flesh; stomach; strength; vigor, sexual; vision

dimness → senses; vision

disappearance → appetite(s); pulse(s)

discharge → anus; bile, yellow; blood; chest; ear(s); eye(s); feces; flesh; larynx; lung(s); nose; nostrils; stool(s); urine; windpipe
dry ~ **Med** VI.37
~ of feculent matter **Rul** 72
mucous ~ **Med** II.8; IX.6; XXIV.11
seropurulent ~ **Med** XXI.42
watery ~ **Com** III. 31 (137)

discomfort → stomach

disease(s) → anus; bile, black; bile, yellow; bladder (, urinary); blood; bone(s); brain; chest; cold; esophagus; eye(s); head; intestines; kidney(s); liver; lung(s); nerve(s); organ(s); phlegm; skin; soul; spleen; stomach; uterus
acute ~ **Ast** V.3; VII.4; **Med** II.25; VI.13, 40; VII.11, 14; X.21; **Com** I.4 (31), 6 (33), 7 (34), 12 (39), 24 (51); II.19 (71), 23 (75); IV.23 (160); V.31 (251); VI.14 (306), 54 (346); VII.1 (353)
autumnal ~ **Com** III.4 (110)
~ occurring to children **Com** III.29 (135)
chronic ~ **Ast** N.1; I.1; VIII.2; XIII.45; X.21; **Hem** VI.1; **Med** VI.4, 69; VII.11, 14; VIII.19, 73; X.21; XIII.40; **Reg** II.9; **Com** I.4 (31), 12 (39); III.29 (135); IV.23 (160)
cold ~ **Med** XXI.46; **Reg** II.11; **Com** III.3 (109)
endemic ~ **Med** XXIII.15
epidemic ~ **Med** XXI.26; XXIII.16
evil ~ **Rul** 86; **Com** IV.36 (173)
fatal ~ **Med** VI.94; XXI.52
gassy ~ **Med** VII.53; IX.44
grave ~ **Ast** VII.1; XIII.38; **Hem** II.2
~ caused by heat **Com** I.2 (29)
hot ~ **Reg** II.11; **Com** VII.1 (353)
human ~ **Med** XXV.59, 69
inflammatory ~ **Med** VII.38
lengthy/long ~ **Rul** 20; **Med** XIII.40; **Com** II.28 (80); IV.36 (173)
malignant ~ **Med** VI.77, 87
mild ~ **Ast** XIII.7; **Reg** IV.5
nonfatal ~ **Med** VI.94
pestilential ~ **Med** XXI.52
prolonged ~ **Med** VI. 80, 87, 90; VII.11; **Com** I.12 (39); IV.37 (174), 40 (177), 56 (193)
protracted ~ **Com** VII.61 (413)
serious ~ **Ast** VII.1; IX.9; XIII.38; **Hem** I.4; **Med** XII.20; **Com** II.27 (79)
severe ~ **Hem** I.1; **Med** VIII.28; XI.3; XII.20; XXV.59; **Com** I.9 (36); II.13 (65)
short ~ **Com** I.12 (39)
spring ~ **Com** III.20 (126)
summer ~ **Com** II.25 (77); III.21 (127), 22 (128)

ulcerous ~ **Med** XXIII.49
winter ~ **Com** III.23 (129)
woman's ~ **Com** V.29 (249)
dislocation → hip joint; joint(s); thigh bone
dissolution → abdomen, lower; body; fat; flesh; navel; nerve(s); spleen
distension **Ast** V.1; **Med** IX.91
→ colon; intestines; nerve(s); organ(s); stomach
distortion → eye(s); eyebrow; lip; nose
distress **Ast** N.2; V.6; VIII.2, 4; IX.6; **Hem** VI.1; **Rul** 30; **Med** IX.42, 79; X.64; XIII.47; XX.8, XXIII.82; **Reg** II.7; III.3, 16; **Com** II.30 (82); V.61 (281)
→ soul
melancholic ~ **Ast** V.6
disturbance (in the body) **Rul** 18; **Med** IX.24; XVII.11; **Com** II.13 (65); IV.5 (142); VII.33 (385)
→ activity; brain; intestines; mind; pulse(s); respiration; sensation; sleep; speech; stomach; taste; vision
anomalous ~ **Med** VI.86
dizziness **Med** VI.34; IX.3; XV.14; XXV.11; **Com** II.37 (89); III.23 (129), 31 (137); IV.17 (154)
dog, domestic/mad → bite
dripping → ulcer(s)
dropsy **Ast** VII.4; XIII.36; **Rul** 50; **Med** VI.45, 48; IX.58, 62, 63, 65, 66; IX.94, 99; XI.5; XII.42; XV.7; XX.39, 69; XXII.24; XXIV.16; **Reg** IV.20; **Com** I.12 (39); III.22 (128); VI.8 (300), 12 (304); VI.14 (306), 27 (319), 35 (327), 43 (335); VII.5 (357), 47 (399)
dry ~ **Med** XXIII.50; **Com** IV.11 (148)
→ tympanites
~ of the flesh → anasarca
drunkenness **Ast** VII.1; **Med** I.27, 38, 39; VI.31; **Reg** IV.15, 16; **Com** V.5 (225)
drying (of the body) **Ast** X.8
→ belly; blood; bowels; heart; nerve(s); organ(s); sperm; windpipe
dryness (of the body) **Rul** 58, 83; **Med** VIII.56; XV.33; XX.61; XXV.43; **Com** II.26 (78)
→ abdomen; eye; liver; organ(s); organs, respiratory; skin; spasm(s); stomach; stool(s); uterus
extreme ~ **Med** XXV.43
severe ~ **Poi** 91
dubayla (cystic abcess) **Med** XXIII.39a, **Com** VII.8 (360)
dullness → senses; understanding
dying → limb(s)
dyscrasia **Rul** 27, 28, 30, 35; **Med** XVII.9; XIX.19, 26; XX.31; XXI.43; XXIII.13, 17; XXV.3, 7, 21, 28, 72; **Elu** 21–23, 25
→ heart
dysentery **Med** XXI.11; XXII.20, 60, XXIII.89, 93; **Com** III.11 (117), 12 (118), 16 (122), 22 (128); IV.24 (161), 26 (163); V.65 (285); VI.3 (295), 43 (335), 48 (340); VII.5 (357), 23 (375)
→ intestines: ulceration of the
chronic ~ **Com** VI.43 (335)
severe ~ **Poi** XIII.10; **Reg** IV.8
dyspepsia **Med** II.24; VI.21; XXIII.80
dyspnea **Med** XXIII.79
dysuria **Com** III.5 (111), 31 (137); VI.36 (328); VII.48 (400)

ear(s) → earhole
abscess beneath the ~ **Med** VIII.53
abscess in the roots of the ~ **Med** III.85, 86
discharge from the ~ **Med** IX.3; **Com** III.24 (130)
illnesses of/obstruction in the ~ **Med** XXII.58
pain in/of the ~ **Med** IX.26, 27; XXI.94; XXII.12; **Com** III.21 (127)
→ earache
black pustule behind the ~ **Med** VI.71
tumors beneath the ~ **Med** X.44
tumors at the roots of the ~ **Med** XI.15
ulcers in the ~ **Rul** 65
earache(s) **Med** XXII.58; **Com** III.21 (127)
→ ear(s): pain in the
earhole
affliction in the inner ~ **Med** VI.94
eczema **Com** III.20 (126)
edema (soft swelling) **Med** XXIII.52
→ swelling(s)
elbow(s)
arms cut off below the ~ **Reg** IV.8
pain descending from the back to the ~ **Com** VI.22 (314)

elephantiasis **Rul** 56; **Med** II.16; III.94; IX.98, 107, 108; XIII.20, 30; XX.68; XXII.59; XXIII.47; **Elu** 28
  suppurating ~ **Poi** 83
emaciation (of the body) **Rul** 13, 16, 35; **Med** III.32; VII.16, 18, 36; IX.116; XIX.13; XX.39, 68, 71; XXIV.17; XXIII.21; XXV.43; **Coi** 1; **Com** I.14 (41), 17 (44); II.7 (59), 28 (80); III.12 (118)
  → abdomen, lower; breast(s); intestines; limb(s); liver; navel; organ(s)
emesis (involuntary) **Med** X.31; XI.14; XVII.37; XXII.36; XXIII.82; XXV.35
  → bile
emphysema (inflation) **Med** XXIII.52
emprosthotonos (forwards spasm) **Com** IV. 57 (194); V.6 (226)
empyema **Com** V.8 (228), 10 (230), 15 (235); VI.27 (319); VII.44 (396)
energy
  lack of ~ **Med** XI.17
enlargement → lung(s); spleen; tumor(s)
enterocele **Med** XXIII.57
epilepsy **Ast** V.6; **Hem** II.2; **Med** VII.29, 37; VIII.19; IX.1, 13, 23; XI.2; XII.22; XVIII.7; XXI.96; XXII.3, 18, 27, 36, 56, 59; XXIII.61; XXIV.58; XXV.11, 22, 27, 28, 45; **Com** II.45 (97); III.16 (122), 20 (126), 22 (128), 29 (135); V.7 (227)
  → fit; illness: divine; spasm(s)
  chronic ~ **Med** VIII.19
epiplocele **Med** XXIII.57
epiploenterocele **Med** XXIII.57
erection
  lack of ~ **Coi** 8
erosion → uterus; vessel(s) (, blood)
eructations
  acid/sour ~ **Med** VI.52; **Com** VI.1 (293), 33 (325)
eruptions
  ulcerative ~ **Com** III.20 (126)
erysipelas **Med** II.25; III.110; IX.106; X.2; XV.50; XXIII.41, 42; **Com** II.6 (58); V.23 (243), 43 (263); VI.25 (317); VII.19 (371), 20 (372)
  → *ḥumra*
  hard ~ **Med** XXIII.42
  soft ~ **Med** XXIII.42
  → swelling(s)
  true ~ **Med** X.2
eschar **Med** XV.9; XXIII.38
esophagus
  spitting of blood from the region of the ~ **Med** IX.37
  diseases of the ~ **Med** XXII.51
  illness of the ~ **Med** VI.56
  redness/swelling in/of the ~ **Med** IX.32
  tumor in the ~ **Med** III.105
  ulcer in the ~ **Rul** 64
excess → exultation; eye(s); flesh; organs, respiratory
excessiveness → blood, menstrual
excrescence(s) **Hem** N.1; II.1
  → anus; hemorrhoids; nose
  fleshy ~ **Med** XXII.25
exertion **Med** VII.37, 41; VIII.28; **Coi** 2
  lack of ~ **Med** XVI.9
exfoliation → bone(s)
exhalation
  difficult ~ **Med** I.30
exhaustion **Ast** X.9; XIII.36; **Med** X.18
  severe ~ **Med** IV.29
expectoration **Med** IX.83; XXIII.32; **Com** I.12 (39); V.8 (228)
  → bile; blood; hailstones; lung(s)
  livid ~ **Com** IV.47 (184)
  ~ of small pieces of matter **Med** XXIV.37
extension **Med** XXIII.69
  → cataract
extremities
  cold(ness) in/of the ~ **Med** X.11–13; XXIII.26; **Com** VII.1 (353), 26 (378)
  pallor of the ~ **Med** X.13
exultation
  excess of ~ **Reg** III.11
eye(s) → cataract; chemosis; conjunctivitis; eyebrow; eyelid(s); leucoma; pterygium; trachoma
  affliction in the ~ **Med** VI.94
  collection/formation/originating of pus behind the cornea/horn-like tunic/in the ~ → *kumna*
  difficulty of movement of the ~ **Com** III.17 (123)
  discharge from the ~ **Med** VI.37; **Com** III. 31 (137)

~ disease **Ast** IX.10
distortion of the ~ **Com** IV.49 (186)
dryness of the ~ **Com** VI.31 (323), 52 (344)
excess flesh in the inner angle of the ~ **Med** XV.21
extracted ~ **Ast** XIII.10; **Reg** IV.8
illnesses of the ~ **Med** XII.38; XXV.11; **Com** I.1 (16)
pain in the ~ **Med** IX.22, 26; XII.36; XXI.94; **Com** V.53 (273); VI.31 (323); VII.46 (398)
pain in the roots of the ~ **Med** XVI.5
redness of the ~ **Com** VI.3 (355)
roughness in the ~ **Med** XXV.8
seeing sparks before one's ~ **Med** IX.8
stinging of the ~ **Com** III.17 (123)
sunken ~ **Ast** X.8; **Reg** III.9
acid tear[1] streaming from one ~ **Med** VI.37
tumors in/of the ~ **Rul** 65; **Med** IX.126
eyebrow
distortion of the ~ **Com** IV.49 (186)
eyelid(s)
hailstone in the ~ → chalazion
hardening of the ~ **Med** XXIII.71
heaviness of the ~ **Reg** III.9

face → nerve, facial; paresis; radiance
callous hardenings on the ~ → *naḥīlāt*
loss of the radiance of the ~ **Reg** III.9
fainting **Ast** V.3; X.9; XIII.33, 34, 35, 36; **Poi** 11; **Rul** 18, 26, 28, 37; **Med** III.113; IV.20; VII.2, 3, 13; X.11, 64; XII.7, 23; XIV.11; XV.53; XX.70; XXIV.32; **Com** I.23 (50); II.36 (88), 37 (89), 41 (93); V.16 (236), 56 (276); VI.27 (319); VII.8 (360)
→ syncope
frequent ~ **Com** II.41 (93)
fatigue **Rul** 23; **Med** III.66; IX.112; **Com** IV.31 (168), 32 (169); IV.74 (211)
→ fever(s)
~ (pain) **Com** IV.33 (170)
severe ~ **Med** IX.112
spontaneous ~ **Com** II.5 (57)
ulcerous ~ **Med** XII.23
fat(ness) (of the body) **Ast** N.1; VI.3; **Rul** 12; **Med** IX.101; XII.5; XIII.38; XXIV.17; **Com** II.44 (96); III.25 (131); V.45 (266)
dissolution of the ~ **Med** V.19; VII.4
fear **Ast** VIII.2; **Med** VI.3, 15, 16; VII.12, 36; **Reg** III.9, 10, 12, 15, 16; **Com** IV.67 (204); VI.23 (315), 53 (345)
prolonged ~ **Com** VI.23 (315)
feces
discharge of ~ **Med** VII.62, 63
obstruction of ~ **Med** XXIII.93
retention of ~ **Ast** IX.9
vomiting of ~ **Med** XXIII.93
feebleness (of the body) **Med** VIII.34; XVII.8; **Com** I.20 (47)
→ digestion
feeling → sickness
~ of pressure → lung(s); stomach, cardia of the
feet
illness occurring in the ~ **Med** XXIII.14
→ podagra
swelling of the ~ **Med** XVI.6
tumor(s) in/on (the) ~ **Med** III.90; IX.126
fetus
heavy/large ~ **Com** IV.1 (138)
→ miscarriage
undernourishment of the ~ **Com** V.52 (272)
weak(ness of the) ~ **Med** XVI.36; **Com** IV.1 (138); V.52 (272)
fever(s) **Ast** XII.1; XIII.11; V.6; VII.4; XI.4; XII.1, 2, 7; XIII.11; **Hem** VI.1; **Rul** 17, 18, 20, 23, 28–30, 33, 36, 45; **Med** II.17, 19, III.27, 49, 58, 59, 77, 82; IV.23, 34, 35, 41; V.1, 8, 12; VI.10, 22, 24, 33, 39, 41, 43, 55, 58, 63, 64; VII.8, 42, 53, 58; VIII.3, 12, 24, 27, 30; IX.42, 43, 47, 68, 88, 89, 92; X.1, 2, 4–7, 11, 15–18, 25, 26, 28–32, 36, 41, 44, 52, 53, 62, 67, 68; XI.10, 14, 17; XII.6, 25, 26, 44; XIII.25, 27, 28, 47; XV.2; XIX.11, 26, 29, 35, 37, XX.30; XXI.94; XXIII.19, 30, 31, 32, 62, 67, 68, 79; XXIV.38, 49; XXV.5, 23, 24, 33; **Reg** I.22; II.7, 9; III.5; IV.9; **Elu** 6, 11, 13; **Com** I.11 (38), 16 (43), 17 (44), 19 (46), 24 (51); II.12 (64), 13 (65), 19 (71), 26 (78), 28 (80), 47 (99); III.6 (112), 7 (113), 25 (131), 30 (136); IV.17 (154), 20 (157), 21 (158), 27 (164), 29–31 (166–168), 34–37 (171–174), 43 (180), 44 (181), 45 (182), 49 (186), 51–53 (188–

190), 55–58 (192–195), 61–67 (198–204), 69 (206), 70 (207), 72 (209), 73 (210); V.5 (225), 17 (237), 31 (251), 55 (275), 61 (281), 64 (284), 70 (290); VI.3 (295), 26 (318), 40 (332), 44 (336), 50 (342), 51 (343), 53 (345), 54 (346); VII.1 (353), 6 (358), 31 (383), 37 (389), 42 (394), 52 (404)
→ fatigue; paroxysm
abating ~ **Med** XXV.23, 24
acute ~ **Ast** X.9; **Med** VI.37, 54; VII.26; X.13, 14, 43; XII.15; XIX.25; XXIII.38; **Elu** 13; **Com** I.14 (41); III.7 (113), 11 (117), 14 (120), 29 (135), 60 (197), 66 (203); V.64 (284)
ardent ~ **Med** II.15; VI.6, 19, 33; VI.51; VII.30, 37, 38; VIII.22, 34; X.40, 42–49, 52, 63; XI.14, 25; XVI.5; XXIII.20, 67; XXV.12; **Elu** 6; **Com** I.23 (50); II.26 (78); III.21 (127), 30 (136); IV.29 (166), 54 (191), 57 (194), 58 (195); VI.26 (318)
~ attack(s) **Rul** 20; **Med** III.103; IV.22, 24; VII.44, 45; VIII.29; IX.48; X.6–9, 12, 22, 24, 25, 27–30, 37–39, 50, 55, 65–68, 71; XI.6; XII.25; XIII.29; XXIII.26, 31; **Elu** 18; **Com** I.7 (34), 11 (38), 12 (39), 17 (44), 19 (46); II.1 (53), 30 (82); IV.48 (185)
attacking ~ **Med** XXV.23, 24
blood ~ **Rul** 33
choleric ~ **Ast** XIII.33, 34
chronic ~ **Rul** 33; **Med** XI.15; XX.83; **Com** III.16 (122); V.64 (284)
chymous ~ **Med** XIX.31
~ associated with mental confusion (phrenitis) **Com** III.30 (136)
continuous ~ **Ast** XIII.33, 34, 35; **Rul** 37; **Med** X.15, 20, 21, 31, 54, 63, 65, 69, 70; XI.29; XII.21; XIII.41; XX.7; XXIII.30; XXV.5, 23, 24, 47; **Com** III.21 (127); IV.43 (180)
~ associated with fatigue **Com** IV.74 (211)
ephemeral ~ **Rul** 29, 31–33; **Med** IV.23, 35; IX.56; X.10, 31, 65, 66; XIX.32; **Reg** I.22; **Com** IV.55 (192); VII.42 (394)
hectic ~ **Ast** IX.8; **Rul** 33, 34; **Med** III.27; IV.23, 35; VI.69; X.57, 58, 60; XIX.2, 31, 36; XXIII.20; XXV.45
~ arising from the putrefaction of the humors **Med** XXV.23, 33, 47, 48
~ illness **Com** IV.30 (167)
intermittent ~ **Med** X.19; XI.29; XIX.37; XXV.23; **Com** IV.43 (180)
long lasting ~ **Com** III.27 (133)
low ~ **Com** V.64 (284)
malignant ~ **Ast** II.2; **Med** II.25; X.23; XVII.15; **Elu** 11
non-malignant ~ **Med** X.23
marasmic ~ **Med** X.60–62
mixed (irregular) ~ **Med** X.34; XXIII.31; **Com** III.22 (128)
perpetual ~ **Med** XXIII.30
pestilential ~ **Med** X.59
phlegmatic ~ **Med** X.24, 53; XX.83; XXV.48
protracted ~ **Com** IV.44 (181)
putrefying ~ **Med** IV.22, 35; V.2; XIX.31
putrid ~ **Med** X.3, 10, 22, 65; XIII.41; XXV.48; **Reg** I.22; **Com** VII.42 (394)
non-putrid ~ **Med** X.22
quartan ~ **Med** II.16, 25; VII.30, 45; VIII.65; IX.42, 43, 47; X.19, 20, 23–25, 29, 34, 37; X.56; XI.25, 29; XII.41; XVIII.16; XIX.23; XXV.23, 48; **Reg** IV.24; **Com** I.12 (39); II.25 (77); III.22 (128); IV.59 (196), 63 (200); V.70 (290)
quintan ~ **Med** X.39; XXV.23
quotidian ~ **Med** VIII.65; X.19, 20, 25, 30, 39; X.54; XXV.23; **Com** I.12 (39)
recurrent ~ **Reg** IV.15
severe ~ **Rul** 18; **Med** X.47; **Com** IV.37 (174)
~ associated with sleeplessness **Com** III.30 (136)
synochous ~ **Rul** 33; **Med** X.54, 63–65; XXIII.30
tertian ~ **Med** VII.45; X.19, 20, 23–25, 28, 29, 33–35, 37–39, 53; XI.29; XIX.33; XXV.23; **Com** III.21 (127); IV.43 (180), 59 (196), 63 (200)
semi-tertian ~ **Com** IV.43 (180)
uninterrupted ~ **Com** IV.46 (183)
unremitting ~ **Com** IV.43 (180), 46–50 (183–187)
wasting ~ **Med** VII.11, 14; X.62
fingers
cold ~ **Med** VI.69

black tumor on the ~ **Med** VI.24
horripilation of the hair on one's ~ **Med** XXIV.46
fissure → bone(s)
anal ~ **Hem** V.2
fistula **Med** XV.44
→ anus
chronic ~ **Med** XXII.63
lachrymal ~ **Med** XV.29
→ *gharab*
fit
epileptic ~ **Med** IX.12; XXV.45
flaccidness → penis; stomach, cardia of the
flatulence **Ast** III.3, 9, 10; V.6; XII.7; **Hem** VII.1; **Rul** 50; **Med** VI.66, 86; IX.47; XVII.30; XX.44; XXI.5, 39; XXV.49, 50; **Coi** 4, 5; **Reg** I.15; **Elu** 45; **Com** V.64 (284), 72 (292); VII.34 (386); VII.52 (404)
→ wind(s)
~ generated by mixed wine **Elu** 2
flatworms **Com** III.26 (132)
→ worms
flesh → muscle(s); ulcer(s)
blackening of ~ from mortification **Com** V.17 (237), 20 (240)
corrosion of the ~ **Med** XXIII.39a, 49, 101
corruption of the moist ~ **Med** VII.4
degeneration of part of the ~ of a nerve/ligament/sinew **Rul** 55
diminution of the ~ **Coi** 1
discharge of something similar to pieces of ~ **Com** IV.26 (163)
dissolution of the (soft) ~ **Rul** 61; **Med** XIII.47; XXIII.101; **Com** II.7 (59)
dissolution in the ~ (of the organs) **Med** V.19
dissolution in the ~ (of the spleen) **Med** V.19
excess ~ in the inner angle of the eye **Med** XV.21
formless ~ that a woman produces in the uterus → *raḥā*
illness in the ~ **Med** IX.98
inflammations in the soft ~ in the groin and armpits **Med** XXIII.56
lividness of the color of the ~ **Com** VII.2 (354)
pain of the ~ **Med** VI.62
small pieces of ~ → urine
softening of the ~ **Com** V.16 (236)
swelling of the ~ **Med** III.27
swelling in the soft ~ of the groins → bubo
tumor in the soft ~ **Rul** 31; **Med** X.10, 31; XV.19
→ scrofula
ulcer in the ~ → *ākila* (canker)
flow → breast(s)
flowing out
~ of foul-smelling matter **Com** VII.44 (396)
~ of turbid matter **Com** VII.44 (396)
fluid
accumulation of ~ → *jamʿ al-māʾ*
urination of thin, watery ~ **Med** V.11
flux **Com** VII.16 (368)
female ~ → *nazf*
food(s) → aversion; craving
forearm(s)
broken ~ **Med** XV.62
rigor in the ~ **Com** V.69 (289)
forehead
pain in the ~ **Med** XVI.5
perspiration on the ~ **Med** VI.21
foreskin
severed ~ **Com** VI.19 (311)
forgetfulness **Ast** X.8; **Med** VII.26, 48; IX.35; XXIII.58, 60
foulness → putrefaction; smell
fracture **Rul** 84, 85; **Med** XV.66, 69
→ bone(s); leg(s)
fright (nightmares) **Com** III.24 (130)
furuncle **Med** XXIII.39a
fury **Com** VI.23 (315)

gallbladder
~ stones **Ast** I.1
gangrene(s) **Med** XXIII.41, 51
→ ulcer
gash → brain
genitals
ailment of the ~ **Com** V.22 (242)
putrefaction in the ~ **Com** III.21 (127)
gharab (lacrimal fistula) **Med** XXIII.72
gland(s)
suppuration of the ~ **Med** IX.118
swelling of a ~ **Med** IX.117, 118; X.10

swelling of the ~ (in the groin or armpit) **Med** XIX.32
gluttony **Med** XVII.3; XXIV.57
gout **Ast** I.1; **Med** II.25; IX.121; XXII.57, 67; **Com** V.25 (245); VI.28–30 (320–322)
→ affection; illness(es)
grief **Reg** III.16; **Com** VI.23 (315)
greenness → *ḥumra*; sputum; stool(s); urine
groin(s)
inflammations in the soft flesh in the ~ and armpits **Med** XXIII.56
swelling in the ~ **Com** IV.55 (192)
swelling in the soft flesh of the ~ → bubo
swelling of the glands in the ~ or armpit **Med** XIX.32
swelling in the hollow of the ~ **Med** XVI.5
tumor in the ~ **Med** X.31
growth → tongue; tooth/teeth
gums
irritation in the ~ **Com** III.25 (131)
tumors in the ~ **Med** IX.123
gut
inflation/protrusion of the ~ **Rul** 79

ḥaban (anasarca) **Med** XXIII.50
→ anasarca
hailstone(s)
expectoration of something resembling ~ **Med** XXIV.37
~ in the eyelid → chalazion
hair → urine
horripilation of the ~ (on one's fingers) **Med** XXIV.46
loss of ~ **Med** XXIII.71; **Com** V.11 (231), 12 (232), 14 (234); VI.4 (296)
→ alopecia
hallucinations
acoustic ~ **Med** VI.37
hands
tumor(s) in/on (the) ~ **Med** III.90; IX.126
hangover **Med** XX.26
hardening(s) → eyelid(s); hypochondrium; *naḥīlāt*; nerve(s); pulse(s); skin; spleen; stool(s); testicles; vessel(s) (, blood); windpipe
hardness → bowels; breast(s); hearing; kidney(s); liver; organ(s); organs, respiratory; sensation; skin; spleen; stool(s); tumor(s); ulcer(s); understanding
harming → vision
head → bone(s): of the head (skull)
burning of the ~ **Med** XIX.19
congestion in the ~ **Med** IX.67; **Reg** II.8
damage to the head ~ **Com** V.5 (225)
defluxion in the ~ **Rul** 70
diseases of the ~ **Med** XI.15
heaviness in/of the ~ **Ast** V.6; X.8; **Med** III.84; VI.35; IX.25; XI.17; XVII.14; XX.25; XXV.50, 52; **Com** III.5 (111), 17 (123); V.22 (242), 28 (248)
illnesses of the ~ **Med** XII.38
illness affecting the entire ~ **Med** XXIII.66
→ *bayḍa*; *khūdha*
inflammation in the ~ **Med** XX.79
pain in the ~ **Med** XII.23; XVI.5; **Com** V.64 (284); VI.10 (302)
→ headache
pain in the back of the ~ **Med** VI.37; **Com** V.68 (288)
rigor in the ~ **Com** V.69 (289)
sores on the ~ **Com** VI.34 (326)
tension in the ~ **Med** XII.23
tumor of one of the parts of the ~ **Med** III.90
ulcers in the ~ **Med** XXV.15
headache **Ast** I.1; III.9; **Rul** 17, 40; **Med** III.84; VI.59; IX.9, 21, 25; XI.17; XVII.39; XIX.19; XX.54, 55; XXII.26; XXV.52; **Coi** 5; **Reg** II.8; **Elu** 41; **Com** III.23 (129); IV.70 (207); V.28 (248), 64 (284); VI.10 (302)
→ *bayḍa*; head: pain in the; *khūdha*; migraine
chronic ~ **Med** XXIII.66
~ affecting the whole head **Med** XV.14
~ caused by inebriety **Med** IX.21
inveterate ~ **Med** VI.60
mild ~ **Ast** XIII.5; **Reg** IV.3
one-sided ~ **Med** VI.60
severe ~ **Med** III.84; VIII.34; IX.25; XV.14; **Com** III.13 (119)
sudden ~ **Com** VI.51 (343)
hearing
hardness of ~ **Com** III.5 (111), 17 (123), 31 (137)

loss of ~ **Com** IV.49 (186)
weakening of ~ **Med** VI.94
heart → cardialgia; heartburn; palpitation(s)
affliction of the ~ **Med** X.60
coldness of the ~ **Ast** VIII.2
coldness/drying of the body of the ~ **Med** IV.27
dyscrasia of the ~ **Med** XXV.72
inflammation of the ~ **Ast** VII.4
pain in the ~ **Med** III.98
tear[2] in the ~ **Com** VI.18 (310)
throbbing of the ~ **Elu** 20
weak(ness of the) ~ **Elu** 25, 26; **Com** IV.52 (189)
heartburn **Ast** III.10; IV.3; V.6; **Med** VIII.36; **Com** IV.17 (154), 65 (202)
→ cardialgia
heat → disease(s); sensation; urine
heat-spots **Com** III.21 (127)
heaviness (of the body) **Med** XVI.5; **Com** I.23 (50); IV.1 (138)
→ brain; eyelid(s); fetus; head; knees; liver; loins; organ(s); sensation; side, right; stomach; stomach, cardia of the
hemiplegia **Ast** XIII.36; **Med** XX.69; XXII.38, 43; **Reg** IV.18, 27; **Com** V.31 (251); VI.56 (348), 57 (349)
hemoptysis **Med** IX.61; XXV.53; **Com** III.29 (135); VII.15 (367)
chronic ~ **Med** XII.22
hemorrhage(s) **Rul** 74–76; **Med** IV.29; IX.2; XV.47; XIX.4; XXV.71; **Com** III.20 (126); V.16 (236), 19 (239), 23 (243), 24 (244); VII.21 (373)
severe ~ **Med** XV.46
~ caused by corrosion **Med** XV.40
~ (from the blood vessels) in the omentum **Rul** 79; **Med** I.60
~ caused by putrefaction **Med** XV.40
~ from the jugular veins **Med** XV.47
~ from a pulsatile vessel **Med** XV.40, 46
~ from a non-pulsatile vessel **Med** XV.46
hemorrhoids **Hem** N.1, II.1; IV.1, 2, 6, 7; V.1–4; VI.1, 3, 8, 9; VII.1, 3; **Med** II.25; XIII.39; XV.21; XX.79; XXII.43, 62, 67; XXIII.47; **Com** III.30 (136); IV.25 (162) VI.11 (303), 12 (304), 21 (313)
→ anus: excrescences on the
chronic ~ **Com** VI.12 (304)
external ~ **Hem** IV. 7
internal ~ **Hem** IV.7; **Med** XXII.66
obstructed/open ~ **Hem** II.2
painful ~ **Hem** V.4; VI.1, 9
protruding (part of the) ~ **Hem** VI.1, 3
hernia **Med** IX.102, 123; XXIII.57
scrotal ~ **Med** XX.80
~ enclosing water → hydrocele
herpes **Med** XXIII.49; **Com** V.22 (242)
hiccups **Poi** 91, **Med** IV.20; VI.48, 88; VII.32, 55; IX.40, 52; XX.86; XXIV.19, **Com** V.3 (223), 4 (224), 35 (255), 58 (278); VI.13 (305), 39 (331); VII.3 (355), 10 (362), 17 (369), 18 (370), 41 (393)
hip(s)
pain in the ~ (sciatica) **Com** III.22 (128); V.53 (273); VI.60 (352)
→ sciatica
tumor in the parts next to the ~ **Med** XII.29
hip joint
dislocation of the ~ **Com** VI.59 (351), 60 (352)
illness occurring in the ~ **Med** XXIII.14
→ ischias
hoarseness **Med** XX.81; XXII.45; **Reg** IV.21; **Com** II.40 (92); III.5 (111), 13 (119), 20 (126), 23 (129)
→ throat: rawness of the
"honeycomb" (scalp infection with honey-comb-like masses secreting substance resembling honey; favus (honeycomb ringworm)) **Med** XXIII.54
→ ulcer
horripilation → fingers; hair; skin
humors
ailment caused by cold ~ **Com** II.40 (92)
corruption of the ~ **Ast** III.4, 7, 42; **Med** VIII.10; XX.34; **Reg** III.1; **Elu** 28, 44; **Com** I.17 (44); V.11 (231)
pain caused by ~ **Med** VII.19
putrefaction of ~ **Rul** 20; **Med** II.6, 30; V.2; VII.58; X.2, 6, 7, 19, 42, 65, 68; XXXIII.68; XXV.23, 24, 33, 47, 48; **Reg** III.5; IV.17; **Com** V.11 (231)
→ fever(s)
putrefaction of ~ (in the (major) vessels/viscera) **Med** XXV.23

humpback **Com** VI.46 (338)
ḥumra (erysipelas) **Med** XV.51
blackness/greenness/lividness of the inflammation known as ~ **Med** XV.50
→ erysipelas
hydrocele (hernia that encloses water) **Med** IX.102; XV.36; XXIII.57
hydrophobia **Poi** 54, 63
hydrops
dry ~ **Com** IV.11 (148)
hypersensitivity **Med** XVII.39
hypochondria **Reg** III.10
hypochondrium → hypochondria; illness(es); melancholia/melancholy
affliction in the ~ **Med** VIII.51
contraction of the ~ **Med** VI.53
hardening of the ~ **Com** IV.64 (201)
illness in the ~ **Med** VI.66
pain in the ~ **Com** VI.40 (332)
rumbling in the ~ **Com** IV.73 (210)
burning sensation in the ~ **Med** VI.52
stretching in the ~ **Med** VIII.50; **Com** I.24 (51)
swelling in the ~ **Med** VIII.50; X.30; **Com** I.24 (51); IV.73 (210); V.64 (284)

ileus (severe colic) **Med** XXIII.93; **Com** III.22 (128); VI.44 (336)
illness(es) → abdomen; arm(s); bile, black; bladder (, urinary); brain; chest; collar-bone; esophagus; eye(s); feet; fever(s); flesh; head; hip joint; intestines; joint(s); kidney(s); leg(s); liver; lung(s); mouth; neck, nape of the; nerve(s); organ(s); phlegm; skin: of the head; spleen; stomach; stomach, cardia of the; throat; uterus; vein(s); vessel(s) (, blood); womb
acute ~ **Med** XI.24, 25; **Com** II.19 (71); III.9 (115); IV. 10 (147), 30 (167); V.6 (226); VII.1 (353), 32 (384), 35 (387)
~ with a long/short beginning **Med** XXV.45
chronic ~ **Ast** XIII.36; **Hem** N.1; **Med** III.75, 76; VIII.40; XII.38; XIII.30; XXII.58; XXIV.49; **Com** IV.30 (167); VII.6 (358)
"divine ~" **Med** XXIII.61
→ epilepsy
fatal ~ **Med** X.50; **Com** III.9 (115); IV.67 (204)
flatulent ~ **Med** XXIII.66
gout-like ~ **Com** VI.49 (341)
"hypochondriac ~" **Med** XXIII.66
→ hypochondria; hypochondrium
incurable ~ **Med** VIII.43
lengthy/long(-lasting) ~ **Com** IV.40 (177), 51 (188); VII.34 (386)
malignant ~ **Med** VIII.48
melancholic ~ **Com** VI.56 (348)
→ melancholia/melancholy
mental/psychic ~ **Med** XXV.59; **Reg** III.10
painful ~ **Med** VI.56
physical ~ **Med** XXV.59
prolonged ~ **Med** III.32; V.3, 18; VI.54, 63; XXV.11; **Com** IV.72 (209)
protracted ~ **Ast** XIII.10; **Reg** IV.8; **Com** VII.31 (383)
rare ~ **Med** XXIV.37, 39, 40
severe ~ **Med** VIII.48; XI.11; XII.20; XV.6; XXV.11, 35; **Reg** II.6; **Com** II.17 (69); IV.23 (160), 42 (179); VI.5 (297), 16 (308); VII.18 (370)
strong ~ **Med** VIII.48
~ of young people **Com** V.9 (229)
→ phthisis
illusion(s) **Med** XXIV.22; **Com** III.24 (130)
→ imagination(s)
imagination(s)
frightening ~ **Com** III.24 (130)
→ illusion(s)
loss of ~ **Med** XXIII.64
→ catalepsy; torpor
impotence → erection: lack of
indigestion(s) **Ast** V.3, 6; VI.3; XIII.10, 33, 34; **Rul** 11, 31, 32, 38; **Med** VII.45, 52; VIII.50, 51, 56; IX.43, 44, 47, 48, 56, 57; X.9, 18, 67; XII.5, 11; XXII.21; XXIII.84; **Reg** N; I.2, 14; IV.8, 16; **Com** I.24 (51)
fatal ~ **Reg** I.2
indisposition **Ast** V.6
→ stomach; stomach, cardia of the
indolence **Ast** V.6; **Med** XI.17; XXIII.26; **Coi** 3; **Reg** III.1; **Com** III.5 (111)
induration → spleen
inebriety → headache
inequality → pulse(s)

inertia **Reg** I.1
infection → lung(s)
inflammation(s) **Ast** VII.4; **Poi** 89; **Rul** 63; **Med** IX.89; X.58; XII.29, 36; XV.2; XV.17, 27, 50, 69; XIX.26; XX.7, 31; XXI.84, 95; XXII.67; XXIII.38, 39a, 40, 42, 70, 89; XXV.11, 19, 20; **Com** I.23 (50); V.43 (264), 65 (285); VI.25 (317); 40 (332), 49 (341); VII.19 (371), 22 (374)
→ armpit(s); bile, yellow; bladder (, urinary); body; brain; carbuncle(s); diaphragm; disease(s); erysipelas; flesh; groin(s); head; heart; *ḥumra*; intestines; liver; lung(s); muscle(s); navel; nerve(s); organ(s); phlegmon; pus; rectum; ribs; spleen; stomach; swelling(s); throat; tonsils; tumor(s); uvula; viscera
blackening of ~ **Com** V.23 (243)
large ~ **Med** XXV.20; **Com** I.23 (50)
~ that tend to red **Com** V.23 (243)
severe ~ **Med** IX.85; XV.2; **Com** V.58 (278); VII.18 (370)
uterine ~ → uterus: inflammation(s) of the
inflation **Med** VII.55; XXIII.52
→ emphysema; gut; wind(s)
ingestion → poison; spasm(s)
inhalation
difficult ~ **Med** I.30
injury/injuries **Med** XV.68, 69; XXIV.34
→ artery/arteries; brain; limb(s); nerve(s); spinal cord; vein(s)
inqilāb (upset stomach) **Med** XXIII.87
insanity **Hem** II.2; **Med** XVI.38
insensibility **Med** XXIII.41, 43
insolence → behavior
insomnia **Ast** V.6; **Med** III.28
interruption → voice
intestine, large
ulcer in the ~ **Rul** 64; **Med** III.93
wound(s) in/to the ~ **Rul** 77; **Med** III.93
intestine, small
tumor in the ~ **Med** XXIII.93
ulcer in the ~ **Med** III.93
wound(s) in/to the ~ **Rul** 77; **Med** III.93
intestines → rumbling; wind(s); worms
abrasion of the ~ **Med** VI.90; XXI.22, 27; **Coi** 10; **Reg** II.7; III.3; **Com** III.30 (136); IV.24 (161); VI.3 (295)
abscess in the ~ **Med** IX.8
affliction of the ~ **Med** X.60
spitting of blood from the region of the ~ **Med** IX.37
burning in the ~ **Med** XIII.53
corrosion/wounds in the ~ **Com** VII.23 (375)
disease of the ~ **Med** VI.82
distension of the part of the ~ called "colon" **Med** VII.65
disturbance in the ~ **Med** XIII.47
emaciation in the ~ **Com** VI.3 (295)
illness in/of the ~ **Med** VIII.15, 37
inflammation of the ~ **Com** IV.24 (161)
irritation of the ~ **Rul** 31
lientery of the ~ **Med** XXIII.94
pain in the ~ **Ast** V.6; **Med** IX.92; XIII.47; **Com** IV.66 (203); VI.7 (299)
protrusion of the ~ **Rul** 80
putrefaction of the ~ **Med** XXIV.34
severing of one of the smaller ~ **Com** VI.24 (316)
stones in the ~ called "colon" **Med** VI.92
swelling in one of the ~ **Com** IV.55 (192)
tear[2] in one of the smaller ~ **Com** VI.18 (310)
tumor in the ~ **Med** III.105; **Com** IV.26 (163)
ulcers in the ~ **Rul** 64; **Med** VI.71, 72, 83; IX.90; XIII.37, 43; XXII.16, 60, 61
ulceration of the ~ **Med** XXIII.89, 93
→ dysentery
intoxication **Poi** 88; **Reg** IV.23; **Elu** 2; **Com** V.5 (225); VII.7 (359)
irregularity → breath(ing); pulse(s); respiration
irritation → bile, black; gums; intestines; liver; organ(s); stomach, cardia of the
ischias (illness) **Med** IX.122; XII.30; XXIII.14
itch(ing) **Poi** 88; **Med** II.25; VI.7, 8; XXIII.40; XXIV.19; **Com** VI.9 (301)

jamʿ al-māʾ (accumulation of fluid; ascites) **Med** XXIII.50
jamr (carbuncles) **Med** XXIII.39
jaundice **Med** II.19; IX.60, 61; XIII.30; XX.84; XXII.11, 58; **Com** IV.62 (199), 64 (201); V.72 (292); VI.42 (334)

jaw
abscess near to the ~ **Com** IV.31 (168)
broken **Med** XV.62
severed delicate part of the ~ **Com** VI.19 (311)
jejunum
ulcer in the ~ **Med** III.93
wound(s) to the ~ **Rul** 77; **Med** III.93
joint(s) → hip joint
abscess in the ~ **Com** IV.31 (168), 74 (211)
dislocation of a ~ **Med** XV.46
illness occurring in/spreading into all ~ **Med** XXIII.14
→ arthritis
pain in the ~ **Ast** V.6; **Med** VIII.19; IX.121; XXI.96; XXII.26, 27; **Com** IV.44 (181), 45 (182); V.25 (245)
swellings in the ~ **Com** V.25 (245)
tumor(s) in the ~ **Com** IV.44 (181), 45 (182)
wounds to the ~ **Rul** 77
joy
frequent ~ **Med** VII.4
lack of ~ **Reg** III.10

khafaqān (burning sensation in the cardia of the stomach) **Com** IV.65 (202)
khūdha ("helmet;" illness affecting the entire head) **Ast** I.1; **Med** XXIII.66
khurāj (abscess) **Com** VII.8 (360)
kidney(s) → nephritis
abscess in a ~ **Med** IX.95
affliction of the ~ **Med** X.60
~ ailment **Med** V.11
bursting of a vessel in the ~ **Com** IV.78 (215)
chilling of the ~ **Reg** IV.20
~/renal diseases **Med** III.91; VII.66
hardness of the ~ **Med** III.91, 92
illness(es) of the ~ **Med** XXIII.94; **Com** V.58 (278); VI.6 (298); VII.34–36 (386–388)
pain in the ~ **Med** II.25; XI.25; XXII.26, 59
sickness of the ~ **Med** VIII.15
~ stones **Ast** I.1; III.2; **Med** VI.92; XIX.13; XX.69; XXII.38, 39, 48, 66, 69
suppuration of the ~ **Com** V.58 (278)
tear[2] in the ~ **Com** VI.18 (310)
tumor(s) in the ~ **Med** III.105; XII.29, 34
ulcers in the ~ **Rul** 64; **Med** IX.95
ulceration in the ~ **Com** IV.75 (212)
weak(ness of the) ~ **Med** VIII.15; IX.64, 94
knee(s)
heaviness in the ~ **Com** IV.20 (157)
pain in the ~ **Com** V.53 (273)
tumor of the ~ **Med** XXII.23
kumna (collection/formation/originating of pus behind the cornea/horn-like tunic/in the eye) **Med** XV.25; XXIII.71

labor
difficult ~ **Com** V.35 (255)
→ childbirth; delivery
lack → activity; appetite(s); comprehension; energy; erection; exertion; joy; lust; pus; sperm; thirst; thought
lameness (of the body) **Com** VI.60 (352)
larynx
closure of the ~ **Com** IV.34 (171)
discharge/spitting of blood from the ~ **Med** IX.34, 37
redness/swelling in/of the ~ **Med** IX.32
laying bare → bone(s); nerve(s)
laziness **Ast** V.5; X.8; **Med** XVII.2; **Reg** I.1
leanness (of the body) **Ast** N.1; VI.3; X.8; XII.5; XIII.44; **Rul** 12, 13; **Med** VII.31; VIII.56; XII.2, 5; XIII.38; XVII.14, 17; XXV.43; **Coi** 1; **Reg** 28; **Com** I.17 (44); II.7 (59), 44 (96)
→ abdomen, lower; cheeks; navel
leg(s)
broken ~ **Med** XV.62
~ cut off below the knee **Ast** XIII.10; **Reg** IV.8
fracture of the ~ **Med** XV.68
illness in the ~ **Med** IX.118
numbness/pain in the ~ **Med** VII.66
thickening of the ~ **Med** XV.23
trembling of the ~ **Med** VII.36
wasting away of the ~ **Com** VI.60 (352)
leprosy **Med** II.16, 25; III.94
→ skin: peeling of the
lethargy **Ast** V.6, **Med** IX.17, 20; XXIII.59, 68
chronic ~ **Med** IX.19
leucoma (white opacity of the eye) **Med** IX.30; XXII.69, 70

leucophlegmasia **Med** XXIII.50
→ anasarca
lice **Med** XXII.54
lientery **Med** XXII.36; XXIII.80, 90, 93; **Reg** IV.22; **Com** III.22 (128), 30 (136); IV.12 (149); VI.1 (293), 43 (335)
→ intestines; stomach
chronic ~ **Com** VI.1 (293)
ligament
degeneration of part of the flesh of a ~ **Rul** 55
limb(s)
blackening of a ~ **Med** XV.10
crushing of a ~ **Com** II.6 (58)
dying of a ~ **Med** XV.10, 12
emaciation of a ~ **Med** XV.66
injury of a ~ **Med** XV.69
pain of the ~ **Ast** X.6; **Med** IX.103; XXII.26
paralysis of a ~ **Com** VII.40 (392)
putrefaction of a ~ **Poi** 61; **Med** XV.12
tumor of a ~ **Med** XXII.17
weak ~ **Ast** X.6, 7; **Poi** 61
limpness (of the body) **Com** I.20 (47)
lip
distortion of the ~ **Com** IV.49 (186)
lisp **Com** VI.32 (324)
liver
abrasion of the ~ **Med** VI.90
abscess in the ~ **Ast** VII.4; **Com** I.12 (39)
~ affection **Med** V.11
affliction of the ~ **Med** XX.31; **Com** IV.62 (199)
~ ailment **Med** IX.41; XXIII.88
coldness of the ~ **Ast** XII.6; Med IX.65
~ complaint **Com** IV.48 (185)
corruption of the blood of the ~ **Med** VI.58
damage/emaciation of the ~ **Reg** III.5
~ disease(s) **Med** VI.82; XXII.39
dryness of the ~ **Med** III.14
hardness of the ~ **Med** II.25; III.91, 92; VII.30; IX.72; XII.45; **Com** VI.42 (334)
heaviness in the region of the ~ **Med** XIX.39
illness of the ~ **Med** VI.58; IX.66; XXIII.88
illnesses (in the parts) above/below the ~ **Med** XII.28; XXV.11
illness in the substance of the ~ **Med** IX.65
inflammation in/of the ~ **Med** VI.55, 57; XII.22; XXI.7; **Com** V.58 (278); VII.17 (369), 18 (370)
irritation of the ~ **Ast** IV.3
obstruction in/of the ~ **Ast** III.1; **Med** I.16; IX.67, 70; XIX.39; XX.54, 79, 84; XXI.22, 37; XXII.58
obstruction of the passages of ~ **Med** XX.88
pain in the (region of the) ~ **Ast** V.6; **Med** X.30; XIX.39; **Com** VII.52 (404)
pain where the ~ is connected to the diaphragm **Med** XXIV.7
pus in (the membrane of) the ~ **Com** VII.45 (397)
rigidness in the substance of the ~ **Med** VII.30
stretching of the ~ **Med** III.33
swelling of the ~ **Reg** IV.22
tear[2] in the ~ **Com** VI.18 (310)
tension in the region of the ~ **Med** XIX.39
tumor(s) in/of the ~ **Rul** 23, 24, 45; **Med** III.113, VI.47, 48, 50; VII.54; IX.62, 68–70, 74, 75, 126; X.71; XI.5, 14; XII.29, 33; XIII.28; XXV.55
watery vesicles in (the membrane surrounding) the ~ **Med** IX.89; **Com** VII.55 (407)
weak(ness of the) ~ **Ast** XIII.36; **Med** III.89; VI.51, 78; VII.5, 56; IX.64, 70; X.71; XXI.45; XXII.54
weakening of the ~ **Med** VI.55; **Reg** III.5; **Com** VI.43 (335)
wound in the lobes of the ~ **Med** XXIV.54
lividness → expectoration; flesh; *ḥumra*; tooth/teeth
loins
pain in the ~ **Med** XII.23; XVI.5; **Com** III.23 (129); IV.11 (148), 20 (157)
rigor in the ~ **Com** V.69 (289)
sensation of heaviness in the ~ **Med** XIX.13
tension in the ~ **Med** XII.23
loneliness **Reg** N
looseness (of the body) **Com** III.17 (123)

→ bowels; skin; stool(s)
loss → activity, mental; appetite(s); blood; consciousness; face; hair; hearing; imagination(s); memory; movement(s)/moving; pulse(s); reason(ing); sensation; speech; strength; tongue; touch; vision; voice
lung(s) → pneumonia; stenosis
abscess in the ~ **Med** XXIV.9
bursting of a vessel in the ~ **Com** VI.12 (304)
catarrh filling the cavities of the ~ **Reg** IV.22
coldness of the ~ **Med** I.17
decay of the ~ **Med** IX.39
discharge/spitting of blood from the ~ **Rul** 72; **Med** IX.34, 37
diseases of the ~ **Med** VI.4; XI.14; XXII.51
enlarged ~ **Com** VI.46 (338)
expectoration of pieces of putrefied ~ **Med** XXIV.37
illnesses of the chest and ~ **Com** V.9 (229)
infection of the ~ **Com** I.12 (39)
→ phthisis
inflammation of the ~ **Med** XII.22
obstruction of the (pulsatile) vessels in the ~ **Med** VII.49; XXIV.38
pain in the ~ **Med** XIX.26; XXI.17
feeling of pressure in the ~ **Ast** XI.2
pressure of the pulsatile vessels in the ~ **Med** XXIV.38
pus (in the area/cavity) between the chest and the ~ **Med** XV.4; **Com** VI.27 (319); VII.44 (396), 54 (406)
tightness of the ~ **Com** VI.46 (338)
tumor in the ~ **Rul** 45; **Med** VI.47; X.42; XII.29, 33
ulcer(s) in the ~ **Rul** 64, 67, 69, 70, 72; **Med** VI.51; IX.39; XV.7; XXIII.17; XXV.18
→ phthisis
ulceration of the ~ **Com** V.15 (235)
lust
~ for food **Med** XVII.3
→ gluttony
lack of ~ **Reg** IV.8
weakening of the ~ (for sexual intercourse) **Coi** 3, 5
madness **Med** VI.3; VI.32, 94; XXIII.62; **Com** III.20 (126), 22 (128); V.40 (260), 65 (285); VI.21 (313), 53 (345), 56 (348); VII.5 (357)
makhba (absconsio) **Med** XXIII.37
mālankhūliyā → melancholia/melancholy
malnutrition **Med** VII.42
mange **Med** II.16; III.94; IX.98
marasmus **Med** III.95, 100; VI.50; VIII.58; IX.100; X.57, 60–62; XIX.2, 34, 36; XX.74; XXI.12; XXII.44; XXIII.19; XXV.43
→ fever(s)
burning/cold/syncopal ~ **Med** XXIII.20
complex ~ **Med** XXIII.19
meagerness (of the body) **Coi** 1
melancholia/melancholy (*mālankhūliyā*) **Hem** II.2; **Med** II.25; VI.15, 16, 94; VII.30; XII.22; XXIII.63; **Elu** 24; **Com** VI.11 (303); 23 (315)
→ bile, black; delusion; distress; illness(es)
hypochondriac ~ **Med** VI.52; XXII.49
"member, male" → penis
membrane(s) → bone(s); brain; liver; ribs; skin
membrane, abdominal (peritoneum) → abdomen
membranes, pleural
stretching of the ~ **Med** VII.54
memory
loss of ~ **Ast** XIII.3; **Reg** IV.1
short-term ~ loss **Med** VI.37
menses/menstruation → blood, menstrual
retention of the ~ **Med** XII.42; XVI.1, 5, 16; XXIV.17
stopping of the ~ **Med** XII.42
micturition → blood; pus; urine
migraine **Ast** I.1; **Med** VI.35; IX.4; XV.14; XX.68; XXII.26; XXV.52
pain of ~ **Med** XXV.52
mind
benumbing/weakening of the ~ **Com** V.16 (236)
corruption(s) of the ~ **Med** XXII.49, 54
derangement of the ~ **Med** VIII.34
disturbance of the ~ **Med** VI.94
dullness/slowness of the ~ **Ast** V.6
sluggishness of the ~ **Ast** V.6; **Med** XVII.26

miscarriage **Med** XVI.26, 27, 30; XXIV.24; **Com** III.12 (118); IV.1 (138), 23 (160); V.30 (250), 34 (254), 37 (257), 44 (264), 45 (265), 53 (273); VII.27 (379)
dangerous ~ **Com** V.55 (275)
missing → respiration
mortification **Med** XII.14; XXI.57; XXIII.41; **Com** 22 (242); VII.50 (402)
blackening of flesh from ~ **Com** V.17 (237), 20 (240)
~ of the solid parts of the body **Med** XXIII.51
→ gangrene; sphacelus
mouth → taste
illness in the ~ **Poi** 8
fetid odor from the ~ **Med** XXII.68
bad smell from the ~ **Med** XXII.56
tumor(s) in/of the ~ **Med** III.105; IX.123, 126; XII.33
tumor in the upper part of the ~ **Med** III.105
ulcers in the ~ **Rul** 64, 65; **Com** III.21 (127)
→ aphthae
movement(s)/moving (of the body)
difficulty of ~ **Med** XXIII.23; **Com** III.5 (111), 17 (123)
→ eye(s); tongue
diminishment of ~ → vessel(s) (, blood)
loss of ~ **Med** XXIII.22
missing of ~ → respiration
weakening of ~ **Med** III.9; XXIII.27; **Reg** IV.18
weakness of ~ **Reg** I.1
muscle(s)
damage of a nerve in the ~ **Med** III.54
inflammations in the ~ of the ribs **Med** XXIII.32
obstruction of the vessels of any ~ **Med** III.64
pain in the ~ in the back **Com** VII.36 (388)
severing of the internal/external ~ **Med** I.26
stretching of the ~ **Com** V.6 (226), 31 (251)
stretching of the ~ (on the spinal column) **Med** XVI.15
swelling in the fleshy part of any ~ **Med** IX.78
swelling of the ~ of the throat **Com** III.26 (132)
tension in the ~ **Med** XIII.32
weak(ness of the) ~ **Med** I.31, 32; VIII.44; **Com** VII.43 (395)
mūzaraj (prolapse) **Med** XXIII.71

naḥīlāt (callous hardenings on the face) **Med** XXIII.72
nakhs → stinging
namla (shingles; ulcer on the skin) **Med** XXIII.35
→ shingles
narrowness → chest
nāṣūr ("polypus;" tumor that forms inside the nose; sinuous ulcer) **Med** XXIII.36, 37, 74
→ nose: tumors in the; ulcer(s)
nausea **Ast** V.6; IX.6; **Med** VI.34, 57; IX.51, 55; XIII.6, 54; XIX.28; XX.81; XXI.14; XXIII.82, 86, 87; **Elu** 10; **Com** V.61 (281)
navel
dissolution/emaciation/leanness/thinness/ weakness of the parts around the ~ and the lower abdomen **Com** II.35 (87)
inflammation of the ~ **Com** III.24 (130)
pain around the ~ **Com** IV.11 (148)
nazf (female flux) **Med** XVI.7
neck
pain in the ~ **Med** XII.23; XVI.5
perspiration on the ~ **Med** VI.21
tension in the ~ **Med** XII.23
tumor of one of the parts of the ~ **Med** III.90
twisting of the ~ **Com** IV.35 (172)
neck, nape of the
illness in the ~ **Med** XII.34
neck, vertebrae of the
curvature of the ~ **Com** III.26 (132)
nephritis **Med** XXV.45; **Com** III.31 (137)
nerve(s) → spasm(s)
affliction of a ~ **Med** IX.115
affliction of the fine ~ distributed in the skin **Med** XXV.37
damage to a ~ **Med** XXV.17
damage of a ~ in the muscle **Med** III.54

damage to the substance of the ~ **Med** IX.120
degeneration of (part of the flesh of) a ~ **Rul** 55
diseases of the ~ **Reg** IV.27, 28
dissolution of the substance of the ~ **Com** V.16 (236)
distension of the ~ **Com** IV.66 (203)
drying of the ~ **Com** IV.66 (203)
hardening of the ~ **Med** III.83
illness affecting the ~ **Med** XXV.16
inflammation of the ~ **Com** V.2 (222)
inflammation in the beginning of the ~ (brain) **Com** VII.3 (355)
injury of a ~ **Rul** 48
laying bare of a ~ **Med** XV.34
obstructions of the hollow ~ **Reg** IV.28
~ pain **Med** VI.60
puncturing a ~ **Rul** 82; XV.46
putrefaction of a ~ **Rul** 82; **Med** XV.17
severed ~ **Com** VI.19 (311)
stretching of (the) ~ **Med** I.6; VII.39; **Com** IV.66 (203)
stretching of the ~ (on the spinal column) **Med** XVI.15
tumors in/of the ~ **Rul** 83
weakening of the ~ **Com** V.16 (236)
weakening of the ~ that move the chest and the diaphragm **Com** IV.50 (187)
weakness of the ~ **Com** VII.43 (395)
~ wounds **Rul** 77; **Med** XV.32–34
nerve, facial
paralysis of the ~ **Reg** IV.18, 27
→ paresis
nerve, sciatic
pain in the ~ **Com** VI.59 (351)
nightmares → fright
nose → nosebleed; nostrils
discharge from the ~ **Med** IX.6
distortion of the ~ **Com** IV.49 (186)
excrescence in the ~ **Med** XV.23; XXIII.74
tumors in the ~ **Med** III.76; XXIII.74
→ *nāṣūr*; polypus
ulcers in the ~ **Rul** 65
nosebleed **Rul** 73; **Med** VI.17, 37, 38; VIII.18; IX.2, 5, 14; IX.114; X.48, 64; XI.14; XII.22, 37, 42; XVII.37; XIX.4, 28; XXII.8; XXIV.22; **Com** I.2 (29); III.27 (133); IV.60 (197), 74 (211); V.33 (253)
nostrils
discharge from the ~ **Com** III. 31 (137)
numbness **Med** XXII.38, 43; XXIII.22, 23; **Com** V.25 (245)
→ leg(s); torpor

obesity (of the body) **Rul** 13; **Med** VII.18; XXIV.17; **Com** V.46 (266)
obstruction **Ast** III.10; IV.2, 3, 8; IX.15; XII.7; **Rul** 15; **Med** III.84; IV.40; VII.13–15, 53; VIII.45; IX.4, 25; X.2, 3, 16; X.66, 68; XII.22; XIII.44; XV.35; XIX.22; XXV.52; **Com** IV.68 (205); V.28 (248); VI.40 (332); VII.48 (400)
→ artery/arteries; brain, ventricles of the; ear(s); feces; hemorrhoids; liver; lung(s); muscle(s); nerve(s); organ(s); spleen; uterus; vein(s); vessel(s) (, blood)
pain caused by an ~ **Com** VI.40 (332)
~ of the passages **Ast** II.1; **Med** VII.43; XII.8; **Com** I.24 (51); III.5 (111)
odor **Med** XXIII.8
→ smell
fetid ~ → mouth
omentum → hemorrhage(s)
bursting of water into the ~ **Com** VII.55 (407)
protrusion of the ~ **Rul** 79, 80, **Com** VI.58 (350)
putrefaction of the ~ **Com** VI.58 (350)
ophiasis **Med** XXIII.53
ophthalmia **Med** IX.31; XII.22, 25; XIX.16; XXII.39; XXIV.20; **Com** III.11 (117), 16 (122), 21 (127); VI.17 (309)
dry ~ **Com** III.12 (118), 14 (120)
opisthotonos (backwards spasm) **Com** IV. 57 (194); V.6 (226)
organ(s)
cold ~ **Med** IX.104; XXV.43
compression of an ~ **Med** IV.47
corrosion of the ~ **Med** VI.25; VII.19; XV.41
damage to the ~ **Med** IV.25
degeneration of an ~ **Rul** 53, 54
diseases of the internal ~ **Poi** 91

dissolution in the flesh of the ~ **Med** V.19
dissolution of the solid ~ **Com** II.7 (59)
dissolution of the substance of ~ **Med** VII.11
distension of an ~ **Ast** V.1; **Reg** I.1
drying of the vital ~ **Ast** X.8
dryness of the ~ **Com** VI.2 (294)
emaciation of the ~ **Com** II.7 (59)
hardness in the/of an ~ **Rul** 43; **Med** IX.72
heaviness in an ~ **Med** III.8
illness of the ~ **Med** IX.104
inflammation(s) in an/the ~ **Med** XII.47; XXIII.79
irritation of the ~ **Med** VII.62; **Com** IV.22 (159)
obstruction of the ~ (arteries) **Med** IV.47
obstruction in the very solid ~ **Med** I.69
pain in the ~ **Med** I.69; IX.104
pressure occurring to an ~ **Med** IV.40
pressure on the ~ lying on the spinal column **Med** XVI.16
putrefaction of the ~ **Rul** 54
rigidness in the ~ **Rul** 43
roughness of the ~ **Med** VII.25, 67
loss of sensation of the ~ hidden beneath the skin **Med** XXV.37
softness of the ~ (arteries) **Med** IV.39
stretching of the ~ **Med** XV.26
swelling of the (internal) ~ **Reg** IV.22
tumor in an ~ **Med** XIII.28
tumor in the internal ~ **Med** XXI.26
tumors in the internal ~ that are not noble **Med** III.79
tumor in the major ~ **Med** XI.10
tumors in the noble ~ **Med** III.76
weakening of an/the ~ **Med** III.58; X.54
weak(ness of an/the) ~ **Ast** I.1, 2; II.1; VIII.2; IX.13; **Rul** 20, 24, 30, 38, 40; **Med** III.8; VII.62; XII.4; XXIII.1
weakness of one of the major ~ **Ast** V.7
weakness of a noble ~ **Rul** 28
weakness of the receiving ~ **Reg** IV.22
organs, digestive
ulcers in the ~ **Rul** 63
wounds to the ~ **Rul** 77
organs, respiratory → affliction
abscess in the ~ **Med** VI.41
dryness/hardness of the ~ **Com** VI.54 (346)
excess of gaseous superfluity in the ~ **Ast** VIII.2
tumor in the ~ **Rul** 45
ulcers in the ~ **Rul** 63, 64; **Med** VI.41
weakness of the ~ **Ast** VIII.2
orthopnea **Ast** N.2; XIII.36; **Med** III.76; XXIII.79; XXIV.38; **Reg** IV.22
asthmatic ~ **Med** XXIV.38

pain **Ast** N.1; I.1; XIII.5; **Poi** 9, 45, 59, 64; **Hem** N.1; II.3; V.4; VI.3, 8, 9; **Rul** 15, 25, 80; **Med** I.38, 69; II.25; III.13, 64, 82, 84, 85, 98, 111; VI.10, 35, 54, 57, 60, 61; VII.6, 7, 12, 14, 27, 33; VIII.27, 31, 37–39, 41, 42, 54, 60; IX.4, 22, 25, 36, 95, 103, 104, 111, 115, 117, 118, 121; X.5; XII.5, 38, 47; XIII.30; XV.15, 16; XV.22, 26, 45, 47; XVI.15, 18; XIX.16; XXI.62; XXII.47; XXIII.32, 43, 101; XXV.21, 52; **Reg** IV.3; **Elu** 1, 35; **Com** I.7 (34); II.1 (53), 30 (82), 46 (98), 48 (100); III.24 (130), 25 (131); IV.11 (148), 32 (169), 33 (170), 67 (204), 73 (210); V.25 (245), 31 (251), 53 (273); VI.5 (297), 7 (299), 22 (314), 31 (323), 40 (332), 52 (404), 54 (406)
→ anus; artery/arteries; back; belly; bite; bladder (, urinary); bone(s); brain; breast(s); chest; colic; collarbone; colon; diaphragm; ear(s); elbow(s); eye(s); flesh; forehead; head; heart; hemorrhoids; hip(s); humors; hypochondrium; illness(es); joint(s); kidney(s); knee(s); leg(s); limb(s); liver; loins; lung(s); migraine; muscle(s); navel; neck; nerve(s); nerve, sciatic; obstruction; organ(s); pubes; ribs; shoulders; side(s); side, right; skull; sleep; spleen; stomach; stomach, cardia of the; suppuration; throat; tooth/teeth; vessel(s) (, blood); wind(s)
abdominal ~ → abdomen: pain in the
biting ~ **Med** XII.7; XII.36; XXIII.93; XXV.31
~ deep in the body **Med** VI.60

~ in the middle part of the body **Med** X.11
~ in the tumorous part of the body **Med** III.109
burning ~ **Ast** V.3, 6; **Med.** II.21; XXIII.87
chronic ~ **Med** VI.44; XIII.30; XXII.26; **Com** VI.60 (352); VII.22 (374)
external/internal ~ **Med** VIII.76; **Com** VII.36 (388)
intestinal ~ → intestines: pain in the
labor ~ **Med** XVI.21, 29
pricking ~ **Med** XII.23; XXIII.91
pulsatile ~ **Med** XXV.19, 20
sensation of ~ **Med** III.64; VI.35; VIII.39; **Com** II.46 (98)
severe ~ **Poi** 39, 77; **Hem** N.2; **Rul** 26, 82; **Med** II.6; VI.10, 24, 60; VII.2; VIII.35, 38; IX.4, 22; X.11; XII.25, 36; XV.17; XVI.16, 21; XXII.57; XXIII.66, 91; XXV.52; **Com** I.7 (34), 23 (50), 46 (98); V.65 (285); VI.5 (297), 7 (299), 10 (302); VII.21 (373), 26 (378), 52 (404)
stretching ~ **Med** XII.47
uterine ~ → uterus: pain in the
pallor **Med** VI.91
→ extremities
palpitation(s) **Med** VI.34, 49; VII.38, 40, 55; IX.113; XXI.96; **Elu** 20, 25; **Com** IV.17 (154), 65 (202)
→ bile, black
paralysis **Ast** XIII.36; **Med** III.66; VI.36; XX.69; XXII.43; XXIII.22, 23; XXIV.58; **Com** VII.58 (410)
→ limb(s); nerve, facial; paresis
paresis
facial ~ **Med** XX.69
→ nerve, facial; paralysis
paroxysm **Med** III.103; XXV.23, 24; **Com** I.12 (39); II.13 (65); IV.30 (167)
~ of the fever **Com** II.13 (65); IV.30 (167)
peeling → skin
penis
flaccidness/weakening of (the activity of) the "male member" (~) **Coi** 2
tumor in the ~ **Med** III.105
ulcers in the ~ **Rul** 65
perforation → brain, ventricles of the; chest
perishing → bone(s); vision
peritoneum (abdominal membrane) → abdomen
perspiration **Med** X.31; XI.14, 28; XXI.4; XXIII.8; **Reg** I.19; **Com** I.2 (29), 20 (47); IV.36 (173)
→ chest; forehead; neck; sweat(ing)
cold ~ **Poi** 87
pharynx
redness/swelling in/of the ~ **Med** IX.32
roughness of the ~ **Med** VI.41
phlegm
diseases caused by ~ **Com** III.20 (126)
→ fever(s); tumor(s)
illness caused by inflamed ~ **Elu** 6
putrefaction of ~ **Med** X.23, 37, 53; XXV.48
phlegmon **Med** XXV.19
phrenitis **Med** VI.11, 37, 53; IX.17, 19; XXIII.62, 67; **Com** I.12 (39); III.30 (136); VI.11 (303); VII.12 (364)
→ brain: inflammation of the membranes of the; confusion: mental
phthisis (infection of the lungs) **Rul** 50; **Med** VI.45, 51; VIII.58; XXII.44, 70; XXIII.17; **Com** I.12 (39); III.10 (116), 13 (119), 16 (122), 22 (128), 29 (135); IV.8 (145); V.9 (229), 11 (231), 12 (232), 14 (234), 15 (235), 64 (284); VI.12 (304); VII.16 (368)
plague **Med** XXI.51; XXIV.27
bloody ~ spots **Med** XX.89
pleurisy **Med** IV.42; V.1; VI.40, 44, 54; VII.54; IX.81–84; XI.25; XII.22, 36; XIX.25, 26; XX.84; XXI.18, 26; XXIII.32; XXV.45; **Reg** IV.22; **Com** I.12 (39); III.23 (129), 30 (136); IV.48 (185); V.8 (228), 15 (235); VI.16 (308), 33 (325); VII.11 (363)
malignant/severe ~ **Med** VI.44
pneumonia **Med** VI.40; XI.25; XIX.25, 26; XXI.18; XXV.45; **Reg** IV.22; **Com** I.12 (39); III.23 (129), 30 (136); IV.48 (185); VI.16 (308); VII.11 (363), 12 (364)
podagra **Med** IX.103; XII.22; XXII.26; XXIII.14
chronic ~ **Med** XXIII.14
poison **Med** XXI.35, 36, 48, 49, 51–53; XXII.45, 52
animal ~ **Med** VII.12; XXI.42, 51

collection of deadly ~ (in the body) **Med** III.65
consumption of ~ **Med** XXIV.51
fatal ~ **Med** XXI.34, 48; XXII.64
ingestion of ~ **Poi** 64, 65, 67, 76, 80, 81, **Med** VII.14
~ of the scorpion/snakes **Med** XXI.96
polydipsia **Med** XXIII.94
→ diabetes; polyuria
polypus **Med** XXIII.74
→ *nāṣūr*; nose: tumors in the
polyuria **Med** XXIII.94; XXIV.39
→ diabetes; polydipsia; thirst
pores
obstruction in the ~ (of the body) **Med** X.65; XXI.92
porousness (of the body) **Rul** 26; **Med** III.6
→ skin
pressure → artery/arteries; lung(s); organ(s); spinal column; stomach; stomach, cardia of the; vessel(s) (, blood)
prolapse → *mūzaraj*; uterus
anal ~ **Med** XXII.60
protrusion → gut; hemorrhoids; intestines; omentum; uterus
pruritus (of the body) **Med** VII.21, 22; **Com** III.31 (137)
pterygium **Med** XV.24; XXIII.70
ptilosis → *sulāq*
pubes
pain in the lower part of the abdomen and ~ **Com** IV.80 (217)
pain in the region of the anus and ~ **Com** VII.39 (391)
pulse(s)
abolishment of the ~ **Med** VI.94
alteration of the ~ **Med** XXV.4
ant-like ~ **Med** IV.33, 34
cessation/disturbance of ~ **Med** VI.94
~ compression **Med** XXIII.26
denseness of the ~ **Med** IV.38, 41, 42
dicrotic ~ **Med** IV.46
disappearance of the ~ **Med** XXIII.27
faint ~ **Med** IV.11, 14; XXIII.28
finished ~ **Med** XXIII.27
fragmented ~ **Med** IV.48
hardened ~ **Med** IV.35
irregular(ity of the) ~ **Med** IV.7, 16, 17; X.30; XXIII.78; XXIV.38, XXV.44
loss of the ~ **Med** XXIII.27
mouse tail('s) ~ **Med** IV.11; XXIII.28
rapidness of the ~ **Med** IV.5, 13, 20–22, 30; X.58
rarity of the ~ **Med** IV.6, 15, 20, 24, 30
serrated ~ **Med** VI.54
slowness of the ~ **Med** IV.6, 13, 21, 24, 30, 45
smallness of the ~ **Med** IV.6, 11, 17, 19–21, 23, 24, 30, 33, 38, 41, 42, 45; VI.37, 91; X.18; XXIII.28; **Reg** III.9
softness of the ~ **Med** IV.25
spasmodic ~ **Med** IV.12, 15, 17, 20, 30, 33; XXV.53
undulatory ~ **Med** IV.29, 33, 39, 41
unequal ~ **Med** IV.7–10, 15–17, 19, 29, 31, 40; X.18,30; XXIII.26, 78, XXV.44
vermicular ~ **Med** IV.15, 33, 34, 39
vibratory ~ **Med** IV.12, 37
weak(ness of the) ~ **Med** IV.6, 17, 20, 23, 26, 33, 38, 40; VI.91; XXIII.26, 28
weakening of the ~ **Med** IV.27
puncturing → arm(s); nerve(s)
pus **Med** III.31, 48, 86; VI.10, 66; IX.95; XV.8, 25, 35, 44, 45, 48; XXIII.32, 39a; XXIV.4, 26; **Com** II.47 (99); IV.47 (184); V.15 (235), 22 (242); VI.10 (302), 27 (319), 41 (333)
→ chest; liver; lung(s)
accumulation of ~ **Med** III.96
collection/formation/originating of ~ behind the cornea/horn-like tunic/in the eye → *kumna*
development of ~ **Med** XXI.63; XXIV.5
~ in an inflammation **Med** XXIII.32
lack of ~ **Rul** 60
micturition of ~ **Med** IX.95
spitting of ~ **Com** VII.15 (367), 16 (368)
thin ~ **Rul** 60
urination of ~ **Com** IV.75 (212), 81 (218)
pustule(s) **Med** XXIII.40; **Com** II.15 (67); VI.9 (301)
black ~ **Med** VI.71
→ ear(s)
broad ~ **Med** XXIII.40; **Com** VI.9 (301)
putrefaction(s) (of the body) **Ast** VII.4; IX.9, 15; X.4; XIII.11; **Rul** 11, 32, 48, 49, 56, 65, 76; **Med** III.59, 63; VI.85, 91; IX.70; X.3, 15–17, 19, 54, 63, 66; XIII.24, 37;

xv.9, 19, 20, 41, 48, 65; xix.2; xx.31, 48; xxi.42; xxiii.11, 75, 109; xxiv.11; xxv.23; **Reg** iv.9; **Com** iii.16 (122); v.11 (231); vii.20 (372)
→ bile, black; bile, yellow; blood; carbuncle(s); chest; genitals; hemorrhage(s); humors; intestines; limb(s); lung(s); nerve(s); omentum; organ(s); phlegm; sperm; stomach; sweat(ing); ulceration; vein(s); vessel(s) (, blood); viscera
foul ~ **Med** vi.89
stinking ~ **Med** iii.31

rabies **Poi** 54
radiance → face
raḥā (formless flesh that a woman produces in the uterus) **Med** xxiii.97
rapidness → pulse(s)
rarity → pulse(s)
rattling → chest
raving (mild delirium) **Med** xxiii.58a; **Com** vii.9 (361)
rawness → chest; throat
reason(ing)
loss of ~ (power) **Med** viii.27; xxiii.64
→ amentia
rectum
inflammation in the ~ **Com** v.58 (278)
ulceration of the ~ **Med** xxiii.91
→ tenesmus
reddishness → urine
redness → body; chest; esophagus; eye(s); inflammation(s); larynx; pharynx; tongue
relaxation (weakness) **Com** iii.5 (111)
→ uvula
respiration → organs, respiratory
bad ~ **Med** vi.42; vii.47
broken ~ **Com** vi.54 (346)
cessation of ~ **Med** vi.2, 94
change (in the rhythm) of ~ **Med** vi.43; **Elu** 36; **Com** iv.68 (205)
deep ~ **Med** vi.37, 53
difficult(y of) ~ **Med** xvi.16; xxiv.32; **Com** iv.50 (187)
disturbance of ~ **Med** vi.94
fast/superficial ~ **Med** xxiii.32
~ in great gasps **Med** vii.48
~ similar to groaning **Med** vi.53
intermittent ~ **Med** vi.37
~ in intervals **Med** vii.48
irregular ~ **Med** xxiv.45
missing of the movement of the ~ **Med** vi.1
shallow ~ **Med** vi.53, 54
small ~ **Med** xxiii.41
restlessness **Com** ii.13 (65); iii.24 (130)
retention → blood, menstrual; feces; menses/menstruation; sperm, female; urine
rheum **Rul** 31; **Med** xix.35; xxi.19, **Reg** iv.21; **Com** iii.13 (119), 20 (126), 23 (129)
chronic ~ **Com** iii.14 (120)
rhyas → *dam'a*
rhythm → respiration
ribs
broken ~ **Med** xv.62
inflammations of the membrane covering the ~ **Med** ix.85
inflammations in the muscles of the ~ **Med** xxiii.32
pain in the ~ **Com** iii.5 (111); vi.5 (297)
pain in the ~ (of the back) **Med** vi.56
ri'da (tremor) **Med** xxiii.21
rigor(s) **Med** vi.7, 8, 12, 64; vii.23, 43–46; x.29–31, 34, 37, 53; xx.54; xxiii.92; **Com** iv.29 (166), 46 (183), 58 (195), 63 (200); v.17 (237), 22 (242), 69 (289); vii.7 (359)
→ back; forearm(s); head; loins; thighs
cold ~ **Med** x.36
feverish ~ **Com** v.20 (240)
malignant ~ **Med** x.37
mild ~ **Med** x.29
severe ~ **Med** x.28, 34, 37
tremor of the ~ **Com** iv.46 (183)
rigidness → liver; organ(s); spleen
ri'sha (tremor) **Med** xxiii.21
roughness → eye(s); organ(s); pharynx; tongue; trachea
roundworms **Med** ix.93; **Com** iii.26 (132)
rumbling → hypochondrium
intestinal ~ **Med** vii.55; xxi.5, 7, **Com** iv.73 (210); v.64 (284)
rutaylā' (tarantula) → bite; sting

sadness **Ast** viii.2; **Med** vi.52; viii.32; ix.44, 110; **Coi** 2; **Reg** iii.6, 16

sa'fa **Med** XXIII.54
→ cradle cap
sarcocele (hardening of the testicles) **Med** XXIII.57
→ testicles
satiation **Ast** V.1, 4, 5; **Med** XVII.2; **Reg** I.1–4, 14; **Com** II.4 (56)
scabs → bladder (, urinary)
scales
urination of ~ **Com** IV. 81 (218)
scalp → skin: of the head
sciatica **Med** XI.25; XII.31; XXV.45; **Com** III.22 (128)
→ hip(s): pain in the
scirrhus (a hard tumor) **Med** XXIII.41
→ *skirros*
scorpion → bite; poison; sting
scrofula (hard tumor in the soft flesh) **Rul** 48; **Med** XV.19; XXIII.56; **Com** III.26 (132)
sediment(s) → urine
semen
very thin (watery) ~ **Com** VI.2 (294)
senility **Med** III.1; VII.26; XVII.35; **Com** I.13 (40)
sensation → choking; cold(ness); loins; pain; side, right; skin; ulceration
~ of crawling ants **Med** XXII.25
benumbing of the ~ (of pain) **Com** V.25 (245)
burning ~ **Poi** 65; **Rul** 31
→ hypochondrium
~ of a severe burning **Med** X.50, 51
burning ~ in the cardia of the stomach → *khafaqān*
difficulty of ~ **Med** XXIII.23
disturbance of ~ **Med** VI.94
false ~ (of hunger) **Ast** VI.3
hardness of ~ **Med** XVIII.9
~ of (severe) heat **Med** X.36; **Com** IV.65 (202)
~ of heaviness **Med** VI.55; XIX.13; XXV.52
loss of ~ **Med** XXIII.22, 23
loss of ~ (of the organ hidden beneath the skin) **Med** XXV.37
loss of the ~ of touch **Med** VI.37
pricking ~ **Med** XII.38; **Com** VI.5 (297)
~ of needle pricks **Med** X.28
slowness of ~ **Med** XVIII.9
senses → taste
benumbing of the ~ **Rul** 25
damage to the ~ **Med** XXV.16
dimness of the ~ **Com** III.5 (111)
dullness of the ~ **Reg** III.8
weakening of the ~ **Reg** IV.18
sensitivity
excessive/extreme ~ **Med** III.93; VII.62; **Com** III.24 (130)
→ hypersensitivity
severing → bone(s): of the head (skull); brain; cartilage; head; foreskin; intestine(s); jaw; muscle(s); nerve(s)
shingles **Med** II.25; IX.105, 106; XXII.25; XXIII.35
→ *namla*
corrosive ~ **Med** XXV.54
shivering **Ast** V.6, **Med** VI.7, 8; VII.41, 44, 45; IX.42, XVI.5; XIX.7, 37; XX.54; XXII.16; XXIII.26; **Com** II.1 (53); III.5 (111); V.61 (281); VII.4 (356), 56 (408)
shortness → breath; memory
shoulders
pain between the ~ **Med** VI.56
sickliness **Med** III.71; **Com** III.12 (118)
sickness → kidney(s); bladder (, urinary)
feeling of ~ **Med** VIII.36; XXIII.87
side(s) (of the body)
pain in the ~ **Med** VI.54; XIX.26; **Com** III.5 (111), 23 (129); V.65 (285)
tumor in the ~ **Med** XII.29
side, right (of the body)
pain in the ~ **Med** VI.55
sensation of heaviness in the ~ **Med** VI.55; XIX.13
ulcer in the ~ **Med** VI.55
sinew
degeneration of part of the flesh of a ~ **Rul** 55
skin
affliction of the fine nerve distributed in the ~ **Med** XXV.37
corrosion of the ~ **Med** XXIII.46
diseases of the ~ **Med** IX.98
disease in which the ~ peels off **Med** II.16; III.94
→ leprosy
dry ~ **Com** V.71 (291)
hard ~ **Com** V.71 (291)

hardening of the ~ **Com** V.20 (240)
horripilation of the ~ **Reg** IV.17
illness occurring on the ~ of the head (scalp) **Med** XXIII.54
→ "honeycomb"
looseness of the ~ of the front part of the body **Com** V.69 (289)
pain in the membrane that lies under the ~ **Med** VI.60
peeling of the ~ **Med** II.25; IX.98; **Com** III.20 (126); VI.4 (296)
→ leprosy
porous ~ **Com** V.71 (291)
abolishment of the sensation of the ~ **Med** XXV.37
loss of sensation of the organ hidden beneath the ~ **Med** XXV.37
softness of the ~ **Com** V.71 (291)
stretched ~ **Med** III.48; **Com** V.71 (291)
swelling on the ~ of the head (scalp) **Med** XXIII.54
tightness of the ~ **Rul** 31
ulcer on the ~ → *namla*
ulceration of the ~ **Med** XXIII.46
ulceration on the ~ of the head (scalp) **Med** XXIII.55
→ cradle cap

skirros (a hard tumor) **Med** VIII.59
→ scirrhus

skull → bone(s): of the head
pain on the outside of the ~ **Med** VI.35
→ migraine

sleep → walking
deep ~ **Med** IX.24
disturbance of ~ **Med** VI.37; **Com** II.13 (65)
→ sleeplessness
excessive ~ **Med** III.69
harmful ~ **Ast** X.1; **Med** VIII.29
lethargic ~ **Med** IX.38
pain caused by ~ **Com** II.1 (53)

sleeplessness **Ast** XI.2; **Rul** 11, 29; **Med** VI.37, 48; VII.2, 4, 12, 14, 37, 58; VIII.23, 36, 38, 41; IX.10, 17, 18, 23, 24; X.68; XI.17; XII.5; XV.15; XXIII.58, 59; XXIV.58; **Coi** 2; **Com** II.3 (55), 30 (82); III.24 (130), 25 (131), 30 (136), 31 (137); VII.18 (370)
→ fever(s); sleep: disturbance of

slowness → mind; pulse(s); sensation; understanding

smallness → pulse(s)

smell → odor
bad/terrible ~ → mouth; stool(s); urine
foul ~ **Med** XXIII.11
→ flowing out; sputum; urine

snake(s) → bite; poison

sneezing **Med** VI.4, 48, 95; VII.32; IX.7, 9, 20; XXIV.19; **Com** V.35 (255); VI.13 (305); VII.51 (403)

softening → brain; flesh

softness → artery/arteries; brain; organ(s); pulse(s); skin; stool(s); soul; tooth/teeth; voice

sore(s) → head
cankerous ~ **Med** XXIII.89
→ canker
ulcer(ous) ~ **Med** XXIII.49
→ canker; ulcer

sorrow(s) **Coi** 2, 3; **Com** VI.53 (345)

soul
affections of the ~ **Med** VII.2; VIII.31; **Coi** 3
affliction of the ~ **Med** XXI.51
constriction of the ~ (anxiety) **Reg** III.10, 16
diseases caused by harm inflicted on the ~ **Med** XVIII.2
distress of the ~ **Med** VIII.32
softness of the ~ **Reg** III.11
upsetting of the ~ **Med** IX.51, 55, 79; XXIII.82
weak ~ **Med** XXIV.58

sparks → eye(s)

spasm(s) **Ast** XIII.10; **Rul** 77, 83; **Med** III.10, 77, 83; IV.35; VI.70; VII.30, 37–39; IX.127; XII.5, 24; XV.15, 46; XVI.18; **Reg** IV.8, 27; **Com** I.12 (39); II.26 (78); IV.16 (153), 57 (194), 68 (205); V.3–5 (223–225), 17 (237), 20 (240), 22 (242), 31 (251), 56 (276), 65 (285), 70 (290); VI.39 (331), 54 (346), 56 (348); VII.3 (355), 9 (361), 10 (362), 13 (365), 18 (370), 25 (377)
→ pulse(s); uterus
backwards ~ → opisthotonos
~ caused by dryness **Med** XVI.15; **Com** II.26 (78)

epileptic ~ **Med** IX.23, 24; IX.43
→ epilepsy
forwards ~ → emprosthotonos
~ occurring as a result of the ingestion of white false hellebore **Com** V.1 (221)
~ occurring because of the filling of the nerves **Com** V.5 (225)
~ due to overfilling → epilepsy
sudden ~ **Med** IX.43; **Reg** IV.18
~ occurring as a result of a wound **Com** V.2 (222)

speech
abolishment/disturbance/loss/weakness of ~ **Med** VI.94
→ speechlessness

speechlessness **Com** V.5 (225)
→ speech

sperm
annulling the production of ~ **Coi** 5
drying of the ~ **Coi** 2, 5
lack of ~ **Coi** 8
putrefaction of the retained ~ **Med** IX.110
spoiled ~ **Com** V.62 (282)

sperm, female
corruption/retention of the ~ (in the uterus) **Med** XVI.17

sphacelus (mortification of the solid parts of the body) **Med** XXIII.51; **Com** VII.50 (402)
→ bone(s)

spinal column
pressure on the organs lying on the ~ **Med** XVI.16
stretching of the nerves and muscles on the ~ **Med** XVI.15

spinal cord
concussion of the ~ **Com** VII.58 (410)
injury of the ~ **Med** XX.80

spine
curvature of the ~ **Com** VI.46 (338)

spine, lower
stretching of the parts in the region of the ~ **Com** IV.73 (210)
swelling in the region of the ~ **Com** IV.73 (210)

spitting → bile; blood; chest; larynx; lung(s); pus; windpipe

spleen
abscess in the ~ **Ast** VII.4
affection of the ~ **Med** IX.44; XII.35; XIX.17; **Com** III.22 (128)
calcification of the ~ **Med** XXIII.89
~ disease **Med** VI.51; XXII.34
dissolution in the flesh of the ~ **Med** V.19
enlarged ~ **Ast** III.2; **Med** VII.16
hardening/hardness of the ~ **Ast** III.2; **Med** II.25; III.91, 92; VII.30; IX.77, 78; XII.45; **Com** VI.43 (335)
illness(es) in/of the ~ **Med** VIII.65; IX.66, 78, 79; XII.34; **Com** I.12 (39); VI.43 (335), 48 (340)
induration of the ~ **Med** XXIII.89
inflamed ~ **Med** XXI.7
obstruction in the ~ **Med** XXI.22, 37, 40
obstruction of the vessels of the ~ **Med** XX.88
pain in the ~ **Ast** V.6
rigidness in the substance of the ~ **Med** VII.30
swelling of the ~ **Med** XXII.13
thickness of the ~ **Med** II.16
tumor(s) in/of the ~ **Med** VI.47; IX.66, 76, 78, 80; XII.29; XXI.40; XXII.23; XXV.55
weakness of the ~ **Ast** III.2; **Med** VII.56

sputum
black/green ~ **Med** VI.77
(expectoration of) foul-smelling ~ **Com** V.11 (231), 14 (234)

squeezing → stomach, cardia of the

stenosis
~ of the pulsatile vessels in the lungs **Med** XXIV.38

sting (of a poisonous animal) **Poi** 10, 16, 31
~ of a honey bee/wasp **Poi** 50, 51
~ of a scorpion **Poi** 4, 44, 48; **Med** IX.109; XX.83; XXIV.36
~ of a *rutaylā'* (tarantula) **Poi** 4, 43
~ of vermin **Med** XXI.50; XXII.64, XXIV.51

stinging (*nakhs*) **Com** IV.17 (154); VI.5 (297)
→ eye(s)

stomach → stomach, cardia of the
abscess in the ~ **Com** I.12 (39)
acidity in the ~ **Elu** 45

~ ailment **Med** IX.41; XXIII.87
spitting of blood from the region of the ~ **Med** IX.37
burning in the ~ **Rul** 31; **Med** II.21; IX.57; XIII.53
coldness of the ~ **Ast** IX.14; **Med** III.81
colic in the ~ **Com** V.41 (261)
cramps in the ~ **Ast** XII.9
diminishment of the strength of the ~ **Med** XXI.5
discomfort in the ~ **Med** VII.55
disease(s) affecting/of the ~ **Med** XVI.24; XXII.39, 48
distension of the ~ **Ast** V.1; **Reg** I.1, 2, 4
disturbance in the ~ **Ast** IX.13; **Med** VIII.26; XIII.47
dryness of the ~ **Com** IV.19 (156)
heaviness in the ~ **Ast** IX.13; X.8; **Med** XXIII.86
illness(es) in/of the ~ **Med** VIII.65; IX.50; XXIII.88; XXIV.25
indisposition of the ~ **Med** VII.52
inflammation of the ~ **Ast** VII.4; **Com** VII.3 (355), 37 (389)
lientery of the ~ **Med** XXIII.94
pain in the ~ **Ast** X.8; XII.9; **Poi** 77, 78; **Rul** 17; **Med** II.21; VII.65; IX.93; XIII.47; XVII.14
pressure in/on the ~ **Med** XVI.16; XXIII.86
putrefaction of yellow bile in the ~ **Med** X.48; XXV.12
stretching of the ~ **Hem** I.2
swelling of the ~ **Reg** IV.22
tear² in the ~ **Com** VI.18 (310)
tumor(s) in the ~ **Rul** 23, 24, 45; **Med** III.90, 105, 113; VI.50; IX.68, 74; X.71; XII.29; XXIII.86
ulcer in the upper part of the ~ **Rul** 64
upset ~ **Med** IX.51, 79; XXIII.86, 87
→ *inqilāb*
weak(ness of the) ~ **Ast** XIII.36; **Med** III.89; VIII.44; IX.51; X.71; XIII.35
weakening of the ~ **Ast** V.1; VII.3; X.18; XIII.35; XX.25; XXI.5; **Elu** 3, 9
wound in the ~ **Med** XXIV.54
stomach, cardia of the
burning sensation in the ~ → *khafaqān*
cold of the ~ **Med** XXIII.85
compression/squeezing of the ~ **Med** IV.20
flaccidness of the ~ **Ast** X.8
feeling of heaviness in the ~ **Med** XXIV.32
illness ascending to/of the ~ **Med** XVI.24; XXV.28; **Com** VI.3 (295)
indisposition of the part of the stomach beneath the ~ **Med** VII.52
irritation of the ~ **Ast** VI.3; XIII.33; IX.43; XIV.4; XIX.14; **Reg** I.9
pain in/of the ~ **Ast** V.3; **Med** IV.20; X.30; XII.5; XX.88
pressure at the ~ **Med** IV.20
feeling of pressure in the ~ **Med** X.9; XXIV.32
putrefaction of yellow bile in the ~ **Med** X.48
ulcer in the ~ **Rul** 64
weakening of the ~ **Ast** XIII.33
weakness of the ~ **Ast** XIII.34; IX.55
stone(s) **Med** III.76; VIII.38; XXIV.3, 11, 54; **Com** III.26 (132)
→ bladder (, urinary); colon; gallbladder; hailstone(s); intestines; kidney(s)
stool(s) → constipation
black ~ **Med** VI.77, 84, 89; **Com** IV.21 (158), 23 (160)
coarse ~ **Med** VI.76
~ with different colors **Med** VI.87
discharge in the ~ **Med** VI.78–80, 83
dry(ness of the) ~ **Ast** IX.1, 6; XIII.5; **Hem** II.3; **Med** VI.74; **Reg** N; III.1, 7; IV.3
excessive ~ **Ast** V.6
foamy ~ **Med** VI.86
greasy ~ **Med** VI.85
green ~ **Med** VI.77, 84
hardening of the ~ **Hem** I.4
hard(ness of the) ~ **Ast** IX.7; **Hem** IV.1; **Reg** N; III.3; **Elu** 39; **Com** II.53 (105)
looseness of the ~ **Com** II.53 (105)
putrid ~ **Med** VI.85
retained ~ **Reg** III.1
small (quantity of) ~ **Med** VI.75; **Com** IV.83 (220)
~ with a bad smell **Med** VI.80; **Com** II.14 (66)

soft ~ **Ast** V.6, IX.4; XIII.5; **Med** VI.74–76; XXIII.90; **Reg** IV.3
→ diarrhea
solid ~ **Ast** IX.6
unmixed ~ **Com** VII.6 (358), 23 (375)
viscous ~ **Med** VI.85
deep yellow ~ **Med** VI.84
stopping → menses/menstruation
stoutness (of the body) **Com** I.3 (30)
straining → vertebra, dorsal
strangury **Com** III.16 (122), 22 (128), 31 (137); IV.80 (217); V.58 (278); VI.44 (336); VII.39 (391), 48 (400)
strength (of the body)
collapse of ~ **Rul** 18; **Med** III.113; XII.42; XV.35; XX.27, 70; **Com** VI.27 (319); VII.8 (360)
damage of the ~ **Med** VIII.40; **Com** IV.46 (183)
diminished ~ **Ast** X.4; XIII.10; **Med** III.28, 79; IV.5; VII.2; XX.27; **Reg** III.9; IV.8
→ stomach
loss of ~ **Com** I.23 (50)
→ tongue
weakening of the ~ **Rul** 18; **Med** VII.2, 47; VIII.12, 46; XIII.26; XX.27; **Com** IV.10 (147)
weakness of ~ **Ast** VI.2; **Rul** 20; **Med** VIII.10, 29; XII.16, 47; XIII.33; XVII.29; XIX.28, 31; XX.12; XXIII.21; **Com** II.28 (80), 39 (91); IV.49 (186); V.12 (232); VI.16 (308), 52 (344)
stretching → anus; diaphragm; hypochondrium; liver; pain; membranes, pleural; muscle(s); nerve(s); organ(s); skin; spine, lower; stomach; uterus; vena cava; vessel(s) (, blood); viscera
stroke **Med** I.38; VI.36, 94; IX.12
light/mild ~ **Med** VI.94; **Com** II.42 (94)
severe ~ **Med** VI.94; **Com** II.42 (94)
stupefaction **Reg** III.1
stupidity **Ast** X.8
stupor **Med** III.77; XXIII.58, 58a, 68; **Com** VII.14 (366)
→ attack(s)
stuttering **Med** XX.77
substance → brain; nerve(s); urine
suffocation **Reg** IV.22; **Com** IV.34 (171); VI.35 (327), 46 (338)
hysterical ~ **Poi** 39; **Med** XVI.15, 16, 18; XXI.96; XXIV.58; **Com** V.35 (255)
sudden ~ **Com** IV.34 (171)
sulāq (ptilosis) **Med** XXIII.71
suppuration **Med** XV.52; XXI.95; **Com** V.20 (240), 22 (242), 65 (285); VI.20 (312), 41 (333); VII.20 (372), 22 (374), 38 (390)
→ elephantiasis; gland(s); kidney(s); tumor(s); urethra; uterus; wound(s)
internal ~ **Com** I.12 (39)
pain without ~ **Com** V.20 (240)
swallowing
difficulty of ~ **Com** IV.35 (172)
sweat(ing) **Med** III.115; IV.29; VI.13, 65; VII.3; XXIV.4, 22; **Reg** II.9; IV.17; **Com** I.12 (39); III.6 (112); IV.38 (175); V.71 (291); VII.4 (356), 62 (414)
→ perspiration
cold ~ **Med** VI.63; X.14; XXIV.32, 36; **Com** IV.37 (174), 42 (179); VII.62 (414)
copious ~ **Com** IV.41 (178), 42 (179)
hot ~ **Com** IV.42 (179); VII.62 (414)
profuse ~ **Med** X.64; XIX.4; **Reg** IV.17
putrefaction of ~ **Med** XX.80
swelling(s) (of the body) **Ast** VII.4; **Poi** 47, 88; **Hem** VI.1, 3, 8, 9; **Rul** 49, 50, 61; **Med** IX.15, 125; X.18; XVI.6; XXIII.40, 51, 54, 77; XXV.72; **Elu** 1; **Com** II.47 (99); IV.35 (172); V.65–67 (285–287)
→ armpit(s); bubo; brain; chest; esophagus; feet; flesh; gland(s); groin(s); hemorrhoids; hypochondrium; intestines; joint(s); larynx; liver; muscle(s); organ(s); pharynx; skin: of the head; spine, lower; spleen; stomach; testicles; throat; tonsils; uvula
hard ~ **Med** VI.66; IX.78; **Com** V.67 (287)
hot ~ **Med** III.27; **Com** V.43 (263)
→ inflammation(s)
inflamed ~ **Med** VI.66
internal ~ **Com** IV.55 (192)
large ~ **Com** VI.27 (319)
phlegmatic ~ **Med** III.27; XXIII.60
red ~ **Com** V.65 (285)
soft ~ **Rul** 50; **Med** XXIII.42, 52
→ edema; erysipelas

severe ~ **Med** IX.33
→ angina
syncope **Rul** 26, 40; **Med** III.97; VI.91; VII.8–15, 42; VIII.21, 41, 76; IX.42, 43, 49, 53; IX.100, 116; X.11, 18; XII.15, 19; XIV.4; XV.35; XIX.4, 28; XXIII.20, 85, 87; **Reg** IV.15, 19
→ fainting

tapeworms **Med** VII.31; IX.93; XXII.9
tarantula (*rutaylā'*) → bite; sting
taste
bitter ~ (in the mouth) **Com** IV.17 (154)
disturbance of the sense of ~ **Med** I.45
tear[1] → eye(s)
tear[2] → bladder (, urinary); brain; heart; intestine(s); kidney(s); liver; stomach
tenesmus **Med** XXIII.91; Com VII.27 (379)
→ rectum: ulceration of the
tension **Med** VI.35; XIII.19; XXV.52
→ back; chest; head; liver; loins; muscle(s); neck; vessel(s) (, blood)
convulsive ~ **Com** VI.5 (297)
testicles
cutting off the ~ **Med** XXV.26
hardening of the ~ **Med** XXIII.57
→ sarcocele
swellings (in the area) of the ~ **Med** VII.48; XXIII.57
→ hernia
thickening of the ~ **Med** XV.23
tetanus **Com** IV.57 (194); V.6 (226), 17 (237), 20–22 (240–242), 65 (285); VII.13 (365)
thickening → blood; leg(s); testicles
unnatural ~ **Com** V.65 (285)
thickness → blood; spleen
~ (obstruction) of the passages **Com** III.5 (111)
→ obstruction: of the passages
thigh(s)
broken ~ **Med** XV.62
→ thigh bone
rigor in the ~ **Com** V.69 (289)
ulcer(s) in/on the ~ **Rul** 65; **Med** XV.59
thigh bone
dislocation of the ~ **Com** VI.59 (351)
thinness (of the body)
→ abdomen, lower; navel; urine; voice
extreme ~ **Com** V.44 (264)
thinning → breast(s)
thirst
constant ~ **Med** X.46
false ~ **Reg** I.9
intense ~ **Com** V.27 (247)
lack of ~ **Med** VI.37
severe ~ **Rul** 16; **Med** VI.41, 55, 57, 71; VII.57; VIII.24; XXIII.94; XXIV.39; **Reg** IV.20; **Com** V.27 (247)
→ diabetes; polyuria
thought
lack of ~ **Coi** 2
throat
illness of the ~ **Med** IX.32
→ angina
inflammation(s) in/of the ~ **Med** XXII.19–21; XXV.11; **Com** III.26 (132)
pain in the ~ **Com** II.15 (67)
rawness of the ~ **Com** III.5 (111)
→ hoarseness
swelling in/of the ~ **Med** IX.123; XXIII.77; **Com** IV.34 (171)
→ angina
swelling of the muscles of the ~ **Com** III.26 (132)
swelling on the outside of the ~ **Com** VI.37 (329)
tumor in the ~ **Med** III.105
throat, sore **Com** III.5 (111)
throbbing → heart; wound(s)
tightness → lung(s); skin
tongue
black ~ **Med** VI.51, 55
difficulty of movement of the ~ **Med** XXV.56
severe dryness of the ~ **Med** VI.19
growth on the ~ **Med** VI.24
loss of the strength of the ~ **Com** VII.40 (392)
red ~ **Med** VI.55
roughness of the ~ **Med** VI.37
tumor of the ~ **Med** III.105
tonsils
inflammation of the ~ **Med** XXII.19
swelling of the ~ **Med** IX.123
tooth/teeth
breaking of ~ **Med** VII.34
corrosion of ~ **Med** VII.34; XXI.10; XXII.53

decayed ~ **Poi** 8
lividness of the color of the ~ **Med** VII.34
pain/weakness of the ~ **Med** XXII.7
pain following the extraction of a painful ~ **Med** VII.33
pain from the growth of the ~ **Med** XXII.6
softness of the ~ **Med** VII.34

torpor **Med** IX.11, 12, 17, 18, 23, 24, 35, 43; XXIII.22, 58, 64, 68; XXIV.45
→ imagination(s): loss of; numbness
heavy ~ **Med** VIII.27

touch
loss of the sensation of ~ **Med** VI.37

trachea
roughness of the ~ **Med** VI.41

trachoma **Med** XV.24

transudation → blood

trembling **Med** VII.36, 43; XXII.38, 43, 70
→ arm(s), leg(s)
~ from weakness **Reg** III.9

tremor(s) **Med** VI.48; VII.36, 42, 43; XXII.70; XXIII.21; XXIV.16; **Reg** IV.27, 28; **Elu** 2; **Com** VI.26 (318)
→ *riʿda*; rigor(s); *riʿsha*

tumor(s) **Hem** I.2; **Rul** 15, 20, 30, 46, 51, 52, 78, 82; **Med** III.13, 48, 59, 61, 63, 85, 90, 92, 95, 99, 110, 113; IV.31; VI.28, 39, 40, 68; VII.7, 35, 54; VIII.22, 30, 35, 59, 67; IX.99; X.10, 44; XI.15; XV.13, 35; XXI.11, 20; XXIII.40, 41, 45, 46, 87, 88; XXV.33; **Elu** 1; **Com** II.1 (53), 6 (58); III.20 (126), 26 (132), 31 (137); IV.44 (181), 45 (182)
→ anus; bladder (, urinary); brain; breast(s); cancer; chest; diaphragm; ear(s); esophagus; eye(s); feet; fingers; flesh; groin(s); hands; head; hip(s); intestine, small; intestines; joint(s); kidney(s); knee(s); limb(s); liver; lung(s); mouth; *nāṣūr*; neck; nerve(s); nose; organ(s); organs, respiratory; penis; polypus; side(s); spleen; stomach; throat; tongue; urethra; uterus; viscera; vulva
benign ~ **Med** VI.68
black ~ **Med** VI.24
bloody ~ **Med** VII.53; X.31
→ blood
cancerous ~ **Med** IX.107; XXIII.47
→ cancer
chronic ~ **Med** III.48
cold ~ **Med** III.96; IX.17
enlarged ~ **Med** XV.13
external ~ **Med** VIII.27
hard(ness of the) ~ **Rul** 46, 47; **Med** III.106; VII.54; VIII.59; IX.62, 63, 66, 120, 125; X.2; XI.5; XV.19; XXI.40, 64; XXII.15, 17, 23, 24; XXIII.41, 43, 45, 93; **Com** VI.46 (338)
→ scirrhus; scrofula; *skirros*
hot ~ **Rul** 15, 46; **Med** III.8, 48, 82, 83, 92, 96, 108; **Com** II.6 (58)
inflamed ~ **Med** VI.50; VII.28, 30, 35, 53, 54; VIII.30, 34, 35, 50; IX.42, 57, 123, 125; X.2, 11, 15, 42, 68, 71; XI.10, 14; XII.18, 24, 29, 33, 34, 46; XV.52, 53; XXI.19; XXII.14; XXV.23; **Com** I.24 (51); V.23 (243); VI.36 (328)
internal ~ **Med** VIII.27; XI.14; **Com** II.1 (53)
phlegmatic ~ **Med** III.88
scirrhous ~ **Med** XXIII.45
→ scirrhus; *skirros*
soft ~ **Med** X.2
suppurating ~ **Med** VI.68; **Com** IV.82 (219); VII.57 (409)

tunic, horn-like
collection/formation/originating of pus behind the cornea/~/in the eye → *kumna*
corrosion of the ~ **Med** XXIII.71
ulceration of the ~ **Med** XXV.17

twisting → neck

tympanites (dry dropsy) **Med** XXIII.50; **Com** IV.11 (148)

ulcer(s) **Rul** 57–63, 66, 69; **Med** III.76; VII.62; IX.98, 117; XV.2, 18, 40, 43, 46, 54, 55, 57, 59, 66; XXII.25, 35; XXIII.44, 89; XXIV.33; **Com** V.20–23 (240–243); VI.4 (296), 8 (300), 45 (337)
→ anus; cancer; carbuncle(s); chest; disease(s); ear(s); esophagus; fatigue; head; intestine, large; intestine, small; intestines; jejunum; kidney(s); lung(s); mouth; nose; organs, digestive; organs, respiratory; penis; side, right; stomach;

stomach, cardia of the; thighs; ulceration; vagina; womb(s)
abdominal ~ **Med** XV.38
~ in the fleshy parts of the body **Med** VII.25
cancerous ~ **Med** IX.111
corruption of an ~ **Med** XXIII.48
deep ~ **Med** XV.54, 55
dirty ~ **Med** XV.54
~ dripping **Med** XXI.11
external ~ **Rul** 66
fresh ~ **Med** XV.38
gangrenous ~ **Med** XXIII.44
→ gangrene(s)
hardness of the lips of the ~ **Rul** 61
honeycomb-like ~ **Med** XXIII.55
indurated ~ **Med** XXV.13
inflamed ~ **Med** XV.38
internal ~ **Rul** 66, 69; **Med** VI.72; IX.89
intestinal ~ → intestines: ulcers in the
inveterate ~ **Med** XXII.20
malignant ~ **Med** IX.90; XV.6, 9; XXIII.44
moist ~ **Med** XV.54
putrefied ~ **Med** IX.39; XV.9
putrid ~ **Med** XIII.37; XV.1; **Com** IV.47 (184)
sinuous ~ **Med** XV.45; XXIII.36, 37
→ *nāṣūr*
virulent ~ **Poi** 8
ulceration **Com** V.23 (243), 25 (245); VI.38 (330)
→ bladder (, urinary); eruptions; intestines; kidney(s); lung(s), rectum; skin; skin: of the head; tunic, horn-like
deep ~ **Med** XXV.17
~ with/without putrefaction **Med** XXIII.89
sensation of ~ **Med** VI.7
undernourishment → fetus
understanding
dullness of ~ **Ast** XIII.3; **Reg** IV.1
hardness/slowness of ~ **Med** XVIII.9
unresponsiveness
~ to questions **Med** VI.37
upsetting → stomach; soul
urethra
tumor in the ~ **Com** IV.82 (219); VII.57 (409)
bursting of a tumor in the ~ **Com** IV.82 (219); VII.57 (409)
suppuration of a tumor in the ~ **Com** IV.82 (219); VII.57 (409)
urination → blood; fluid; pus; scales; urine
urine → micturition; urination
black ~ **Med** V.15; VI.77
bubbles of gassy spirit accumulating in the ~ **Med** V.3
bubbles on the surface of the ~ **Com** VII.34 (386)
clear ~ **Med** V.10
cloud in the ~ **Med** V.15; XI.9
black cloud in the ~ **Med** V.16
red cloud in the ~ **Med** XI.9; **Com** IV.71 (208)
white cloud in the ~ **Com** IV.71 (208)
~ having a fine consistency **Med** XI.8
dark/reddish ~ **Med** XVI.5
discharge in the ~ **Med** VI.78–80
fatty/oily ~ **Med** V.12, 16
small pieces of flesh in the ~ **Com** IV.76 (213)
green ~ **Med** VI.77
hair-like bodies/substance in the ~ **Med** XXIV.8; **Com** IV.76 (213)
extremely severe heat of the ~ **Med** VIII.50; **Com** I.24 (51)
heterogeneous ~ **Com** VII.33 (385)
~ resembling mud **Com** IV.69 (206)
~ containing particles **Med** V.16, 19; **Com** IV.77 (214)
retention of the ~ **Ast** IX.9
(bad) sediment(s) in the ~ **Med** II.17; III.45, 59; V.8, 9, 16, 18; XI.9; **Com** VII.31 (383), 32 (384)
sandy sediment in the ~ **Com** IV.79 (216)
→ bladder (, urinary): stone(s)
~ with a bad/terrible smell **Med** V.16; VI.80
foul-smelling ~ **Com** IV.81 (218)
~ covered with a greasy substance **Com** VII.35 (387)
thick ~ **Med** V.18; **Com** IV.69 (206), 76 (213), 77 (214)
thin ~ **Med** V.10, 18, 20; X.45; **Com** IV.69 (206)
transparent/white ~ **Com** IV.72 (209)

turbid ~ **Med** V.10; XI.8; **Com** IV.70 (207)
~ resembling water **Med** V.10, 13
pale yellow/bright yellowish red ~ **Med** XI.8

uterus
affliction of ~ **Med** X.60; **Com** V.35 (255)
ailment of the ~ **Com** V.22 (242)
burning/dryness of the ~ **Com** V.62 (282)
bursting of vessels in the (neck of the) ~ **Med** XII.32; XVI.19
cold ~ **Com** V.62 (282)
contraction of the ~ **Med** XVI.3
corruption of the female sperm in the ~ **Med** XVI.17
dense ~ **Com** V.62 (282)
diseases of the ~ **Med** XXII.66
erosion at the neck of the ~ **Med** XVI.7
formless flesh that a woman produces in the/illness developing in the ~ → *raḥā*
inflammation(s) of the ~ **Med** I.65; XVI.13; **Com** V.58 (278)
obstruction in/weakness of the ~ **Med** XVI.3
pain in the ~ **Med** I.69; XVI.18
prolapse/protrusion of the ~ **Med** XVI.21
spasm(s) of the ~ **Med** XVI.15, 18
stretching of the ~ **Med** XVI.15, 16
suppuration of (an external site of) the ~ **Com** V.47 (267)
tumor(s) in the ~ **Med** III.105; XII.29, 34

uvula
inflammations of the ~ **Med** XXV.11
extreme relaxation of the ~ **Med** XV.27
swelling of the ~ **Med** IX.123; XXII.19
tumors in the ~ **Med** IX.123

vagina
ulcers in the ~ **Rul** 65

vein(s)
illnesses in the ~ **Med** V.1
→ fever(s)
injury of a ~ **Rul** 48
obstruction in the ~ **Ast** II.1; III.1; **Med** III.59
putrefaction of blood in the ~ **Ast** VII.4
varicose ~ **Med** XXIII.47; **Com** VI.21 (313), 34 (326)
weakness of the ~ **Med** VIII.44
widening of the ~ **Com** VI.21 (313), 34 (326)

veins, jugular → hemorrhage(s)

vena cava
stretching of the vessel known as ~ **Med** VII.54

vermin → bite; sting

vertebra → neck, vertebrae of the

vertebra, dorsal
straining a ~ **Com** IV.35 (172)

vertigo **Med** VI.34; IX.3; XV.14; XXV.11; **Com** III.17 (123)

vesicles, watery → liver

vessel(s) (, blood) → hemorrhage(s); stenosis; vena cava
bursting of ~ **Med** X.48; XII.10; XV.39; **Com** I.3 (30); VII.37 (389)
bursting of a ~ (in the kidneys) **Com** IV.78 (215)
bursting of a ~ (in the lungs) **Com** VI.12 (304)
bursting of ~ (in the (neck of the) uterus) **Med** XII.32; XVI.19
diminishment of the movement of the pulsatile ~ **Med** XXIII.27
dry ~ **Med** XXIV.45
erosion of the ~ **Med** XII.32
hardening of a pulsatile ~ **Med** VII.30
illness in the non-pulsatile ~ **Med** IX.98
obstruction of the ~ (of any muscle) **Med** III.64
obstruction of the (pulsatile) ~ (in the lungs) **Med** VII.49; XXIV.38
obstruction of the ~ (of the spleen) **Med** XX.88
pain in a ~ **Med** VI.62; IX.117
pressure of the pulsatile ~ (in the lungs) **Med** XXIV.38
putrefaction in the (large/major) ~ **Med** X.10, 15
putrefaction of yellow bile in the ~ **Med** XXV.12
putrefaction of humors in the (major) ~ **Med** XXV.23, 24
stretching/widening of the ~ (of the anus) **Hem** II.1
tension of a ~ **Med** IX.117
weakening of the ~ **Med** XIII.14
weakness of the ~ **Med** XIII.14; XVI.3

widening of the ~ **Med** IV.41
wounds to the ~ **Rul** 77
vigor
weak(ness of) ~ **Rul** 24; **Com** I.17 (44)
weakening of ~ **Reg** I.1; **Com** I.23 (50)
vigor, sexual
diminishment of ~ **Coi** 2
viper → bite
viscera
inflammation in the ~ **Med** X.4
putrefaction (of humors) in the ~ **Med** X.10; XXV.23
stretching of the ~ **Med** XVI.15
tumor(s) in (one of) the ~ **Med** VIII.29, 34, 50, 51; IX.63; X.11; **Com** I.24 (51)
vision
darkening of ~ **Med** VI.13; XXIII.70
diminishment of the clarity of ~ **Med** VII.69
dimness of ~ **Com** III.5 (111)
disturbance of ~ **Med** VI.94
harming of ~ **Med** VII.69
loss of ~ **Med** VI.94; **Com** IV.49 (186)
perishing of the faculty of ~ **Med** VI.13
weak ~ **Med** XX.83; XXII.5
weakening of ~ **Med** VI.94
voice → hoarseness; throat
interruption/thinness of the ~ **Med** VII.49
loss of the ~ **Com** VI.51 (343)
soft ~ **Reg** III.9
weakening/weakness of the ~ **Reg** III.9
vomiting (involuntary) **Poi** 77; **Rul** 40; **Med** II.14; IV.20, 29; VI.23, 25, 52; VII.53; XIII.54; XVI.23; XX.73, 81; XXIII.83, 87; XXV.39; **Elu** 10; **Com** I.2 (29); III.21 (127), 24 (130); VII.3 (355), 8 (360), 10 (362)
→ bile; bile, yellow; blood; blood, menstrual; feces
vulva
tumor in the ~ **Med** III.105

walking
~ while asleep **Med** I.33, 38; XXIV.21
wart(s) **Med** XXII.25; **Com** III.26 (132)
wasp → sting
wasting **Med** III.14
wasting away (of the body) **Med** XX.62; XXIII.17; XXIV.37, 58; XXV.43; **Com** I.14 (41)
→ leg(s)
weakening (of the body) **Ast** XIII.5; **Med** III.3; VI.94; VII.36; XII.5, 6; XV.7; XIX.3; XX.46; XXI.7; **Reg** IV.3; **Com** IV.23 (160), 46 (183)
→ brain; chest; diaphragm; digestion; hearing; liver; lust; mind; movement(s)/moving; nerve(s); organ(s); penis; senses; stomach; stomach, cardia of the; strength; vessel(s) (, blood); vigor; vision; voice
weakness (of the body) **Ast** XIII.36, 43; **Rul** 38, 58; **Med** I.27; III.10, 70; IV.24; VI.31; VII.3, 61; VIII.6, 13, 40; XII.18; XVII.34; XX.8, 9, 12; XXIII.13; XXIV.25; **Reg** III.9; **Elu** 18; **Com** I.20 (47); II.49 (101); III.5 (111), 12 (118); IV.5 (142), 49 (186); VII.62 (414)
→ abdomen; lower; appetite(s); artery/arteries; bladder (, urinary); brain; breathing; chest; digestion; fetus; heart; kidney(s); limb(s); liver; movement(s)/moving; muscle(s); navel; nerve(s); organ(s); organs, respiratory; pulse(s); relaxation; soul; speech; spleen; stomach; stomach, cardia of the; strength; tooth/teeth; trembling; uterus; vein(s); vessel(s) (, blood); vigor; vision; voice
weariness **Hem** N.2; **Med** XI.17
weasel → bite
widening → anus; vein(s); vessel(s) (, blood)
wind(s) **Rul** 16, 25, 32, 50; **Med** XX.85, XXI.39; **Com** IV.73 (210); V.41 (261), 72 (292); VII.51 (403), 52 (404)
→ flatulence
cold ~ **Med** VIII.54
external/internal ~ **Med** XX.62
flatulent ~ **Med** IX.92; XXI.22, 38, 94
~ generated by mixed wine **Elu** 2
inflating ~ **Rul** 25; **Med** VII.17; VIII.42, 54
intestinal ~ **Med** XX.25
pain caused by/originating from ~ **Med** VI.35; XXV.52; **Com** VI.40 (332)
thick ~ **Med** VII.17, 40; VIII.54; XXI.38; **Com** VI.51 (343); VII.34 (386)

vaporous ~ **Med** VIII.37

windpipe

discharge/spitting of blood from the ~ **Med** IX.34, 37

drying/hardening of the ~ **Ast** IV.3

wine → flatulence; wind(s)

womb(s)

illnesses occurring from the side of the ~ **Com** V.57 (277)

ulcerous ~ **Med** XIII.39

worms → flatworms; roundworms; tapeworms

abdominal ~ **Med** VI.21; IX.93; XXII.46

Guinea ~ **Med** XXIV.8

intestinal ~ **Med** XXIV.8; **Com** III.26 (132)

→ flatworms

vinegar ~ **Med** IX.93

worry/worries **Ast** VIII.2, 4; **Med** VI.3; VII.37; X.68; **Coi** 2, 3; **Reg** III.11, 16; **Com** VI.53 (345)

constant ~ **Reg** III.10

wound(s) **Poi** 8, 9, 49, 63; **Rul** 49, 52, 75–81, 85; **Med** III.13, 78; XII.24; XV.8, 15, 38, 39, 47, 56; XXI.51; **Com** I.1 (16); II.6 (58); V.22 (242), 65 (285), 66 (286); VI.9 (301); VII. 37 (389)

→ belly; brain; breastbone; chest; diaphragm; intestine, large; intestine, small; jejunum; joint(s); liver; nerve(s); organs, digestive; spasm(s); stomach; vessel(s) (, blood)

abdominal ~ **Med** XV.37

corrosive ~ **Com** V.22 (242)

deep ~ **Med** XXIV.54; **Com** VI.18 (310), 19 (311)

large ~ **Med** III.19; XXIV.54; **Com** VI.18 (310)

moist ~ **Med** XXI.29

putrid ~ **Com** VI.3 (295)

suppuration of a ~ **Com** V.22 (242)

violent throbbing in ~ **Com** VII.21 (373)

yawning **Med** IX.42; XXIV.20; **Com** VII.56 (408)

yellowness → complexion; stool(s)

Index of Medicinal Products, Dishes, and Their Ingredients and Components (Including Poisons and Antidotes)

abū ṣūfa ("father of wool") (a tarantula species) **Poi** 48
acacia tree (fruit) – *Acacia nilotica* (L.) Delile **Med** XV.56
aconite – *Aconitum napellus* L. **Med** XXIII.101
acorn (oak – *Quercus* sp. L.) **Poi** 66; **Med** XX.60; XXI.73; XXIV.31; **Com** I.1 (25)
aeonium, tree – *Aeonium arboreum* (L.) Webb & Berthel. (Arab. *ḥayy al-ʿālam*) **Poi** 51; **Med** IX.106; XXI.84
agarikon – *Laricifomes officinalis* (Vill.) Kotl. & Pouzar **Ast** XII.8, 9; XIII.41; **Poi** 27, 36, 52, 80; **Med** XXI.33, 69; **Reg** II.7
agarwood (, Indian) – *Aquilaria malaccensis* Lam. **Med** XXI.75; XXII.56; **Reg** III.8; IV.20; **Elu** 21, 25
agrimony, common – *Agrimonia eupatoria* L. **Poi** 25; **Med** IX.88; XXI.30, 40, 69
ajowan – *Trachyspermum ammi* (L.) Sprague (Arab. *nānakhwāh*) **Poi** 42; **Med** IX.88; XX.49; XXI.80
alkali plant **Poi** 45
almond – *Prunus dulcis* (Mill.) D.A. Webb **Ast** III.10; IV.2, 3, 4, 6; VI.4; IX.3; XII.2, 3, 8, 9; **Hem** III.1, 2; IV.3; **Med** XIII.44, 51; XX.51, 77; XXI.72; XXII.41, 55; **Coi** 4, 7, 8; **Reg** I.22; III.3, 7, 8; **Elu** 13, 30
almond, bitter – *Prunus dulcis* (Mill.) D.A. Webb **Ast** XII.3, 5; **Poi** 57; **Med** XXI.18
aloe – *Aloe vera* (L.) Burm. f. **Rul** 62, 65; **Med** IX.46, 50; XIII.13; XV.47; XVII.38; XXI.29, 43, 75; XXII.54
aloe, Socotra – *Aloe perryi* Baker **Med** XXII.63
amaranth, purple – *Amaranthus blitum* L. **Med** IX.108; XX.47, 84; XXI.79; **Reg** III.2; **Elu** 30
amber (black poplar – *Populus nigra* L.) **Rul** 69; **Med** XXI.80; **Elu** 20, 21, 25
ambergris **Ast** XII.6; **Coi** 10; **Med** XXI.75; **Reg** II.11; **Elu** 21, 25
ammoniac → gum ammoniac; sal ammoniac
amylum → starch
anise – *Pimpinella anisum* L. **Ast** III.10; IX.15; XII.3, 8; **Poi** 16, 29, 37, 44, 49; **Hem** III.2; IV.1, 3, 4; **Med** XIII.6; XIII.44; XX.86; XXI.80; **Coi** 5; **Reg** III.7, 8
ant **Med** IV.33; XXII.25
ant, yellow **Coi** 9
antimony – *Sb* **Med** XXI.87
antula (yellow monkshood – *Aconitum anthora* L.) **Reg** III.8
apple – *Malus pumila* Mill. **Ast** III.10; IX.5, 13; **Poi** 65; **Rul** 15, 63, 69; **Med** IX.53, 69; XX.52, 74; XXI.73, 96; XXII.64; **Coi** 8, 25; **Reg** III.2; **Elu** 8, 10, 20, 23, 25, 26
apricot – *Prunus armeniaca* L. **Ast** III.9; IX.13; **Hem** VI.4, 9; **Med** IX.123; XX.61; XXI.79; **Reg** I.22; **Elu** 11
aqiṭ (type of milk) **Med** XXIII.107
arar tree (resin) – *Tetraclinis articulate* (Vahl) Mast. (Arab. *sandarūs*) **Hem** VII.1, 2; **Med** XXI.69
arsenic – *As* **Ast** XII.6; **Poi** 81; **Rul** 76; **Med** II.5; XXI.88; XXIII.101
artichoke – *Cynara cardunculus* L. **Med** XXI.80; XXII.56
arum – *Araceae* sp. Juss. **Med** XXII.62
ʿaṣā al-rāʿī → knotgrass, common
asafetida (gum resin) – *Ferula assa-foetida* L. **Poi** 12, 13, 33, 42, 53, 55, 57, 80, 84; **Rul** 83; **Med** XIII.3; XXI.80; XXII.19
asarabacca – *Asarum europaeum* L. **Med** IX.46; XXI.65, 80
ash tree (fruit) – *Fraxinus excelsior* L. **Med** XXI.77; **Coi** 8; **Reg** III.8
ʿasīda (porridge) **Hem** VI.3
asparagus – *Asparagus officinalis* L. **Ast** III.8; **Poi** 49; **Med** XX.85; XXI.65, 68; **Coi** 4, 8; **Reg** II.6; III.8

asphodel – *Asphodelus ramosus* L. **Med** IX.88, 123; **Elu** 22
ass, wild **Reg** IV.28

bābūnaj → camomile, German; camomile, Roman
balsam of Mecca (Mecca myrrh – *Commiphora opobalsamum* (L.) Engl.) **Poi** 26, 30; **Med** IX.88; XXI.75; XXII.52
balsam wood (Mecca myrrh – *Commiphora opobalsamum* (L.) Engl.) **Ast** XII.1; **Poi** 26; **Med** IX.46; **Elu** 23
bamboo – *Bambusa bambos* (L.) Voss **Med** XXI.83; **Elu** 20
banana – *Musa × paradisiaca* L. **Med** XX.88; XXI.72
barberry – *Berberis vulgaris* L. **Med** XXI.78; **Reg** III.3; **Elu** 7
barley – *Hordeum vulgare* L. **Ast** III.2, 4, 9; IV.4, 5; IX.3, 13; XI.4; XIII.44; **Poi** 90; **Rul** 11, 15, 27, 33, 35, 69, 71, 72; **Med** VIII.25, 26, 36; IX.21, 69, 70, 81, 100, 105, 108; X.5, 66; XIII.5, 6, 36, 42, 43; XIV.6; XV.51, 52, 55; XVI.34; XVII.22, 38; XX.58, 62; XXI.8, 9, 15, 24, 61, 73, 93, 95; XXII.23; XXIII.33, 100; **Reg** II.6; III.2; IV.25; **Elu** 9, 28, 38, 44, 45; **Com** I.4 (31)
baṣaliyya (onion dish) **Poi** 73
basil, bush – *Ocimum minimum* L. **Med** XXI.70; **Reg** II.11
basil, sweet – *Ocimum basilicum* L. (Arab. *bādharūj*; *faranjamushk*; *rayḥān*; *al-rayḥān al-qaranfulī*) **Med** XX.49; XXI.75; XXV.14; **Elu** 8, 21
basil, wild (Arab. *faranjamushk*; *al-rayḥān al-qaranfulī*) **Med** XXI.75; **Elu** 21
bat **Med** XXII.4
baṭrasālinūn (seed) (mountain parsley – *Peucedanum Oreoselinum* (L.) Moench) **Med** XX.49
bdellium (, blue) (gum resin) (African myrrh – *Commiphora africana* (A. Rich.) Engl.) **Ast** XII.8, 9; **Poi** 12; **Hem** IV.2, 3, 5; V.1, 2, 3; VI.4, 8, 9; VII.2; **Med** XIII.13; XXI.45, 64, 80
bean, broad – *Vicia faba* L. **Ast** III.3; IX.13; **Poi** 59; **Hem** II.3; **Rul** 71; **Med** IX.115; XV.11, 55; XXI.61, 73; XXII.54; XXIII.3, 100; **Coi** 4; **Reg** IV.23
bean, mung – *Vigna radiata* (L.) R. Wilczek (Arab. *māsh*) **Med** XXI.73
bear **Med** XXI.91; XXIV.28
bee, honey **Poi** 50, 51; **Med** XV.33
beef (meat) **Hem** II.3; **Med** XX.9, 14; XXII.58
beetroot – *Beta vulgaris* L. **Ast** IV.1; IX.3, 4, 7; XII.7; **Hem** II.3; VI.2; **Med** II.4; XX.18; XXI.73, 74; XXV.55; **Reg** III.2
behen, red (possibly Mediterranean sea lavender – *Limonium vulgare* Mill.) **Med** XXI.77; **Coi** 8; **Reg** III.8; **Elu** 21
behen, white – *Centaurea behen* L. **Med** XXI.77; **Coi** 8; **Reg** III.8; **Elu** 21, 25
ben oil (ben oil tree – *Moringa oleifera* Lam.) **Ast** XII.6; **Coi** 10; **Reg** IV.23
ben seed (ben oil tree – *Moringa oleifera* Lam.) **Med** XXI.80
betel nut – *Areca catechu* L. **Med** XXI.83
bezoar (a calculus or concretion found in the stomach or intestines of certain animals, especially ruminants, formerly reputed to be an effective remedy for poison) **Poi** 20, 21, 22, 23, 79
bindweed, field – *Convolvulus arvensis* L. (Arab. *lablāb*) **Ast** IX.2; **Med** XVII.38; XXI.69
bird **Ast** III.4, 9; IX.13, 108; **Med** XX.58; XXI.91
birthwort – *Aristolochia clematitis* L. **Ast** XII.8; **Poi** 43; **Hem** IV.3; **Rul** 62; **Med** IX.88; XXI.75
birthwort, long – *Aristolochia longa* L. **Ast** XII.6; **Poi** 27, 32; **Hem** VII.1
bisnaga – *Ammi visnaga* (L.) Lam. (Arab. *nānakhwāh*) **Poi** 42; **Med** IX.88; XX.49; XXI.80
biṭṭīkh → melon, common; watermelon
bitumen of Judea (Arab. *ḥumar*; *kufr al-yahūd*) **Med** XXI.75
blackberry – *Rubus fruticosus* L. **Med** IX.105; XX.49; XXI.31, 65, 73
bole, Armenian **Rul** 62, 63, 69
borage – *Borago officinalis* L. **Ast** VII.2; XII.1, 9; **Hem** IV.1, 3, 4; **Med** XXI.72; **Coi** 8, 10; **Reg** II.6; III.3, 6, 7, 8; **Elu** 2, 8, 17, 21, 25, 26, 37, 40, 44
borax (sodium borate) – $Na_2B_4O_7{\cdot}10H_2O$ **Ast** XII.7, 10; **Poi** 13, 80, 84, 90; **Med** VIII.58; XXI.75; IX.70; XXI.75

borax, Armenian **Ast** XII.10

boxthorn – *Lycium* sp. L. **Med** XXI.78

bread **Ast** III.1, 2; IV.5, 6; VI.4; IX.13; **Poi** 47, 60, 64, 75; **Hem** I.2; **Rul** 11, 16; **Med** VI.21; IX.4, 53, 116; XV.52; XVII.14, 21, 22, 30; XIX.18; XX.15, 16, 17, 50, 58, 60, 62, 76; XXI.9, 95; XXII.10, 21, 62; XXIV.26b, 31, 50; XXV.55, 64; **Reg** I.3, 12, 13, 22; II.6, 10; **Elu** 27

broth **Ast** IX.13; XI.4; XIII.44; **Poi** 74; **Rul** 11, 69; **Med** VIII.26; XXI.29; XXII.31; **Elu** 28

buckthorn, Mediterranean – *Rhamnus lycioides* L. (Arab. *ḥuḍaḍ*) **Rul** 62, 65; **Med** XXI.87

buckthorn, rock – *Rhamnus saxatilis* Jacq. (Arab. *ḥuḍaḍ*) **Rul** 62, 65; **Med** XXI.87

bull → cow

bunduq → hazelnut

būrī → mullet, black

bustard **Med** XXII.48

busr → date (unripe)

butter **Poi** 8, 45, 64, 65, 76, 87, 89; **Hem** IV.6; VI.9; **Rul** 55; **Med** XXI.18; XXII.67; XXIII.105, 108; XXV.30, 31; **Coi** 6; **Reg** I.16

buttermilk (*dūgh*) **Med** XXIII.107

cabbage – *Brassica oleracea* L. **Ast** III.8; **Poi** 52, 66, 80, 84; **Hem** II.3; **Med** IX.21; XX.49, 60, 81; XXI.29, 69; XXII.45; XXV.13, 14; **Reg** I.20

cadmia **Rul** 62; **Med** XXI.87

calamint, lesser – *Clinopodium nepeta* ssp. *glandulosum* (Req.) Govaerts (Arab. *ḥāshā*) **Ast** XII.1, 3; **Med** XX.49; XXI.80

caltrop – *Tribulus terrestris* L. **Poi** 79; **Med** XXI.73

camel **Ast** V.2; **Med** XX.41, 43, 73; XXII.3; XXV.9, 30; **Reg** I.15

camel grass – *Cymbopogon schoenanthus* (L.) Spreng. **Med** IX.88; XXI.42, 69

camelthorn – *Alhagi maurorum* Medik. **Ast** XII.1; **Hem** IV.1

camomile, German – *Matricaria chamomilla* L. (Arab. *bābūnaj*) **Ast** XII.1; **Hem** VI.3; **Med** XXI.69; XXIII.99

camomile, Roman – *Anthemis nobilis* L. (Arab. *bābūnaj*) **Ast** XII.1; **Hem** VI.3; **Med** XXI.69; XXIII.99

camphor (resin – $C_{10}H_{16}O$) (camphor tree – *Cinnamomum camphora* (L.) J. Presl) **Ast** XII.6; **Poi** 51; **Med** XXI.83; **Elu** 21, 23, 25, 43

cantharide → Spanish fly

caper berry (caper tree – *Capparis spinosa* L.) **Med** XIX.13; XXI.37, 40, 80

caper tree (root) – *Capparis spinosa* L. **Med** IX.77; XXI. 40

caraway – *Carum carvi* L. **Ast** IV.7; **Med** IX.77; XXI.80; **Coi** 5

cardamom, black – *Amomum subulatum* Roxb. **Med** XXI.69; **Reg** III.8; **Elu** 21

cardamom, common – *Elettaria cardamomum* (L.) Maton (Arab. *hāl*) **Med** IX.88; XXI.80; **Elu** 21, 25

carnelian (silica) – SiO_2 **Med** XXII.53

carob – *Ceratonia siliqua* L. **Rul** 62; **Med** XXI.73; **Reg** I.21; **Com** I.1 (25)

carrot, wild – *Daucus carota* L. **Ast** III.8; XII.5; **Poi** 28; **Med** IX.88; XXI.65, 75, 80; XXII.42; **Coi** 4, 6, 8, 9; **Reg** III.8

cassia, purging – *Cassia fistula* L. **Ast** XII.7, 8; XIII.41; **Hem** IV.1; **Med** XXI.68; **Reg** II.7; III.3, 7

castor oil plant – *Ricinus communis* L. **Hem** IV.6; V.1; **Med** VI.24

castoreum **Ast** XII.7; XIII.15; **Poi** 13, 39; **Hem** VI.9; **Med** VII.40; IX.92; XXI.19, 80; XXII.16; **Reg** II.5; IV.13; **Elu** 21, 23, 42

cat (fur) **Reg** IV.27

cataplasm **Rul** 25; **Med** VIII.42; IX.33; XV.2; XXII.26; **Elu** 1

caterpillar, stinging or urticating, of the pine-woods **Med** XXIII.101

cauliflower – *Brassica oleracea* L. **Med** XXI.69

celandine, greater – *Chelidonium majus* L. **Med** XXI.80

celery – *Apium* sp. L. **Ast** III.8; XII.8; **Poi** 28; **Hem** I.2; IV.6; **Med** IX.47; XVII.32; XXI.65, 80; XXV.22; **Reg** II.6

celery, wild – *Apium graveolens* L. **Med** XX.49

centaury, common – *Centaurium erythraea* Rafn **Ast** XII.1, 7; **Med** IX.70; XXI.80

cerate **Med** XV.65

ceruse **Rul** 62; **Med** XXI.87

charcoal **Med** XVI.23; XXI.55; **Elu** 44

chard – *Beta vulgaris* L. **Ast** III.8; **Rul** 55; **Reg** III.2; **Elu** 30

cheese **Ast** III.4; IX.12; **Hem** II.3; **Med** VI.17; XX.41, 42, 45, 60; XXI.29; XXV.30, 31; **Reg** I.16

cherry – *Prunus avium* (L.) L. **Med** XX.61; XXI.74; **Reg** II.6

cherry, Mahaleb – *Prunus mahaleb* L. **Med** XXI.71

chestnut, sweet – *Castanea sativa* Mill. **Med** XX.51, 60; XXI.73; **Com** I.1 (26)

chevon (meat) **Ast** III.3; **Hem** II.3

chicken (also: cock; hen; rooster) **Ast** III.4, 9; IV.1, 3, 4; IX.7, 13; XII.6, 7; **Poi** 10, 66, 67, 76, 77; **Hem** III.1; VI.2, 3, 5; **Rul** 11, 16; **Med** IX.47, 92, 116; XIII.6; XX.20, 58, 68, 71, 83; XXI.91; XXII.28; **Coi** 4, 6; **Reg** I.12; II.10; III.2, 3, 4; **Elu** 30, 38

chickpea – *Cicer arietinum* L. **Ast** IV.1; VII.2; **Hem** III.2; IV.1; **Med** XXI.72; XXII.42, 57; **Coi** 4, 6, 7

chicory – *Cichorium intybus* L. (Arab. *hindibā'*) **Ast** XII.1, 6; **Poi** 50, 65; **Rul** 15; **Med** IX.71, 106; XXI.74; **Reg** II.6; **Elu** 3, 4, 21, 26, 44

chrysocolla – $(Cu,Al)_2H_2Si_2O_5(OH)_4{\cdot}nH_2O$ **Med** XXIII.101

cinnamon – *Cinnamomum verum* (L.) J. Presl **Ast** IV.7; VI.4; VII.2; **Poi** 14, 27, 87; **Med** IX.46, 88; XIII.6; XXI.42, 80; **Coi** 8; **Reg** III.8; **Elu** 15, 21

cinnamon, Chinese – *Cinnamomum cassia* (L.) D. Don **Med** IX.88; XXI.42, 80, 96; **Coi** 5, 6, 8; **Elu** 21, 30

citron – *Citrus medica* L. (Arab. *utrujj*) **Ast** IX.1, XII.1; **Poi** 12, 18, 22, 42, 79; **Med** XX.88; XXI.68; XXII.40, 52; XXV.34; **Coi** 10; **Reg** II.6; III.6, 8; IV.20; **Elu** 20, 23, 30

clove – *Syzygium aromaticum* (L.) Merr. & L.M. Perry **Ast** IV.7; **Med** XXI.80; XXII.40; **Coi** 5, 6, 8, 10; **Reg** III.8; IV.20, 23; **Elu** 40

cocculus indicus (seed) (Levant nut – *Anamirta cocculus* (L.) Wight & Arn.) **Med** XXI.85

cock → chicken

coconut – *Cocos nucifera* L. **Hem** III.2; V.1; **Med** XXI.77; **Coi** 4, 8

collyria **Med** XXII.48

colocynth – *Citrullus colocynthis* (L.) Schrad. **Ast** IX.5; XII.7, 8, 9; XIII.15; **Poi** 42; **Hem** VII.1; **Med** III.112; IX.70, 122; XIII.13, 50, 51; XX.13; XXI.80; XXII.54; **Reg** II.5; IV.13

colostrum **Med** XXIII.108

copper – *Cu* **Med** XXI.88; XXII.29

coral **Rul** 69; **Med** XXI.73; **Elu** 21, 25

coriander – *Coriandrum sativum* L. **Ast** IV.7; **Poi** 50, 51; **Med** XXI.69; **Elu** 10, 20, 30, 38

corundum (aluminium oxide) – Al_2O_3 **Med** XXI.69

costus (root) – *Saussurea costus* (Falc.) Lipsch. **Ast** XII.6; **Poi** 27, 33, 39; **Med** XXI.80

cotton – *Gossypium* sp. L. **Hem** VII.1; **Med** XXII.67

cow (also: bull) **Ast** III.3; **Poi** 12, 13; **Med** XXI.91; XXII.7, 8, 9, 13, 23; XXIII.99

cowry **Med** XXII.60

crab, river **Poi** 29, 55, 56, 66; **Med** XXII.15, 29; **Elu** 21, 25

crab, sea **Med** XXII.29

cress, garden – *Lepidium sativum* L. (Arab. a.o. *shīṭaraj*) **Ast** III.8; **Hem** IV.3; **Med** XIII.52; XX.49; XXI.85; XXV.14

crocodile **Med** XXI.54; XXII.16

crocus, autumn – *Colchicum autumnale* L. **Med** XXI.75; XXII.67

cubeb – *Piper cubeba* L. **Med** IX.88; XXI.80; **Reg** III.3; **Elu** 21

cucumber – *Cucumis sativus* L. (Arab. a.o. *faqqūs*; *khiyār*) **Ast** III.9; XII.1; **Poi** 50, 65; **Hem** I.2; **Med** VII.15; XX.14, 48, 61, 87; XXI.79; **Coi** 5; **Reg** I.20; II.6; **Elu** 6, 21, 25

cucumber, squirting – *Ecballium elaterium* (L.) A. Rich. **Ast** XII.8; XIII.15; **Med** IX.88; **Reg** IV.13

cucurbit – *Cucurbitaceae* sp. Juss. **Elu** 9, 30

cumin – *Cuminum cyminum* L. **Ast** III.9; XII.7; XIII.46; **Poi** 29, 38; **Med** IX.47; XVII.40; XXI.80; **Coi** 5

cumin, black – *Nigella sativa* L. **Poi** 38, 49, 55, 68; **Med** IX.88; XV.58; XXI.80; XXII.19; **Coi** 5

cyclamen, European – *Cyclamen purpurascens* Mill. **Med** XXIII.99

cypress, Mediterranean – *Cupressus sempervirens* L. **Med** XXI.69

dādhī → St. John's wort, bearded; St. John's wort, perforate
dam al-akhawayn → dragon's blood
daphne, February – *Daphne mezereum* L. **Med** XXI.85
darnel – *Lolium temulentum* L. (Arab. *shaylam*) **Med** XV.11; XXIII.102
date (date palm – *Phoenix dactylifera* L.) **Ast** III.9; **Hem** II.3; V.2, 3; **Med** XX.54, 55, 79, 89; XXI.69
date (unripe) (date palm – *Phoenix dactylifera* L.) (Arab. *busr*) **Med** XX.54
deer (also: stag) **Ast** III.7; **Poi** 20, 68; **Med** XXII.7, 50
devil's trumpet – *Datura metel* L. **Poi** 87, 88
dill – *Anethum graveolens* L. **Ast** IX.13; XII.7; **Poi** 76; **Hem** VI.3; **Med** VIII.25; IX.108, 112; XX.86; XXI.55, 65, 80; **Elu** 44
dittany, Cretan – *Origanum dictamnus* L. **Poi** 13, 14; **Med** XVI.2
dodder – *Cuscuta epithymum* (L.) L. **Ast** XII.8; **Med** XVII.40; XXI.70, 80; **Elu** 13, 21, 22
dog **Med** XXII.20
donkey **Ast** V.2; **Rul** 35; **Med** XX.41, 42, 43; XXI.12; XXII.34, 70; XXV.9, 30
dough **Ast** III.1; **Med** XX.15; **Reg** I.13
dragon's blood (red resin) (Socotra dragon-tree – *Dracaena cinnabari* Balf. f.) (Arab. *dam al-akhawayn*; *qāṭir*; *shayyān*) **Rul** 62; **Med** XXI.83
duck **Ast** III.4; XII.7; **Poi** 12; **Hem** VI.3, 5, 8; **Med** IX.47, 92
duckweed, common – *Lemna minor* L. **Poi** 51; **Med** IX.106; XXI.79; XXV.54
dūgh → buttermilk
dullāʿ → melon, common; watermelon
dung (also: excrements) **Poi** 12, 13, 76; **Med** IX.30; XXII.2, 10, 20, 22, 23, 25, 26, 28; **Reg** IV.27
dung beetle **Med** XXII.12

earth, sealed → *terra sigillata*
earth almond (yellow nutsedge – *Cyperus esculentus* L.) (Arab. *fulful al-sudān* (Sudanese pepper); *ḥabb al-zalam*) **Med** XXI.82; **Coi** 4, 8
earthworm **Med** XXII.10, 11, 32
egg (also: egg shell; egg white; yolk) **Ast** III.4; VI.4; **Poi** 80; **Hem** I.2, 4; III.1; VI.5, 8; **Rul** 11, 15; **Med** IX.26, 30, 116; XV.47; XX.58, 60, 72; XXII.61; XXIII.105; XXV.8; **Coi** 4, 6, 8; **Reg** I.12; II.10
egg fritter → omelet
egg shell → egg
egg white → egg
eggplant – *Solanum melongena* L. **Ast** III.8; **Hem** I.2; II.3; V.1; **Med** XX.81; XXIV.13, 14, 15; **Reg** I.20; **Elu** 12
elecampane – *Inula helenium* L. (Arab. *janāḥ*; *rāsan*) **Ast** XII.1, 5; **Med** XXI.81, 96
emerald – $Be_3Al_2(SiO_3)_6$ **Poi** 19, 22, 23, 78, 79; **Med** XXII.36; **Elu** 16
emmer wheat – *Triticum dicoccum* Schrank (Arab. *khandarūs*) **Med** VI.17; IX.100, 116; XX.58
endive – *Cichorium endivia* L. (Arab. *hindibāʾ*) **Ast** XII.1, 6; **Poi** 50, 65; **Rul** 15; **Med** IX.71, 106; XXI.74; **Reg** II.6; **Elu** 3, 4, 21, 26, 44
eryngo, field – *Eryngium campestre* L. **Med** XXI.26, 73; XXII.46; **Reg** II.6
excrements → dung

falanja **Med** XXI.75, 80
falanjamushk → basil
falcon **Med** XXII.5, 49
fānīdh (pulled taffy; chewy sugar-candy) **Ast** III.10; IV.8; VI.4; XII.4; **Hem** III.2; **Coi** 8
faqqūs → cucumber
farbiyūn → spurge, resin
fat **Ast** III.7; IX.7; XII.6, 7; **Hem** VI.3, 5, 8, 9; **Med** IX.47, 92; XXI.54; XXII.14, 16, 50
faṭīr (pancake) **Hem** II.3; **Reg** I.13
fennel – *Foeniculum vulgare* Mill. **Ast** III.8; IV.4; XII.1, 3, 5, 8; **Hem** IV.4; **Med** IX.88; XIII.6; XX.49; XXI.65, 80; **Coi** 4; **Reg** II.6; III.3, 7; **Elu** 30
fennel, giant – *Ferula communis* L. **Coi** 8
fenugreek – *Trigonella foenum-graecum* L. **Ast** IX.7; XII.3, 5; **Hem** VII.1; **Rul** 15; **Med** IX.22; XXI.76

fern, hart's-tongue – *Asplenium scolopendrium* L. (Arab. *sqūlūfandriyūn*; *ʿuqrubān*) **Ast** XII.1, 5; **Med** XXI.40, 75
fern, maidenhair – *Adiantum capillus-veneris* L. **Ast** VII.2; XII.1, 3, 5; **Poi** 52; **Med** IX.88; XXI.68; **Reg** II.6; III.3
fern, male – *Dryopteris filix-mas* (L.) Schott **Med** IX.73; XXI.70
fern, rusty-back – *Ceterach officinarum* Willd. (Arab. *sqūlūfandriyūn*; *ʿuqrubān*) **Ast** XII.1, 5; **Med** XXI.40, 75
fig – *Ficus carica* L. **Ast** III.9, 10; IX.2; XII.1, 3; **Poi** 13, 34, 53, 64, 65, 84, 89; **Hem** III.2; **Med** XV.52; XVII.31, 38, 40; XX.51, 56; XXI.34, 61, 76; XXII.54; **Coi** 8; **Reg** I.21, 22; **Elu** 28, 38
fig, white – *Ficus virens* W.T. Aiton **Poi** 35
fish **Ast** III.4, 5; IX.13; **Poi** 66; **Rul** 11, 16, 69; **Med** VIII.25; IX.100, 108; XX.58, 60; **Reg** I.18
flatworm **Com** III.26 (132)
flax, common (seed) – *Linum usitatissimum* L. **Ast** IX.7, 8; XII.5; **Poi** 42; **Hem** VI.3; **Med** XXI.61, 71
fleawort (seed) – *Plantago psyllium* L. **Ast** XII.4; **Poi** 89; **Med** IX.106; XIII.6, 53; XXI.78; XXV.54; **Elu** 8
flour (also: meal) **Ast** III.1, 2; XII.3; **Poi** 52, 57, 60; **Rul** 54, 62, 71; **Med** IX.115; XV.11, 51, 52, 55; XXI.61, 63, 95; XXII.23, 62; XXIII.100; **Reg** I.13; **Elu** 28, 38
fowl **Ast** III.4; IV.2; **Poi** 64, 66, 73
fox **Ast** III.7; **Reg** IV.27; **Med** XXII.30
francolin **Ast** III.4; **Poi** 66; **Med** XX.58; **Reg** I.12; **Elu** 28
frankincense – *Boswellia sacra* Flueck. **Poi** 45, 56; **Rul** 62; **Med** XV.47, 48, 55; XXI.61, 76; XXII.29; **Elu** 25; **Com** V.59 (279)
frog **Med** XXV.56
fulful al-sudān (Sudanese pepper) → almond, earth
fumitory, common – *Fumaria officinalis* L. **Med** XXI.70; **Reg** III.6; **Elu** 22, 44
fungus, Maltese **Rul** 62

galangal, greater – *Alpinia galanga* (L.) Willd. **Med** XXI.80; XXII.66; **Coi** 5, 8; **Reg** III.8
galbanum (gum resin) – *Ferula gummosa* Boiss. **Ast** XII.6; **Poi** 53; **Med** XIII.3; XXI.80
galia (a perfume prepared from different ingredients, with amber, musk, and ben oil as basic ingredients) **Coi** 10
galingale, common – *Cyperus longus* L. **Med** XXII.66
gallnut **Rul** 62, 63; **Med** XV.56; XXI.78; XXII.61
garlic – *Allium sativum* L. **Ast** III.3; IX.12; **Poi** 12, 13, 26, 36, 42, 64, 65, 66, 73; **Hem** I.2; **Med** IX.100; XIII.46; XX.49; XXI.35, 39, 80; XXIII.99; XXV.14, 22; **Reg** I.20
garum (condiment) **Med** XVII.32, 33
gazelle **Ast** III.7; **Med** XX.70; **Reg** IV.28
gentian, great yellow – *Gentiana lutea* L. **Poi** 27, 36, 38, 55, 56; **Med** IX.88; XXI.80; XXII.29
gentian, Roman **Poi** 32
geranium grass – *Cymbopogon martini* (Roxb.) W. Watson (Arab. *qaṣab al-dharīra*) **Med** XXI.42
germander, felty – *Teucrium polium* L. **Med** XXI.65, 75
ginger – *Zingiber officinale* Roscoe **Ast** IV.7; VII.2; IX.14, 15; XII.8; **Poi** 27, 36; **Med** XXI.81; **Coi** 5, 8; **Reg** III.8; **Elu** 23
ginger, bitter – *Zingiber zerumbet* (L.) Sm. **Ast** IV.7; **Med** XXI.75; **Coi** 5; **Elu** 21, 25
"glass of Pharaoh" **Med** IX.30
gnat **Med** VII.69
goat **Ast** III.3; **Poi** 12, 68; **Rul** 35; **Med** IX.47; XIII.32, 53; XX.41, 43; XXI.11, 91; XXII.23; **Reg** I.15
gold – *Au* **Med** XXI.68; XXII.39, 68; **Elu** 16; 21
goose **Ast** III.4; **Med** XXII.14
gram, black – *Vigna mungo* (L.) Hepper (Arab. *māsh*) **Med** XXI.73
grape (grapevine – *Vitis* sp. L.) **Ast** III.9; XII.4, 5, 8; **Med** VIII.35; IX.112; XX.51; XXI.61; XXII.32; XXIII.6, 103; XXV.49; **Coi** 4; **Reg** I.21, 22; **Elu** 11; **Com** I.1 (25)
grape (unripe) (grapevine – *Vitis* sp. L.) **Ast** IX.4; **Poi** 50; **Rul** 65; **Med** XX.73; **Reg** IV.25

grape, glossy forest – *Rhoicissus rhomboidea* (E. Mey. ex Harv.) Planch. (Arab. *ḥamāmā*) **Med** IX.88; XXI.80
grapevine – *Vitis* sp. L. **Med** IX.105; XXI.31; **Poi** 13, 52
gruel **Ast** III.4, 9; IV.4, 5; IX.3; **Poi** 90; **Rul** 23, 35, 72; **Med** IX.100, 108; X.5; XIII.5, 36, 42, 43; XIV.6; XVI.34; XX.58; XXI.8, 15, 24, 61; **Reg** II.6; III.2; IV.25; **Elu** 9; **Com** I.4 (31)
Guinea worm **Med** XXIV.8
gum ammoniac (ammoniakum – *Dorema ammoniacum* D. Don) **Med** IX.78; XIII.3; XXI.64, 80
gum Arabic **Ast** XII.4; **Rul** 63; **Med** XIII.13; XXI.78
gum tragacanth (milkvetch – *Astragalus* sp. L.) **Ast** XII.4, 8, 9; **Rul** 63; **Med** III.112; XIII.44; XXI.78
gysophila – *Gypsophila struthium* Loefl. (Arab. *kundus*) **Med** XXI.85

ḥabb al-zalam → almond, earth
hāl → cardamom, common
ḥamāmā → grape, glossy forrest
ḥandaqūq → lotos
hare **Poi** 24, 79, 80, 84; **Med** XV.47; XXI.75; XXII.44; XXIII.107; **Reg** IV.28
ḥarīra (a kind of soup, silk-smooth and flowing in consistency) **Ast** III.1; **Reg** I.13
harīsa (a certain wheat (grain) preparation, or smooth porridge cooked with meat and grains such as rice or wheat) **Ast** III.1; **Hem** II.3; **Coi** 6; **Reg** I.13
hartwort, Massilian – *Seseli tortuosum* L. **Ast** XII.5; **Med** XX.49; XXI.65
hawk **Med** XXII.49
hayūfārīqūn → St. John's wort, bearded; St. John's wort, perforate
ḥayy al-ʿālam → aeonium, tree; houseleek, common
hazelnut (common hazel – *Corylus avellana* L.) (Arab. *bunduq*; *jillawz*) **Ast** III.10; **Poi** 64; **Med** XX.56; XX.88; XXI.75; **Coi** 4, 8
ḥāzir (type of milk) **Med** XXIII.107
hedgehog **Ast** III.7; **Med** XXII.50; 59
hedgenettle, common – *Stachys officinalis* (L.) Trevis. **Reg** III.8
hellebore – *Helleborus* sp. L. **Ast** XIII.15; **Med** XIII.32, 51; XX.13; XXI.33, 80; **Reg** II.5; IV.13; **Com** IV.13 (150), 14 (151), 15 (152), 16 (153), V.1 (221)
hellebore, black – *Helleborus niger* L. **Ast** XIII.15; **Med** IX.70; **Reg** II.5; IV.13
hellebore, white false – *Veratrum album* L. **Ast** XII.10; XIII.15; **Med** XXI.33; **Reg** II.5; IV.13; **Com** V.1 (221)
hemlock, poison – *Conium maculatum* L. **Poi** 39, 86; **Med** XXI.83
hemp – *Cannabis sativa* L. **Med** XXII.58
hen → chicken
henbane, black – *Hyoscyamus niger* L. **Poi** 39, 86; **Hem** VII.1; **Med** XXI.83
henna – *Lawsonia inermis* L. **Med** XXI.87
hiera (a name used for a number of compound medicines) **Ast** XIII.41; **Reg** II.7
hiera picra (the most common hiera with aloe as main component) **Ast** XII.8, 9; XIII.41; **Poi** 80; **Rul** 19; **Med** IX.45, 46; XVI.2; XVII.38, 39
hindibāʾ → endive; chicory
hippopotamus (skin) **Med** XXII.15
honey **Ast** III.1; IV.4, 5; VI.4; VII.2; IX.2, 6, 7, 13, 14, 15; XII.1, 3, 4, 5, 10; **Poi** 12, 27, 30, 32, 33, 36, 38, 42, 43, 45, 51, 57, 60, 64, 82, 91; **Hem** I.2; VII.2; **Rul** 35, 72; **Med** IX.13, 70, 71, 77, 105, 115; XV.11, 45, 47, 52; XVII.32; XIX.13; XX.35, 41, 42; XXI.8, 10, 14, 17, 18, 22, 23, 40, 61, 75, 96; XXII.2, 4, 5, 9, 21, 57, 62; XXIII.100; XXIV.42; XXV.35; **Coi** 8, 10; **Reg** I.17; II.6; III.8; **Elu** 20, 21, 22, 33
horehound, white – *Marrubium vulgare* L. **Ast** XII.1; XII.3, 5, 8; **Med** XXI.75, 80
hornpoppy, blackspot – *Glaucium corniculatum* (L.) J.H. Rudolph (Arab. *māmīthā*) **Med** XXI.78
hornpoppy, yellow – *Glaucium flavum* Crantz (Arab. *māmīthā*) **Med** XXI.78
horse (also: mare) **Ast** V.2; **Med** XX.43; XXI.11; XXII.34; XXV.62, 64, 67
houseleek, common – *Sempervivum tectorum* L. (Arab. *ḥayy al-ʿālam*) **Poi** 51; **Med** IX.106; XXI.84
ḥuḍaḍ → buckthorn, Mediterranean; buckthorn, rock

ḥumar → bitumen of Judea
ḥuwwārā (white flour) **Reg** I.13; **Elu** 27
hydromel **Ast** VI.5; IX.3; XII.8, 10; **Rul** 23, 66, 72; **Med** IX.100; XIII.36, 41; XIV.6; XV.45; XVI.2; XXI.15, 16, 24; XXIII.106; **Coi** 4; **Reg** II.6; **Elu** 33, 36, 39; **Com** I.4 (31); V.41 (261)
hyena (gall) **Med** XXII.5
hyssop – *Hyssopus officinalis* L. **Ast** XII.1; **Med** IX.88; XXI.8, 80

indigo – *Indigofera tinctoria* L. **Med** II.3
iris, Florentine – *Iris germanica* var. *florentina* (L.) Dykes **Ast** XII.1, 3, 5, 8; **Poi** 28; **Rul** 62; **Med** IX.88; XV.55; XXI.61, 76; XXII.5
iron – *Fe* **Med** XIII.39; XV.6; XXII.20; XXV.46; **Coi** 10
ironwood, Ceylon – *Mesua ferrea* L. **Med** IX.88
isfīdabāj (pl. *isfīdabājāt*) (stew) **Ast** IV.1; **Hem** III.1; **Elu** 30
iṭrīfal (electuary containing myrobalans) **Reg** II.7; **Elu** 39, 42
iṭrīfal, great **Reg** III.8; **Elu** 19
iṭrīfal, small **Hem** IV.2
iṭriya (vermicelli) **Reg** I.13
ivy, common – *Hedera helix* L. (Arab. *lablāb*) **Med** XXI.69

jacinth (red zircon) – $ZrSiO_4$ **Elu** 16, 21, 24, 42, 43
janāḥ → elecampane
jarārāt → scorpion
jasmine, Arabian – *Jasminum sambac* (L.) W.T. Aiton (Arab. *yāsamīn*; *zanbaq*) **Hem** V.1; **Med** XXI.75; **Coi** 9
jasmine, white – *Jasminum officinale* L. (Arab. *yāsamīn*; *zanbaq*) **Hem** V.1; **Med** XXI.75; **Coi** 9
jillawz → hazelnut
jūdhāb (pl. *jūdhābāt*) (cereal pudding with meat juice) **Hem** III.1
jujube, Christ's thorn – *Ziziphus spina-christi* (L.) Desf. **Ast** III.10; **Poi** 51; **Med** XXI.73; **Reg** I.21
jujube, common – *Ziziphus jujuba* Mill. **Ast** XII.1, 2; **Hem** IV.1; **Med** XXI.72; XXII.51; **Elu** 3
julep **Ast** VII.2; XII.1; **Poi** 89; **Rul** 72; **Med** XIII.6; **Reg** III.8; **Elu** 26
juniper, savin – *Juniperus sabina* L. **Med** IX.88, 123; XVI.2; XXI.80

kaʿk (something baked; rusk, biscuit, or the like) **Ast** III.1
kāmakh (pl. *kawāmikh*) (vinegar dressing) **Ast** IX.12; **Hem** I.2; **Reg** IV.24
karafs al-māʾ ("water celery") → waterparsnip, wideleaf
kashk (type of milk) **Med** XXIII.107
khabīṣa (pudding) **Ast** IV.8
khandarūs → emmer wheat
khawkh → plum
khilāf → willow, Egyptian
khilāṭ (type of milk) **Reg** I.16; IV.24
khīrī → stock, hoary; wallflower
khiyār → cucumber
kid (meat) **Rul** 16; **Med** VI.17; XX.19, 70; XXV.10; **Reg** I.14; **Elu** 15, 28, 32
kite **Med** XXIV.57
knotgrass, common – *Polygonum aviculare* L. (Arab. *ʿaṣā al-rāʿī*; *qaḍāb*) **Med** IX.106; XXI.84; XXV.54
kubab (small balls of meat pounded with vegetables) **Hem** I.2
kufr al-yahūd → bitumen of Judea
kundus → gysophila; sneezewort; soapwort

labdanum (resin) (rockrose – *Cistus* sp. L.) **Med** XXI.71
lablāb → bindweed, field; ivy, common
lac dye (from lac insects) **Med** XXI.75
lākisha (vermicelli) **Reg** I.13
lamb (meat) **Rul** 16; **Med** VI.17; XX.19; XXV.10; **Reg** I.14; **Elu** 28
lambskin **Med** XXII.44; **Reg** IV.27
lanolin (wool fat) **Med** XXIII.49, 89
lapis lazuli **Med** XXI.75; **Elu** 13, 21
lark **Med** XX.69; XXII.31
latex plant **Poi** 82; **Med** XIII.3
laurel, bay – *Laurus nobilis* L. **Med** XIII.50; XXI.80
laurel berry (bay laurel – *Laurus nobilis* L.) **Poi** 32
lavender, French – *Lavandula stoechas* L. **Ast** XII.1, 9; **Poi** 36; **Med** XXI.69; **Reg** III.6, 8; **Elu** 21

lawr (type of milk) **Med** XXIII.108
laymūniyya (lemon chicken stew) **Poi** 73; **Hem** I.4; II.3; **Reg** III.2
lead – *Pb* **Med** XXI.87
leek – *Allium porrum* L. **Ast** III.3; IX.13; **Hem** III.1; IV.5, 6; VII.1, 2; **Med** II.4; VIII.25; IX.108; XX.49; XXI.85; XXV.14, 22; **Reg** I.20
lemon – *Citrus × limon* (L.) Burm. f. (Arab. a.o. *utrujj*) **Ast** III.9; IV.4; IX.1, 3, 14, 15; XII.1, 3; **Poi** 12, 18, 22, 42, 67, 79; **Hem** I.2; **Med** XX.88; XXI.68; XXII. 40, 45, 52; XXV.34; **Coi** 10; **Reg** II.6; III.2, 6, 8; IV. 20, 25; **Elu** 20, 23, 30, 31, 38, 44
lemon balm – *Melissa officinalis* L. **Poi** 42, 49; **Med** XXI.69; **Elu** 8
lemon grass – *Cymbopogon citratus* (DC.) Stapf (Arab. *qaṣab al-dharīra*) **Med** XXI.42
lentil – *Lens culinaris* Medik. **Ast** III.3; **Hem** II.3; VI.3, 8; **Med** V.19; IX.21, 105; XX.14, 60; XXI.68; **Coi** 5
leopardbane, great false – *Doronicum pardalianches* L. **Med** XXI.80; **Coi** 8; **Reg** III.8; **Elu** 21, 25
lettuce, cultivated – *Lactuca sativa* L. **Ast** III.8; **Poi** 49, 50, 65; **Med** IX.21, 106; XX.47; XXI.79; XXV.54; **Coi** 5; **Elu** 6, 25, 30
lichen, usnea cartilage – *Ramalina usnea* (L.) R. Howe **Med** XXI.73; XXII.66
licorice – *Glycyrrhiza glabra* L. **Ast** VII.3; IX.3; XII.1, 2, 3, 4, 5; **Med** XIII.44; XXI.74; **Reg** II.6; III.3, 7
linen (common flax – *Linum usitatissimum* L.) **Rul** 23; **Med** IX.2, 123; XVII.14; **Reg** III.7; IV.17
litharge (lead oxide) – *PbO* **Poi** 81; **Rul** 62; **Med** XXI.87
lizard **Med** IX.30
lotos (Arab. *ḥandaqūq*) **Poi** 52
louse **Med** XXII.54; XXV.64
lucerne – *Medicago sativa* L. **Coi** 8
lupine, white – *Lupinus albus* L. **Med** XX.83; XXI.69; XXII.21; XXIII.100
lycium, Indian **Poi** 55; **Hem** VI.7

mace (aril) (nutmeg – *Myristica fragrans* Houtt.) **Ast** IV.7; VII.2; XII.6; **Hem** IV.1, 3, 4; **Med** XXI.68; XXII.40; **Reg** IV.23; **Elu** 40
madder, common – *Rubia tinctorum* L. **Ast** XII.1; XII.3, 5; **Med** XXI.69
maḍīra (curdled milk stew) **Poi** 73; **Coi** 6
malabathrum, Indian (Indian bark – *Cinnamomum tamala* (Buch.-Ham.) T. Nees & Eberm.) **Elu** 21
mallow – *Malva sylvestris* L. **Ast** III.8; **Poi** 51; **Hem** II.3; VI.2; **Med** IX.108; XXI.74
māmīthā → hornpoppy, blackspot; hornpoppy, yellow
mandrake – *Mandragora officinarum* L. **Poi** 15, 27; 88; **Med** XXI.83
manna (camelthorn – *Alhagi maurorum* Medik.) **Ast** XII.1; **Hem** IV.1; **Med** XXI.68, 71; **Coi** 8; **Reg** II.6; **Elu** 21
marcasite (iron sulfide) – FeS_2 **Med** XXII.17
mare → horse
marjoram – *Origanum majorana* L. **Med** IX.88
marking nut – *Semecarpus anacardium* L. **Poi** 82; **Med** XXI.85
marshmallow, common – *Althaea officinalis* L. **Ast** IX.3; XII.1; **Poi** 13, 50; **Hem** VI.3, 8; **Med** XIII.6; XXI.69, 95; XXIII.99; **Reg** II.6; III.3, 7
māsh → bean, mung; gram, black
maṣl → whey
māst (type of milk) (also: *rā'ib*) **Med** XXIII.107; **Reg** I.16
mastic (gum resin) (Mediterranean mastic tree – *Pistacia lentiscus* L.) **Ast** VII.2, 3; XII.6, 8, 9; **Hem** IV.3; **Med** III.112; IX.46, 68, 126; XIII.44; XXI.75; XXII.39; **Reg** III.7, 8; IV.20; **Elu** 15, 21, 30
maṣūṣ (sour stew prepared mostly with meats other than quadrupeds, such as birds and shrimp) **Ast** IV.4
meal → flour
meat **Ast** III.3, 4, 6, 7; IV.2, 4; **Poi** 64, 66, 73, 80; **Hem** I.3; II.3; III.1; **Med** VI.17, 78; IX.101; XVII.21, 34; XX.9, 18, 19, 20, 21, 22, 23, 58, 60, 69, 70; XXI.29; XXII.38, 42, 59; XXIV.28, 43; **Coi** 6, 8; **Reg** I.3, 12, 14; II.10; IV.24, 27, 28; **Elu** 12, 28, 31, 32
medlar, common – *Mespilus germanica* L. **Ast** III.10; **Med** XXI.73; **Reg** I.21

melilot – *Melilotus officinalis* (L.) Pall. **Poi** 23; **Hem** VI.3; VI.8; **Med** IX.22; XII.41; XXI.69
melon, common – *Cucumis melo* L. (Arab. *biṭṭīkh; dullāʿ*) **Ast** III.9; IX.13; **Med** VII.15; XX.14, 48, 53, 61; XXI.79; XXII.39; **Coi** 5, 7; **Reg** I.20; II.6; **Elu** 11, 13, 25
mercury (quicksilver) – *Hg* **Med** XXV.46
milk **Ast** III.4; IV.6; IX.12; **Poi** 15, 16, 26, 49, 50, 64, 76, 86, 89, 90; **Rul** 35, 66; **Med** VI.17; VII.15; IX.100, 111; XIII.32, 39, 52, 53; XVII.30; XX.40, 41, 42, 43, 44, 45, 61, 73; XXI.10, 11, 12, 13, 14, 17, 35; XXII.16, 20, 54, 70; XXIII.105, 107, 108; XXV.9, 30, 31; **Coi** 4, 6, 8; **Reg** I.15, 16; IV.23; **Elu** 28, 38; **Com** V.64 (284)
milk, sour **Poi** 65; **Hem** 27; **Med** XXI.10; XXIII.105
millet – *Panicum miliaceum* L. **Med** IX.92; XXI.94; XXIII.33, 102
mint – *Mentha* sp. L. **Ast** III.8, 9; XII.1, 7; XIII.46; **Poi** 13, 14, 33, 79; **Med** VII.23; IX.53, 70, 88; XVI.2; XXI.80; XXII.40
mint, mountain **Ast** XII.3; **Med** XX.49
mint, water – *Mentha aquatica* L. **Ast** VII.2; XII.3; **Poi** 12; **Med** IX.86; XVI.2; XX.49
Mithridates (an antidote ascribed to Mithridates VI. Eupator, king of Pontus (reg. 120–63)) **Ast** XIII.38; **Poi** 3, 8, 32, 52, 78; **Reg** II.5, 8
moghat (root) – *Glossostemon bruguieri* Desf. (Arab. *mughādh; mughāth*) **Med** XXI.77
mole **Med** VII.73
monkshood, yellow → *antula*
morning glory, ivy-leaded – *Ipomoea nil* (L.) Roth **Med** XXI.80
mouse **Med** XXII.2, 10
mughādh/mughāth → moghat
mugwort – *Artemisia vulgaris* L. **Med** XXI.80; XXIII.33
mulberry – *Morus nigra* L. **Ast** III.9; **Poi** 49, 84, 86; **Rul** 65; **Med** XX.53, 61; XXI.73; XXIII.6
mullet **Ast** III.5
mullet, black (Arab. *būrī; rāy*) **Reg** I.18
mūmiyā (bitumen) **Med** XXI.80
murrī (condiment sauce) **Ast** IX.12, 13; **Poi** 73; **Hem** II.3
murrī al-naqīʿ, al- (condiment sauce) **Med** XXII.46
mushroom **Poi** 90; **Rul** 70; **Med** XX.60; XXIV.32
musk **Med** IX.30; XIII.49; XXI.75, 96; **Coi** 8, 9, 10; **Reg** II.11; III.6; IV.20; **Elu** 20, 21, 22, 25, 42, 43
mustard – *Brassica* sp. L. **Ast** IV.6; XII.10; **Poi** 13, 68; **Hem** I.2; **Rul** 70; **Med** IX.20; XX.49; XXI.85; XXII.47; XXV.22; **Coi** 5, 9
mustard, hedge – *Sisymbrium officinale* (L.) Scop. **Coi** 8
mustard, Syrian – *Euclidium syriacum* (L.) W.T. Aiton **Ast** IV.6
mutawakkaliyya (dish named after the Caliph al-Mutawakkil) **Poi** 73
mutton (meat) **Ast** III.3, 6; IV.1, 2; **Hem** I.4; **Med** XX.85; **Coi** 4, 6; **Reg** I.12, 14, 22; IV.27; **Elu** 28
myrobalan **Ast** XII.8, 9; XIII.41; **Hem** IV.1; **Reg** III.7, 8
myrobalan, beleric – *Terminalia bellirica* (Gaertn.) Roxb. **Hem** IV.1, 3, 5; **Reg** III.8
myrobalan, chebulic – *Terminalia chebula* (Gaertn.) Retz. **Hem** IV.1, 3, 5; **Med** XXI.73; XXII.52; **Reg** II.6; III.7, 8
myrobalan, emblic – *Phyllanthus emblica* L. **Hem** IV.1, 3, 4, 5; **Med** XXI.73; **Reg** III.7, 8
myrobalan, Indian (unripe fruit) – *Terminalia chebula* (Gaertn.) Retz. **Med** XXI.73; **Reg** III.7, 8
myrobalan, yellow (citrine) – *Terminalia citrina (Gaertn.) Roxb. ex Flem.* **Med** XXI.73
myrrh – *Commiphora* sp. Jacq. **Ast** XII.3, 5, 6, 8; **Poi** 32, 33, 38, 39, 56; **Rul** 62; **Med** XXI.80; **Com** V.59 (279)
myrrh, Mecca – *Commiphora opobalsamum* (L.) Engl. **Ast** XII.1; **Reg** III.8
myrrh, sweet – *Opopanax chironium* (L.) Koch **Med** XV.55; XII.61
myrtle – *Myrtus communis* L. (Arab. a.o. *rayḥān*) **Poi** 49; **Rul** 63, 66, 72; **Med** VIII.77; IX.123; XIII.6; XV.48; XXI.73; **Reg** II.11; **Elu** 8, 38

nabīdh (intoxicating drinks) **Ast** VII.1; IX.13; **Coi** 8, 10
nabiq (fruit) (Christ's thorn jujube – *Ziziphus spina-christi* (L.) Desf.) **Ast** III.10; **Med** XXI.73; **Reg** I.21
nalta jute – *Corchorus olitorius* L. **Med** XX.47; XXI.72
nānakhwāh → ajowan; bisnaga
narcissus – *Narcissus* sp. L. **Med** XIV.8; XXI.75; XXII.56
natron (sodium carbonate) – $Na_2[CO_3]{\cdot}10H_2O$ **Ast** IX.6; XII.7, 10; **Poi** 80, 84, 87; **Med** IX.70
nettle, Roman – *Urtica pilulifera* L. **Ast** XII.5, 8; **Poi** 53; **Med** IX.70, 88; XXI.75; XXV.49; **Coi** 8
nightshade, black – *Solanum nigrum* L. **Poi** 91; **Med** IX.106; XXI.78
nīlūfar → water lily, blue Egyptian; water lily, European white; water lily, yellow
noodles **Ast** III.1
nut, king's → walnut
nutmeg – *Myristica fragrans* Houtt. **Med** XXI.75; **Coi** 5; **Elu** 23
nux vomica → poison nut

oleander – *Nerium oleander* L. **Hem** IV.7
olive (olive tree – *Olea europaea* L.) **Med** XX.56
olive oil (olive tree – *Olea europaea* L.) **Ast** IV.6; IX.3, 6, 7; XII.7; **Poi** 8, 11, 13, 21, 42, 47, 59, 64, 76, 87; **Hem** IV.7; **Rul** 32, 50, 83; **Med** III.61; V.12; VIII.25; IX.47, 55, 68, 92, 108; X.52; XIII.41; XV.33, 34, 65; XVII.32, 33, 38; XXI.68, 92; XXII.12, 47; **Reg** I.13; II.6; III.2; **Elu** 44
olive tree (resin) – *Olea europaea* L. **Med** XXII.63
omelet (egg fritter) **Poi** 80; **Coi** 6
omphacine oil **Med** XIX.19
onion – *Allium cepa* L. **Ast** III.3; IX.12, 13; **Poi** 57, 60, 64, 66; **Hem** I.2; **Med** II.4; IX.101; XIII.54; XX.49, 72; XXI.85; XXIII.99; XXV.14, 22; **Coi** 4, 6; **Reg** I.20
opercula → *ungues odorati*
opium (opium poppy – *Papaver somniferum* L.) **Poi** 36, 39, 43, 68, 82; **Hem** VI.9; **Elu** 21
opopanax (resin) (sweet myrrh – *Opopanax chironius* W.D.J. Koch) **Ast** XII.7, 8; XIII.15; **Poi** 53; **Rul** 62, 83; **Med** XIII.3; XV.33; XXI.80; **Reg** IV.13
orach, garden – *Atriplex hortensis* L. **Ast** III.8; **Med** IX.108; XX.47, 84; XXI.74; **Coi** 5; **Reg** II.6; III.2; **Elu** 6
oregano – *Origanum vulgare* L. **Ast** III.8; XII.9; **Med** XX.49, 83; XXI.80
ostrich **Med** XXII.48
ox **Ast** XII.6; **Poi** 80; **Med** XXV.62, 64; **Coi** 8
oxymel **Ast** IX.13, 14, 15; XII.1; XIII.33, 44; **Poi** 50, 65, 90; **Rul** 23, 33; **Med** VIII.25, 26, 69; XIV.6; XV.11; XXI.7, 15, 21, 22, 23, 24, 25, 26, 27; XXII.13, 59; XXIV.32; **Reg** II.6; III.4, 5; **Elu** 7, 33, 34, 39, 42

pancake **Ast** III.1
parsley – *Petroselinum crispum* (Mill.) Fuss **Med** XX.49
parsley, mountain – *Peucedanum oreoselinum* (L.) Moench **Med** XX.49; XXV.22
partridge (Arab. *ṭayhūj*) **Ast** III.4; **Poi** 66; **Med** XX.58, 68; **Coi** 4; **Reg** I.12; **Elu** 28
pea, black-eyed – *Vigna unguiculata* ssp. *unguiculata* (L.) Walp. **Ast** III.3 **Hem** II.3; **Med** XXI.72; **Coi** 4
pea, Indian – *Lathyrus sativus* L. **Ast** III.3; **Hem** II.3; **Coi** 5; **Reg** IV.23
peach – *Prunus persica* (L.) Batsch **Ast** III.9; **Med** XX.61; XXI.79; XXII.46, 63; **Reg** I.22; **Elu** 11, 13, 15, 31
pear – *Pyrus communis* L. **Rul** 33; **Med** IX.55; XX.52, 75; XXI. 73; **Reg** I.22; III.2; **Elu** 11
pearl **Elu** 20, 21, 25
pellitory (root) – *Anacyclus pyrethrum* (L.) Lag. **Poi** 33, 43; **Med** XXI.85; **Coi** 9
pennyroyal – *Mentha pulegium* L. **Med** IX.53
peony – *Paeonia officinalis* L. **Med** XXI.70; XXII.18, 56
pepper (, black) – *Piper nigrum* L. **Ast** IV.7; **Poi** 33, 36, 43, 87, 90; **Rul** 32; **Med** VII.23; XXI.8, 38, 85; **Coi** 5; **Elu** 23
pepper, long – *Piper longum* L. **Poi** 36; **Med** XIII.44; XXI.38, 85; **Coi** 5, 8; **Reg** III.8
pepper, Sudanese (*fulful al-sudān*) → earth almond

pepper, white (black pepper – *Piper nigrum* L.) **Ast** IX.15; XII.3; **Poi** 36, 38, 39
peppermint – *Mentha* × *piperita* L. (Arab. *naʿnaʿ*; *fūdhanj bustānī*) **Ast** III.8, 9; IV.4; VII.2; **Poi** 57; **Med** XVI.2; **Coi** 4
pepperwort – *Lepidium latifolium* L. (Arab. *shīṭaraj*) **Hem** IV.3; **Med** XXI.85
pheasant **Med** XX.58
pig (also: piglet) **Poi** 72; **Med** XXI.91; XXIV.29; XXV.56
pigeon **Ast** III.4, 9; IX.13; **Poi** 10, 12, 13, 66; **Med** XX.58, 68, 72; XXII.26, 42, 43; **Coi** 4, 6; **Reg** IV.27
pigeon, domestic **Med** XX.69; XXII.43
piglet → pig
pine nut (pine tree – *Pinus* sp. L.) **Ast** III.10; IV.8; XII.3, 5; **Med** VII.59 IX.112; XX.60; XXI.71; **Coi** 4, 7, 8; **Reg** III.8
pine tree (resin) – *Pinus* sp. L. **Poi** 42; **Med** XXI.88; **Com** IV.70 (207)
pistachio nut – *Pistacia vera* L. **Ast** III.10; IV.8; VI.4; XII.8, 9; **Poi** 64; **Hem** III.1; **Med** IX.88; XIII.44, 51; XX.78; XXI.69; **Coi** 4, 7, 8; **Reg** I.22; III.7, 8; **Elu** 30, 36, 38;
pitch **Poi** 13; **Rul** 12; **Med** IX.115; XXI.88; **Com** IV.70 (207)
plantain, broadleaf – *Plantago major* L. **Med** IX.105; XXI.78
plum – *Prunus domestica* L. (Arab. a.o. *khawkh*) **Med** XVII.32; XX.61; XXI.74; **Reg** I.22; II.6; **Elu** 3, 9, 30
poison nut (*nux vomica*) (strychnine tree – *Strychnos nux-vomica* L.) **Reg** II.5
polypody, common – *Polypodium vulgare* L. **Ast** XII.8; **Med** IX.70; XXI.80; **Reg** III.7
pomegranate – *Punica granatum* L. **Ast** III.9; IX.4; **Poi** 50, 65; **Rul** 15, 23, 33, 62, 63, 66; **Med** IX.21, 55, 69; XV.56; XX.76; XXI.73, 78; XXIII.6; **Reg** III.2; IV.20, 25; **Elu** 10, 11, 25, 40
poplar, black – *Populus nigra* L. **Med** IX.88
poppy, opium – *Papaver somniferum* L. **Ast** XII.4, 5; **Poi** 3; **Rul** 66; **Med** IX.18; XX.50; XXI.86; XXII.57; **Elu** 9, 44
pork (meat) **Med** VI.17; IX.53; XX.19, 62; XXI.11; XXIV.10, 43; XXV.10
port wine → tawny
"potion of angels" **Med** XXI.96
poultry (meat) **Hem** I.4
pumpkin, field – *Cucurbita pepo* L. (Arab. *qarʿ*) **Ast** III.8; **Med** VII.15; **Med** IX.93, 108; XX. 53, 61; XXI.79; **Elu** 25
purple-fish **Med** XXII.19
purslane, common – *Portulaca oleracea* L. **Poi** 50, 89; **Med** IX.106; XX.47, 84; XXI.84; XXII.57; XXV.54; **Reg** II.6; **Elu** 6, 10, 22, 25, 30

qaḍāb → knotgrass, common
qāhiriyya (a sort of candy; sweets) **Ast** IV.8
qarṭāsī (striped garment; short and light linen dress; garment made from papyrus) **Reg** IV.27
qaṣab al-dharīra → geranium grass; lemon grass
qaṭā'if (delicate sweet crepes stuffed with sugar and nuts and drenched in perfumed syrup) **Ast** III.1; **Hem** II.3
qāṭir → dragon's blood
qilyun (potash or soda) **Poi** 13
quail **Med** XIII.32; XX.69
quartz – SiO_2 **Med** XXII.70
quicklime (calcium oxide) – *CaO* **Poi** 13
quince – *Cydonia oblonga* Mill. **Ast** III.10; IX.4, 5, 15; XII.4, 6; **Rul** 63, 68, 69, 72; **Med** IX.21, 47, 55, 57, 68, 126; XVII.39; XX.87; XXI.73, 96; XXII.45; XXIII.6; **Reg** I.22; III.2; IV.25; **Elu** 7, 10, 11, 25
qurrat al-ʿayn → waterparsnip, wideleaf

rabbit **Ast** III.7
radish – *Raphanus sativus* L. **Ast** III.8; IX.12, 13; XII.10; **Poi** 90; **Hem** I.2; IV.6; **Med** XIV.6; XX.18, 49; XXI.80; XXII.45; **Coi** 8, 9; **Reg** I.20; II.6
radish, wild – *Raphanus raphanistrum* L. **Poi** 73
rā'ib (type of milk) → *māst*
raisin (grapevine – *Vitis* sp. L.) **Ast** III.10; IV.2, 3; VI.4; IX.2, 4; XII.1, 3; **Hem** III.2; **Med** XIII.46; XX.57, 73, 78; **Coi** 8; **Reg** I.22; III.5; **Elu** 30, 36, 39, 42
rāsan → elecampane
rāy → mullet, black
rayḥān → basil, sweet; myrtle
rayḥān al-qaranfulī, al- → basil

rhubarb (, Chinese) – *Rheum palmatum* L. **Ast** IX.1; XII.8; XIII.41; **Med** IX.88; XXI.30, 75; **Reg** III.2, 7; **Elu** 4, 13, 43

rhubarb, Syrian – *Rheum ribes* L. **Rul** 63; **Med** XXI.78

rice – *Oryza sativa* L. **Ast** III.3; **Hem** II.3; **Med** XXI.69

rocket, garden – *Eruca vesicaria* (L.) Cav. **Med** XX.49; XXI.77; XXII.61; **Coi** 7, 8; **Reg** III.8

rockfish **Rul** 11; **Med** VIII.25, 108; XVII.25

rooster → chicken

rose – *Rosa* sp. L. **Ast** IV.4; IX.13, 14; XII.6; XIII.33, 41; **Poi** 30; **Hem** IV.4; V.2; VI.5, 6, 7, 8, 9; **Rul** 50, 54, 62, 68; **Med** VIII.35; IX.17; XIII.53; XIX.19; XXI.19, 51, 73, 93; XXII.14, 39, 40, 55; **Reg** II.6, 11; III.2, 3, 4, 6, 7, 8; IV.20; **Elu** 20, 21, 22, 25, 30, 34, 36, 39, 40, 42

rose, dog – *Rosa canina* L. **Med** XXI.75; **Reg** IV.23

rose water (rose – *Rosa* sp. L.) **Ast** XII.6; **Poi** 51; **Hem** VI.6; **Reg** IV.23; **Elu** 2, 26, 31, 37

roundworm **Med** IX.93; **Com** III.26 (132)

rue (, common) – *Ruta graveolens* L. **Ast** III.9; XII.7; **Poi** 33, 34, 35, 52, 64, 79; **Rul** 32, 50; **Med** IX.47, 88; XXI.34, 80; **Coi** 5

rue, Syrian – *Peganum harmala* L. **Hem** VII.1; **Med** XXI.80

rummāniyya (pomegranate stew cooked mostly with chicken) **Poi** 73; **Hem** I.4

rutaylā' (tarantula) **Poi** 4, 43, 47, 48, 49

safflower (seed) – *Carthamus tinctorius* L. **Ast** IV.4; IX.2, 3; **Hem** II.3; VI.2; **Med** IX.70; XVII.38, 40; XXI.75; **Reg** III.2

saffron – *Crocus sativus* L. **Ast** IV.7; VII.2; XII.3, 5; **Hem** V.3; VI.3, 5, 8; **Rul** 54, 69; **Med** IX.46; XX.86; XXI.41, 47, 76; **Elu** 21, 22, 25, 32

ṣafṣāf → willow, Egyptian

ṣaḥna (condiment made by salting small river fish or locusts) **Reg** IV.24

sagapenum (gum resin) (Persian giant fennel – *Ferula persica* Willd.) **Ast** XII.7, 8; **Poi** 13, 53; **Hem** VI.9; **Med** IX.88; XIII.3; XV.33; XXI.80; **Reg** II.5

sal ammoniac (ammonium chloride) – *NH_4Cl* **Med** XXI.88

salep (root) (orchid – *Orchis* sp. L.) **Coi** 8

salsify, meadow – *Tragopogon pratensis* L. **Rul** 63; **Med** XXI.73

salt **Ast** III.9; VI.4; IX.2; XII.10; **Poi** 12, 13, 34, 35, 42, 47, 51, 57, 64, 66, 90; **Hem** II.3; **Rul** 12, 50; **Med** VIII.25, 58; XII.34; XIII.37, 44; XV.11; XX.41, 42; XXI.14, 35, 55, 75, 95; XXII.61, 62; XXIII.33, 107, 108; **Coi** 6, 8; **Reg** I.15; **Elu** 38, 44

samīdh (white flour) **Reg** I.13

sandalwood – *Santalum* sp. L. **Ast** XII.6; **Med** XXI.26, 83; **Elu** 3, 6, 22

sandalwood, Indian – *Santalum album* L. **Elu** 44

sarcocolla (gum resin) – *Astragalus sarcocolla* Dymock **Ast** XII.8; **Rul** 62; **Med** XXI.69

sawīq (semolina) **Med** IX.105; XXI.9, 93

scammony – *Convolvulus scammonia* L. **Ast** IX.5; XII.8, 9; **Med** XIII.3, 13, 32; XX.13; XXI.80; **Reg** II.5

scorpion (Arab. *jarārāt*) **Poi** 4, 16, 21, 41, 42, 43, 44, 45, 46, 48, 54, 64, 68; **Med** IX.109; XX.83; XXI.96; XXII.10; XXIV.36

sea squill – *Drimia maritima* (L.) Stearn **Ast** IV.5; IX.14; XII.3; **Poi** 72; **Med** XVII.24; XXI.25, 65, 80; **Coi** 8

sebesten (Assyrian plum – *Cordia myxa* L.) **Ast** IX.3; XII.1; **Med** XXI.68

sekakul parsnip – *Pastinaca sekakul* DC. **Med** XXI.72; **Coi** 8; **Reg** III.8

semolina → *sawīq*

Senegal gum (acacia tree – *Acacia nilotica* (L.) Delile) **Rul** 63; **Med** IX.123; XXI.73

senna – *Senna* sp. Mill. **Med** XXI.69

senna, wild – *Senna tora* (L.) Roxb. **Med** XXI.77; **Coi** 8

senna of Mecca **Reg** III.7; **Elu** 13, 22

serpent root (a species of melilot that has pods resembling tails of scorpions and was employed against the sting of this animal) **Poi** 23, 79

service tree, true – *Sorbus domestica* L. **Med** XXII.54, 65

sesame – *Sesamum indicum* L. **Ast** III.10; XII.7; **Hem** III.1; V.2; VI.3; **Med** III.1; V.2; VI.3; XX.50, 80; XXI.72; XXII.62; **Coi** 4, 6, 7, 8

sharāb → wine
shaylam → darnel
shayyān → dragon's blood
sheep **Ast** III.3; **Hem** III.1; **Med** XX.41, 42, 43; XXI.11, 91; XXII.4, 6; XXII.25; XXV.30; **Coi** 6; **Reg** I.12, 14
shīrāz (type of milk) **Reg** I.16
shīṭaraj → cress, garden: pepperwort
shrimp **Med** XXII.9
silk **Poi** 45, 47; **Hem** IV.1, 4; **Rul** 76, 79; **Med** IX.88; XXI.69; **Reg** III.6; **Elu** 21, 25
silver – *Ag* **Elu** 16
ṣīr (small salted fish) **Ast** IX.12; **Hem** I.2; **Reg** IV.24
skink **Hem** VI.9; **Med** XXII.61; **Coi** 6, 8
smearwort – *Aristolochia rotunda* L. **Ast** XII.3, 5; **Poi** 38, 52
snail **Med** XXI.29
snake **Ast** XIII.38; **Poi** 52, 68; **Hem** VII.1; **Med** IX.93; XXI.53, 96; XXV.64
sneezewort – *Achillea ptarmica* L. (Arab. *kundus*) **Med** XXI.85
snow, Chinese (potassium nitrate) – KNO_3 **Med** IX.30
soapwort – *Saponaria officinalis* L. (Arab. *kundus*) **Med** XXI.85
sorghum – *Sorghum bicolor* (L.) Moench **Med** XXIII.102
sorrel, common – *Rumex acetosa* L. **Med** XXI.29, 73; **Reg** III.6; **Elu** 8, 40
soup **Ast** III.4; IV.4; VI.4; XI.4; XII.6; **Poi** 29, 66, 67, 73, 77; **Hem** III.1; VI.2; **Rul** 72; **Med** IX.33; XIII.6; XX.68, 69, 83; XXI.61; **Reg** II.10
Spanish fly (cantharide) **Poi** 89
sparrow **Med** XX.68; XXII.42; **Coi** 4, 6
sparrow, mountain **Med** XX.58
spicknel – *Meum athamanticum* Jacq. **Med** XXI.42
spider **Poi** 47
spikenard (, Indian) – *Nardostachys jatamansi* (D. Don) DC. **Ast** IV.7 VII.2; XII.1, 5, 6; **Hem** IV.3; V.1; **Rul** 68, 69; **Med** IX.46, 68, 126; XVII.39; XXI.42, 46, 70; **Reg** III.7, 8; **Elu** 15, 21, 30, 44
spikenard, Celtic – *Valeriana celtica* L. **Poi** 25; **Med** XXI.46
spinach – *Spinacia oleracea* L. **Hem** II.3; VI.2; **Rul** 33; **Med** XX.84; XXI.74; **Coi** 5; **Reg** III.2; **Elu** 6, 30
spurge, caper – *Euphorbia lathyris* L. **Med** XXI.85
spurge, resin – *Euphorbia resinifera* O. Berg (Arab. *farbiyūn*; *tākūt*) **Rul** 83; **Med** XXI.85; XXIV.59; **Coi** 9
squash, winter – *Cucurbita maxima* Duchesne (Arab. *qarʿ*) **Ast** III.8; **Med** VII.15; IX.93, 108; XX.9, 53, 61; XXI.79; **Elu** 25
squirrel (fur) **Reg** IV.27
sqūlūfandriyūn → fern, hart's-tongue; fern, rusty-back
St. John's wort, bearded – *Hypericum barbatum* Jacq. (Arab. *dādhī*; *hayūfārīqūn*) **Med** IX.88; XXI.80; XXII.66
St. John's wort, perforate – *Hypericum perforatum* L. (Arab. *dādhī*; *hayūfārīqūn*) **Med** IX.88; XXI.80; XXII.66
St. Thomas lidpod – *Operculina turpethum* var. *turpethum* (L.) S. Manso **Ast** IX.5; XII.8, 9; **Med** XIII.50; XXI.80; **Reg** II.7
starch (amylum) – $(C_6H_{10}O_5)_n+(H_2O)$ **Ast** III.10; IV.8; XII.4, 5; **Rul** 63, 71, 72; **Med** VI.17; XX.17
stavesacre – *Delphinium staphisagria* L. **Med** XXI.80
stock, hoary – *Matthiola incana* (L.) R. Br. (Arab. *khīrī*) **Med** IX.88; XXI.75
stomachic **Rul** 32; **Med** IX.47; XVII.40; **Coi** 8
stone, Armenian **Elu** 13, 21
stone, Jews' **Med** XXI.65, 69
strawberry tree (fruit) – *Arbutus unedo* L. **Poi** 36
styrax, liquid (resin of drug snowbell – *Styrax officinalis* L.; Oriental sweetgum – *Liquidambar orientalis* Mill.; or sweetgum – *Liquidambar styraciflua* L.) **Ast** XII.6; **Hem** VI.4, 9; **Med** XXI.64, 71
styrax, solid (*see above*) **Med** XXI.64, 71; **Com** V.59 (279)
sugar **Ast** III.1, 10; IV.4, 5; VI.4; IX.3, 15; XI.4; XII.1, 2, 4, 9; **Poi** 50; **Hem** I.2; II.3; III.1; IV.1, 4; VI.2; **Rul** 35, 66; **Med** IX.123; XIII.6; XX.78; XXI.69; XXII.40; **Coi** 7, 8; **Reg** II.6; III.2, 3, 4; IV.20; **Elu** 10, 20, 26, 30, 33, 34, 38, 40, 43

sulfur – *S* **Poi** 12, 13, 42, 53, 68; **Rul** 76; **Med** VII.59; VIII.58; XXI.89; XV.33; XXI.89
suet (hard fat) **Elu** 28
sumach, tanner's – *Rhus coriaria* L. **Ast** IX.4; **Hem** II.3; **Rul** 23, 63, 65; **Med** XXI.78; XXII.61; XXV.43; **Reg** IV.25
summāqiyya (meat stew soured with sumach juice) **Ast** IX.4; **Poi** 73; **Hem** I.4
sweet flag – *Acorus calamus* L. **Poi** 27; **Med** IX.88; XXI.65, 80

tabasheer (bamboo – *Bambusa bambos* (L.) Voss) **Med** XXI.83; **Elu** 20, 22, 23, 25
tākūt → spurge, resin
tamarind – *Tamarindus indica* L. **Ast** IX.1; **Hem** IV.4; **Rul** 33; **Med** XXI.83; **Reg** II.6; III.2; **Elu** 3, 15, 30, 43
tamarisk, French – *Tamarix gallica* L. **Poi** 49; **Med** IX.88; XXI.69
tapeworm **Med** VII.31; IX.93; XXII.9
tar **Poi** 13; **Med** XII135; XXI.89
tarantula → *abū ṣūfa*; *rutaylā'*
taro, wild – *Colocasia esculenta* (L.) Schott **Ast** III.8; **Hem** I.2; **Med** XX.86
tawny (port wine) **Med** XVII.28
ṭayhūj → partridge
tellin shell **Med** XXII.60
terra sigillata (sealed earth) **Poi** 19; **Rul** 69
thapsia – *Thapsia garganica* L. (Arab. a.o. *yantūn*) **Med** XXI.82
tharīda/thurda (meat dish with bread) **Poi** 64, 76; **Hem** II.3
Theodoretus (compound medicine, from Greek Theodoros) **Ast** XIII.38; **Reg** II.5
theriac (compound drug, used as a panacea or universal antidote to poison) **Ast** XIII.38, 41, 43, 46; **Poi** 3, 4, 8, 31, 32, 33, 34, 36, 37, 42, 43, 52, 54, 56, 78; **Rul** 69, 70; **Med** IX.103; X.56; XVII.41; XXI.39, 51, 52, 53; XXII.36; XXIV.26; **Reg** II.5, 8
theriac, great **Ast** XIII.38; **Poi** 3, 8, 19, 26, 32, 34, 52, 78; **Med** IX.86; XXI.50
thistle – *Cirsium* sp. Mill. **Med** XXI.73
thistle, soldier – *Picnomon acarna* (L.) Cass. **Med** XXI.73
thurda → *tharīda*
thyme, broad-leaved – *Thymus pulegioides* L. **Poi** 50; **Med** IX.88; XXI.19, 80
thyme, creeping – *Thymus praecox* ssp. *arcticus* (Durand) Jalas (Arab. *ḥāshā*) **Ast** XII.1, 3; **Med** XX.49; XXI.80
trotters (dish) **Rul** 69
truffle **Poi** 90; **Med** XX.60; XXI.79
tubāla (dish) **Coi** 6
turmeric – *Curcuma longa* L. **Med** XXI.80
turnip – *Brassica rapa* L. **Ast** III.8; **Med** XX.47, 72, 85; XXI.75; XXII.41, 42; **Coi** 4, 5, 6, 8
turpentine resin (turpentine tree – *Pistacia terebinthus* L.) **Ast** IX.2; XII.6; **Rul** 83; **Med** IX.70; XV.33; XVII.38; XXI.45, 61
turpentine tree – *Pistacia terebinthus* L. **Hem** IV.6; **Med** XXI.75; **Coi** 8
turtle dove **Poi** 66, 67; **Med** IX.30; XX.58, 68; **Reg** I.12; **Elu** 28
ṭuṭmāj (vermicelli) **Reg** I.13
tutty **Rul** 62; **Med** IX.111; XV.55; XXI.87
tutty, Indian **Med** IX.30

ungues odorati (opercula) **Med** XXI.96
'uqrubān → fern, hart's-tongue; fern, rusty-back
utrujj → citron; lemon

valerian – *Valeriana officinalis* L. **Med** XXI.65
varan **Coi** 8
veal (meat) **Med** XX.19; XXV.10
venison (meat) **Ast** III.7
verdigris (basic copper carbonate) – $Cu_2CO_3(OH)_2$ **Poi** 81; **Rul** 76; **Med** XV.57; XXI.89
vermicelli **Ast** III.1
vermin **Poi** 7, 8, 52, 68, 69; **Med** XXI.50; XXII.64; XXIV.51
vetch, bitter – *Vicia ervilia* (L.) Willd. **Poi** 52, 57, 60; **Rul** 54, 62; **Med** V.19; VI.24; XV.11, 55; XXI.61, 70; XXIII.33, 100
vinegar **Ast** III.9; IV.2, 3, 4, 5, 6, 7; IX.13, 15; **Poi** 11, 13, 14, 15, 16, 24, 28, 42, 51, 52, 79, 80, 86, 90; **Hem** I.2; II.3; III.1; **Rul** 43, 50, 62, 72; **Med** II.14; IX.13, 17, 53, 77, 78, 88, 115, 120, 126; XV.11; XVII.24; XIX.13; XX.56, 58; XXI.19, 23, 25, 28, 35, 40, 65, 73, 93; XXII.2, 3, 17, 23, 24, 25, 28, 46, 58, 61, 68; XXIII.33, 109; **Coi** 5; **Reg** III.4, 5; IV.25; **Elu** 30, 33, 44; **Com** IV.23 (160)

vinegar worm **Med** IX.93
violet – *Viola odorata* L. **Ast** XII.1, 4; **Poi** 8; **Med** XXI.74; **Reg** II.6, 11; III.7; **Elu** 5
viper **Poi** 16, 52, 53, 54; **Med** III.65; IX.108; XXI.53, 54, 55; XXII.2, 16, 19, 64; XXIV.26a, 26b
vitriol **Med** XV.9, 41; XXI.88; XXV.46
vitriol, green (iron(II) sulfate) – $FeSO_4{\cdot}7H_2O$ **Rul** 50, 62, 76; **Med** XXI.75; XXV.46
vitriol, red (cobalt(II) sulfate) – $CoSO_4{\cdot}7H_2O$ **Med** XXV.46
vitriol, yellow **Med** XV.9; XXV.46

wallflower – *Erysimum × cheiri* (L.) Crantz (Arab. *khīrī*) **Med** IX.88; XXI.75
walnut – *Juglans regia* L. (also: king's nut) **Poi** 34, 35, 57, 64, 65; **Hem** IV.6; **Rul** 65; **Med** XX.51, 56, 77; XXI.34, 76; XXIII.102; **Coi** 8
wasp **Poi** 50, 51
water **Ast** III.1, 4, 10; IV.1, 6; V.1; VII.2, 3, 4; VIII.1; IX.1, 2, 6, 7, 13, 15; X.2, 4, 5; XII.2, 3, 4, 7, 10; XIII.1, 4, 11, 15, 18, 19, 32; **Poi** 15, 16, 18, 19, 23, 26, 27, 29, 42, 49, 50, 55, 56, 65, 73, 74, 76, 87, 91; **Hem** I.4; IV.3, 4; V.4; VI.3, 6; **Rul** 1, 11, 12, 16, 27, 30, 31, 34, 50, 66, 72, 79, 82; **Med** II.19; V.4, 10, 13, 16; VI.6, 78; VIII.22, 24, 25, 34, 58, 69, 76; IX.21, 22, 33, 39, 42, 46, 47, 58, 69, 70, 101, 108, 126; X.2, 4, 28, 47, 52, 63; XI.8; XIII.6, 46, 47, 53; XIV.4, 11; XV.8, 17, 20, 36, 39, 58; XVII.27, 41; XIX.6, 7, 8, 9, 11, 12, 15, 19, 32, 33, 34, 36, 37; XX.22, 24, 25, 30, 32, 33, 34, 35, 36, 37, 38, 64; XXI.3, 5, 6, 7, 28, 50, 63, 93, 95; XXII.8, 29, 36, 39, 43, 70; XXIII.6, 15, 16, 20, 33, 106; XXIV.48; XXV.31, 62, 64, 72; **Coi** 8, 9, 10; **Reg** I.1, 9, 18; II.5, 9, 10; III.2, 6, 7, 8; IV.1, 2, 9, 13, 17, 18, 20, 24, 25; **Elu** 1, 27, 28, 30, 34, 44; **Com** N (8); IV.11 (148), 48 (185); V.21 (241), 25 (245), 26 (246), 27 (247); VI.10 (302), 14 (306), 27 (319), 31 (323); VII.42 (394), 46 (398), 55 (407), 56 (408)
"water celery" → waterparsnip, wideleaf
water lily, blue Egyptian – *Nymphaea nouchali* var. *caerulea* Savigny (Arab. *nīlūfar*) **Ast** XII.1; **Med** IX.106; XIII.51; XXI.74; XXV.54; **Coi** 5; **Reg** II.11; **Elu** 13, 17
water lily, European white – *Nymphaea alba* L. (Arab. *nīlūfar*) **Ast** XII.1; **Med** IX.106; XIII.51; XXI.74; XXV.54; **Coi** 5; **Reg** II.11; **Elu** 13, 17
water lily, yellow – *Nuphar lutea* (L.) Sm. (Arab. *nīlūfar*) **Ast** XII.1; **Med** IX.106; XIII.51; XXI.74; XXV.54; **Coi** 5; **Reg** II.11; **Elu** 13, 17
waterfowl **Ast** III.4; IX.108; **Hem** II.3
watermelon – *Citrullus lanatus* (Thunb.) Matsum. & Nakai (Arab. *biṭṭīkh*; *dullāʿ*) **Ast** III.9; IX.13; **Med** VII.15; XX.14, 48, 53, 61; XXI.79; XXII.39; **Coi** 5, 7; **Reg** II.6; **Elu** 11, 13, 25
waterparsnip, wideleaf – *Sium latifolium* L. (Arab. *karafs al-māʾ* ("water celery"); *qurrat al-ʿayn*) **Med** XX.49
wax **Hem** VI.6, 7; **Med** VIII.35; IX.47; XXI.87, 93; **Com** IV.70 (207)
weasel **Poi** 10; **Med** XXI.54; XXII.3, 16
wetiqa (dish made with flour, olive oil, and salt) **Ast** III.1
wheat – *Triticum aestivum* L. **Ast** III.1, 2; IV.8; IX.7; XII.2; **Poi** 59; **Rul** 23; **Med** XX.40; XXI.63, 71, 95; XXIII.7; **Reg** I.12, 13; **Elu** 28, 38
whey (Arab. *maṣl*) **Med** IX.108; XXI.29; XXIII.107; **Elu** 13
willow, Egyptian – *Salix aegyptiaca* L. (Arab. *khilāf*) **Med** XXI.73
willow, silver – *Salix mucronata* Thunb. (Arab. *ṣafṣāf*) **Med** XXI.73
wine (also Arab. *sharāb*) **Ast** VI.4, 5; VII.1, 2; IX.13; XIII.38; **Poi** 8, 15, 18, 23, 25, 27, 28, 29, 33, 36, 37, 39, 43, 44, 45, 49, 50, 52, 53, 57, 64, 65, 74, 79, 87, 90; **Hem** IV.1; **Rul** 16, 23, 27, 51, 54, 63, 66, 72, 79, 80; **Med** II.7, 15; III.61; VI.3, 78, 81; VII.1, 69; VIII.34; IX.4, 42, 49, 87, 126; XIII.43, 50; XV.45, 55, 65; XVII.14, 24, 26, 28, 32, 33, 41; XIX.12; XX.24, 25, 26, 27, 28, 29, 30, 31, 35; XXI.3, 4, 6, 10, 15, 20, 25, 35, 50, 51; XXII.21; XXIII.106, 109; XXV.22; **Coi** 4, 6, 7, 10; **Reg** I.19; II.10; **Elu** 2, 29, 30, 31, 33, 34, 37, 38, 39, 40, 41, 43, 48; **Com** II.18 (70), 21 (73); IV.22 (159); V.5 (225); VI.31 (323), 53 (345); VII.46 (398), 48 (400)
wolf **Med** XXII.22; **Reg** IV.27

woodpecker, green **Med** XXV.56
wool fat → lanolin
wormwood, absinth – *Artemisia absinthium* L. **Ast** XII.8; **Med** IX.68, 77, 126; X.33, 56; XIII.44; XVII.39; XXI.16, 40, 44, 70; XXIV.25

yantūn → thapsia
yāsamīn → jasmine, Arabian; jasmine, white
yeast **Med** XX.15, 16; XXI.95; XXII.62
yolk → egg

zalābiyya (fried dough with honey or syrup) **Reg** I.13
zanbaq → jasmine, Arabian; jasmine, white
zarnab (also: *falanja*) **Med** XXI.80
zedoary – *Curcuma zedoaria* (Christm.) Roscoe **Elu** 21
zīrbāj (stew) **Ast** IV.4; IX.13; **Hem** III.1
zircon, red → jacinth

www.ingramcontent.com/pod-product-compliance
Lightning Source LLC
Chambersburg PA
CBHW031318230926
51848CB00001B/4